Management and Welfare of Farm Animals

UNIVERSITIES FEDERATION FOR ANIMAL WELFARE

About UFAW

The Universities Federation for Animal Welfare (UFAW) is an international independent scientific and educational animal welfare charity. UFAW's vision is a world where the welfare of all animals affected by humans is maximised through a scientific understanding of their needs and how to meet them. UFAW promotes an evidence-based approach to animal welfare by funding scientific research, supporting the careers of animal welfare scientists and by disseminating animal welfare science knowledge both to experts and the wider public.

UFAW improves animal welfare worldwide

- through our programme of awards, grants and scholarships;
- by educational initiatives, especially at university and college level;
- by providing information in books, videos, reports;
- by publishing our scientific journal Animal Welfare;
- by providing expert advice to governments and others, including for legislation and 'best practice' guidelines and codes;
- and by working with animal keepers, scientists, vets, lawyers and all those who care about animals

UFAW relies on the generosity of the public through legacies and donations to carry out our work improving the welfare of animals now and in the future. For further information about UFAW and how you help promote and support our work, please visit our website or contact us at the address below.

Universities Federation for Animal Welfare
The Old School, Brewhouse Hill, Wheathampstead, Herts AL4 8AN, UK
Phone: +44 (0)1582 831818; Website: www.ufaw.org.uk
Email: ufaw@ufaw.org.uk

UFAW's aim regarding the UFAW/Wiley-Blackwell Animal Welfare book series is to promote interest and debate in the subject and to disseminate information relevant to improving the welfare of kept animals and of those affected in the wild through human agency. The books in this series are the works of their authors, and the views they express do not necessarily reflect the views of UFAW.

Management and Welfare of Farm Animals

The UFAW Farm Handbook

Edited by

John Webster
University of Bristol, Somerset, UK

Jean Margerison
Walnut Collage, Loughborough, UK

Sixth Edition

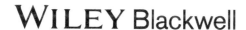

This edition first published 2022
© Universities Federation for Animal Welfare 2022

Edition History
5e © 2011 Universities Federation for Animal Welfare
4e © 1999 Universities Federation for Animal Welfare
3e © 1988 Baillière Tindall
2e © 1978 Baillière Tindall
1e © 1971 Churchill Livingston

The right of John Webster and Jean Margerison to be identified as the authors of the editorial material in this work has been asserted in accordance with law.

Registered Office
John Wiley & Sons Ltd, The Atrium, Southern Gate, Chichester, West Sussex, PO19 8SQ, UK

Editorial Office
9600 Garsington Road, Oxford, OX4 2DQ, UK

For details of our global editorial offices, customer services, and more information about Wiley products visit us at www.wiley.com.

Wiley also publishes its books in a variety of electronic formats and by print-on-demand. Some content that appears in standard print versions of this book may not be available in other formats.

Library of Congress Cataloging-in-Publication Data
Names: Webster, John, 1938- editor. | Margerison, Jean, editor.
Title: Management and welfare of farm animals: The UFAW Farm Handbook / edited by John Webster, University of Bristol, Somerset, UK, Jean Margerison, Walnut Collage, Loughborough, UK.
Description: Sixth Edition. | Chichester, West Sussex, UK ; Hoboken, NJ : John Wiley & sons, 2022. |
Series: UFAW animal welfare | Includes bibliographical references and index.
Identifiers: LCCN 2021061385 (print) | LCCN 2021061386 (ebook) | ISBN 9781119532484 (paperback) | ISBN 9781119532491 (pdf) | ISBN 9781119532460 (epub)
Subjects: LCSH: Livestock--Great Britain--Management. | Livestock--Great Britain--Handbooks, manuals, etc.
Classification: LCC SF61 .M23 2022 (print) | LCC SF61 (ebook) | DDC 636--dc23/eng/20220103
LC record available at https://lccn.loc.gov/2021061385
LC ebook record available at https://lccn.loc.gov/2021061386

Cover images: © Suslov Denis/Shutterstock; © Delpixel/Shutterstock; © PHATTARAWATOUM/Shutterstock; © Mai.Chayakorn/Shutterstock
Cover design by Wiley

Set in 9.5/12.5pt STIXTwoText by Integra Software Services Pvt. Ltd, Pondicherry, India

SKY54137855-DBF8-410A-978E-C0F2C17A1D81_052422

Contents

Preface to Sixth Edition

The Universities Federation for Animal Welfare (UFAW), founded in 1926, is an internationally recognized animal welfare charity concerned with promoting high standards of welfare for farm, companion, laboratory and captive wild animals. One of the most important ways by which it works to improve animals' lives is through the promotion of education in animal care and welfare. This includes the publication of books, videos, articles, technical reports and the journal *Animal Welfare*.

Through successive editions, *Management and Welfare of Farm Animals* has become internationally recognized as a classic introductory textbook for university and college students of agriculture and veterinary science. Each edition has adhered firmly to the principles originally put forward by Charles Hume, UFAW's founder, in his forward to the first edition, namely: 'This book ... seeks to put forward the case for the humane treatment of farm animals in as rational a way as possible. UFAW does not necessarily support all the procedures that are described. However, it is acknowledged that farming is a business and that in the face of intensive competition, improved and more humane techniques can be brought about only if consumers will pay more for the food that they buy.'

Recent years have seen many changes in what is deemed acceptable practice in regard to the husbandry and welfare of animals. The European Union in the 1997 Treaty of Amsterdam acknowledged that since animals are sentient beings, members should pay full regard to their welfare requirements. The UK Animal Welfare Act (2006) imposed a duty of care on responsible persons to provide for the basic needs of their animals (both farmed animals and pets). Specific laws have been passed to prohibit practices such as the confinement of laying hens and pregnant sows in, respectively, barren cages and individual stalls. Although, to date, there have been no such changes in USA federal law, an increasing number of individual states are passing state laws to ban these and other practices that arouse public concern. The legal definitions of acceptable practice are in a state of continuous flux. Moreover, there has been an upsurge of consumer demand for alternative methods and improved standards in the production of food from animals that can be seen to give due respect to animal welfare and, increasingly, to the conservation and welfare of the living environment. In recent years, the impact of public pressure, expressed through the medium of consumer choice, has had a far greater impact on these things than that which has been achieved through legislation.

Our primary aim is to provide a comprehensive introductory textbook for young people requiring professional, technical or vocational education in the management and welfare of farm animals. However, we have, in many ways, sought to broaden our remit. Although much of the book deals, as before, with the large-scale commercial rearing of animals for food (rightly so, since this affects the welfare of the great majority), authors have been asked to give special attention to alternative farming systems. One example is the commercial farm that seeks to meet the market for added-value products from consumers seeking higher standards of animal welfare. Another is the small-scale, non-industrialized farm in which animals are likely to be cared for on an individual basis, whether these are traditional family farms in the developing world, or 'hobby farmers' in the Western world who wish to practice good husbandry and ensure welfare on a more intimate scale. However, in all circumstances – the industrial farm mass-producing a commodity, the specialist 'high welfare' farm producing added-value food for discerning consumers, the family farm producing food as a rewarding hobby or as the only realistic alternative to starvation – the health and welfare needs of the animal are the same.

Successive editions of *Management and Care of Farm Animals* have been published at approximately 12-year intervals. In each edition, management and welfare have been described on a species-by-species or a group-by-group basis by authors with internationally recognized experience as teachers, scientists and consultants. The previous, fifth, edition (2011) was considerably more ambitious in scope than what had gone before. For a start, it was twice as long as its predecessor. It also introduced three conceptually new chapters to reflect new understanding of animal welfare science, ethics and the role of society in helping to ensure and improve standards of animal welfare. These chapters considered general principles of good husbandry and its impact on animal welfare, animal behaviour as an indicator of welfare, and the assessment, implementation and promotion of high standards of animal welfare in practice.

This latest edition is essentially similar in scope to its predecessor. However, some of the chapters have new authors and nearly all contain significant new material that reflect advances in knowledge and our increasing concern for the welfare of not just the farm animals but the whole of life on earth. Each chapter concludes with a brief list of specific references and general suggestions for further reading. Many of the latter refer to books and articles of broad interest so not quoted in reference to specific items within the text for further reading. In recognition of the googlification of knowledge transfer many of these are links to web sites.

Writing as editors, we must express our thanks to all the authors who have found time within their busy careers to write these comprehensive and authoritative chapters. Your reward will, we hope, be found in the knowledge that you have contributed to the production of something of real value to a lot of sentient and sapient creatures. These include, of course, students undertaking courses in agriculture, animal science, veterinary science and nursing, biosciences, animal welfare and care, companion and equine studies, animals and the environment. We hope that these chapters will prove especially valuable as a basis for courses taught in English within the developing world, because of the breadth of information they convey within a single book. We also suggest that they may prove useful to those wishing to learn the elements of animal welfare and good husbandry on a more informal basis, perhaps as a prelude to keeping farm animals for themselves. Finally, and critically, our book is addressed to the animals themselves. There is an international groundswell of public concern for farm animal welfare and, in principle, this has to be a good thing. However, caring *about* animals is not enough. Caring *for* them is what matters. This requires compassion, knowledge, understanding and a great deal of skill. These things cannot be gathered from any single source, but what we offer here is, we hope, a useful beginning.

John Webster
Jean Margerison

Contributors

Joy Becker BSc, PhD
School of Life and Environmental Sciences
University of Sydney
Camden, NSW
Australia

Cristian Bonacic MV, MSc, DPhil
School of Agriculture and Forestry Science
Pontificia Universidad Catolica de Chile
Casilla 306
Correo 22, Santiago
Chile

Andy Butterworth, BSc(Hons), BVSc, PhD, DipECAWBM, FLS, MRCVS
14 Stonewell Lane
Congresbury
N Somerset
BS49 5DL

Cathy Dwyer BSc, PhD
SRUC, Roslin Institute Building
Easter Bush
Midlothian EH25 9RG

Bernadette Earley
Teagasc, Animal Bioscience Department
Grange Research Centre
Dunsany
Co. Meath
Ireland

Sandra Edwards
School of Agriculture, Food and Rural
Development
Newcastle University
Newcastle on Tyne NE1 7RU

Patrick Garland
Premier Nutrition
Brereton Business Park
Rugeley, Staffordshire WS15 1RD

Pete Goddard
Macaulay Land Use Research Institute
Craigiebuckler
Aberdeen AB15 8QH

Laura Griffin BSc Hons
School of Biology and Environmental Sciences
University College
Dublin
Ireland

Alison Hanlon BSc, MSc, PhD
UCD School of Agriculture, Food Science
and Veterinary Medicine
University College
Dublin
Ireland

Stephen Lister BSc, BVet Med, Cert PMP,
DiplECPVS, MRCVS
Crowshall Veterinary Services
1 Crowshall Lane
Attleborough
Norfolk

Jean Margerison BSc, PhD, PGCE, NDAg
Associate Professor of Ruminant Nutrition
School of Bioscience
Division of Animal Science
University of Nottingham
Sutton Bonington, LE12 5RD

Alan Mowlem
Water Farm, Stogursey
Bridgwater
Somerset TA5 1PS

Christine Nicol MA, DPhil
Royal Veterinary College
South Mimms
London

Cormac O'Shea B.Agric.Sc1, PhD PGCIE
Division of Animal Sciences
University of Nottingham

School of Biosciences
Sutton Bonington Campus
Loughborough LE12 5RD

Graham Scott BSc, PhD
48, Hampton Drive
Newport
Shropshire
TF10 7RE

John Webster MA, VetMB, PhD, DVM (Hon),
MRCVS
Old Sock Cottage
Mudford Sock
Yeovil
Somerset B22 8EA

David Welchman MA, VetMB, PhD, MRCVS
VLA -Winchester
Itchen Abbas
Winchester SO21 1BX

Helen (Becky) Whay
NUI Galway
Ireland

1

Husbandry and Animal Welfare

John Webster

KEY CONCEPTS

1.1 Introduction

The broad aim of this book, as in earlier editions, is to provide an introduction to the management and welfare of farm animals through the practice of good husbandry within the context of an efficient, sustainable agriculture. Successive chapters outline these principles and practices for the major farmed species within a range of production systems, both intensive and extensive. This chapter opens with a description of concepts in animal welfare that may be applied to any sentient farm animal, then progresses to general principles that may be applied to their management. These general principles are illustrated by specific examples relating to animal species and production systems (e.g. broiler chickens, dairy cows). For those of you who are new to the study of animal management and animal welfare, some of these examples may make sense only when you have read the chapter on the species to which they refer.

Management and Welfare of Farm Animals: The UFAW Farm Handbook, Sixth Edition.
Edited by John Webster and Jean Margerison.
© Universities Federation for Animal Welfare 2022. Published 2022 by John Wiley & Sons Ltd.

I also suggest that, when you have read, learned and inwardly digested a chapter on a particular species, you might refer back to this opening chapter and consider how well (or not) current management practices for that species meet the general criteria for good husbandry and welfare within the categories outlined here.

The purpose of farming is to use the resources of the land to provide the people with food and other goods. For most of the history of agriculture and, even now, throughout most of the world, the role of the farmer has been straightforward: to produce food to meet the needs of the people. If they could produce it, we would buy it. Today, in developed, affluent, urbanized society, consumers have much greater freedom in their choice of food and their decisions will range beyond the direct elements of price and nutritive value to include issues such as provenance, animal welfare and environmental cost. An increasing number, ovo-lacto-vegetarians, reject meat. Vegans will not eat or wear anything of animal origin. To succeed, modern farmers must combine a knowledge and understanding of how to care for the life of their land with a shrewd awareness of the needs and wants of their consumers to obtain the best possible value from what they have to sell. Successful livestock farmers are those who also have the best understanding of the needs and wants of their animals.

Successive chapters will consider the special needs of different farmed species and provide practical advice as to how to meet these needs within the context of viable production systems. The aim of this opening chapter is to introduce principles of husbandry and welfare as they apply to the feeding, breeding, management and care of animals throughout their lives on farms large and small, and in times of special need such as during transport and at the point of slaughter. Most of the meat, milk and eggs for sale to the public in the developed world come from highly intensive systems in which very large numbers of animals are confined and 'managed' by very few people. However, farm animals in most of the world are still reared within traditional communities where animals are more likely to be cared for on an individual basis. At the time of writing the previous edition, the big concern for livestock farmers was the growing movement to reject industrialized farming methods and return to systems that appear to afford more care and respect to farm animals as individuals. This has been expressed both by those who seek organic, high-welfare or trusted local produce in the shops and by those who wish to farm, whether full- or part-time, to such standards. Today, our concerns are not just for high standards of farm animal welfare through skilled and sensitive animal husbandry but also for the sustainability of the living environment through skilled and sensitive planet husbandry that takes into account wildlife, soil and water conservation, and the contribution of agriculture to climate change.

This new edition addresses these issues from first principles, on the basis that the fundamental welfare needs of an animal such as a chicken are the same, whether it is scavenging for food in an African village or confined in a controlled environment building containing 100,000 birds. The ethical challenge in either circumstance is how to reconcile the welfare needs of the animals, the needs of the farmers to obtain a fair return for their investment and labour, the needs of the people for safe, high-quality, affordable food and last (but not least) the need to preserve the quality of the living environment.

1.1.1 Traditional Agriculture

Agriculture, past, present and future, can be defined by four eras: traditional, industrial, value-led and one-planet. Traditional agriculture, as practised for most of history, and still practised in much of the world today, was low output but sustainable, not least because most of the animals looked after themselves. Sheep and goats consumed fibrous food, unavailable to humans, commonly grazing land the farmer did not own. Chickens and pigs (where culturally acceptable) were fed or scavenged leftovers, and food that humans failed to harvest or elected not to eat. In many traditional communities, chickens also fulfilled a valuable community service, consuming ticks and other pests of humans and animals. A dairy cow justified more attention from the farmer (or more likely his wife) who would cut, cart and conserve her feed since she (the cow) was a source of real income through sale of milk. The system seldom generated great riches but it was usually sustainable, partly because it imposed a minimal drain on capital reserves such as fossil fuels, but mainly because nothing was wasted. The use of food and other resources by humans and farm animals was complementary rather than competitive.

1.1.2 Industrial Agriculture

It is easy for the well-educated, well-fed citizen of the developed world to paint a rosy picture of traditional agriculture. However, it provided little more than subsistence for most farmers, most of the time, and could not meet our modern expectations for a wide variety of good, safe, cheap food in all seasons. This has been achieved through an industrial revolution in farming that began less than 100 years ago, and only in the industrialized world. In undeveloped countries, it has hardly started. The key distinction between the traditional and the intensive livestock or poultry farm is that nearly all the inputs to the latter system – power, machinery and other resources (e.g. food and fertilizers) – are bought in. Until recently, output from these farms has been constrained only by the amount that the producer can afford to invest in capital and other non-renewable resources and the capacity of the system to process them. Such livestock enterprises can rightly be designated as 'factory farms' on the basis that most, or all, of the feed and other resources necessary to rear the animals in confinement do not come from the farm itself but arrive by truck. Now, the first constraint on expansion of these intensive units is the need to dispose of slurry, manure and other wastes without causing pollution.

The key objective of industrialized livestock production can be summed up in a single phrase: to control the environment in the immediate vicinity of the animal. The overall impact of industrialized agriculture has had the opposite effect: it has disrupted the balance of nature that had been sustained for millennia. Controlled environment, precision farming is based on three principles. Feeding involves the provision of a nutritionally balanced ration in optimal quantities and at least cost. Housing is designed partly to provide animals with comfort and security, but mainly to maximize income relative to the costs of building and labour. Control of health is achieved through attention to biosecurity and hygiene. These general principles will be developed below and applied to the various species of farm animals in successive chapters.

Figure 1.1 outlines the genealogy of the intensive livestock farm, as typified by modern intensively housed pig and poultry units (Webster 2005). Some feed for pigs and poultry (e.g. cereals)

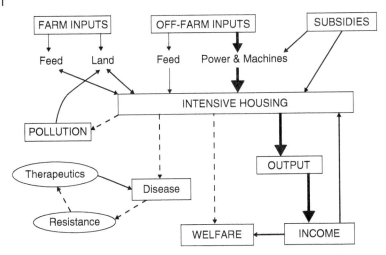

Figure 1.1 Factors influencing the development of industrialization in livestock farming. Potentially adverse effects are indicated with broken lines (from Webster 2005).

may be grown within the farm enterprise, but this, along with purchased feed supplements to ensure a balanced diet, is trucked onto the unit and dispensed to animals in controlled environment houses by mechanical feeding systems. Mechanical and electrical power is used to control temperature and ventilation, to dispense feed and to remove and disperse the manure. Factory farming was born when it became cheaper, faster and more efficient to process feed through animals using machines than to let the animals do the work for themselves. Once the high set-up costs had been met, the input of cheap energy and other bought-in resources was able to increase output and reduce running costs. In consequence, poultry meat from chickens and turkeys, once the food of family feasts, is now the cheapest meat on the market.

Potential (although avoidable) harmful outputs from intensive livestock systems (hatched lines in Figure 1.1) include increased pollution, infectious disease and abuse of animal welfare. Bringing animals off the land and into close confinement inevitably increases the risks of infectious disease. To combat this increased risk, it has been necessary to introduce strict new strategies to eliminate, or at least reduce, exposure to infection. The key to elimination in an intensive pig or poultry unit is biosecurity. This requires strict controls on the movement of animals and stock-keepers who shower and don protective clothing before entering the unit. This will normally ensure the health of the animals (one essential element of welfare), but there are obvious limits to the expression of natural behaviour in a large isolation hospital. The key element of hygiene is to minimize contact between animals and their excreta.

Where exposure to infection cannot be eliminated through exclusion or hygiene, it is necessary to develop routine disease control measures that include vaccines, antibiotics and antiparasitic drugs. If access to cheap power had been all that was necessary for the success of intensive livestock farming, then this industrial revolution would have happened in the 1920s. In fact, the greatest rate of expansion was delayed until the 1950s when antibiotics effective against the major endemic bacterial diseases of housed livestock became cheap and freely available. Alternative, subtler approaches to disease control, such as the development of specific vaccines and strains of animals genetically resistant to specific diseases, have also contributed to the commercial success of intensive systems, especially in the case of poultry. However, it is fair to claim that industrialized farming of pigs and poultry has, for the last 50 years, been sustained by the routine use of antibiotics, coccidiostats and other chemotherapeutics to control endemic diseases. In some cases these diseases could be life-threatening. In most cases, however, chemotherapeutics have been used routinely to increase productivity by reducing the effects of chronic, low-grade infection.

In Europe there is now a ban on the routine use of antibiotics and many other chemotherapeutic 'growth promoters', mainly on the basis of concern that the development of microbial resistance to antibiotics used as growth promoters will pose an increasing risk to human health. The scientific evidence in support of this legislation is inconsistent. However, on balance, and in time, it has to be a good thing, for both the animals and ourselves, to restrict the routine use of antibiotics in livestock agriculture. It is an unequivocal insult to the principle of good husbandry to keep animals in conditions of such intensity, inappropriate feeding or squalor that their health can only be ensured by the routine administration of chemotherapeutics.

Although the industrial farming of livestock and poultry does present opportunities, assessed in terms of animal health and welfare, it also presents inherent threats. It is obviously impossible to care for each chicken as an individual within a poultry house containing over 100,000 animals. Any individual that falls behind the average by virtue of ill health, impaired development or reluctance to compete at the feed trough has little chance of being nursed back to normality through sympathetic stockmanship.

1.1.3 Value-led Agriculture

The main impact of industrial agriculture has been to provide an ample supply and wide, year-round choice of food that is reliable, safe and cheap, looks and tastes good. This is what most of the people have wanted most of the time. However, in recent years and within societies that can afford such morals, consumers have begun to display an increasingly compassionate concern for other, less tangible, elements of food quality, especially animal welfare and the quality of the environment. Farmers and retailers involved in livestock production have responded to this demand by developing alternative husbandry systems that give increased attention to animal welfare and environmental sustainability through developments and improvements to husbandry. The development of such alternative systems will be a feature of this book.

1.1.4 One-planet Agriculture

The aim of good husbandry has always been twofold: to provide good food and other products for humans, while at the same time sustaining the quality of the land and the life of the land. In the future, the pressure on agriculture throughout the world, intensive and extensive, will increasingly be driven by the need to sustain the living environment. This may challenge our current, comfortable feelings of compassion for other sentient creatures, farm animals, wildlife and poor people. The challenge will be to sustain improvements in animal welfare within the context of animal production systems that are efficient in use of resources, do not pollute the soil and waterways, and restrict the production of greenhouse gases, especially from ruminants. However, the amount of care that farmers can give to the welfare of both their animals and the land is constrained by what they can afford. If society wishes to give added value to such things as animal welfare and the environment, then society must pay for it.

For many years agricultural support within the EU in the form of subsidies to farmers has been determined almost entirely by the size of the farm with little attention paid to the difference between the supply of private goods (food and clothing) and public goods (e.g. conservation of soil, management of water resources, respect for wildlife). There is now growing recognition of the principle that public money in the form of farm subsidies should be directed wholly, or in major part, towards these public goods. The corollary to this is that there should be little or no public subsidy to support the business of food production per se. There are, at present, penalties for pollution, and some constraints on the production of excessive amounts of nitrogenous wastes, e.g. from intensive dairy farms in the Netherlands. In the near future, taxes, similar to the carbon tax, may be imposed on factory farms to offset their negative impact on the environment.

This book outlines the basic principles that define our duty of care to farm animals and the practices that contribute to their management. However, these principles and practice can never be divorced from the primary need to ensure the economically competitive production of food and other goods, while sustaining the productivity and quality of the living environment. This being so, compromise is inevitable. An ethical approach to such compromise is presented in the closing section of this chapter.

1.2 Concepts in Animal Welfare

The expression 'animal welfare' has two distinct meanings. The first is a description of the physical and mental state of an animal as it seeks to meet its physiological and behavioural needs. This is a measure of welfare as perceived by the animal itself and something that we can study through careful observations of animal behaviour and the disciplines of welfare science. This approach is considered in detail in Chapter 2. The second concept of animal welfare is as an expression of moral concern. It arises from the belief that animals can experience feelings that we would interpret as pain and suffering, so that we have duty to protect animals in our care from these things. A concern for animal welfare is obviously a virtue. It is good that we should care about animals. Caring *for* animals, however, involves more than virtue; it requires a sound understanding of the principles of husbandry and welfare and these things can only be acquired through education and practical experience. This book is aimed mainly at those who will have direct responsibility for the care of farm animals. However, the moral responsibility to provide a duty of care does not apply only to those directly involved with animals on the farm, in transport and at the place of slaughter. The responsibility must be shared by all who, directly or indirectly, derive any value from the exploitation of animals to suit our ends, whether for food, clothing, sport or companionship. These responsibilities may be outlined as follows:

1) to acknowledge and understand the concepts of welfare, sentience and suffering in farm animals
2) to breed and manage farm animals to promote good welfare and avoid suffering throughout their working lives
3) to increase public awareness of the welfare needs of farm animals, within a context that also recognizes the needs of farmers to produce good food and maintain a decent living through the practice of good husbandry: the competent and caring management of the land and the life of the land
4) to work towards improved standards of farm animal welfare through the parallel development of improved husbandry systems and increased public demand for food and other goods produced to these higher standards.

1.2.1 Sentience, Welfare and Wellbeing

Animal welfare has been defined as 'the state of an animal as it attempts to cope with its environment' (Fraser and Broom 1990). The definition may be applied to any animal from an ant to an ape. Farm animals, however, have been classified, at least within the European Union, as 'sentient creatures', and there are currently moves within the UK to extend the recognition of sentience to a wide range of species, domestic and wild, vertebrate and invertebrate.

The current debate on the nature of sentience in animals (at least in legal minds) asks a simple either/or question. Is this species sentient or is it not? This approach conflicts with reality. Is a lobster, or an earthworm, sentient or not? If sentient, does that put it in the same class as an elephant and so worthy of equal respect?

The most satisfactory *scientific* exposition of the varied nature of sentience within the animal is, to my mind, that contained within Buddhist philosophy. This recognizes five categories: *skandhas* which are present to a greater or lesser degree in all living creatures. It recognizes all animals as sentient but some more sentient than others. The five skandhas of sentience are matter, sensation, perception, mental formulation and consciousness. These are illustrated in Figure 1.2, which also presents estimates, based on evidence relating to animal behaviour and motivation, of the degrees of sentience involved in the interpretation of primitive sensations like hunger and pain and expressions of more complex behaviours and emotions such as companionship, altruism, hope and despair. These are considered in some detail in a new book, *Animal Welfare Understanding Sentient Minds and Why It Matters* (Webster 2022). Here, in brief:

Matter describes living organisms as defined by their structure, chemical composition and the processes that enable them to operate within a complex environment. This category embraces all plants and animals. It includes the ability to react to environmental stimuli, like the movement of sunflowers towards the sun, or the movement of amoebae away from an acid solution, without necessarily involving sensation as we would define it.

Sensation describes the ability of living creatures to experience feelings, and the intensity of feelings that take them out of their comfort zone. These include pain, severe heat and cold, hunger and fear. At this level of sentience, animals interpret these sensations as unpleasant (aversive), pleasant (attractive) or unimportant (indifferent) and these sensations will

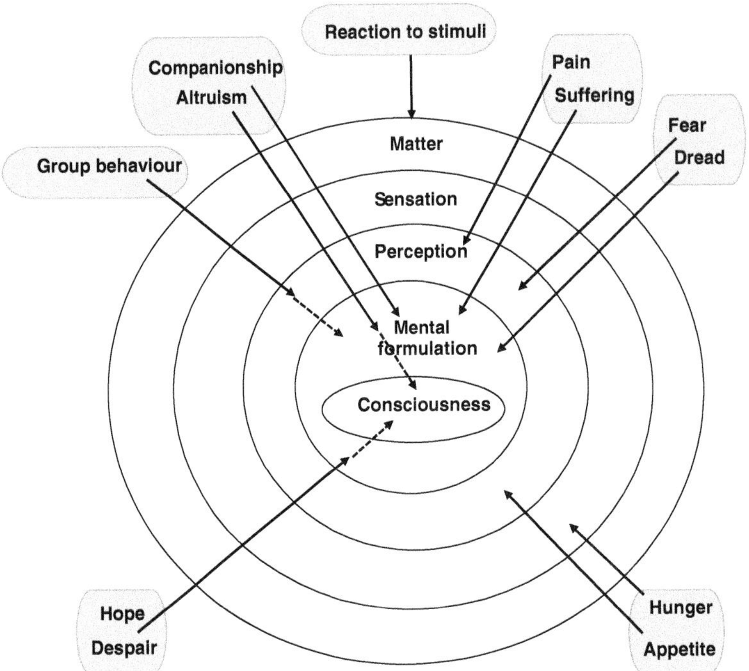

Figure 1.2 The five skandhas or circles of sentience. The solid arrows indicate the known extent of sentience involved in different forms of experience and social behaviour. Dotted lines indicate possible but unproven extension of sentience into the inner circles. For further interpretation see text (from Webster 2022).

motive them to take action, if necessary, to adjust how they feel. According to current EU legislation for farm animals, this property is sufficient to define them as sentient.

Perception describes the ability to register, recognize and remember objects, experiences and emotions. Simple examples of recognition and remembrance include 'this food is good to eat', 'this electric fence caused me pain, I shall avoid it in future'. Animals with the property of perception do not just react to stimuli as they occur; they can learn from experience. This carries the important message that they do not just live in the present. This enhances their capacity to cope with the challenges of life but increases the potential for suffering if the challenges are too severe, too prolonged, or if they are in an environment that restricts their ability to perform coping behaviour.

Mental formulation describes the ability to create mental pictures (or diagrams) that integrate and interpret complex experiences, sensations and emotions. This improves the ability of animals to learn from experience by gaining some understanding of the mechanisms of cause and effect. This further increases their capacity to cope with challenge but, equally, increases the potential for suffering if they find themselves unable to cope.

Consciousness: In the Buddhist skandhas, the word 'consciousness' is restricted to the deepest circle of sentience and equates to human consciousness, best described as 'being aware that we are aware'. This carries the potential for advanced forms of social behaviour, both good and bad, such as empathy, compassion and cheating.

It should become clear from reading this book (if it is not clear already) that the animals we farm and kill for the production of food and other goods all meet at least the three outer circles of sentience, matter, sensation and perception, and probably have a considerable capacity for mental formulation. It follows from this that respect for their welfare demands more than freedom from pain and physical suffering but must also respect their mental capacities and how important these are in contributing to their quality of life. Welfare may therefore be defined as 'the state of body and mind of a sentient animal as it attempts to cope with its environment'. This definition covers the full spectrum of welfare from healthy to sick, pain to pleasure. The aim of the sentient animal is to achieve a state of good welfare, or *wellbeing*, defined simply as *fit and happy* or *fit and feeling good* (Webster 2005). For the body. This implies sustained health; for the mind it implies, at least, an absence of suffering from such things as pain, fear and exhaustion. It should also embrace a sense of positive wellbeing (*feeling good*) achieved by such things as comfort, companionship and security.

The most simple and concise definition of sentience is *feelings that matter* (Webster 2005). Marian Dawkins (1990) has pioneered the study of motivation in animals by seeking to measure how hard animals will work to achieve (or avoid) a resource or stimulus that makes them feel good (or bad) (see Chapter 2). This definition recognizes that the behaviour of animals is motivated by the emotional need to seek satisfaction and avoid suffering. Many of these emotions are associated with primitive sensations such as hunger, pain and anxiety. Species with the property of perception and mental formulation will also experience 'higher feelings' such as friendship and grief at the loss of a relative. However, we should not assume that the distress caused to animals by the emotions of hunger, pain and anxiety is any less intense because they are primitive.

Figure 1.3 illustrates how sentient animals perceive their environment and how this motivates their behaviour (Webster 2022). The 'control centres' in the central nervous system (CNS) constantly receive information from the external and internal environment. Much information, e.g. the perception of how an animal stands and moves in space, is processed at a subconscious level. However, any stimulus that calls for a conscious call for action must involve some degree of interpretation. Motivation scientists observing the response of sentient animals may define a stimulus as positive, aversive or neutral. In simpler words, the animal, when presented with the stimulus, will experience feelings that are good, bad or indifferent. This is an emotional (i.e. sentient) response to the stimulus. The sentient animal (within which category we must include *Homo sapiens*) may or may not also interpret the incoming information in a cognitive fashion, i.e. apply reason. However, all sentient animals are usually and most powerfully motivated by how they feel.

This psychological concept of mind makes a clear distinction between the reception, categorization and interpretation of incoming stimuli. Although it may appear abstract it is soundly based in neurobiology. Kendrick (1998) has made recordings from nerve centres involved in these processes. When a sheep is presented with grain or hay (or photographic images of these

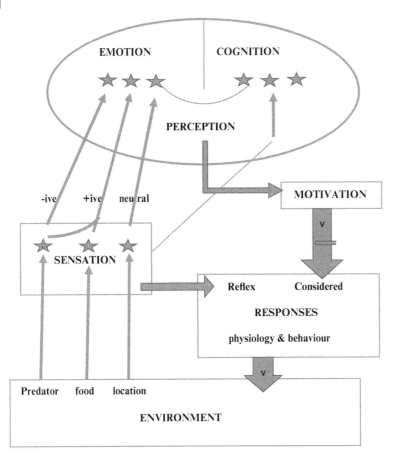

Figure 1.3 The sentient mind:sensation, perception and motivation. For further explanation, see text (from Webster 2022).

things) this triggers signals in a family of neurones that convey the generic information 'food'. A second set of stimuli or images, e.g. dogs and men, form another generic category of information that we may call 'predator'. The information 'food' then proceeds to a second processing centre where it stimulates a family of neurones that transmit a positive emotion (good). The information 'predator' passes to another centre that transmits the negative emotion (bad). However, if the sheep is now presented with a picture of a human carrying a sack of food, two categories of information (food and predator) are passed to the emotion centre, evaluated together and in this case passed on as a single, unconfused emotional message, namely 'good'.

The sentient animal is then motivated to respond according to how it feels (good, bad or indifferent) about the information it has received. Moreover, the interpretation is not a simple yes/no decision. The intensity of its feelings will vary. It will, for example, feel more or less hungry, more or less afraid, and this will determine the strength of its motivation to respond in positive or negative fashion. By studying the strength of motivation of an animal to seek or avoid the feelings it associates with certain sensations and experiences, we can measure not only what an animal senses as good and bad but also how much these feelings matter.

Having behaved in a way designed to achieve a satisfactory emotional state, an animal with the capacity of perception will then review the consequences of its action. If it has been effective, it will feel better and it will gain the assurance that it knows what to do next time. If its action fails, either because the stress was too great, or because it was constrained in such a way that it was unable to do what it felt necessary in order to cope, then it is likely to feel worse and be more anxious for the future. Such animals, which include all those mammals, birds and fish that we farm for food, do not live only in the present: their mood and understanding are modified in the light of experience.

1.2.2 Stress and Suffering

The fact that the emotional response of an animal to stimuli is governed by its past experience carries obvious survival advantages in a challenging environment and forms an essential contribution to the survival of the fittest. The interpretation of past experience is equally important to a domestic animal since it is a key indicator of the animal's success, or otherwise, in coping with stress. To illustrate this point, consider the difference between fear and anxiety (Figure 1.4). Fear is an emotional response to a perceived threat that acts as a powerful motivator to action designed, where possible, to evade that threat. It is also an educational experience, since the memory of previous threats, the action taken in response to those threats and the consequences thereof ('was it less bad than I feared or worse?') will obviously affect how the animal feels next time around. Thus fear, like pain, is an essential part of sentience. These emotions have evolved as key elements for

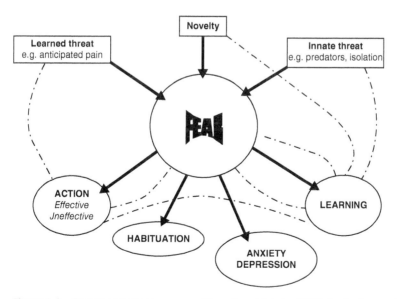

Figure 1.4 Causes and consequences of fear (from Webster 2005; for further explanation see text).

survival. An animal that has no sense of pain or fear, for itself or its offspring, is at a profound disadvantage in the struggle for existence. So too is an animal that cannot remember what gave rise to pain or fear in the past and how well or badly it coped.

Stress and suffering are not the same. Animals are equipped to respond and adapt to challenges in circumstances that permit them to make an effective response. If so, then they learn that they can cope. An animal is likely to suffer when it fails to cope (or has extreme difficulty in coping) with stress:

- because the stress itself is too severe, too complex or too prolonged (e.g. a dairy cow worn out by the sustained complex stresses of metabolic overload and chronic pain from lameness); or
- because the animal is prevented from taking the constructive action it feels necessary to relieve the stress (e.g. a sow in the extreme confinement of an individual pregnancy stall).

1.3 Principles of Husbandry and Welfare

1.3.1 The Five Freedoms and Provisions

The essence of good farm animal husbandry is to provide the resources and management necessary to ensure the economic production of food and other goods in a way that does not compromise the health and welfare of the animals (and the environment). Since wellbeing has been defined as 'fit and happy', provision must be made to promote both the physical and psychological elements of good welfare. These aims have been expressed according to the principles of the 'five freedoms and provisions' (Farm Animal Welfare Council 1993) as set out in Table 1.1. The 'five freedoms' identify the elements that define an ideal state of wellbeing as perceived by the animals. The 'five provisions' define the husbandry and resources required to promote, though possibly never achieve, this ideal state. This requires proper attention to physiological needs through good nutrition, good housing and attention to health and hygiene. It also requires attention to the psychological needs of sentient animals to avoid fear and stress and achieve satisfaction through the freedom to express normal, socially acceptable behaviour. The five freedoms should not be interpreted as a counsel of perfection but as a set of standards for compliance with acceptable principles of good welfare and a

Table 1.1 The five freedoms and provisions.

1) *Freedom from thirst, hunger and malnutrition* – by ready access to fresh water and a diet to maintain full health and vigour
2) *Freedom from discomfort* – by providing a suitable environment including shelter and a comfortable resting area
3) *Freedom from pain, injury and disease* – by prevention or rapid diagnosis and treatment
4) *Freedom from fear and distress* – by ensuring conditions which avoid mental suffering
5) *Freedom to express normal behaviour* – by providing sufficient space, proper facilities and company of the animal's own kind

Source: Farm Animal Welfare Council (1993).

Table 1.2 An outline comparison of the welfare of laying hens in the conventional battery cage, in the enriched cage and on free range.

Factor	Conventional cage	Enriched cage	Free range
Hunger and thirst	Adequate	Adequate	Adequate
Comfort, thermal	Good	Good	Variable
Comfort, physical	Bad	Adequate	Adequate
Fitness, disease	Low risk	Low risk	Increased risk
Pain	High risk (feet and legs)	Moderate risk	Variable risk (feather pecking)
Stress	Frustration	Less frustration	Aggression
Fear	Low risk	Low risk	Aggression, agoraphobia
Natural behaviour	Highly restricted	Restricted	Unrestricted

Source: Webster (2005).

practical, comprehensive checklist from which to assess the strengths and weaknesses of any husbandry system, whether within the context of international standards for production systems or at the level of the individual farm.

Application of the five freedoms to the evaluation of standards for production systems is illustrated by Table 1.2, which considers alternative husbandry systems for laying hens: the conventional barren battery cage that constitutes the environment for most hens worldwide, the 'enriched' cage, that will become the minimum standard for Europe in 2012, and the 'free range' system. These systems are reviewed in detail in Chapter 7. Here they are briefly compared using the evaluation structure provided by the five freedoms. Thus:

- Adequate freedom from hunger and thirst can be achieved in all systems.
- Thermal comfort can be maintained in all cage systems. On free range it will be variable. However, since hens can choose whether to be indoors or out, then thermal comfort is likely to be satisfactory most of the time.
- Physical comfort is unacceptably bad in the conventional barren battery cage when the floor space allowance for hens is only 450 cm^2. To give two examples only: the birds damage their feet on the wire floors and they are unable by virtue of restricted space and the barren environment to perform natural comfort behaviours such as wing flapping, grooming and dust bathing. In the enriched cage, which provides a perch, a scratching surface and more space, some of these comfort behaviours become possible. Outdoors, on free range, the bird has both the freedom and the resources necessary to perform comfort behaviour.
- Control of bacterial and parasitic infections is easier in cages, mainly because the birds are kept out of contact with their own excreta, and that of passing wild birds. This assumes great importance when there is a risk of their contracting a disease such as bird flu, especially strains that may also infect humans.
- Osteoporosis leading to chronic pain from bone fractures is likely to be a problem with all laying birds in the extreme confinement of the barren cage stocked at 450 cm^2 per bird. This is because one of the major predisposing factors to osteoporosis is extreme, enforced

inactivity. The enriched cage permits more movement and some increase in bone strength. Active birds on free range have denser bones but are at greater risk of damage, e.g. to the sternum or keel bone as they fly to roost.

- There is good evidence that laying hens experience extreme frustration in the barren cage, most especially the frustration associated with their inability to select a suitable nesting site prior to laying their daily egg. The enriched cage and the free-range unit are both equipped with nest boxes.
- A laying hen may be less likely to experience fear when confined in a group of three or four birds within a caged system, than when in a group of 10,000 birds on a free-range unit. Fear in free-range birds may result from experience of aggression, or it may simply involve agoraphobia, i.e. fear of open spaces. Note, however, that while fear may be a stress, it may lead to adaptation rather than suffering if the birds learn to cope. On free range, birds have greater freedom of action and opportunities for education. They can take action (e.g.) to avoid the consequences of aggression. They can also habituate to the experience of being outdoors, i.e. learn that it is not a cause for alarm but a source of satisfaction.
- According to the fifth of the freedoms, the freedom to express normal behaviour, the free-range unit wins by a distance.

Application of the five freedoms and provisions to the evaluation of animal welfare on an individual farm is illustrated in Table 1.3. In this example, the five provisions create a structure for the identification of risks and hazards, and thus the application of a programme for the monitoring and control of animal welfare at farm level according to internationally recognized HACCP (hazard analysis and critical control point) principles. This approach is considered in more detail in Chapter 17. Hazards characterized as inadequate provision of nutrition

Table 1.3 Application of the 'five provisions' to the identification of risks and hazards to farm animal welfare.

Provision	Hazard	Risk	Examples
1. Nutrition	Under-feeding	Hunger	Out-wintered sheep
	Unbalanced diets	Metabolic disease	High-yielding dairy cows
2. Housing	Concrete floors	Discomfort	Lameness in cows and pigs
	Cages	Injury and pain	Bone fractures in hens
3. Health care	Poor hygiene	Infectious disease	Mastitis in cows
	No vaccination policy		Respiratory diseases in poultry
	Lack of foot care	Pain	Lameness in cattle, sheep
4. Security	Barren environment	Injury	Tail-biting in pigs
	Poor stockmanship	Anxiety	Rough handling
5. Choice	Extreme confinement	Frustration	Sow stalls
	Barren environment	Learned helplessness	Barren cages for hens

include underfeeding, e.g. in out-wintered sheep, creating a risk of hunger, possibly amounting to starvation. The category also includes the feeding of nutritionally imbalanced diets creating a risk of metabolic disease, e.g. in high-yielding dairy cows. The other hazards and risks within the categories of housing, health care, security and choice should now be self-explanatory. As one further example, I would cite freedom from fear and stress, here expressed by the single word, security. Hazards include barren environments for growing pigs that can increase the risk of tail-biting and aggression, and poor stockmanship, especially rough handling, that can provoke increased anxiety in farm animals when in the presence of humans.

These examples are presented here in brief to illustrate the central logic of the five freedoms. The welfare of animals in any system must be assessed according to all the paradigms. It is not sufficient to claim that the free-range system is superior simply because the birds are free to express normal behaviour. If mortality, preceded by a period of malaise (i.e. feeling unwell) on a free-range unit is shown to be significantly greater than in a caged system, then this must be taken into account, not just on economic grounds, but also because it is an important measure of poor welfare. Different individuals and different societies rank the importance of the five freedoms differently when passing judgement in matters of animal welfare. For example, the long-term housing of pregnant sows in individual stalls is prohibited within the European Union but currently permitted in the USA by federal law.[1] The fact that legislators within the two communities reviewed the same scientific evidence but came to opposing conclusions reflects the fact that, while such decisions may claim to be based on science, they are in fact value judgements influenced not only by science but also by pressure, on the one hand, from consumers in the current will of society. However, whatever may be the overall judgement on animal welfare on an individual farm or within a production system; it must include reference to all the freedoms. The best judgement is likely to be that which assesses the importance of the different freedoms in a way that most closely approximates to the animal's own measure of these things. This requires a profound understanding of the nature of animal motivation and animal behaviour (Chapter 2).

1.3.2 Good Feeding

So far as the animals are concerned, the first provision of good husbandry is to ensure freedom from hunger and thirst. Freedom from thirst is achieved by provision of water fit for drinking from natural sources, containers (e.g. water troughs) or dispensers (e.g. nipple drinkers) that allow each individual to satisfy its needs. Provision of food for farm animals is a much more complex affair. In most livestock production systems animal feed is the major cost to the farmer. Thus the first essential for economic production is to maximize the efficiency of conversion of animal feed into saleable animal produce (meat, milk or eggs). The terms 'food conversion efficiency' (FCE) and 'food conversion ratio' (FCR) are used both by farmers and throughout this book. FCE is the proper description of efficiency (i.e. output: input). However,

---

1 Individual states within the USA (e.g. California, Maine, Michigan) have passed state laws to ban pregnancy stalls for sows and barren cages for laying hens.

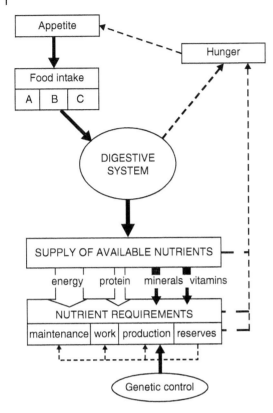

Figure 1.5 Factors affecting the supply and demand for digestible nutrients in animals.

FCR (input:output) is in more common use. A broiler production unit may report an FCR of 1.56. In this case it is the ratio of total of feed consumption by a flock of birds relative to the weight of birds sold for slaughter.

Figure 1.5 outlines the steps involved in the conversion of animal feed to animal product as seen by both the animal and the farmer. Consider the case of intensive pig and poultry systems where machines are used to mix and dispense a 'compound' ration usually based on a cereal such as barley combined with a protein source (e.g. soya bean meal) and other supplements to provide a balanced supply of nutrients. This feed mixture (illustrated for simplicity in Figure 1.5. by ingredients A, B and C) is broken down in the digestive tract to supply nutrients available for metabolism: energy, protein (as amino acids), minerals and vitamins to meet the animals' requirements for maintenance and production of saleable produce such as meat, milk or eggs. Feed required to sustain maintenance of body tissues generates no output (i.e. FCE at maintenance is zero). As output increases relative to maintenance FCE increases, although as nutrient supply approaches the genetic capacity of the animal to produce milk, meat or eggs, increasing amounts of energy will be stored as fat in adipose tissue. These fat reserves can, of course, be called on in times when nutrient demand exceeds supply. This can occur when supply of digestible nutrients is restricted, as is the case for grazing animals during the winter in higher latitudes or during the dry season in the tropics. It can also occur when the productive capacity of the animal exceeds its capacity to consume and digest feed, as is the case for many high-yielding dairy cows in early lactation.

An animal's motivation to eat is driven by hunger and appetite. These two things are not quite the same. The conscious appetite of an animal may be stimulated by the sight or smell of good food, or the foreknowledge that feeding time is approaching. If it has not eaten for some time its appetite will be increased by a sense of hunger. If it has recently eaten a large meal, it will be satiated and its appetite will be less. The internal sensations of hunger and satiety are determined partly by sensations from the digestive tract (e.g. a full stomach) and partly by a sense of 'metabolic hunger' stimulated (e.g.) by a low blood concentration of an essential substrate such as glucose. An animal that is unable to meet its dietary requirements for maintenance and production will experience metabolic hunger. As indicated above, this can occur in a sheep kept outside over winter where the quantity and quality of the food are insufficient to meet maintenance needs. It can also occur in a high-yielding dairy cow when her nutrient requirements for lactation exceed her capacity for digestion. In these circumstances she can be both 'hungry and full-up'. She experiences the simultaneous discomfort of metabolic hunger and digestive overload.

A 'good feed' for farm animals should meet four criteria:

- It should provide a balanced supply of nutrients for the needs of maintenance and production (work, growth, pregnancy and lactation).
- It should promote efficient, healthy digestion.
- It should provide oral satisfaction.
- It should do no harm.

The provision of a ration containing a balanced supply of nutrients has been introduced already. It is equally important that the feed should be provided in a form that matches the digestive function and digestive capacity of the animal. This is particularly important when feeds are prepared for natural grazers such as ruminants. The rumen of cattle and sheep has evolved to permit the anaerobic microbial digestion of cellulose and other fibres within a large well-stirred fermentation vat. Most compound rations for ruminants at high levels of production (e.g. the dairy cow) supply energy from a mixture of fibrous grasses, fresh or conserved as silage or hay, and starchy cereals. If the ratio of starch to digestible fibre is too high, fermentation may proceed too rapidly, leading to indigestion and acidosis within the rumen, with complications such as painful inflammatory laminitis within the feet. If the ratio of highly digestible starch to less digestible fibre is too low, the dairy cow will be unable to consume and digest enough feed to meet her nutrient requirements for lactation. She will then draw excessively on her body reserves, leading to loss of body condition, infertility and increased predisposition to injury and disease.

The feed should provide oral satisfaction. This is particularly important in housed adult animals such as horses and pregnant sows fed rations well below the limits of their appetite and given little to occupy their time. It is natural for a grazing animal such as the horse to nibble at food for 8–10 hours a day. It is natural for a pig to root in the ground for nuts, worms and other attractive food sources. Offered only a highly digestible, high-energy diet, a horse or pig may be able to consume enough nutrients to meet its needs within 10 minutes. It is then likely to become hungry and frustrated for the rest of the day. This frustration can lead to profoundly disturbed, stereotypic behaviour (Chapter 2) such as bar-chewing in sows, crib-biting and wind-sucking in horses. The oral satisfaction provided by a diet that includes hay or chaff for a horse, or by an environment that allows a sow to root in the earth, can prevent these behavioural disturbances and the frustration that they reveal.

The fourth essential of a good diet is that it should do no harm. It should not contain poisonous weeds or other toxic substances such as heavy minerals. Furthermore, it should be free from infectious agents, such as pathogenic bacteria or fungal toxins acquired during improper storage. Any feed of animal origin must be demonstrably free from prions responsible for the transmission of spongiform encephalopathies (TSEs), most notably responsible for 'mad cow disease'.

1.3.3 Housing and Habitat

Farm animals are housed mainly for the convenience of the farmer. Pigs and poultry are confined in houses to save land and reduce the cost and labour involved in feeding and handling. Cattle are brought off pasture in the winter more to protect the pasture than to protect the animals. It is, however, good husbandry, and usually good economics, to design housing and other facilities so as to meet the environmental requirements of the confined animal. The four most important environmental requirements of farm animals are comfort, security, hygiene and freedom to perform behaviours intended to achieve these things. In Table 1.4, freedom of behaviour is described by the single word, 'choice'. Freedom from thermal discomfort is achieved by providing an environment that is neither too hot nor too cold, where hot and cold cannot be defined simply by air temperature but must take into account all factors that determine heat transfer between an animal and the environment; especially air movement, precipitation and solar radiation. Provision of an optimal thermal environment is

Table 1.4 Major environmental requirements of farm animals (adapted from Webster 1995).

Comfort, thermal	Neither too hot nor too cold
Comfort, physical	A suitable resting area
	Space for grooming, limb-stretching, exercise
Security	Of food and water supply
	From death or injury due to predation, aggression, floods etc.
	From fear of predation or aggression
Hygiene	To reduce the risk of disease
	To avoid the discomfort of squalor
Choice	To permit coping behaviours
	To allow animals to acquire security through experience and adaptation to the normal sights and sounds of farm activity

dealt with on a species-by-species basis in subsequent chapters. As a general rule, most intensively farmed pigs and poultry are kept in controlled environment buildings, mainly to minimize feed energy requirement for maintenance and so maximize FCE. For most grazing animals, shelter from excessive sun, wind and rain is usually sufficient to ensure both adequate welfare and efficient production. For a fuller description of factors affecting the heat exchanges of farm animals, see Wathes and Charles (1994).

The most important requirement in terms of physical comfort, security and hygiene is a good resting area. The relative importance of the different criteria necessary to define a suitable resting area is summarized in Table 1.5. Poultry, for example, do not require a soft bed or a yielding mattress. They prefer to rest on perches. Chickens are motivated to perch at night by an innate fear of predators operating at ground level. This has been essential to their survival in the wild. Although there be may no real risk of predation in a controlled environment poultry house, the innate fear persists, so their selection of resting area is driven primarily by the need to experience a sense of security. The need to achieve a real (rather than imagined) degree of security is important for laying hens, who can and will injure one another, but not for young broilers, who do not.

The requirements of the large, bony, heavy dairy cow may be placed at the opposite end of the spectrum from those of the laying hen. Her greatest need is for a bed that is soft and yielding when she lies down, but does not impede her movement when in the act of standing up and lying down. Bare concrete fails on both counts. Rubber mats are barely adequate. Deep straw is comfortable but may fail on grounds of hygiene and increase the risk of mastitis. Deep, dry sand is close to ideal in terms of both comfort and hygiene (see Chapter 3). Most of the other rankings in Table 1.5 should now be self-explanatory and all will be considered in more depth in subsequent chapters. However, note all the reasons why it is important to provide a suitable resting area for neonates, especially when they have been removed from their mothers. Hygiene and warmth are particularly important, the former to reduce the risk of exposure to infection, the latter to reduce the risk of thermal stress leading to a loss of resistance to infection.

Table 1.5 The relative importance of the different criteria necessary to define a suitable resting area for farm animals (adapted from Webster 1995). Importance is ranked from 0 (unimportant) to ''' (highly important).

	Hygiene	Dryness	Softness	Warmth	Security
Poultry, broilers	*	***	0	*	0
Poultry, layers	*	**	0	0	**
Pigs, weaners	**	**	*	**	*
Pigs, dry sows	*	**	**	**	***
Cattle, young calves	**	***	**	**	0
Cattle, dairy cows	**	**	***	0	**
Sheep, adult ewes	*	**	*	0	*
Horses, adult	**	**	**	0	*
Neonates, general	***	***	*/0	***	***

The last, but not the least, environmental requirement listed in Table 1.4 is defined as 'choice'. Sentient animals make decisions that enable them to cope with environmental challenges and improve the way they feel. As explained earlier, an animal such as a sow in the extreme confinement of an individual pregnancy stall may suffer because it is prevented from taking any constructive action it feels necessary to relieve its frustration. This is an extreme example (and in Europe, illegal). However, as a general rule, farm buildings and confinement areas should be designed and managed so as to allow the animals to acquire a sense of security through experience and adaptation to the normal sights and sounds of farm activity. This requirement is clearly stated in the UK *Codes of Welfare for Farm Animals* (DEFRA 2003).

1.3.4 Fitness and Health

The third of the five freedoms (Table 1.1) is 'freedom from pain, injury and disease, by prevention or rapid diagnosis and treatment'. The aim of good husbandry should go beyond this: it should be to breed, feed and manage farm animals so that they can sustain productivity and maintain physical fitness throughout a profitable working life. Since most animals reared for meat are killed at a very young age, this concern relates mostly to adults, breeding sows, laying hens and lactating cows. Here physical fitness implies more than just freedom from pain, injury and disease; it includes the maintenance of fertility and body condition. To give an extreme example, too many emaciated dairy cows are culled for infertility after a working life of less than three lactations. This is not only a measure of poor welfare for the cows, it also represents a loss to the farmer from animals that might have been highly productive at the start of their first lactation but failed to achieve an economically satisfactory lifetime performance.

Farm animals are susceptible to a wide range of diseases for which the primary cause is infection with pathogenic viruses or bacteria, or infestation with parasites. Farm animals may also act as carriers of infections that cause them little or no harm but can cause serious diseases in humans. The most important of these are bacterial infections with certain strains of *Campylobacter*, *Escherichia coli*, *Salmonella* and *Listeria* species. Thus control of infection and disease on farms is essential not only for the health and welfare of the animals but also for the protection of the general public. The strategies adopted for the prevention and control of farm animal diseases are outlined in Table 1.6. The surest way to protect farm animals from a specific pathogen is to adopt a strategy of total exclusion: i.e. ensure that the animals never come into contact with the infectious agent. This strategy can operate at national level, e.g. the UK policy to exclude and eliminate foot and mouth disease. It can also operate at farm level. Many pig farms are designated as carrying Minimal Disease, or Specific Pathogen Free (SPF) herds. In this case, the animals are protected from infection by a rigid programme of biosecurity. Animals live in controlled environment buildings protected from contact with possible disease carriers such as wild animals and birds. Stock-keepers have to wear protective clothing and shower in and out. Any new animals brought onto the site (e.g. breeding sows) must come from a farm operating to the same standards of SPF control. The exclusion approach is highly effective so long as it works. However, if there is a breach of biosecurity and disease enters the country, or the farm, the next step is draconian: slaughter all animals infected or exposed to infection, disinfect, leave the buildings unoccupied until safe to re-enter, then start again.

Table 1.6 Strategies for the prevention and control of infectious diseases in farm animals.

Strategy	Examples
Exclusion	National exclusion and eradication: e.g. foot and mouth disease
	Biosecurity at farm level: e.g. swine pneumonia
Vaccination	Poultry: Newcastle disease, coccidiosis
	Sheep: clostridial diseases
Hygiene	Dairy cattle: contagious and environmental mastitis
	Sheep, horses: parasite control through pasture management
Drug therapy	Pigs: antibiotic control of post-weaning diarrhoea
	Sheep, horses: parasite control through routine worming
Natural immunity	Calves: controlled exposure to endemic infections
	Pigs: reducing weaning stresses

For many infectious diseases of farm animals, the most effective means of prevention is to promote a lasting immunity through vaccination. Poultry in controlled environment buildings are vaccinated *en masse* against Newcastle disease (fowl pest), an infection that would otherwise cause catastrophic losses in an environment where so many birds are confined in a small space. Vaccination is the only effective method for control of clostridial diseases (see Chapter 5) in sheep at pasture because the bacteria that cause these diseases can survive for many years in the soil. Unfortunately many diseases of farm animals are not controlled by vaccination, because the vaccine does not exist, is limited in its effect or is too expensive.

Prevention of infectious disease through exclusion or vaccination is highly effective but only for those diseases for which such a strategy is possible. Since these methods are effective, these diseases are usually under control. It follows that most of the infectious disease problems on modern commercial farms are those associated with endemic organisms that cannot be eliminated from the environment and where absolute immunological protection is unfeasible. Examples include parasitic infections in grazing cattle and sheep, mastitis in dairy cows, and many respiratory diseases. With this category of diseases, it is not possible to exclude the possibility of infection. Indeed, infection is the natural state: the aim of the farmer must be to create an environment wherein the balance between the challenge from the pathogens and the immune and other defence mechanisms of the animal is shifted in favour of the animal.

The three strategies for control of endemic diseases where vaccination is not an option are hygiene, use of chemotherapeutics (antibiotics and antiparasitic drugs) and promotion of natural immunity. In each case the aim is not to eliminate infection but to reduce the risk that infection will proceed to disease. Hygiene is designed to reduce the magnitude of the challenge. Examples presented in Table 1.6 include the control of mastitis in dairy cattle through good hygiene in the milking parlour, and the control of parasitic worm infestation through pasture management. These practices are admirable but not infallible. It is customary, and usually good husbandry, to reinforce the practice of good hygiene with the controlled use of chemotherapeutics (antibiotic or antiparasitic drugs) to keep the pathogen burden under control. However this approach can be abused. To take but one example: it has been common practice to dose growing pigs routinely and regularly with antibiotics. This was done initially to prevent catastrophic losses from diarrhoea and pneumonia. However, it was discovered that animals that were apparently healthy (to a casual eye) grew more efficiently (FCE was improved) when dosed regularly with antibiotics, which then acquired the name of 'growth promoters'. The reasons for this are complex but one of the reasons was a reduction in low-grade infection. This practice gave rise to public concern, mainly relating to the public health risks of increasing antibiotic resistance in bacteria pathogenic to humans. The use of antibiotics as growth promoters for farm animals is now banned in Europe. However, it is still possible for veterinarians to prescribe antibiotics for all the animals in a piggery when only a few appear to be sick. Thus the practice has not gone away. The use of chemotherapeutics for the prevention of disease in populations, rather than the treatment of individuals, is something that has to be considered on a case-by-case basis and in accordance with fundamental principles of good husbandry. It is, for example, good practice to incorporate regular worming of horses and sheep (especially the young animals) as part of an overall strategy for parasite control. It is good practice to control mastitis in dairy cows through dry cow therapy (Chapter 3). It is *not* good practice to rely on antibiotics as a strategy for keeping calves, pigs or poultry alive in conditions of squalor.

Last but not least among the strategies for prevention and control of infectious disease is to design systems that enhance natural immunity and so reduce the risk that exposure to infection will proceed to losses and ill thrift due to clinical disease. Natural immunity can cope with many infections when the challenge is not too severe and the immune mechanisms are not impaired by stress. Weaning is a particularly stressful time for young animals and can precipitate outbreaks of diarrhoea in pigs or pneumonia in calves. The aim should be to minimize weaning stresses and ensure that these do not coincide with increased exposure to infection (e.g. not moving weaned calves directly into a building containing older animals who are likely to be carriers of respiratory viruses).

Some of the most important diseases and disorders of farm animals are described as 'production diseases'. This description acknowledges that the prevalence and severity of these diseases are profoundly influenced by the standards of feeding, housing and hygiene imposed by the husbandry system. Table 1.7 lists some of the more common production diseases. These include infertility, mastitis and lameness in dairy cows, diarrhoea and wasting in weaner pigs, osteoporosis and bone fractures in laying hens, and lameness and hock burn in

Table 1.7 Some common production diseases of farm animals.

Animal	Disease
Dairy cattle	Infertility, mastitis, claw lameness, digital dermatitis
Beef cattle, finishers	Rumen acidosis, liver abscess, laminitis
Pigs, weaners	Diarrhoea and wasting
Laying hens	Osteoporosis, bone fractures
Broiler chickens	Lameness, hock burn

broiler chickens. Diarrhoea in weaner pigs, and mastitis and digital dermatitis in dairy cattle, involve infectious agents, but their cause and control are largely down to management. Other conditions such as lameness in broiler chickens and osteoporosis in laying hens can be attributed entirely to the way the animals are bred, fed and housed.

Infectious diseases and injuries that cause pain and lameness compromise both the success of the farm enterprise and the welfare of the affected animals. The aim is to control these things, ideally by prevention, but when they occur, by early diagnosis and treatment. The first aim of treatment is to attack the causative agent, e.g. by administration of an appropriate antibiotic in the event of bacterial infection. It is also necessary to address the welfare of the sick or injured animal through symptomatic treatment and nursing. To give two examples: the welfare of a lame cow will be improved if she is not required to stand on concrete but can be moved to a box with a comfortable straw bed. The welfare of a calf or foal suffering the chills of a pneumonic fever will be improved if it is allowed to lie under a heat lamp.

1.3.5   Freedom from Fear and Distress: The Art of Stockmanship

The aim of good husbandry is to promote freedom from fear and distress by ensuring conditions which avoid mental suffering (Table 1.1). In all but the most extensive farming systems (e.g. hill sheep) the animals come into regular contact with humans. The essence of good stockmanship is therefore to do all that is possible to avoid causing fear and distress and to strive to instil in the animals a sense of security. The principles of good stockmanship as applied to the different farm species are excellently set out in the DEFRA (2003) *Codes of Recommendations for the Welfare of Livestock*. Daily routines should be carried out calmly and consistently with the aim of accustoming the animals to the normal sights and sounds of farm activity. Farm animals, in common with most sentient creatures, are neophobic; they have an innate fear of novelty (Figure 1.4). Once the sights and sounds become routine, they habituate and acquire a sense of security.

There are, however, some occasions when the imposition of fear and distress is inevitable. These include procedures such as castration, de-horning, foot trimming, sheep dipping, transport and the routine administration of medicines. The use of anaesthetics is required by law for many painful procedures such as castration. Even procedures unlikely to cause pain (e.g. foot trimming, loading on to a lorry) can cause distress because they are novel, and because the animals are severely restrained, or forced in a direction they don't want to go. These procedures are likely to cause the most distress to extensively reared animals like sheep coming off the hill for the first time. The best way to minimize distress in animals that need to be moved or handled is through the design of facilities that permit the animals to move naturally with minimal disturbance and in the company of their own kind. The best exposition of the principles and practice of good livestock handling and management is that of Temple Grandin (1993).

1.4   Breeding for Fitness

Evolution through natural selection involves the survival of the fittest. Those animals whose genetic make-up is better suited to a particular environment are those more likely to breed successfully and pass on their genetic superiority (in that environment) to their offspring.

By domesticating animals and controlling their breeding to suit our own purposes, we have redesigned their phenotypes to produce more of the things we want and at greater efficiency: more milk per cow, more eggs per hen, faster growth and leaner carcasses in pigs and poultry, improved FCE. Controlled breeding of farm animals has been conspicuously successful at achieving these aims and, in the case of growth rates, milk yields and FCE, the evidence would suggest that the rate of progress can be sustained.

If a trait, such as growth rate, is heritable, then that trait can be 'improved' through genetic selection at a rate that is determined by its heritability. However, the consequences of selection are not limited to the trait or traits included in the selection programme, and some of these correlated responses to selection may compromise fitness and welfare. Thus, selection for increased milk yield in dairy cows has led to correlated increases in infertility (Simm 1998); selection for increased growth rate in broiler chickens has led to an increase in the prevalence of limb disorders (Kestin et al. 1992). The principles and practice of genetic selection in farm animals are too complex to consider here in any detail: for an excellent introduction see Simm (1998). There is, however, one general truth that needs emphasis. The traits that carry the highest heritability, such as coat colour, growth rate, and proportion of meat in the most expensive cuts, tend to be those which carry little or no benefit to the animals themselves within the Darwinian context of fitness. The traits that really matter to the animal, like mothering ability and viability of the offspring, carry a very low heritability.

The impact of genetic selection on production and production efficiency has been most conspicuous in the intensive poultry and pig industries. This does not automatically imply that these industries are more advanced. The first reason for the high response to selection is that these animals are kept securely in controlled environment houses with all the high-quality feed they need. The second reason is that selection has been directed almost entirely at 'improved' traits in animals destined directly for slaughter (e.g. growth rate, carcass quality, FCE) with little regard for traits that may affect the fitness of the breeding animals. Table 1.8 outlines some of the key factors that determine the efficiency of production in meat animals

Table 1.8 Factors affecting the efficiency of meat production: allocation of food energy to the breeding and slaughter generations in broiler chickens, pigs, sheep and suckler beef cattle.

Inputs and outputs	Broilers	Pigs	Sheep	Beef cattle
Weight of breeding females (kg)	3	180	75	450
Progeny/year	240	22	1.6	0.9
Carcass yield from each meat animal (kg)	1.5	50	18	250
Total carcass yield/weight of dam	120	6.2	0.38	0.50
Proportion of feed energy/year				
to slaughter generation	0.96	0.80	0.32	0.48
to breeding generation	0.04	0.20	0.68	0.52

Source: Webster (2005).

and their implications for genetic selection. The most important single factor is the prolificacy of the breeding female. A broiler breeder that produces 250 chicks/year, slaughtered for meat at an average weight of 1.5 kg, can produce 120 times her own weight in the form of saleable meat per annum. At the other extreme, a ewe that produces 1.6 lambs per year yielding on average 18 kg of saleable meat/lamb only yields 32% of her own weight. In the case of broilers, 96% of feed is eaten by the slaughter generation; in pigs it is 80%, in sheep only 32%, i.e. 68% of feed is eaten by the breeding generation. Thus the improvements in efficiency (output: input) achieved through genetic selection in the pig and poultry industries reflect the fact that the slaughter generation dominates both outputs and inputs. Where the requirements of the breeding generation are relatively high (e.g. suckler beef cattle and sheep) then selection based on simply on growth rate, FCE and so on can drive efficiency in the wrong direction. It would, for example be extremely unproductive to stock the hills of Scotland with Suffolk sheep. In these circumstances breeding policy is typically based on the principle of 'divergent selection'. In sheep this might involve selection for 'meaty' traits in the sire breeds (e.g. Suffolk or Texel) and hardy, low-maintenance traits in the breeding females (e.g. Scottish Blackface). A fuller explanation of breeding strategies in the sheep industry is given in Chapter 5.

Within the global poultry, pig and dairy industries, the phenotype of the ideal production animal is determined by a small number of international companies who constitute the nucleus breeders. They provide the 'superior' male genes (usually in the form of semen) and breeding females and market these products either direct to commercial farms or through 'multiplier' units (Chapter 6). The superior genotypes are developed on the basis of a 'selection index' that nominates multiple traits relating both to productivity and fitness and weights them with the aim of achieving the most efficient compromise, measured in strictly economic terms. This will inevitably put greatest weight on production traits such as growth rate in broilers, even if it leads to a deterioration in the leg strength of growers and the fitness of broiler breeders (Chapter 8). However, breeding companies have, in recent years, come to place increased emphasis on fitness traits, in response to criticism from both producers and consumers that so-called high genetic merit animals were becoming increasingly unable to sustain fitness throughout their productive lives. Thus dairy cow selection in the USA is now based on an 'index of lifetime merit' that still gives 62% weighting to milk fat and protein yield but now allocates 38% to fitness-related traits such as reduced somatic cell count in milk and increased productive life.

In summary, the overall aim of controlled breeding in farm animals is to produce a superior animal, measured mainly in terms of production and productive efficiency. However, genetic superiority is not an absolute concept: it can only be measured in the context of a specific environment and in relation to the criteria used to define superiority. The 'superior' lines of pig or broiler chicken generated from the nucleus breeders for intensive, controlled environment production systems all tend to be very similar because both the selection criteria and the environments for which they have been selected are all much the same. Moreover, traits that may be defined as superior in commercial terms may not be consistent with fitness, especially in breeding adults. One sees the most genetic diversity within extensive livestock systems, where animals have to fend for themselves in a wide range of environments. Where environmental control is not an option, it makes more sense to exploit natural selection and genetic diversity to match animals to the environment, rather than vice versa, and this inevitably implies giving added weight to fitness traits. Paragraph 29 in the Welfare of Farmed Animals (England) Regulations (2000) states: 'No animals shall be kept for farming purposes unless it can reasonably be expected, on the basis of their genotype or phenotype, that they can be kept without detrimental effect on their health or welfare.' The intention of this regulation is admirable but it has yet to be tested in the form of a challenge as to whether any current breeding programme might be detrimental to animal health and welfare.

1.5 Transport and Slaughter

The procedures involved in the transport of farm animals and their handling in abattoirs up to the point of death will inevitably involve some degree of stress. Recent UK orders, the Welfare of Animals (Transport) Order 1997 and the Welfare of Animals (Slaughter or Killing) Regulations 1995, based on European Council Regulations, acknowledge that these procedures are inherently stressful and are designed to minimize the risk that animals will suffer physically as a direct consequence of any of these procedures, or suffer mentally in anticipation of them. The Transport Order sets out regulations concerning vehicle design, journey times and rest periods. The Slaughter Regulations state that 'No person engaged in the movement, lairaging, restraint, stunning, slaughter or killing of animals shall: (a) cause any avoidable excitement, pain or suffering to any animal; (b) permit any animal to sustain any avoidable excitement, pain or suffering.'

This legislation recognizes the range of potentially stressful experiences that an animal might encounter from the moment it is taken from the relative security of the farm environment to the point of death. The humanity of processes involved in the transport and slaughter will be determined by how well these principles are put into practice. Once again the five freedoms may be used as a comprehensive structure that can identify the major problems and point to solutions (Table 1.9).

Table 1.9 Application of the 'five freedoms' to identify welfare problems for farm animals in transport and at the place of slaughter.

	Poultry	Pigs	Cattle	Sheep
Hunger and thirst			Thirst	Thirst
Physical discomfort	Overcrowding[**] Shackling	Overcrowding[*]	Exhaustion	Exhaustion
Thermal discomfort	Heat stress[***] Cold stress[*]	Heat stress[***]		
Pain and injury	Bone fractures		Bruising	Smothering
Infection	Day-old chicks		Young calves[**]	
Fear and stress		Fighting	Fighting	Neophobia

Source: Webster (2005).

Pigs and poultry are much more susceptible to thermal stress (especially heat stress) than cattle and sheep, mainly because of their limited ability to regulate heat loss by evaporation. Pig and poultry transporters are designed, ventilated and sometimes air-conditioned to minimize the risk of thermal stress for the sound commercial objective of preventing animals from arriving dead at the abattoir. Sheep and cattle are unlikely to be killed as a direct consequence of heat stress but it can exacerbate their suffering from severe thirst and physical exhaustion when they are transported long distances. European regulations state that journey times for cattle, sheep and goats should not exceed 14 hours and must be followed by a rest period of at least 1 hour (Council Regulation (EC) 1/2005 on the Protection of Animals during Transport). This recognizes that the main problem for these animals will be exhaustion because they are likely to remain standing throughout the journey for reasons of security. Journey times for pigs may be up to 24 hours provided they have continuous access to liquid. This is because they lie down. Fighting, and injuries caused by fighting, constitute one of the main sources of stress in pigs and cattle, especially in lairage. All farm animals are likely to experience the stress of neophobia when exposed for the first time to the procedures involved in loading and unloading from vehicles. This problem is likely to be greatest for animals such as hill sheep that have had little or no previous experience of contact with humans and hardware. I repeat, the most effective way to minimize stresses in transport and at the place of slaughter is to design facilities that minimize human contact and encourage animals to move naturally and with a sense of security (Grandin 1993). This assumes particular importance when handling animals such as red deer (Chapter 10) where overexcitement and fear can also lead to serious injuries.

This is not the place to review in any detail the methods used for the stunning and slaughter of farm animals. For more information see Gregory (1998) and publications produced by the HSA (http://www.hsa.org.uk). Regulations state that 'animals should be slaughtered instantaneously or rendered instantaneously insensible to pain until death supervenes.' In most cases animals are first stunned to render the animal insensible, then 'stuck' and bled to death. The most common stunning method for cattle involves concussion, using a captive bolt pistol or percussion bolt gun. Pigs and poultry have conventionally been stunned by application of electric currents to induce an epileptic seizure. However, in recent years there has been increasing use of the gases carbon dioxide, argon or mixtures thereof to create insensibility prior to bleeding out.

The 1995 Slaughter Regulations recognize two key stages essential to ensure the humanity of the slaughter process:

- The stunning process should ensure that animals are rendered (almost) instantaneously insensible to pain (and fear) until death ensues.
- All abattoir procedures from the time of the animals' arrival to the time of death should be designed and executed in such a way as to avoid excitement, pain or suffering to any animal.

Incorporation of these principles into abattoir design and management is a complex business but vital in terms of both animal welfare and meat quality, since the two are related (Gregory 1998). The key principle must always be compassion. At an excellent abattoir in Scotland, there is written above the point of animal entry the words 'Quality control starts here. Treat all animals with care and kindness.' That says it nicely.

1.6   Ethics and Values in Farm Animal Welfare

Ethics, or moral philosophy, is a structured approach to examining and understanding the moral life: right thought and right action. There are two classic approaches to addressing moral issues, conveniently abbreviated as 'top-down' and 'bottom-up'. The classical 'top-down' approach asks the question: 'What general moral norms for the evaluation and guidance of conduct should we accept, and why?' The drawback to this approach is that practical issues tend to be given little emphasis or ignored. The alternative 'bottom-up' approach is first to identify a specific practical issue, then construct an analysis of relevant moral issues by a process of induction. Beauchamp and Childress (2001) have developed a powerful and widely adopted 'bottom-up' approach to addressing problems in biomedical ethics which builds upon well-established principles of 'common morality'; i.e. those principles and norms identified as relevant and important by reasonably minded people. These principles have been adapted by Mepham (1996) to livestock farming. The three pillars of common morality are all based on the central principle of respect:

- *beneficence*: – a utilitarian respect for the aim to promote the greatest good and least harm for the greatest number;
- *autonomy*: – respect for the rights of each individual, e.g. to freedom of choice;
- *justice*: – respect for the principle of fairness to all.

Any ethical evaluation of the use of animals by humans is complicated by the fact that the animals cannot contribute to the debate, and no benefit accrues to the individuals used in the process. This applies particularly to the principle of justice. Humans are moral agents and carry moral responsibilities. The animals are 'moral patients'. In this context, therefore, the concept of justice demands that we should always seek a fair and humane compromise between the likely benefits to humans and our moral duty to respect the welfare and intrinsic value of any animal in our care. Respect for the general welfare of individuals and populations is a utilitarian principle; respect for the intrinsic value of every farm animal is in accord with the principle of autonomy. However, no moral judgement regarding animal welfare, nor any action consequent upon this moral judgement, can be made in isolation. It must also consider the farmers who produce our food, consumers, especially those with little money to spend on food, and the overall impact of any decision on the living environment.

The three principles of respect and the four parties commanding respect are brought together in Table 1.10 in the form of an ethical matrix (after Mepham 1996). Farmers and all who work in the food chain have a duty to provide the public with safe, wholesome, affordable food. The utilitarian principle commands that we, the general public, have a duty to help farmers to promote the welfare of their animals and the living environment through our actions and our laws. This help may take the form of financial rewards for food produced to high welfare standards and subsidies for conservation of a living environment that can sustain biodiversity, wildlife and the beauty of the living countryside.

Our moral duties to farmers and their animals may be explained largely in utilitarian terms. They are also motivated by self-interest. Even the duty to sustain the living environment reflects not only our human respect for beauty but our long-term need to preserve the planet

Table 1.10 The ethical matrix as applied to the production of food from animals (adapted from Mepham 1996).

Respect for	Beneficence Health and welfare	Autonomy Freedom/choice	Justice Fairness
Farm animals	Animal welfare	*Telos*	Duty of care
Producers	Farmer welfare	Choice of system	Fair trade and law
Consumers	Safe, wholesome food	Choice/labelling	Affordable food
Living environment	Conservation	Biodiversity	Sustainability of populations

for our own ends. The matrix however recognizes that utilitarianism alone is not enough: our actions should also be motivated by the principles of autonomy and justice. The principle of autonomy commands respect for other living creatures and for the living environment by virtue of their very existence. It is most simply expressed by the maxim: 'Do as you would be done by.' In this context, the most important element of autonomy is equal freedom of choice, for us and for them. Individual consumers should have the right to select their food on the basis of knowledge (or at least trust) of those things that matter to them – price, quality, safety and maybe (if they wish) production methods. Farmers should have the freedom to adopt, or not adopt, production methods of which they may or may not approve, such as hormone implants in beef cattle, or genetically engineered crops.

Respect for the autonomy of the moral patients, farm animals and the living environment is a more difficult concept since it cannot be reciprocated (we may assume that animals feel no moral obligation to us). Nevertheless, the principle encourages us to recognize the *telos*, i.e. the fundamental biological and psychological essence of any animal; in simple terms 'the pigness of a pig'. A pregnancy stall for sows that denies them the freedom to express normal behaviour is an insult to *telos*, even if we cannot produce evidence of physical or emotional stress. If you disagree with this concept (and many do), consider two more extreme possible manipulations of farm animals in the interests of more efficient production: breeding blind hens for battery cages, or genetically engineering pigs to knock out genes concerned with perception and cognitive awareness (in essence, to destroy sentience). A strictly utilitarian argument could be marshalled to defend both practices since it could be argued that blind hens would be less likely to damage one another, and less sentient pigs would be less likely to suffer the emotional effects of discomfort and frustration. I offer these examples in support of the argument that, even when considering non-human animals, utilitarianism is not enough.

The principle of justice implies fairness to all parties. In the context of farm animal welfare the principle of justice imposes on us the duty of care. All those who keep farm animals and all those who eat their products should accept that these animals are there to serve our interests. Their 'purpose' is to contribute to our own good. It is therefore only fair to do good to these animals in a way that is commensurate with the good they do for us. We owe them a duty of care.

This chapter has introduced the major elements of good farm animal husbandry and welfare. Successive chapters describe the practical application of these principles to the management of farm animals in the major production systems. Our understanding of good husbandry is founded on science, technology and, most important of all, generations of practical experience and it is these things that that make up most of this book. Nevertheless, our duty of care to farm animals and to the living, farmed countryside cannot be measured in scientific terms. It can, and should, be informed by science, but it is defined by our sense of *values*. Ethics has been defined as the 'science of values': it offers justification and guidance for right action. The ethical matrix (Table 1.10) has something in common with the 'five freedoms' in that it can operate in practice as a checklist of concerns and an aid to diagnosis in matters of value. I invite you to use both frameworks when evaluating the welfare of farm animals within different production systems. The five freedoms will help you to assess how the animals feel ('fit and happy?'); the ethical matrix will help you to assess how well we meet our duty of care.

References and Further Reading

Beauchamp, T.L. and Childress, J.F. (2001). *Principles of Biomedical Ethics*, 5e. Oxford: Oxford University Press.

Dawkins, M.S. (1990). From an animal's point of view: motivation, fitness and animal welfare. *Behavioural and Brain Sciences* 13: 1–61.

DEFRA. (2003). *Codes of Recommendations for the Welfare of Livestock*. http://www.defra.gov.uk/foodfarm/farmanimal/welfare/onfarm/index.htm#we)

DEFRA (Department for Environment, Food and Rural Affairs). (2003). *Revised Codes for the Welfare of Pigs, Laying Hens, Meat Poultry and Dairy Cattle*. London: HMSO.

Farm Animal Welfare Council. (1993). *Second Report on Priorities for Research and Development in Farm Animal Welfare*. London: DEFRA Publications.

Fraser, D. and Broom, D.B. (1990). *Farm Animal Behaviour and Welfare*. Wallingford: CABI Publishing.

Grandin, T. (ed.) (1993). *Livestock Handling and Transport*. Wallingford: CABI Publishing.

Gregory, N. (1998). *Animal Welfare and Meat Science*. Wallingford: CABI Publishing.

Kendrick, K.M. (1998). Intelligent perception. *Applied Animal Behaviour Science* 57: 213–231.

Kestin, S.C., Knowles, T.G., Tinch, A.E., and Gregory, N.G. (1992). Prevalence of leg weakness in broiler chickens and its relationship with genotype. *Veterinary Record* 131: 191–194.

Mepham, B. (1996). Ethical analysis of food biotechnologies: an evaluative framework. In: *Food Ethics* (ed. B. Mepham), 101–119. London: Routledge.

Simm, G. (1998). *The Genetic Improvement of Cattle and Sheep*. Ipswich: Farming Press.

Wathes, C.M. and Charles, D.R. (1994). *Livestock Housing*. Wallingford: CABI Publishing.

Webster, J. (1995). *Animal Welfare: A Cool Eye Towards Eden*. Oxford: Blackwell Science.

Webster, J. (2005). *Animal Welfare: Limping Towards Eden*. Oxford: Blackwell Science.

Webster, J. (2022) Animal Welfare: understanding sentient minds – and why it matters.

2

Behaviour as an Indicator of Animal Welfare

Christine Nicol

2.1 Introduction

The study of animal behaviour can contribute to the assessment of farm animal welfare in many ways, and this chapter attempts a broad overview, with five major themes:

Section 2.2 describes approaches to the study of the motivation and causation of different activity patterns. This can inform thinking about which behaviours animals need to perform when kept in captive conditions. It is also important to understand how strongly an animal might be motivated to perform different behaviours, and to have insight into its preferences and aversions. Such information obtained from the animal's perspective can be set alongside

Management and Welfare of Farm Animals: The UFAW Farm Handbook, Sixth Edition.
Edited by John Webster and Jean Margerison.
© Universities Federation for Animal Welfare 2022. Published 2022 by John Wiley & Sons Ltd.

knowledge of the long-term health implications of different practices and policies and used to enable better decisions about farm animal housing and management.

Section 2.3 briefly considers the learning and cognitive abilities of farm animals and how these, within limits, can help animals adapt to a wide range of environments. Studies show that farm animals fare better in enriched environments that support flexibility and brain development and that allow opportunities for the expression of individual preferences, agency and control.

Section 2.4 addresses the question of how changes in behaviour can be validated as indicators of pain or disease, and as indicators of specific emotional states such as fear or frustration. The increasing use of technology has increased the range of behaviours that can be used as indicators of welfare at both finer and larger scales than previously possible. Examples include subtle changes in individual facial expression as a marker of pain, kinematic analysis to identify lameness, and changes in overall flock movement as an indicator of disease.

Section 2.5 considers whether there are any valid general markers of whether an animal is in a positive or negative welfare state. This can be addressed by identifying how behavioural and physiological changes are associated with patterns of animal choice. A large body of research is also examining how exposure to positive or negative conditions shifts an animal's general outlook, detected by biases in judgement and decision-making. Results from farm animal studies so far are highly variable. Possible reasons for this are identified.

Section 2.6 recognizes that even within genetically similar groups, animals differ in temperament or personality, with individuals adopting different social roles within groups. Genetic selection that produces animals that form good social relationships and beneficial social structures will be an important future goal.

Box 2.1 contains definitions of the terms used in this chapter.

Box 2.1   Definitions

Affective state – used variably in the literature as (i) a synonym for 'emotion' (ii) a description of long-term cumulative mood states or (iii) a psychological construct which includes (at least) dimensions of valence and arousal (see Figure 2.3).

Allostasis – the process of achieving stability through physiological or behavioural change

Arousal – the degree of activation of the sympathetic nervous system

Aversion – an observed tendency to avoid one resource or environment over another

Behavioural priority – a behaviour for which the animal shows a demonstrably high demand in a given housing environment

Behavioural substrate – an environmental material towards which an animal directs exploratory, foraging or comfort behaviour

Candidate behaviour – a behaviour that may be important for animal welfare in a given housing environment, but for which further evidence is required

Causal factor – an input to the brain's behavioural decision-making centre, derived from changes to the environment (external cues) or from changes to the animal's physiological state (internal cues)

Conditioned place preference (or aversion) – a measure of the amount of time an animal spends in (or avoids) an area that has been associated with an event or a stimulus, from which the valence of the event or stimulus can be inferred.

Conspecific – a member of the same species

Discriminatory cue – a stimulus that informs an animal when to make a response.

Economic demand theory – a method of assessing animals' priorities by establishing how much energy, work or time they will allocate to obtain one resource or behavioural opportunity relative to another. The methods were derived from economists' studies of human consumer behaviour

Habituation – the gradual waning of a response to a repeated event, in the absence of any reward or punishment associated with that event

Motivation – the study of the proximate causes of behaviour; the constantly shifting internal and external factors that result in decisions to change from one behaviour to another at any given time

Preference – an observed tendency to choose one resource or environment over another

Rebound behaviour – a response that indicates that internal causal factors have risen above the level that would normally result in behavioural performance in an unconstrained environment. When the behaviour is permitted after a period of prevention or restriction it occurs more intensely, more frequently or for a longer duration than normal

Resilience (sensu 1) – a measure of short-term adaptive capacity.

Resilience (sensu 2) – a measure of behavioural prioritization.

Robustness – a measure of long-term adaptive capacity.

Stereotypic behaviour – a repetitive and invariant response, that develops when other behavioural responses are frustrated, but eventually becomes emancipated from its original causal factors

Transitive – a property of a set of relations or preferences, such that if a > b and b > c, then a > c.

Utility – a term derived from economics that describes whether an event or stimulus is perceived as positive or negative. It provides a way of representing a preference relationship and can be considered as the common currency that enables animals to make choices between different options. It describes the value obtained (pleasure or satisfaction) from a resource.

Valence – a term derived from psychology that describes whether an event or stimulus is perceived as positive or negative. As with 'utility' it provides a way of representing a preference relationship and can also be considered as the common currency that enables animals to make choices between different options. It may be experienced as pleasant or unpleasant in animals that have conscious experiences. Valence is one dimension of affective state (see Figure 2.3).

2.2 Behaviours That Matter in Captive Environments

2.2.1 Identifying Candidate Behaviours

If a domestic animal is observed in a barren environment doing little other than feeding and resting it is difficult to know whether all is well, or whether something important is missing. The animal might be content, or it might be frustrated because the resources that would allow it to do a wider range of activities are absent. Unless information is available about what the animal *should* perhaps be doing (its candidate behaviours) it is impossible to distinguish these possibilities. The complex and adaptive behaviour of ancestral species provides a good place to start to think about what domestic farm animals may be capable of and what might matter for their welfare. Ancestral species include the European wild boar (*Sus scrofa*), ancestor of the modern pig, and the various sub-species of junglefowl (*Gallus gallus*) that have contributed to the origin of the domestic chicken. Observing wild boar and junglefowl in the wild can provide clues about pig and chicken candidate behaviours but it is not a gold standard for thinking about what domestic breeds need, not least because of the genetic changes that have occurred during domestication. Intense selection for high production has altered some of the behavioural tendencies of modern commercial strains. For example, compared with the red junglefowl, modern chickens have generally lost their capacity for broodiness. They are also less fearful, show altered patterns of social proximity, an increased preference for familiar companions, and a poorer ability to cope with group disruption (e.g. Eklund and Jensen 2011). Similarly, domestic pigs are less aggressive than wild boar.

Another point of comparison comes from the study of domestic animals that have escaped or been released from captivity and now live and reproduce freely with little or no interference from humans. Genetically these feral animals will be very similar to managed domestic breeds. Scientists have sometimes deliberately released domestic animals into semi-natural or highly enriched environments, with the aim of examining their behaviour under unconstrained conditions. In one study, domestic chickens that were released onto a small Scottish island were observed to form small, stable groups, roost at night and select extremely well-hidden nest sites. Stolba and Wood-Gush (1989) released pigs into a semi-natural woodland and observed their unconstrained behaviour. The pigs spent more than 50% of their time rooting and grazing, even when their energy needs were met with concentrate feed rations. Piglets from the same litter formed close social bonds with each other, whilst the maternal behaviour of the feral sows was complex and attentive. Observations of ancestral species and feral animals provide a good starting point for studies aimed at enriching farm animal environments or improving management at key periods, such as weaning. Even where no direct ancestral species now exists, a comparative approach can still be taken. Rorvang et al. (2018), for example, considered the impact of commercial housing and management on the welfare of dairy cows around the time of calving by using the unconstrained behaviour of closely related species as a baseline. Although the most direct cattle ancestor (the aurochs) is now extinct, the authors reviewed the perinatal behaviour of a range of other wild ungulates and feral cattle breeds, and used this to support their view that confinement, high stocking densities and unnatural olfactory stimuli all interfere with dairy cow welfare at this critical time.

2.2.2 How Much Do These Behaviours Matter?

Once candidate behaviours have been identified, the focus shifts to the question of whether domestic animals need to perform these behaviours in captive environments. Many welfare assessment frameworks assert that animals should be allowed full expression of normal behaviour but applying this in practice can be difficult and expensive, and it is worth examining the proposition in more detail.

If normal behaviour is considered to be simple body movements such as stretching, turning and self-grooming (the focus of the original 1965 Brambell Committee report (Brambell 1965) into the welfare of farm animals kept in intensive farming systems) then few would disagree that modern farming systems should be constituted to allow animals to do all of these movements. However, candidate behaviours also include courtship, exploration, foraging and fighting, and some of these may be virtually impossible to accommodate in captivity. Accommodating normal social behaviours can be particularly challenging in modern farming systems. For example, all commercial chicks are reared in hatcheries without their mothers and it is difficult to see how this could change, despite evidence of the benefits of maternal care for chick welfare.

We need to explore the question of desirability in more depth. If we are to maximize animal welfare within whatever economic or political constraints are operating, it is essential to understand how behaviour is motivated. Comparing the behaviour of a captive animal with that of its wild or feral counterpart is not sufficient to draw conclusions about animal welfare. Further information is needed about the cues that elicit different behaviours, about animal preferences and aversions, and information about how much these behaviours *matter* in the captive environments in which farm animals live.

2.2.3 Cues That Elicit Behaviour

Animal behaviour can be studied from different viewpoints, all of which are simultaneously relevant. If we ask 'why does the pig forage?', a valid functional answer would be that foraging is a good method of finding food, and pigs that forage effectively are most likely to survive and reproduce. But the same question can be rephrased to ask, 'why has the pig just stopped doing its current behaviour and switched to foraging?' This addresses the more immediate causes of behaviour. To answer it, the various current internal and external influences on foraging behaviour have to be identified. The study of animal *motivation* takes this causal viewpoint and is concerned with establishing the nature and strength of the cues for each behaviour. For foraging, these cues might include things like the concentration of glucose in the blood and the smell of the litter material on the floor. Studying motivation is highly relevant for animal welfare. If a behaviour is elicited mostly by adverse external *causal factors* then good welfare can be achieved either by allowing the animal to respond appropriately to those external cues *or* by removing those cues completely. Conditions such as excessive heat, noise or the appearance of an aggressive competitor or a predator are all examples of external causal factors that motivate normal adaptive responses such as seeking shelter, fighting or fleeing. In these situations, removing the external causal factors may be the best policy to protect welfare. The management of laboratory rodents provides a good practical illustration. The UK Home Office takes a precautionary approach and advises that rats and mice should not be co-housed within the same airspace, because rats are potential predators of mice. Removing any olfactory cues emanating from rats (the external causal factors) eliminates the motivation of the mice to hide or flee and reduces their anxiety. Since partridges (ground-living and foraging birds related to chickens) have recently been shown to avoid olfactory cues from potential predators, similar consideration should be applied to poultry housing.

However, the motivation for many other behaviours cannot be removed just by altering the environment. Although the underlying physiology is not always clear, many behaviours are motivated by internal cues that increase in strength during periods when the behaviours are not performed. Animals become hungrier, thirstier, more tired and more cramped if they are housed in systems that prevent feeding, drinking, lying or exercise. Removing food does not remove the desire to feed and restricting space does not remove the desire to move. When laying hens, rabbits or calves are released from confinement they show exceptionally high ('rebound') levels of movement and play, whilst dairy cows show a pronounced rebound in lying behaviour when deep-bedding is freely provided after a period of deprivation or difficult access.

Many other behaviours (e.g. sexual responses, nesting behaviours) are motivated by complex interactions between external and internal cues. Hens and sows, for example, continue to build nests even if they are given a perfect pre-formed nest, unlike gerbils which show a notably reduced motivation to dig if a pre-formed burrow is provided. For these reasons, nest-building in sows and chickens is sometimes described as a behavioural need as the provision of the ultimate goal does not remove the internal motivation to perform the behaviour.

2.2.4 Preference

Once something is known about the causation of a behaviour, the next step is to obtain an overview from the animals' viewpoint about which environments, resources or substrates they like or dislike. Choice tests are a good way of obtaining such information because animals appear to have evolved a general reward system to evaluate options both within and between motivational systems. Costs and benefits can be compared across different motivational systems only if there is some form of common currency for evaluation. The solution produced by natural selection appears to be the development of a general dopamine-based reward system which marks positive outcomes as pleasurable and negative outcomes as aversive. This currency might be called *utility* (by economists) or *valence* (by psychologists). When making a choice a farm animal is therefore likely to be estimating the likely affective consequences in advance.

Preference and aversion tests have been employed in a very broad range of contexts. One important area has been in support of development of valid environmental enrichment resources for pigs, poultry and cattle. In the case of pigs, this area of work has been stimulated by both legislation (notably a European Commission Directive which requires pigs to be given enrichment that enables 'proper investigation and manipulation activities') and the growth in farm animal certification schemes that require enrichment provision. In general, animals seem to prefer substrates that can be manipulated in natural ways, with flexible and destructible components, rather than things that are superficially exciting ('shiny toys') but give no lasting reward. The strong preferences of both growing pigs and sows for materials such as peat, compost, chewable ropes or straw are related to their evolutionary history as animals that chew and root with their snouts, and provision of these materials has the greatest beneficial effect in reducing harmful social behaviours. However, despite clear behavioural evidence showing that indestructible items such as hanging chains are not valued by pigs, many authorities are willing to accept their use rather than insisting on the inclusion of more beneficial forms of enrichment.

Preference tests have also contributed to the debate about the importance of outdoor or pasture access for dairy cows (Smid et al. 2018). At a time when the public is concerned about the growing practice of zero-grazing systems for dairy cows, information from the animals' perspective is important. Preference tests show that cows value access to outdoor areas and pasture but only under certain environmental conditions. If given the choice, cows generally spend most of their time indoors in winter to avoid rain and wind and in summer they spend considerable periods of time indoors to avoid solar radiation and flies. However, on warm summer nights cows choose to spend long periods lying outdoors. In cold or wet countries, where access to full pasture is not always feasible access to a deeply bedded outdoor area adjacent to the house has been trialled. Although these outdoor areas are less preferred than full pasture, they are nonetheless used extensively on summer nights.

Other preference tests have examined the foraging, dustbathing, lighting, and ramp design preferences of chickens as well as the features that contribute to biologically relevant roosting sites. Studies can reveal preference trade-offs, showing for example that the height of a perch is more important than its shape when chickens select roosting sites. Generally, preference is measured as the amount of time the animal spends accessing the available resources whilst remaining free to leave again at any time. More formal preference tests measure the frequency of discrete choices an animal makes for different alternatives and confine the animal for a short period of time after each choice in its chosen environment. This method has been used, for example to detect calf preferences for being brushed by a human caretaker. Although used less often, this latter method is more sensitive in detecting marginal preferences, probably because animal has to weigh up the consequences of its choice, rather than being able to leave at will.

The results from such preference tests are useful only if we believe that experimenters have accounted for perceptual and cognitive constraints and that the preferences expressed in tests are stable and reliable. Animal welfare scientists cannot predict in advance what animals should choose based on evolutionary theory and so confidence in the results is critical. One approach is to compare more than two different choice options against each other, as that can help to reveal the underlying structure of preference and can help us to understand whether animals are ranking the different options on some absolute currency linked to affective state, and hence to welfare. Importantly, the chickens studied by Nicol et al. (2009) made *transitive* choices, in that a bird that preferred A over B, and B over C, was very likely to choose A over C. This matters, because it suggests that the birds had relatively stable preferences over a long period of time and that their preference for one complex environment did not shift with age or the nature of the second environment it was paired with. Such information greatly increases confidence in results from preference tests.

2.2.5 Aversion

Just as animal behaviour experiments can be used to ask what sorts of stimuli or environments animals prefer, they can also be used as a tool to discover what animals find most aversive. Assessing *aversion* generally involves study of the learnt associations formed between stimuli that predict an aversive event and the onset of that same event. This means that animals do not have to be exposed repeatedly to potentially highly unpleasant events. Techniques for studying aversion depend therefore on associative learning.

Active avoidance techniques have been used to assess the aversiveness of pollutant gases such as ammonia in the animal house or of gases used for controlled atmosphere stunning prior to slaughter. In this important work, animals are either allowed to enter or leave a chamber at will, or to insert or withdraw their heads from a feeding station. If the gas being assessed for its potential use as a humane stunning agent is perceived as pungent, irritant or painful, then the animal will withdraw its head or leave much earlier. One method of stunning is to add carbon dioxide to air, which causes rapid acidification of the blood, depressed brain activity and relatively rapid death. However, experiments have shown that poultry perceive carbon dioxide in air to be highly aversive as it causes hyperventilation before brain activity is depressed. A better approach appears to be to use a mix of carbon dioxide within an inert gas (nitrogen or argon) which is less aversive and produces fewer signs of distress before unconsciousness. Similar approaches have been taken to assess the aversiveness of different types of anaesthetics for laboratory fish and it has been suggested that this work should be applied to develop food-grade anaesthetics that could be added to water to reduce distress during the slaughter of farmed fish.

Sometimes, however, animals are unable to mount effective active avoidance behaviours in the presence of highly aversive or frightening stimuli. They can literally become too scared or confused to move. For this reason, passive avoidance techniques have sometimes been used to assess aversion, whereby an animal learns *not* to perform a response, such as walking down a runway, or pecking a key, if it wants to avoid exposure to an aversive event. This aligns much better with the animal's innate response to the event. Passive avoidance has been used to demonstrate that particular handling and transport methods are aversive, including electro-immobilization (illegal in the EU, but still practiced in countries such as Australia), the isolation of sheep from each other during shearing, and some types of motion experienced during transport.

Aversions can also be assessed using conditioned preference testing procedures which rely on animals forming an association between a location (e.g. a distinctively coloured chamber) and an event experienced there. The advantage of conditioned preference tests is that they not only evaluate the aversiveness of various external stimuli (e.g. Paul et al. 2018) but can also be used to assess the aversiveness of internal sensations such as the animal's experience of pain or hunger, or the effectiveness of measures (analgesics or other drugs) designed to alleviate these states.

2.2.6 Assessing Priorities

Information about animal preferences is important, but it is not the whole story. Sometimes it may be difficult or expensive to adapt housing systems or management practices to cater for animal preferences and regulators may query the extent to which increased investment will genuinely increase animal welfare. This has resulted in the development of methods to evaluate the strength of animal motivation. Dawkins (1983) argued that the value animals place on particular behaviour patterns could be explored formally in a variety of ways using techniques derived from *economic demand* theory. By reducing the animal's effective income (its energy or time budget) one can observe how it redistributes its activities. When the total time available for feeding, lying and social contact was constrained, Danish Holstein dairy cows defended lying time at the expense of time spent eating or in social contact, during both early and late lactation (Munksgaard et al. 2005). Lying could therefore be described as the most *resilient* of the behaviours examined. This contrasts with the observation that baboons conserve time spent in social interactions at the expense of time spent resting, meaning that social behaviour is more resilient than resting in these primates.

A related approach is to observe what happens when an animal has to pay a one-off 'entrance fee' to access a resource but can then make use of that resource for as long as it wishes. This is useful to assess demand for resources whose value may depend on duration of access, such as social contact or access to a nest. The currency of the entrance fee is most often effort expended in pushing against a weighted door with adjustable resistance. This method has been used to calibrate the strength of motivation for access to perching, dustbathing and nesting resources in hens, as well as social contact in fish. In dairy cows, Tucker et al. (2018) found that as push-door weight was increased cows proportionally increased their efforts to obtain deep bedding, with a proportion of cows making the maximum effort possible by pushing 40% of their body weight. Others have reported that cows will work as hard to access pasture during the evening hours as for access to fresh feed in the period after milking. When entrance fee tests are employed animals often show compensatory behaviour. As the cost of access increases, animals may reduce the number of times they pay the price whilst increasing the length of time they stay with the purchased resource. From a welfare perspective, the extent of compensation is an important factor to consider alongside the maximum effort the animal will expend.

A more formal approach derived from economic demand theory is to adjust the specific price that an animal has to pay to access a given resource or environment. As the price is adjusted, changes in the animal's demand are observed. This approach has been used to compare the number of panel presses performed by pigs to access either food, partial social contact, or an empty pen (control) (Matthews and Ladewig 1994). Pigs worked for food under both low and high price conditions, increasing their efforts as the price of access was steadily increased to maintain consumption. This defence across price change can be described as an inelastic pattern of demand. In contrast, although pigs worked for social contact at the lower prices their demand tapered rapidly as price increased. Demand for social contact was therefore described as elastic, although it was still demonstrably higher than for the control condition. Despite the theoretical appeal of this approach, and its potential advantage in allowing the importance of different behaviours to be compared independently of whether they occupy a large part of a daily time budget (sleeping) or a very small part (stretching), experimental studies of demand elasticity are time-consuming to perform and are still relatively uncommon in farm animal welfare science. Scientists continue to explore the underlying methodology using food as a standard reward. There are also some studies of demand elasticity for foraging or dustbathing substrates in chickens, partial or full social contact in calves, and lying requirements in heifers.

Another sensitive technique is to allow an animal to work simultaneously for two different resources, providing an integrated assessment of the animals' relative preferences and the motivational strength underlying the preference. The cross point of these double demand curves provides a measure of the relative attractiveness of the two resources whilst the steepness of the line provides a measure of the demand elasticity. This approach has been used to measure the preferences and motivational strengths of pigs' demand for rooting materials (Figure 2.1 from Pedersen et al. 2005) and calf demand for different types of roughage.

Although measuring demand elasticity is an appealing approach, it is not appropriate in all situations. Other measures of motivation such as maximum price paid, total number of

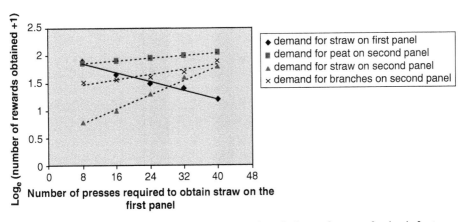

Figure 2.1 The double-demand approach assesses the relative preference of animals for two resources. Here, pigs worked to obtain straw on panel 1, and an alternative substitute (peat, straw or branches) on panel 2. The experiment was designed so that when straw on panel 1 required 8 presses, the alternative substrate required 40 presses; when straw on panel 1 required 16 presses, the alternative substrate required 32 presses, and so on. The pigs' preference for peat was stronger than their preference for the other substrates. Equal amounts of straw and peat were obtained when straw cost 9 presses and peat cost 39 presses (adapted from Pedersen et al. 2005). Used with permission from Elsevier.

responses, speed of choice or the degree of use made of the resource once accessed are also used. The very high number of panel presses made for food by pigs kept under commercial levels of feed restriction is a good indication of their chronic hunger. Similarly, food-restricted broiler breeder chickens will traverse surprising lengths and depths of water to obtain access to foraging materials (Dixon et al. 2014). Birds on the most severe commercial levels of feed restriction were willing to pay a maximum price that was two to three times higher than that for birds on less severe levels of feed restriction, as measured by more frequent and faster crossings of the water and greater use of the foraging material once it was accessed. Such results might suggest that the adverse consequences of food restriction could be avoided by increasing oral satisfaction or the sensation of gut-fill by bulking diets with fibre, or by providing more opportunities to forage. However, such strategies appear only partially effective, and severe food restriction is associated with ongoing metabolic hunger in pigs and broiler breeder chickens. Selection for increased growth potential appears to have altered their hunger regulation mechanisms, and appetite persists even when diets are bulked, and when further eating results in obesity and compromised health (de Jong et al. 2003). In studies of pigs, the maximum price that sows would pay using a panel press response to make social contact with subordinates was relatively low in comparison to the price that the same pigs would pay for a small proportion of their daily feed allowance. However, it should be recognised that assessing demand for social contact is far more difficult than assessing demand for food. Animals, social mammals in particular, are likely to have preferred companions, something not yet factored in to demand experiments.

The original papers proposing the application of economic techniques to animal welfare (e.g. Dawkins 1983) captured the imagination of scientists and these remain some of the most highly cited papers in the field. Despite this, there have been relatively few experimental studies of farm animal demand and the studies that have been conducted have not provided simple answers. Demand experiments cannot answer the difficult question of whether animals 'miss' resources that are currently out of sight (or out of the perceptual range of any other sense organs) or that have never been experienced. In some cases, strong demand in an experiment may be an artefact of the experimental situation itself. Economic demand methodologies are also highly dependent on the precise methodologies employed, and on the background experiences of the animals. They rely on the animal gaining some experience of the resource that they are working for, either during training or testing, and there is a risk that satiation effects can creep in. Whatever the method of assessing motivational strength employed, careful interpretation is essential and still requires a point of comparison. If demand for a resource such as social contact or enrichment is compared against the effort that a very hungry animal will expend to obtain food (a common 'yardstick') this sets a very high bar and risks underplaying the importance of the other resources under investigation. These methods are one of the most important tools in the welfare toolbox, but one of the most difficult to use. A general conclusion might be that the results obtained should be considered alongside other lines of evidence in making an overall judgement about animal welfare.

2.3 Learning and Cognition Support Adaptation and Agency

Animals that have been domesticated are adaptable and flexible. They may thrive in a variety of different management systems or when leading feral lives in a variety of different environments. This is recognized in the concept of allostasis, the idea of 'stability through change'. Good animal welfare is characterized within this framework as a capacity to anticipate and deal with environmental challenges, and it predicts that farm animals will be able to adapt within a relatively broad range of situations. Some have argued that so long as animals are free to make trade-offs and decisions on their own adaptive terms then even situations which superficially appear to be stressful will not cause suffering. If the animal has entered willingly into the situation and has the resources to deal with it, then all will be well. The capacity to adapt may be what is most crucial for animal welfare. Two patterns of environmental challenge and adaptive response have been distinguished. The ability of animals to respond and cope with short-term episodic or situation-specific challenges through their capacity to learn is described as *resilience (sensu 1)*, whilst their ability to thrive in a wide range of stable environments or to acclimatize to slow changes through innate regulatory pathways, is described as *robustness*.

The degree to which initial reactions to stimuli can be modified by learning is a critical component in the animal's ability to cope with many modern housing systems, and learning can sometimes shift an animal's preferences and aversions. A novel noise, for example, may be initially experienced as frightening but through the process of *habituation*, the animal may learn that the noise is harmless and cease to react with innate responses (such as flight or attack). Habituation is stimulus-specific (an animal will continue to react as before to new stimuli – it is not fatigued) and occurs most rapidly if the animal is exposed repeatedly to the irrelevant stimulus, with short intervals between exposures. Specific habituation programs using such principles can successfully reduce negative reactions to new procedures such as machine milking in cows, buffalo or even donkeys, but habituation will also occur naturally if there is genuinely nothing for the animal to fear. Habituation to the presence of people is perhaps the most useful adaptation of farm animals, as well as for wild animals forced into ever-closer proximity with human visitors and tourists. It is crucial to appreciate that habituation takes place *only* to stimuli that are irrelevant. Animals will not habituate to aversive stimuli such as rough handling by humans, repeated chasing (in fish farming) or excessive noise. On the other hand, the effects of habituation can persist through generations. Quail raised by human-habituated mothers do not become generally less fearful, but they do show a specific reduction in fear of humans. The converse of habituation is sensitization, a process whereby animals react more intensively to stimuli that they have encountered repeatedly. In most farming systems this is not a good thing, particularly if the reaction is one of fear or pain. It is well established that early life exposure to acute pain can result in later chronic sensitization or hyperalgesia. In mammals, the high turnover of neural connections during early growth of the brain allows a much greater degree of plasticity than is possible in later life, so early exposure to stress or pain can have profound effects on stress, pain and behavioural responses throughout life. Farm animals, such as sheep and pigs, are routinely subjected to painful husbandry procedures (e.g. tail-docking, castration) soon after birth. In other species, including humans, pain in infancy commonly sensitises the affected regions (Schwaller and Fitzgerald 2014). So, not only are such mutilations a cause for concern on welfare grounds at the time, but for many months or even years afterwards

Associative learning is the other major way in which animals can adapt to their environments. In classical conditioning, animals learn to predict how one event follows another, whilst in instrumental learning, an animal learns to perform a new behaviour. Associative learning occurs primarily when an animal's existing expectations about the world no longer hold true. Learning is thus intimately bound up with the occurrence of the unexpected and serves to establish new expectations based on patterns of events. Common examples of learning within farming systems abound – the use of electric fencing, electronic sow feeders and robotic milking systems all depend on the instrumental learning capacities of farm animals. Sows, for example, can learn to enter a feeding station specifically when they hear their own unique acoustic cue signalling that is their turn to approach and feed (Kirchner et al. 2014).

Farm animals are social creatures, with a capacity for learning from each other and a tendency to attend to and remember social events. Social acquisition of knowledge about where and how to find food has been convincingly demonstrated in chickens, sheep and calves. The influence of same-age companions is important, and farm animals can also learn socially from humans. For example, goats solve a spatial maze task more quickly if they observe a human demonstration. Social memory and extrapolation of social position is generally excellent. Sheep, for example, remember the identity of at least 50 other different sheep faces for more than two years. Sheep also use sophisticated spatial memory strategies to remember the location of preferred foraging patches and integrate this knowledge with an assessment of their own position within the group social structure. Dominant sheep develop their own expectations of where the best food might be found, and also monitor, use and exploit their subordinates' expectations about food. Chickens too assess their own relative social position against a strange bird, by extrapolating information about how the stranger fares in encounters with familiar dominant and subordinate companions.

The young of all of these species learn particularly well from their mothers. Lambs, for example, show a more prolonged tendency to avoid unsafe feeding sites avoided by their mothers, than if they rely purely on their own experience. The role of the mother hen is also hugely important to young chicks. Hens give characteristic food calls and demonstrate the edibility of an item by picking it up and dropping it again in front of their chicks. They increase the intensity of this display when the food is of particularly high quality, or when the chicks move away or fail to respond. Even more remarkably, hens seem to recognize when the chicks make mistakes. This has been investigated in experiments that ensure that the chicks' information about food palatability is different from that of the hen. If the hen perceives that her chicks are wrong, then she increases the intensity of her food-calling display. This cognitive ability is not restricted to the domain of feeding. Hens similarly use their knowledge about potentially dangerous spatial locations (e.g. those associated with the likely occurrence of an air puff) to guide the behaviour of their chicks. If a hen observes her chicks standing in a location that she perceives to be risky she will give a warning display even when

(i) she is herself in a safe environment and (ii) in the absence of any signs of fear or distress in the chicks (who believe the environment to be safe) (Edgar et al. 2013). The hen extrapolates her own knowledge and applies it not just to her own situation, but to that of her relatives.

These studies provide evidence that farm animals have sophisticated learning abilities. Their innate cognitive abilities are also sometimes surprising. Newly hatched chicks have cognitive abilities that are ready-to-use within hours of emergence. For example, young chicks can distinguish numbers up to five in the absence of any other cues (size or surface area), are able to perform simple addition and subtraction operations, and can also order numbers, picking the third, fourth or sixth position in a number line (e.g. Rugani et al. 2009).

From a welfare perspective it is important to consider how best to enhance the learning capacities of domestic animals to improve their *resilience (sensu 1)* and capacity to cope with new events and contingencies. Enriched environments improve both animal welfare and animal learning capacity. Performance in spatial learning and other cognitive tasks is improved in pigs raised in an enriched environment with straw and rooting materials, chickens raised in aviaries rather than barren cages, and calves raised in social groups. There is also evidence that farm animals fare better if provided with the opportunity to use their own agency to gain control over their environment. In natural conditions animals have a high degree of control over many aspects of their lives, including diet selection, social companions and degree of activity. In captivity much of the capacity for control is removed, and animals are often housed in standard environments which do not allow for differing preferences between individuals, or changes in individual preference over time or context. Experiments show that individuals who can choose when to leave or terminate negative situations have better welfare than animals that receive identical stimulation but which lack the opportunity to exercise control. If it is not possible to provide control, then welfare can still be improved in many situations by providing opportunities for animals to predict and prepare for events using their associative learning capacities. Knocking on a door before entering a chicken shed is one example of how stockpersons adopt this approach which can dramatically reduce startle and cardiac responses.

From the perspective of animal welfare it is also worth noting that farm animals will actively seek opportunities for cognitive engagement and to consider that farm animals may, like dogs, gain some pleasure from solving problems. Thus, not only should enrichment be provided because it sustains an adaptive capacity, but also because the opportunity to use learning and cognitive abilities may be considered a need analogous to the need to perform simpler stretching, foraging or locomotor behaviours. Farm animals are adaptable but they are not infinitely flexible, and they will suffer when kept in environments that deprive them of the opportunity to move properly or to forage, where they are separated from bonded companions, or subjected to chronic and unavoidable noise or pollution. These situations exceed their capacity to cope. Similarly, animals that are kept in under-stimulating conditions, unable to build new skills or develop their own agency in the world, may experience mental states that have some similarities with human boredom. Animals kept in barren conditions may even have an altered perception of time due to the monotony of their environment.

2.4 Behaviour as a Welfare Indicator

Animal behaviour can provide a highly sensitive indicator of animal welfare. Against a background of constantly shifting internal state, and variable external environment, an animal must integrate all inputs and produce just one behavioural output at any given time. Very subtle shifts in internal state or external circumstances can therefore produce observable changes in the type of behaviour performed, or the overall structure or patterning of behaviours over time. This section will review the advances made in methods of recording behaviour using automated technologies and will also review the types of changes that may be diagnostic of negative or positive changes in welfare.

2.4.1 Scale of Categorization

Behaviour consists of a continuous stream of movements which must be divided up into discrete units or categories. Traditionally the behaviour of domestic animals has been described using a catalogue of individual activities divided according to their presumed function (feeding, roosting, playing) or their overall gross structure (head extended, back arched). However, the advent of sophisticated technologies has heralded the ability to divide behaviour into much finer categories than previously possible. Small and subtle shifts in movement or facial expression can be captured by camera and have proved meaningful as indicators of pain and other emotional states. Pain grimacing is observed immediately post-surgery or following some other invasive intervention and is reduced if analgesic drugs are provided. Using this information, changes in facial expression such as a semi-closed eyelids and tightened muscles around the eye area, bulging of the nose and flattening of ears have been validated as signifiers of pain in laboratory animals. Many features of the pain grimace a shared across different mammalian species, but more detailed species-specific descriptors have also been validated for lambs, sheep and pigs (e.g. piglet grimace scale, Figure 2.2 Viscardi et al. 2017)

and then used to assess the effectiveness of different analgesic drugs for pain control during procedures such as castration. Farm animals and horses also discriminate between facial expressions linked with emotion that they observe in other animals. Horses, for example, change facial expression when being gently groomed and generally prefer to approach photographs of conspecifics captured under positive conditions. Remarkably, farm animals can also read human facial expressions, with goats preferring representations of happy human faces and horses pre-exposed to photos of angry or happy human faces subsequently reacting more favourably to humans who had appeared happy. Facial expression in poultry has received less attention, but it is possible that signs such as raised feathers on the head may signal emotional state. Other fine categories of behaviour being used in animal welfare

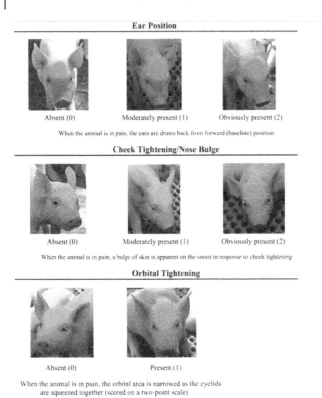

Figure 2.2 Facial expressions indicative of pain in pigs: the piglet grimace scale (from Viscardi et al. 2017).

studies include changes in pupil size (e.g. associated with stereotypic behaviour in pigs and dustbathing in quail) and measures of lateralized use of limbs or snouts.

Video technology also enables the categorization of behaviour of entire groups, herds or flocks of animals, at a very large scale. Video cameras installed overhead in chicken houses can record shifting patterns of brightness that reflect patterns of bird movement within the flock. The rate of change of brightness in each area of an image frame can be analysed across both time and space, using optical flow analysis. Differences in mean or variance measures of optical flow have been linked with feather damage in laying hens, and lameness, dermatitis and Campylobacter infection in flocks of broiler chickens (e.g. Colles et al. 2016). Assessment of flock behaviour at this level of analysis has great potential as a routine surveillance tool to identify emerging flock problems at an early stage, and alert stockpersons so that remedial management steps can be taken. Acoustic technology is also being applied to measure flock behaviour, with sound analysis able to detect changes in bird vocalization linked with thermal comfort, and with flock growth rate and feed intake. Many livestock farmers already use drones to monitor the movement and location of their cattle or sheep, and as costs reduce the use of satellite technology could also be used to monitor aspects of the behaviour of groups of animals in relation to each other and the environment, for example, in monitoring patterns of outdoor range use. Huge growth in the use of surveillance technology on farms is predicted.

2.4.2   Automated Technology for Assessing Individual Animal Behaviour

In addition to changing the scale at which behaviour can be monitored, new technologies are driving rapid changes in the collection of welfare-relevant data in all types of agricultural systems. Some technologies enable the collection of very large amounts of data over periods of days or weeks, during light and dark periods without potentially confounding effects of human presence. Other technologies are honed to improve the detection or measurement of severity of specific welfare problems. Where, as part of the methodology, animals are fitted with tags or required to carry recording equipment it is essential to first assess the baseline impact of the kit on animal behaviour.

Kinematic analysis is an automated approach to the assessment of movement patterns in animals. It uses highly automated video technology to describe the movement of marked points on an animal's body, defining the co-ordinates precisely as the animal moves, and tracking patterns of movement. It can add great value to assessment of lameness or discomfort in cattle, pigs and broiler chickens, and can provide a guide to the space requirements needed for basic locomotion and comfort movements (Mench and Blatchford 2014). Kinematic analysis may also be able to distinguish differing emotional states, particularly those associated with different levels of activity or arousal. One advantage of this method is, apart from some small markers, nothing is attached to the animal.

The movement and location of animals can be monitored by attaching radio frequency identification (RFID) tags to individuals, and by placing readers in relevant locations. In recent years, this technology has been used to monitor the movement of laying hens within multi-tier houses, to describe how factors such as flock size, stocking density, early life experience and bone health influence range use in both broiler chickens and laying hens, as well as to measure the feeding and drinking patterns of growing pigs and sheep and identify animals that show changes in intake that could signify a welfare problem.

Animals can also be fitted with accelerometers to measure basic activity level, to distinguish different types of activity, and to assess the forces that animals may experience when jumping or landing. For humans, computer algorithms have been developed to translate the accelerometer data into a simple readout such as number of steps taken, as recorded by simple pedometers. Pedometers have been widely used with cattle and pigs (and more recently goats, sheep and buffalo) to measure how basic locomotor activity changes with age; pain due to causes including foot lesions, dehorning or castration; disease or parasite load; floor or substrate type, or imminent calving or farrowing. It is more complicated to write algorithms that can distinguish different types of behaviour, but much work is being invested in this area with machine learning techniques applied to validate how the automated read-outs map onto the gold standard observations. Accelerometers can now relatively accurately record lying times in goats, horses and cattle, and they can also distinguish gait types (walk, trot, canter) in horses. Accelerometers have also been used to distinguish locomotor play in calves, nesting behaviour in sows, to assess jumping heights and landing forces in hens, and to measure different patterns of inactivity in hens with and without bone fractures.

For animals kept in extensive systems, GPS tracking has been applied to monitor the distribution and movement of animals and has greatly increased the number of studies evaluating the environmental influences and impacts of livestock movement. GPS tracking is not possible when animals are housed indoors, but Geographic Information System (GIS) approaches (sensors fitted to birds, and beacons installed within the house) have been used to monitor indoor movement.

The challenge for the animal welfare community is to make sense of this burgeoning capacity to collect data. Many of the old questions about the interpretation of animal behaviour as a measure of animal welfare apply to the datasets generated by automated technologies. How can we know that a shift in facial expression, locomotor activity or vocalization is a valid indicator of a welfare state? To answer this we turn now to a growing body of work that is exploring how behavioural signs are altered by manipulations including responses to pharmacological manipulations, a feature of experimentally induced specific emotions, or reliably associated with positive or negative valence.

2.4.3 Behavioural Indicators of Pain, Disease and Stress

Behavioural changes are often the first or most obvious manifestation of the onset of pain or disease. Signs of acute pain include escape attempts, increases or decreases in activity and behaviours directed towards the pain site. An obvious example would be the uneven gait of animals with hoof lesions, joint infections or skeletal abnormalities. In chickens, such signs of lameness are associated with other changes in behaviour. Lame birds re-prioritize their daily activities to minimize movement, making fewer but longer visits to feeders, and they become more sensitive to heat or pressure stimulation. Vocalizations also occur in response to acute pain. For example, although restraint alone prompts a great deal of vocalization in piglets, calls occur more frequently when piglets are castrated, compared with uncastrated controls or with piglets given analgesics. During the actual castration period, the mix of high frequency (>1000 Hz) calls given in response to restraint changes to a less variable 3000 Hz shriek.

Assessing chronic pain can be more difficult. Changes in general level of activity are not very specific, and so hard to interpret. The changes in facial expression reviewed above appear to be more sensitive and specific and much work has now been conducted to validate these as pain responses by testing animals with and without analgesic drugs. But even this approach does not wholly address the question of pain perception as animals may show unconscious but protective responses that are reduced due to anti-inflammatory effects of analgesic drugs. The fact that decerebrate chickens will limp after a noxious injection to the ankle suggests that some pain-related behaviour is controlled at the level of the brainstem. Scientific approaches cannot answer the question of conscious experience in animals, but it can add indirect evidence. For example, studies showing that animals will learn to do novel tasks to manage their own pain demonstrate the involvement of higher brain regions in pain perception. Nasr et al. (2013) found, for example, that hens with healed bone fractures prefer coloured pen locations that have been experimentally associated with pain relief whilst uninjured birds do not show any preference, using a conditioned place preference procedure. This at least increases the likelihood that healed keel bone fractures in hens are associated with residual pain and contributes to the debate about the welfare impact of this common problem in laying hen production.

Infectious diseases can produce adaptive 'sickness behaviour' responses with a reallocation of physiological resources and reserves to help fight the infection, so that the animal spends more time resting and sleeping. But more subtle responses can also be observed, for example, changes in feed preference in chickens infected with salmonella. Generally, across a range of chronic pain or disease conditions it is observed that core behaviours such as drinking persist, but less resilient behaviours (such as exploration, grooming or play) may be reduced or cease entirely. This has been shown in studies where mice developing early signs of Huntington's disease stopped using cage enrichments such as ropes and climbing equipment earlier than their cage-mates. More recently, it has been shown that the use of an automated brush for self-grooming is reduced in dairy cows in the days following artificial insemination, or in cows with metritis or with moderate or severe lameness. The key prediction that needs to be tested in a wider range of contexts is that low *resilience (sensu 2)* behaviours will be more sensitive indicators of early signs of disease or recovery than core behaviours or traditional clinical measures.

2.4.4 Specific Behavioural Indicators of Emotion

2.4.4.1 Emotional Systems in Farm Animals

There has been a rapid rise in studies of animal emotion within the broader field of animal welfare science. The study of animal emotion focuses on understanding the multi-component (behavioural, physiological, cognitive and subjective) responses of animals to events and situations, but navigating this literature is hampered by substantial differences between researchers in their use of the term emotion. One framework is to view farm animal emotions as temporary states with physiological and behavioural features that arise from the appraisal of a situation. Thus, an animal that appraises a situation as sudden and threatening may flee or show startle responses alongside increased heart rate, a pattern of response characteristic of an emotional state of fear. Similarly, a hungry animal unable to access food may perceive the situation as negative, uncontrollable and inconsistent with its prior expectations, resulting in an emotional state of frustration. Situations that an animal perceives to be negative trigger emotional or affective states that are themselves negative valenced (and which may indeed feel bad); whilst situations appraised as positive will trigger emotional states which are positively valenced (and which may feel good). These emotional states have other characteristics including their intensity and duration (Mendl et al. 2010, see Figure 2.3). The extent to which animal emotions can be mapped within a general framework where valence and intensity vary continuously or whether they should be divided into neurobiologically relevant and named emotional categories remains an open question.

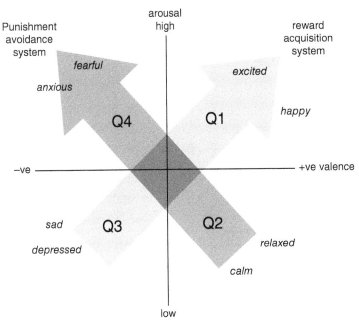

Figure 2.3 Core affect represented in two-dimensional space. Arrows indicate putative biobehavioural systems associated with reward acquisition (Q3–Q1) and punishment avoidance (Q2–Q4) (from Mendl et al. 2010).

Mammals are thought to have many primary emotional systems, each governed by discrete neural circuits but farmed birds such as chickens may possess fewer systems. Certainly, chickens possess both a Fear system and a Seeking system that can result in an emotional state of frustration (when resources are difficult or impossible to access) or deprivation (when resources are absent) but the chicken capacity for other emotional systems associated with Play, Rage or social care, awaits further research. The mammalian emotional system of rage may be limited to brief and momentary attack during the establishment of a dominance hierarchy. Chickens do not show the type of impulsive, violent aggression characterised by high levels of arousal that is sometimes observed in mammals such as cats and rodents. Adult chickens also appear not to form highly specific social attachments to other individuals and so their emotional systems relating to care (including panic or grief if separated from a bonded companion) may be less developed than in mammals.

2.4.4.2 Indicators of Frustration, Deprivation and Anticipation

Behavioural indicators of emotional states linked to Seeking (frustration, deprivation and anticipation) have been widely studied. Behavioural indicators of frustration include displacement behaviour, pacing, and specific vocalisations. Deprivation is harder to study as it concerns the total absence of key resources, and the resource of interest has to remain absent during the experiment. Attempts have been made to assess how hard deprived animals will work to obtain searching or exploratory opportunities e.g. to forage in the absence of reward or to run in a wheel or circular enclosure. There is some evidence that such locomotor behaviour increases in animals deprived of key resources. Another response to resource absence, or its poor quality, is seen when animals redirect their behaviour to an alternative substrate. However, if normal foraging or feeding behaviour is redirected towards companions then severe welfare problems can arise for the recipients. Problems of injurious pecking in laying hens, tail biting in pigs and non-nutritive suckling in calves can be considered within this framework.

Anticipation is another emotional state closely linked to the Seeking system. Farm animals can form expectations and anticipate events in the near future. For example, if a sound signals the arrival of food, then chickens may pace and head-bob near the feeder in anticipation. If the interval between sound and food arrival is very short, the chicken may start pecking the feeder as soon as it hears the sound. However, with longer delays, chickens show more generic anticipatory responses such as increased activity. Regardless of whether the expected event is positive or negative, chickens increase the frequency and intensity of their head movements during anticipatory periods. Sheep also show clear behavioural responses when anticipating a food reward, with increased head orientation towards the location where food is expected to appear, and a more asymmetric ear posture associated with increased right hemisphere cortical activation. Anticipation of a reward is, in humans, often accompanied by a sensation of pleasure and may therefore be a positive welfare indicator. Indeed, it has been suggested that providing signalled periods during which animals would anticipate a positive reward could be a way of improving welfare. However, this is not straightforward. Firstly, an animal with good welfare, living in a complex environment, may show *less* of an anticipatory response to reward than an animal housed in a more barren environment, for whom the occasional reward will carry far more significance. In addition, there is much overlap between anticipatory responses observed for positive and negative events, so many signs of anticipation may simply signal arousal. Lastly, the greater the reward, the greater the possibility that the anticipatory period is experienced as frustrating rather than pleasurable. This has been noted in sheep where brushing by a familiar human was experienced as positive, but the period before brushing was accompanied by signs of agitation and arousal.

Under conditions of frustrated motivation, it is possible that stereotypic behaviour will develop, with its characteristic features of repetition, invariance and apparent lack of function. The role of frustrated motivation is seen as the original behaviour pattern e.g. an attempt to escape from a cage or other enclosure becomes continually repeated, developing an increasingly fixed or unvarying appearance and pattern. This general developmental story has been verified by many different experiments, including work showing that mice direct most of their bar-biting at cage doors which have previously provided exit opportunities. The causation of mouth-based or oral stereotypies also tends to result from frustrated foraging and feeding attempts. The onset of crib-biting may be an adaptive attempt to deal with the uncomfortable digestive consequences of the wrong diet. Crib-biting could be performed initially as a response to visceral pain, as it results in a small release of saliva which may partially alleviate gut acidity problems. However, crib-biting like other stereotypic behaviours, develops its repetitive and invariant nature precisely because the animal's reasonable response does *not* fully succeed in resolving the problem.

The initial stages of stereotypy development are universally associated with frustration or aversion, and thus the appearance of a new stereotypy is generally agreed to be a valid and reliable indicator of poor welfare. But it is less clear whether long-established stereotypies can be regarded as reliable indicators of welfare. The arguments hinge on two issues: (1) whether the development of an established stereotypy allows the animal to cope better with a suboptimal environment than do its non-stereotypic companions; and (2) whether established stereotypies reflect current welfare state at all, or are simply persistent behavioural 'scars' of previous frustration.

Whether or not stereotypies help animals cope with the adversity of the eliciting environment has been a controversial question in applied ethology. Some researchers have found that stereotypies in laboratory animals reduce stress or aversion to a barren environment, but others have failed to find such stress-reducing effects. Oral stereotypies in horses show a rebound in performance after a period of prevention, indicating that these stereotypies may have a functional role, but stereotypic wire-gnawing in mice shows no such rebound. To make sense of this conflicting evidence there is a great need for longitudinal studies that examine baseline differences in the stress responses of animals before they do, or do not, develop stereotypies. Without this background it is impossible to know whether stereotypic animals were more or less stressed than their companions even before they developed the abnormal behaviour.

Mason and Latham (2004) suggest that, for stereotypy to be used as an indicator of welfare one should check that non-stereotypic animals are not faring worse than stereotypic animals housed in the same environment. An environment that gives rise to stereotypic animals can be regarded with great suspicion, as it is likely to be causing severe frustration in some way, and therefore resulting in poor animal welfare. But we cannot assume that it is the stereotypic animals in that environment that are suffering most. The performance of the stereotypy may actually have some benefits, if only in increasing exercise levels. Moreover, steps taken to prevent the appearance of the stereotypy (including surgical operations, electric shock collars) can result in worse welfare outcomes than allowing the stereotypy to persist.

2.4.4.3 Indicators of Fear and Anxiety

Behavioural indicators of fear include both immobility and flight responses and vary between species and between individuals. In some circumstances, the best response is to avoid detection by crouching or freezing, or even to enter a state of complete tonic immobility (playing dead), but in other situations an animal will try to flee or to fight in order to escape. Standardized tests have been developed to measure fear responses in a wide range of farm animal species, and these include the animals' locomotor patterns when placed in a novel arena, or their reactions and approach distances to novel objects or human experimenters. Fear, as a primary emotional state should be detectable using more than one measure, but the best measures should be consistent and capable of detecting fear in a variety of different contexts. In addition, behavioural indicators of fear should ideally be practical to apply on farm. In pigs and cattle, fearfulness measured using time-consuming novel object and human approach tests is strongly correlated with levels of spontaneous home-pen activity, lending itself to assessment using the automated methods reviewed earlier.

2.5   Behavioural and Cognitive Indicators of Valence

The studies reviewed above show that behaviour can provide highly specific and diagnostic information within defined animal contexts – from the head bobbing of a chicken that expects imminent food delivery, to the orbital tightening of a piglet in pain. But are there also patterns of behaviour that could reliably indicate that an animal is in a generally positive or negative affective state across a broad range of situations? Such general markers of the valence dimension of animal emotion could be of enormous use when performing on-farm welfare assessments where the ultimate might be to decide whether an animal was in overall good or poor welfare. One approach to this question has been to use information about animal choice as a gold standard against which to map other behavioural (and physiological) indicators. Research with laying hens has found that, even though different individual birds preferred different environments, certain indicators are reliably and consistently associated with positive or negative choices. Regardless of the *nature* of the chosen environment, positive choices are made for environments where birds had shown lower levels of blood glucose, reduced frequency of head shaking, longer durations of preening and drier faeces (e.g. Nicol et al. 2009).

Other approaches might be to step back from a focus on individual activity patterns and take an overview of the full structural complexity of behaviour. For example, a reduced complexity of behavioural sequences measured over time is observed in sheep with nematode infections and in turkeys with footpad dermatitis. A general increase in the frequency of transitions between activities in a given time period is observed in chickens housed in more stressful or barren conditions giving an impression of general agitation. This would suggest that the appearance of uninterrupted but complex sequences of behaviour could be a general signifier of good welfare, particularly so if complex sequences of play, affiliative social behaviour or exploration are observed. These behaviours demand time and energy and yet their benefits are long-term, so they could be postponed if conditions were difficult. Correspondingly, their appearance in the repertoire may be a reliable indicator of good times and accompanying positive affective state. Play is a good example of a behaviour that is most often observed when environmental conditions are good, when animals are well-nourished housed in enriched environments. It is also more likely to be observed in animals that are not in pain. In calves, the administration of analgesic drugs to counter pain in the immediate postpartum period increases subsequent play. Other pharmacological studies show that morphine increases social play in calves suggesting an association between play and a rewarding experience mediated by brain opioids.

A third approach addresses the possibility that underlying positive or negative affective states may be accompanied by shifts in perception. This theory arises from observations that humans experiencing negative affective states (including anxiety and depression) tend to interpret ambiguous events more negatively than other people, and also may pay more attention to potentially negative or threatening cues in the environment, described as a cognitive bias. A typical protocol based on the original application of this theory to animals (Harding et al. 2004) is to pre-train an animal that a positive cue such as a tone at a given pitch (P) indicates a reward, whilst a negative cue, a tone at a clearly lower or higher pitch (N), indicates no reward or a punishment. The low and high pitches are typically set one octave apart, which equates to a doubling in frequency. Once the animal is reliably and appropriately responding to these cues, it is occasionally presented with ambiguous cues that share features of both P and N, such as a tone at an intermediate pitch. The animal must decide how to respond and must judge whether the intermediate cue is more likely to result in a P or an N outcome. During the test protocol the intermediate cues are generally unrewarded.

The general hypothesis under test is that animals in a negative affective state will judge intermediate cues to share more N features than animals in a positive affective state. A great variety of studies have been conducted to investigate this hypothesis. The better studies provide independent evidence to reinforce the claim that an animal is in a negative or positive affective state during the test procedure, but this is not always done. Without this independent evidence it is impossible to test the basic hypothesis. Despite the difficulties, this approach is of such intuitive interest to experimenters that it has defined the zeitgeist of animal welfare research in the past decade, with hundreds of studies published on farm, laboratory, zoo, companion animals as well as on invertebrate species. Of the 50 or so studies conducted with farm animal species, many have produced results in line with the basic hypothesis, but a large number have found no effect or have reported contradictory findings. As work progresses, it will become possible to assess the influence of procedural factors, such as whether testing takes place during or after the animal has been placed in a negative or positive affective state. Developing a predictive framework that specifies in advance how long any negative or positive effects of affect manipulations are expected to persist will allow clearer experimental predictions.

It is highly probably that this area of work in farm animal welfare science will continue to develop and that other fundamental considerations will need to be addressed. One challenge will be to consider whether cognitive biases are a good general indicator of positive or negative valence across a very wide range of contexts, or an indicator of positive or negative valence in just a handful of *specific types* of context. Interest in cognitive bias arose from observations in humans who have experienced relatively long-term states of depression, anxiety or chronic pain, rather the brief painful or frightening events. More consideration will also need to be directed to the question of relative results. A bias is not an absolute measure and so the selection of *both* treatment and control groups is critical to the ultimate interpretation of results. Pigs from enriched environments may show more optimistic judgements than pigs from barren environments, but this is a relative result and it does not prove that pigs are in a positive affective state. If the same enriched pigs had been compared against a different control group (e.g. pigs living in natural conditions) the same results could be presented as showing a relatively pessimistic judgement. Just as those interested in animal preference, motivational strength and behavioural priorities have had to wrestle with concepts of relative choice, baselines and yardsticks, the same applies to this maturing field of study.

Another area ripe for further investigation will be the reasons for sometimes large differences in judgement biases between individuals treated in the same way. This suggests that individual personality frames the situation within which an animal finds itself. Pigs with more proactive tendencies (Asher et al. 2016) tend to show more optimistic judgements. However, blanket predictions about the nature of this type of interaction are not possible as recent studies show a positive association between fearfulness and optimism in hens, but a negative association between these traits in calves. This suggests that we need to understand more about animal personalities in domestic farm animals.

2.6 Animals with Individual Personalities and Social Roles

The older literature on farm animal behaviour and welfare considered animals as if they were identical group members, with proposals for management practices based on a hypothetical average. It is now known that even genetically similar animals often possess differing behavioural traits and may have differing environmental preferences. Commercial laying hens of the same strain have different physical characteristics that are linked with differing environmental preferences. It could be said that these birds have different personalities, but to be sure we would require more evidence that behaviours were consistently different between individuals, but highly consistent *within* individuals over time and across different contexts. Some traits do show this individually consistency, including boldness, response to novelty and aggression in chickens, and gregariousness in sheep. Pigs show personality differences in aggression, coping style (bold or shy) and vocalization rate. The adaptive value of a personality type will depend upon prevailing environmental or social conditions. For example, under semi-natural conditions with good food availability, 'shy' female wild boar with low aggression and exploratory tendencies raised more offspring than more aggressive and exploratory sows, but this personality advantage vanished under scarcer food conditions.

Many animals benefit from group living. In the right circumstances, the benefits can include protection from predators as group members share the costs of vigilance, insulation from extremes of weather as group members huddle or crowd together, and greatly increased chances of finding food or killing prey. To live in a group the advantages must, on average, outweigh the disadvantages of increased competition, conspicuousness and risks of disease transmission. Simply living in an aggregation, where no social relationships are formed between group members (imagine a fly within a cloud of other flies, or a jellyfish within a large drifting shoal) can confer these benefits. But, in mammals especially, group living involves the formation of social relationships and preferential interactions with certain companions.

Social factors are powerful modulators of both stress response and immune functions and so an animal's social position within a group may be one of the most important determinants of its welfare. In humans, social stress is one of the strongest risk factors for depression and anxiety, and in animals social stress leads to related changes in anxiety, brain structure and survival. Social stress is a recurring factor in the lives of almost all mammals, and conflict in particular can *profoundly* reduce the animal's ability to cope with a variety of environmental challenges. There may be almost nothing worse than being in a bad social situation and being unable to get away. A striking example of the social difficulties faced by a minority of individuals is the presence of 'pariah' birds within flocks of hens. These birds are repeatedly attacked by other birds and tend to shelter under any cover they can find for prolonged periods of time, foregoing food and water intake until the last possible moment. These pariah birds have significantly reduced welfare by almost any measure. Thus, although a non-cage barn or free-range system provides better welfare than a cage for the majority of birds, the welfare of the pariah birds is severely compromised. This highlights a more general issue for farm animal welfare at a time when many production systems are shifting towards reducing physical restrictions such as cages, tie-stalls and crates and housing animals in group-systems. It becomes essential to consider how to avoid negative effects of injurious pecking, aggression or tail-biting. One approach is for animal behaviour scientists to work alongside geneticists so that social genetic effects can be taken into account in breeding programmes. This approach means that animals are selected not just on the basis of individual production traits, but also considering the effect any given individual may have on its conspecifics.

Ideally, such selection programmes could focus not only on negative social interactions, but also on good social relationships. Relationships with preferred partners can provide social support, increasing adaptive capacity, reducing anxiety and probably producing feelings of great pleasure. In piglets the buffering effects of social support have profound effects on the amygdala region of the brain, increasing the capacity of the pig to cope with stressful situations. Perhaps the strongest social bond of all is that between the mother and her offspring. This is a highly selective attachment – the mother essentially falls in love with her own offspring and not just young animals in general. In mammals, this strong attachment is formed during parturition and lactation, processes associated with the release of high concentrations of oxytocin. Indeed, in some species it has been shown that individual differences in the density of oxytocin receptors in the brain's reward areas are correlated with differences in the level of maternal care shown. When the mother and infant are close then stress levels are low, but separation results in extreme anxiety. Despite this, early weaning is a very common, and often unquestioned, practice in Western agricultural systems. Many studies have documented the severe effects of weaning on infants and there is now more attention paid to the importance of providing appropriate social support for newly weaned animals, implementing more gradual weaning protocols or even developing systems that allow dairy cows and calves to stay together.

References

Asher, L., Friel, M., Griffin, K., and Collins, L. (2016). Mood and personality interact to determine cognitive biases in pigs. *Biology Letters* 12: e20160402

Brambell Committee. (1965). Report of the Technical Committee to Enquire into the Welfare of Animals Kept under Intensive Livestock Husbandry. HMSO, London.

Colles, F.M., Cain, R.J., Nickson, T., Smith, A.L., Roberts, S.J., Maiden, M.C.J., Lunn, D., and Dawkins, M.S. (2016). Monitoring chicken flock behaviour provides early warning of infection by human pathogen Campylobacter. *Proceedings of the Royal Society B- Biological Sciences* 283: e20152323

Dawkins, M.S. (1983). Battery hens name their price: consumer demand theory and the measurement of ethological needs. *Animal Behaviour* 31: 1195–1205.

De Jong, I.C., van Voorst, A.S., and Blokhuis, H.J. (2003). Parameters for quantification of hunger in broiler breeders. *Physiology and Behavior* 78: 773–783.

Dixon, L.M., Brocklehurst, S., Sandilands, V., Bateson, M., Tolkamp, B.J., and D'Eath, R.B. (2014). Measuring motivation for appetitive behaviour: food restricted broiler breeder chickens cross a water barrier to forage in an area of wood shavings without food. *PLOS ONE* 9: e102322

Edgar, J.L., Paul, E.S., and Nicol, C.J. (2013). Protective mother hens: cognitive influences on the avian maternal response. *Animal Behaviour* 86: 223–229.

Eklund, B. and Jensen, P. (2011). Domestication effects on behavioural synchronization and individual distances in chickens (*Gallus gallus*). *Behavioural Processes* 86: 250–256.

Harding, E.J., Paul, E.S., and Mendl, M. (2004). Animal behaviour-cognitive bias and affective state. *Nature* 427: 312–312.

Kirchner, J., Manteuffel, C., Manteuffel, G., and Schrader, L. (2014). Learning performance of gestating sows called to the feeder. *Applied Animal Behaviour Science* 153, 18–25.

Mason, G.J. and Latham, N.R. (2004). Can't stop, won't stop: is stereotypy a reliable animal welfare indicator? *Animal Welfare* 13: S57–S69.

Matthews, L.R. and Ladewig, J. (1994). Environmental requirements of pigs measured by behavioral demand-functions. *Animal Behaviour* 47: 713–719.

Mench, J.A. and Blatchford, R.A. (2014). Determination of space use by laying hens using kinematic analysis. *Poultry Science* 93: 794–798.

Mendl, M., Burman, O.H.P., and Paul, E.S. (2010). An integrative and functional framework for the study of animal emotion and mood. *Proceedings of the Royal Society B – Biological Sciences* 277: 2895–2904.

Munksgaard, L., Jensen, M.B., Pedersen, L.J., Hansen, S.W., and Matthews, L. (2005). Quantifying behavioural priorities-effects of time constraints on behaviour of dairy cows, *Bos Taurus*. *Applied Animal Behaviour Science* 92: 3014.

Nasr, M.A.F., Browne, W.J., Caplen, G., Hothersall, B., Murrell, J.C., and Nicol, C.J. (2013). Positive affective state induced by opioid analgesia in laying hens with bone fractures. *Applied Animal Behaviour Science* 147: 127–131.

Nicol, C.J., Caplen, G., Edgar, J., and Browne, W.J. (2009). Associations between welfare indicators and environmental choice in laying hens. *Animal Behaviour* 78: 413–424.

Paul, E.S., Edgar, J.L., Caplen, G., and Nicol, C.J. (2018) Examining affective structure in chickens: valence, intensity, persistence and generalization measured using a conditioned place preference test. *Applied Animal Behaviour Science* 207: 39–48

Pedersen, L.J., Holm, L., Jensen, M.B., and Jorgensen, E. (2005). The strength of pigs' preferences for different rooting materials using concurrent schedules of reinforcement. *Applied Animal Behaviour Science* 94: 31–48.

Rorvang, M.V., Nielsen, B.L., Herskin, M.S., and Jensen, M.B. (2018). Prepartum maternal behavior of domesticated cattle: a comparison with managed, feral and wild ungulates. *Frontiers in Veterinary Science* 5 (e): 45.

Rugani, R., Fontanari, L., Simoni, E., Regolin, L., and Vallortigara, G. (2009) Arithmetic in newborn chicks. *Proceedings of the Royal Society B: Biological Sciences* 276: 2451–2460.

Schwaller, F. and Fitzgerald, M. (2014) The consequences of pain in early life: injury-induced plasticity in developing pain pathways. *European Journal of Neuroscience* 39: 344–352.

Smid, A.M.C., Weary, D.M., Costa, J.H.C., and von Keyselingk, M.A.G. (2018). Dairy cow preference for different types of outdoor access. *Journal of Dairy Science* 101: 1448–1455

Stolba, A. and Wood-Gush, D.G.M. (1989). The behavior of pigs in a semi-natural environment. *Animal Production* 48: 419–425.

Tucker, C.B., Munksgaard, L., Mintline, E.M., and Jensen, M.B. (2018). Use of a pneumatic push gate to measure dairy cattle motivation to lie down in a deep-bedded area. *Applied Animal Behaviour Science* 201: 15–24.

Viscardi, A.V., Hunniford, M., Lawlis, P., Leach, M., and Turner, P.V. (2017). Development of a piglet grimace scale to evaluate piglet pain using facial expressions following castration and tail docking: a pilot study. *Frontiers in Veterinary Science* 4: eUNSP51.

Further Reading

Barnard, C. (2007). Ethical regulation and animal science: why animal behaviour is special. *Animal Behaviour* 74: 5–13.

Burn, C.C. (2017). Bestial boredom: a biological perspective on animal boredom and suggestions for its scientific investigation. *Animal Behaviour* 130: 141–151

Colditz, I.G. and Hine, B.C. (2016). Resilience in farm animals: biology, management, breeding and implications for animal welfare. *Animal Production Science* 56: 1961–1983.

DePasquale, C., Sturgill, J., and Braithwaite, V.A. (2020). A standardized protocol for preference testing to assess fish welfare. https://www.jove.com/v/60674/a-standardized-protocol-for-preference-testing-to-assess-fish-welfare (accessed 14 December 2021).

Ellen, E.D., Rodenburg, T.B., Albers, G.A.A., Bolhuis, J.E., Camerlink, I., Duijvesteijn, N., Knol, E.F., Muir, W.M., Peeters, K., Reimert, I., Sell-Kubiak, E., van Arendonk, J.A.M., Visscher, J., and Bijma, P. (2014). The prospects of selection for social genetic effects to improve welfare and productivity in livestock. *Frontiers in Genetics* 5: e377.

Freire, R. and Nicol, C.J. (2019). A bibliometric analysis of past and emergent trends in animal welfare science. *Animal Welfare* 28. 465–485.

International Society for Applied Ethology. https://www.applied-ethology.org (accessed 14 December 2021).

Korte, S.M., Olivier, B., and Koolhaas, J.M. (2007). A new animal welfare concept based on allostasis. *Physiology & Behavior* 92: 422–428.

Papini, M.R., Penagos-Corzo, J.C., and Perez-Acosta, A.M. (2019). Avian emotions: comparative perspectives in fear and frustration. *Frontiers in Psychology* 9: e2707

Veissier, I., Boissy, A., Desire, L., and Greiveldinger, L. (2009). Animals' emotions: studies in sheep using appraisal theories. *Animal Welfare* 18: 347–354.

Panksepp, J. (2014) The science of emotions: Jaak Panksepp at TEDxRainier. https://www.youtube.com/watch?v=65e2qScV_K8 (accessed 14 December 2021).

3

Dairy Cattle

Jean Margerison

Management and Welfare of Farm Animals: The UFAW Farm Handbook, Sixth Edition.
Edited by John Webster and Jean Margerison.
© Universities Federation for Animal Welfare 2022. Published 2022 by John Wiley & Sons Ltd.

3.1   Introduction

World milk consumption was approximately 190 million, most (81%) of which was produced by dairy cows, which reached a population of 137 million in 2020. There are approx. 150 million households involved in the production of milk in the world, which are largely small family farms in developing countries, including Thailand, compared with large-scale specialized enterprises in developed countries and China. The vast majority of milk is consumed in the region where it is produced in the form of fresh dairy products, including pasteurized and fermented products, along with ultraheat treated (UHT) milk, while solid processed dairy products, such as especially milk powders, cheese, and butter are exported and the consumption of these are closely related to income growth. This and increases in human population are expected to increase global milk and product consumption by 1.6% annually between 2020 and 2029, to reach 997 million tons by 2029. The required increase in milk production is likely to be met by optimization of milk production systems, through improvements in animal health, feeding efficiency and the continued genetic improvement of plants and animals. This will result in an increase in milk yield per cow in most production systems, except for grazing-based systems which are more likely to increase milk yield by increasing the number of cows kept and milk yield per ha. The main challenges faced by the dairy production industry are related to human mortality due to antimicrobial resentence (AMR), climate change and loss of wildlife biodiversity. The industry must lower antibiotic use and be carbon neutral by 2050. This will be achieved by improving animal health and welfare through disease prevention and enhancement of natural microbiome and immunity. While the carbon footprint will be lowered by the adoption of changes in whole farm management practices that lower gas emissions and nutrient leaching, source and selling of products more locally and increase carbon sequestration and wildlife biodiversity on farm.

3.1.1 Milk Production for Human Consumption

The production of milk is monitored through on-farm milk testing and farm assurance schemes, which are based on recording and regular assessment of the production system. The areas assessed include staff training, animal welfare using the five freedoms, food safety using the principles of hazard identification, risk assessment and control, management of animal health through forward planning and disease prevention, the adequacy and appropriateness of animal nutrition and protection of the environment. These are independently assessed by qualified inspectors using accredited systems to monitor dairy farms at regular intervals. These procedures, along with full traceability of the product supply chain, including animals and feeds along with rigorous milk quality testing, are essential for consumer confidence. In developed countries, an increasing emphasis has been placed on animal welfare, environmental protection and now the carbon footprint. The production and supply of milk is dominated by milk buyers, particularly supermarkets, who use individual farm assurance requirements as marketing tools and these standards change more rapidly than and often exceed government legislation. These typically involve additional assessment and requirements related to animal health and welfare, environmental standards, along with monitoring and recording, which reflect the need to market milk staple food product in accordance with consumer perceptions of the dairy industry.

3.1.2 Consumption of Milks and Human Health

The main constituents of milk are water, fats, proteins and lactose (Figure 3.1). It can be consumed as liquid milk or converted by different processes (traditional or modern) into a variety of dairy products and food ingredients and has some industrial uses. The concept of nutrition of humans in developed countries has progressed from the simple provision of adequate nutrients to include longer-term health benefits and risks. Although obesity and diabetes are major modern concerns in the developed, over-fed world, the high nutritive value of dairy products means that they can make a valuable contribution to the daily human diet. Increasing wealth has allowed the consumption of dairy products in many countries. The greatest increases in milk production and consumption of milk are occurring in Asia.

Milk from dairy cows plays a significant role in the human diet in developed and developing countries and the consumption of three portions of dairy products daily has been recommended for a well-balanced human diet and weight control. Cow milk and dairy products are known to be an excellent source of fatty and amino acids, along with bioactive minerals and vitamins and a balanced diet contains three portions of dairy products daily. Unfortunately, in developed countries the consumption of soya and nut milks has become increasingly popular. However, these are nutritionally inferior compared with milk from cows, mainly due to

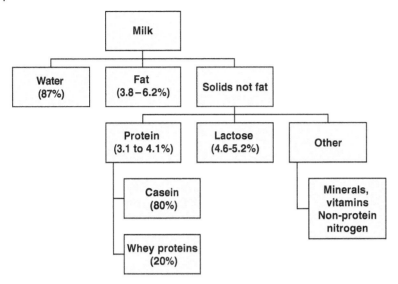

Figure 3.1 Composition of whole milk from differing breeds of dairy cattle.

the relatively poor amino acid profile and porosity of bioactive minerals, particularly calcium. Some of these alternative milks have a high sugar content. These factors make them nutritionally inferior and unsuitable for children and adolescents, especially females who need to consume enough bioavailable calcium to build and maintain good bone density to avoid post-menopausal osteoporosis and potentially meet the demands of pregnancy and lactation.

The consistent consumption of milk products from cows promotes good bone and tooth health, and is an essential source of minerals and vitamins, along with other functional components that include natural antioxidants and anti-carcinogenic agents. The concentration of certain essential fatty acids such as conjugated linoleic acid (CLA) can be affected by the cow's diet and milk from cows consuming grazed and/or fresh pasture contains higher amount of CLA compared with cows consuming conserved grass.

The consumption of cow's milk is not considered suitable as a direct replacement for breast milk in young infants and currently breast feeding is recommended, where possible, for at least the first 6 months of age. This can be ameliorated and eventually replaced by cow or goat milk in most cases. Naturally existing lactose intolerance, due to a lack of suitable intestinal enzymes, exists in a relatively small proportion of the human population and the consumption of goat milk or de-lactosed cow milk products are potential alternatives. People with continued problems should consult their doctor in the first instance, potentially followed by a qualified dietician for suitable and alternative approaches to achieve a well-balanced diet.

In developing countries, dairy products make a great contribution to the improvement of human health, but they can be scarce or prohibitively expensive and or of poorer keeping quality. Due to the importance of milk and dairy products in the development of dense bones, strong teeth and mental ability, especially in children, dairy production in countries such as China and Thailand has been supported greatly by the government. These counties in general consume all home-produced milk and continue to be net dairy product importers, mainly in the form of milk powder. Increasing wealth is resulting in greater dairy product consumption per capita and less lactose intolerance as dairy consumption becomes more common place, while bone pain and poor dentition remains a problem in more senior generations, due to the lack of adequate dairy consumption previously.

3.2 The Global Dairy Industry

Globally there are over 270 million cows producing milk. India has a large population, using both buffalo and dairy cows for milk production, but yield per animal is relatively low (2000 to 3000 L/cow/yr) due to inclement weather conditions and feed quality, but they are increasing the productivity of the national herd using European dairy cows and improving feed resources. The European Union (7346 l/cow/y) is one of the largest milk producers and has approx. 3 (20.5 ex UK) million dairy cows compared with 10 million cows in the USA (10,620 l/cow/y), and there are 5.92 million dairy cows in New Zealand (4,259 l/cow/y) and 1.5 million cows in Australia (6,170 l/cow/y). In South-East Asia dairy cow numbers and milk production continue to increase, including countries that have not traditionally milked dairy cows, such as China (5,803 l/cow/y), which now has over 12 million cows producing milk (Table 3.1), along with Thailand (3000 l/cow/y) and other Asian countries.

Most of the milk is produced from specialized dairy cattle breeds, predominantly the Holstein Friesian, followed by a relatively small percentage of Jersey and even fewer numbers

Table 3.1 Countries with the greatest cow populations (Source Statista 2021).

Country	1,000 head
India	56,450
EU	22,672
Brazil	16,200
USA	9,375
Russia	6,580
Mexico	6,550
China	6,150
New Zealand	4,815
Ukraine	1,840
Argentina	1,610
Belarus	1,495
Australia	1,435
Canada	967
Japan	716

of Brown Swiss, Guernsey and traditional breeds such as Ayrshire and Dairy Shorthorn. The Holstein Friesian represents over 90% of dairy cattle in North America and the EU, with relatively low levels (5%) of Jersey and other breeds. Tropical countries have adopted European breeds, but they have their own specialized dairy breeds that are too numerous to describe, which are often cross-bred with the Holstein and Jersey to increase milk production. European dairy cows, particularly the Holstein Friesian, have actively been selected as a specialist, single-purpose milk-producing animal capable of high volumes of milk production and is easily managed in automated milking systems. The milk yield per cow continues to increase, mainly due to improved genetic merit, nutrition, disease control and prevention. However, infertility of dairy cows continues to be one of the main challenges, this related to the high milk yield of early lactation coinciding with the onset of ovarian activity and need for to generate conception at about 80–100 days post-partum to ensure regular, approximately annual, calving which is an essential contributor to efficient milk production. The selection of cattle for milk production leads to a competition for partitioning of nutrients, which is prioritized towards milk yield, relative to the maintenance of body condition and reproduction. In the past, selection of Holstein dairy cattle and bulls for high milk production, rather than fertility and other important traits consistent with longevity, such as mobility, mammary conformation and health, has been a problem in some countries. More recently there have been changes in genetic selection of dairy bulls and European breeding policies, which place greater emphasis on fertility and health, along with production have been adopted more widely and, most recent has been the addition of feed efficiency traits.

The other main dynamic of dairy production has been the general continued trend towards fewer larger dairy herds, with many dairy units now including thousands and, in some countries, such as China, many thousands of cows on a single dairy unit. This leads to new challenges in herd and personnel management in the dairy industry and the regular use of standard operating practices (SOPs) by farm personnel. Other advances have been the continued application of on-farm quality assurance schemes, for feed manufacturers and milk producers, that ensure the quality, safety and carbon footprint of milk production and for human consumption.

3.2.1 Specialized Dairy Production

Milk production in the USA is dominated by dairy cows, in particular the Holstein Friesian breed. In New Zealand the domination of the Holstein Friesian is less pronounced, as smaller, lighter 'Kiwi' (Frisian, Jersey) cross-breeds are better suited to pasture-based systems. Here, the North American Holstein Friesian represents less than 50% of the dairy cow population, along with an estimated 32% of cows being New Zealand Holstein Friesian cross Jersey and 14% Jersey. This reflects the dominance of pasture-based systems for low-cost milk production, which is facilitated by mild winters, high winter light intensity and sunshine, and relatively consistent rainfall in many areas or irrigation of pastures in others. However, increasing drought frequency and land prices, especially in the North Island, along with greater access to cost-effective by-products and the increased use of forage maize (especially in times of drought) have led to more farmers offering supplementary feeds to dairy cattle.

The production of milk in countries with established dairy industries has continued to be characterized by declining numbers of milk producers, with larger herd sizes (mean > 350 cows) and increasing milk production per cow. More recently, there has been a decline in dairy cow number in the UK (–1.5%) and most EU countries, most notably in Germany (–2.2%), except for southern Ireland (+2.1%) (Table 3.2). The improvements made through genetic selection and breeding have increased the genetic potential of the dairy herds; in particular there has been a dominance of the Holstein Friesian dairy breed. Improved genetics, along with improvements in feed resources, conservation techniques, diet formulation and subsequent nutrition of dairy cattle, has led to substantial increases in milk yield per cow in the last 10 years. One of the most recent changes has been the adoption of differing measures of feed efficiency or feed conversion efficiency, which has long been a characteristic of the pig and poultry industries that has been adopted by the dairy industry to lower the impact on the environment, particularly climate change and deforestation related to animal nutrition.

3.2.2 Developing Milk-producing Countries

In China and Thailand, the importation of the Holstein Friesian has been central to the development of the dairy industry. However, in countries with more tropical climates, the use of imported dairy cattle genetics has been less successful, mainly due to their lack of heat tolerance and resistance to endemic disease. These genetics are often referred to as European, although they are likely to be American or Canadian Holstein which originated from cows bred in Northern Europe. Holstein Friesian, Jersey and Brown Swiss breeds have been used to cross-breed with the 'local' breeds of cattle and this has been a much more successful method of improving milk yield, while retaining some of the desirable characteristics of the local breeds. However, the main problem is the maintenance of the advantages of the cross-breeding and segregation of the phenotype in the following

Table 3.2 EU countries with largest dairy cow population (Source, Eurostat 2021).

	2015	2016	2017	2018	2019	Change %
Germany	4,285	4,218	4,199	4,101	4,012	–2.0
France	3,637	3,637	3,597	3,554	3,491	–2.0
Poland	2,134	2,130	2,153	2,214	2,167	–1.9
Italy	2,057	2,060	2,040	1,939	1,876	–1.9
UK	1,918	1,898	1,904	1,879	1,867	–0.2
Netherlands	1,717	1,794	1,665	1,552	1,590	–1.3
Ireland	1,240	1,295	1,343	1,369	1,426	+ 2.1
Romania	1,191	1,193	1,175	1,158	1,139	–1.5
EU-15	18,353	18,371	18,191	17,804	17,634	–
EU-ex UK	21,652	21,634	21,409	21,029	20,766	–1

generations. In the long term, recording and selective breeding within the local population of dairy cattle offers the opportunity to retain the genetic biodiversity as a future resource. However, the extraction of milk for human consumption from many of the 'local' breeds and crosses with local breeds often requires the presence of the calf in order to aid milk letdown. These systems may also allow the calf to suckle from the cow on a restricted basis, rather than artificially rear the calf (see Section 3.9.3.7). These 'cow-calf' systems are currently being assessed and applied within in Europe mainly due to the poor perception that cow-calf separation by consumers.

3.2.3 Main Milk Product–exporting Countries

The main milk product–exporting countries (% of total world milk exports), where annual milk production exceeds the need of the local population, include New Zealand (21.8 %), the Netherlands (8.4%), the USA (6.7%), followed by Belgium, France, Hong Kong and Australia. The production of milk within the EU, with its expanding number of member states, has been declining, while Australia's milk production has continued to be hampered by drought conditions and water shortages. The size of the New Zealand dairy industry is more or less currently stable, but, with its relatively small human pupation, has a large export capacity for milk products, mainly milk powder, cheese and butter. This lowers transport and processing costs by emphasizing the production of milk solids (fat plus protein, measured in kg; 381 kg of milk solids per cow annually).

In general, within countries, dairying is better suited, but by no means limited, to wetter areas that receive regular rainfall particularly during the drier summer period(s), where animals can graze grass or consume a range of fodder crops or conserved forages. However, the dairy cow, as a ruminant, is well able to utilize a range of forages, feed, food waste and co-product resources to are non-edible directly by humans. A range of cereals, maize, straw and co-products from the food, beverage and biofuel industries also provide feed for dairy cattle, which provide a valuable biological function upgrading the low-quality feeds into valuable essential nutrients for humans. The availability, cost including any transport, storage requirements, nutrient composition, fibre content and anti-nutritional factors of feeds are used as the basis of formulating a cost-effective diet to fulfil the nutrient requirements of dairy cattle. In many countries dairy cattle are housed for six to eight months of the year, during the winter periods when environmental temperature and pasture growth is low. In warmer regions of temperate countries where winter temperatures and sunlight levels are higher, such as New Zealand, some areas of Ireland, the UK, South America and the USA, cows can graze pasture or other forage crops for extended periods and even all year around. In other hot climates, such as Saudi Arabia and areas of the USA, and other countries cows may be cooled using housing, shade, fans and the addition of water as a bath or mist. During periods of low rainfall and drought, when fresh forage growth is limited, the use of conserved forage, fodder crops and/or feed supplements is required to ensure sufficient nutrients are available to maintain an economic level of milk production and body condition or else the output of milk would be much lower.

3.2.4 Milk Sale and Purchase

3.2.4.1 Milk Price, Marketing and Levy Boards

The price of milk is greatly affected by the global production and supply of milk and farmers have little or no control over milk price they receive. Most countries do not protect their national milk markets against imports, and low milk price has been one of the main characteristics of the dairy industry, resulting in the need for greater efficiency, specialized dairy breeds and diversity of milk production systems. There are a few exceptions, most notably Canada and Japan, that protect their national milk production using import restrictions to protect dairy farmers from fluctuations in global milk price and low milk prices. This typically leads to an increase in the milk price and thus cost of liquid milk and dairy products for consumers.

Overall, the production, transport, processing and storage of milk and milk products need to be carefully managed to ensure good milk quality and hygiene. Consequently, many countries have or historically have had milk marketing boards run by the government, which regulate milk production, collection, quality testing, processing and marketing, along with knowledge transfer and extension in some cases. In some countries, these have been replaced by farmer cooperatives or milk processors; some of these have devolved into farmers having individual contracts with milk buyers. In this case farmer may be able to seek out the best milk price and initiate a contract with a localized milk buyer. These individual contracts reflect the requirements of the milk buyer and farmers produce milk that facilitates efficient processing into products such as low-fat liquid milk, cream, cheese and so-called luxury higher-fat dairy products.

Low milk price has led farmers to diversify into the application of differing systems of production, which include calving large numbers of cows in 'blocks', usually spring and/or autumn and calving cows all year round. This either provides large amounts of milk that can be processed into products such as cheddar cheese or provides a relatively consistent level of milk supply that allows processors to control milk supply, maximizing the opportunity to supply the consumer demand, along with use of the processing facilities that minimize the need for investment in expensive processing infrastructure. In all cases, the aim is to produce high-quality milk that is of a suitable composition to achieve the maximum margin between income from milk sales and the cost of producing the milk, according to the payment scheme.

In most countries the differing sectors of the agricultural industry have levy boards that collect money per litre of milk produced or kg of milk solids processed. This money, which is collected directly from the milk processor from farmers' payments, is used for the development of the industry through marketing, research and knowledge transfer. The government of each country is also involved to a greater or lesser extent in research, development, education and extension of technologies within the dairy industry and facilitating the export and import of dairy products and technologies.

More recent developments have included more direct sales of milk and milk products. In more densely populated countries this has seen the return of doorstep deliveries and farmers installing milk dispensing machines on farm, which allow consumers to collect milk directly from the farm and to visit the farm where the milk is produced. These products often use more recyclable materials such as glass bottles, and consumers find this more attractive than the use of plastic containers. Other striking differences between countries is the consumption of refrigerated fresh liquid milk in some countries, notably the USA, Australia, the UK and NZ, while in many other countries the consumption of ultra-heat treated (UHT) milk, which is not required to be refrigerated, is much more common.

3.2.4.2 Milk Quotas and Co-operative Shares

In the EU and UK, quotas had been in place since the mid-1980s, while production quotas have been in place for much longer in other countries such as Canada. These quotas control the amount of milk farmers can produce and are milk fat linked. The EU withdrew milk quotas in March 2015 and milk production has increased subsequently. In New Zealand, while there is no quota system, the majority of farmers sell milk to a farmer-owned dairy cooperative and are required to own shares in order to supply milk to the cooperative, thus controlling the amount of milk supplied for processing. The milk production in New Zealand is highly seasonal, with most of the milk being processed into commodity products such as butter, cheese and milk powder for export. The milk is produced cheaply to meet world market prices and producers block-calve their cows in their spring (July to September) to coincide with the grass-growing season. The lactation length is approx. 280 days and therefore many of the processing factories are closed for a period at the end of the season. There is a small population of milk producers that have cows calving in spring and autumn to allow continued 'winter' milk production for the fresh liquid milk and product market for the relatively small internal human population.

3.3 Animal Breeding

3.3.1 Animal Selection and Genetic Improvement

The selection of dairy cows and sires to increase milk production, animal health and lifetime milk production potential is one of the main tools that have been used to increase economic efficiency. The selection process is based on the assessment of relatively heritable (25 to 50%) milk production and milk composition traits and body conformation (type) traits (7 to 54%), followed by less heritable, but important, traits such as longevity (8%), health (somatic cell counts – SCC: 12%) and fertility (4%). The use of computer-based linear production models (e.g. BLUP; best linear unbiased prediction) has allowed the calculation of relatively complicated indexes including economic weighting for milk components and for each sire and cow. The number of factors included in the index varies from country to country and these have changed considerably in the last 10 years. In some countries there are differing indexes according to the milk product to be produced, such as liquid milk or cheese, or overall 'net' genetic merit.

The traits selected can be described as production, durability and health including fertility (Table 3.3). In the past, many indexes gave the highest proportion (%) of weighting

Table 3.3 Main production, longevity and health traits used in the breeding indexes for dairy cattle.

Category	Selection trait	Measurement criteria
Production	Milk protein	kg or %
	Milk fat	kg or %
	Milk yield	kg or litres
Health and fertility	SCC (mastitis)	Somatic cell count levels and/or incidence of mastitis
	Fertility	Fertility of the cow or her daughter
	Other diseases	Metabolic disease, lameness, etc
Durability	Longevity	Number of lactations completed, daughters lactations
	Feet/legs	Conformation score (legs mid-range of scale), high/sharp foot angle
	Udder traits	High scores for attachment
	Calving ease	High scores (few calving problems or assistance)
	Temperament	High score (good temperament)
	Milking speed	Fast to average milking speed
Other factors	Live weight	Pasture-based systems aim to reduce this

to production traits; however, this resulted in a relatively low number of lactations being completed by dairy cattle due to infertility, mastitis and lameness and reduced dairy margins. Consequently, fertility, disease resistance, particularly to mastitis (e.g. low SCC), and traits related to increased herd life/durability of dairy cattle have increased in their importance in the breeding indexes of most countries. The aim is to produce a more robust cow with an improved lifetime performance, reduced replacement cost and greater farm margins. In a breeding index of selection traits that are given weighting (numerical values) and positive values are given to 'desirable' traits, the higher the value the greater the selection intensity of that specific trait; negative weighting can be applied to reduce undesirable traits. The use of negative weightings (– values) on traits such as animal live weight or milk volume (l) would favour the selection of smaller cows or cows that produce a lower volume of milk. Positive weighting can be applied to increase desirable traits such as kg or % of milk fat or protein, fertility or animal conformation characteristics such as mammary system or foot and leg scores (see Section 3.8.4.1). Overall, most countries are applying a greater proportion (40 to 50%) of their breeding index (+ and highest numerical values) to durability, health and fertility traits and a lower proportion than previously to production traits (50 to 60%).

The pedigree societies in each country use professional personnel to visually assess dairy heifers to give conformation scores (e.g. legs and feet, udder, dairy type). These conformation scores can be used to compare the 'breed quality' of cows and sires within a herd, across herds and more importantly the reliability of a sire's potential transmitting ability (PTA) of traits in other countries (international sire PTAs).

3.3.2   Improved Contemporary Comparisons and Quantitative Trait Loci

The use of artificial insemination and high-quality sires is a key factor in increasing the genetic merit of dairy herds. At present the performance of the daughters of sires in differing herds is defined in terms of 'improved contemporary comparisons' (ICC), accompanied by an expression of reliability (REL), which depends on the number of daughters across the number of herds and has been used to assess the potential transmitting ability of the sire. However, this process is inevitably slow, with sires taking approximately nine months of age to produce semen. There follows nine months of gestation and a two-year growing period before the daughter produces milk and can begin to generate milk production data for the ICCs. In recent years genetic technology has identified an increasing array of quantitative trait loci (QTLs) on the genome that exert a positive effect on the desirable traits and these have now largely replaced ICC in the short term to increase the speed of genetic selection and improvement.

3.3.3   Breeding Herd Replacements and Beef from the Dairy Herd

In practical terms approximately 22 to 25% of the dairy herd requires replacement annually. In commercial dairy herds, the application of sexed semen has become more common place to avoid the production of male dairy calves and allow more cross-bred beef calves to be produced. This sexed semen produces a high proportion of females (well over 90%) that allows the best approx. 25 to 30 % of the dairy herd to be mated to produce heifers, while the rest can be used to produce dairy heifers or cross-bred beef calves for sale to other enterprises. A small selection of sires is generally used (to reduce the risk of inbreeding) at any one time to improve a few specifically selected production and conformation traits in daughters of the better-quality and more productive dairy cattle, based on milk production and conformation records. In this way each herd can increase its genetic merit over time. In pasture-based systems, with the added pressure of seasonal calving, the use of nominated sires for AI may take place at the beginning of the breeding season and this will be followed by the use of beef bulls, so that the calving season is limited to a short period to coincide with spring grass growth for the following season. Some pedigree herds with cows of high genetic merit may breed a large proportion or the entire dairy herd to selected dairy sires in order to produce high-quality dairy replacements for sale to other herds.

3.4   Lactation

The mammary gland of the dairy cow is made up of four separate quarters, with a single teat, orifice and streak canal for each of the four quarters. At birth the gland has few developed structures but starts to develop at a faster rate at puberty, which occurs at approximately 40% mature weight and at approx. four to six months of age depending on the early growth rate of the animal. The gland continues to develop, and a final rapid stage of development occurs

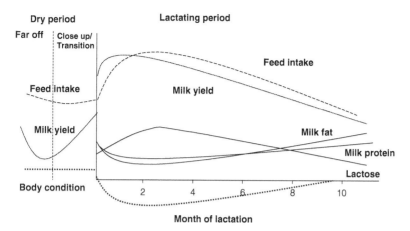

Figure 3.2 Lactation curve of dairy cattle including changes in milk yield, milk composition and body condition.

during pregnancy, during which the milk-secreting epithelial cells within the alveoli develop and colostrum is produced.

Lactation and the secretion of milk are initiated by changes in hormone levels around parturition. The total milk yield per lactation is dependent on the genetic merit of the animal and level of feeding, with yields from 3,500 l being common in pasture/forage-based feeding systems and yields in excess of 10,000 l when cows are offered mixed rations based on concentrated feeds (e.g. cereals) and forage. The level of milk yield and composition of the milk is affected by the stage of lactation, breed and age and nutrition of the cow. The peak milk yield, in early lactation, is associated with a slight decrease in protein and fat concentration, which recovers as lactation progresses. Protein and fat concentration in milk can be manipulated by diet and genetic selection. Lactose, which acts as an osmotic regulator in the mammary gland, follows the pattern of milk yield (Figure 3.2). The somatic cell count of the milk tends to be highest in early and late lactation and may be greater in older cows that have encountered more incidences of mastitis.

3.5 Dairy Farm Infrastructure

The housing of dairy cattle is an important factor contributing to animal welfare and is practices during inclement weather conditions, both to promote the wellbeing of animals and to protect the pastures. Good levels of housing and hygiene are important in providing cows comfort, preventing disease and ensuring the production of high-quality milk for human consumption. The other main important welfare requirements include the separation of calving cows into deep-bedded calving boxes or in calving paddocks, where they still have the sight and smell of other cattle. It is not good practice to allow cows to calve in free stall cubicles.

3.5.1 Dairy Production Systems

In pasture-based systems most dairy units calve cows in spring to coincide with maximum pasture growth rates and these systems are commonly practiced in New Zealand, Australia, areas of South America, Southern Ireland and some areas of Europe and the USA, including a small proportion of the UK dairy herd. These are areas suited to grass growth that allow animals to graze for long periods starting in early spring, often supplemented by fodder crops. The use of housing and amount of concentrate feed offered to the dairy cattle is less than other systems. However, in these systems may require cattle to walk long distance and the provision, design and maintenance of cow tracks (raceways) and, more importantly, the appropriate handling of cattle moving to and from the milking area are of great importance to animal welfare and prevention of lameness. In these pastoral systems, more animal waste is deposited on the land and the leaching of nutrients and fertilizers into ground and surface water can be a considerable problem. These systems may include areas, known as feed pads, often without roofing, that can be used to offer supplementary feeds to dairy cattle and to hold cattle ('stand offs') when pasture conditions are too wet to allow cattle to graze efficiently, thus reducing pasture and soil damage (poaching or pugging).

Milk production systems have diversified in response to market forces, climate and resource availability. Many countries, i.e. New Zealand, Australia and more recently the UK, have classified the relative dairy production systems (1 to 5), according to the amount of grazing and feed supplements cows receive (Australia; NZ) and the calving pattern (UK) (Table 3.4). This is because feed is one of the main costs associated with and affecting the amount of milk produced and grazed grass is less costly than ensiled grass. In the UK, prolonged housing of dairy cows is more common, due to climatic conditions. Block calving is often applied to lower feed costs, by coinciding the time of calving and early lactation with the greater volume of spring grass growth. Alternatively, autumn calving takes advantage of greater milk price to offset the greater expense of autumn and winter feeding. All year-round calving systems either use a combination of grazing and winter-feeding diet formulations, while all year-round systems benefit from greater productivity due to ensiled feed and supplements providing a more consistent diet. A recent evaluation of dairy farms across Great Britain (GB) showing that spring block calving with grazing and all year-round calving and housed

Table 3.4 Dairy system classification in Great Britain according to calving pattern, season, amount of days grazed annually and feed supplement and partial mixed ration (PMR) use.

	Dairy Production System				
Descriptor	**1**	**2**	**3**	**4**	**5**
Calving	Spring	Block/All year	Block/All year	All year	All year
Grazing, d/yr	> 274	183 to 274	91 to 182	0 to 90	0
Supplements	Limited	More	with PMR	Mostly PMR	All PMR

systems were amongst the most efficient, both in terms of whole farm feed use and financially. Interestingly, system 4 in the Australian, New Zealand and GB dairy system categories is the least efficient: the full rational for this is yet to be fully understood. Clearly, low milk price has limited the opportunity for substantial investment into the dairy business, without substantially increasing the risk, which would limit the ability of farmers to invest in housing, allowing them to move from system 4 into system 5.

The application of the 5-system approach allows farm to identify with and apply differing performance indicators relevant to each system. It is essential that farmers compare farm performance against relevant key performance indicators (KPIs) to make efficient management decisions (Table 3.5). In terms of genetic merit, countries have introduced system-based sire evaluation, allowing farmers to select more suitable sires to enhance the herd efficiency when managed in specific systems such as seasonal/block calving and all year-round calving (Table 3.5), along with once and twice daily milking in New Zealand.

3.5.2 Types of Cow Housing

There are some areas of the world where housing is not required or required for very short periods of the year, in which case farms may only have a covered milking unit and few other buildings. These are more typically found in areas such as Central and South America, Mexico, New Zealand and some parts of Australia. Housing can be used to protect animals from extreme cold, shade and cooling, or protect the soil and environment from damage.

Most dairy cattle are housed to some extent during winter, while there is an increasing trend towards housing cows throughout the year (or throughout lactation). In these circumstances fresh and grazed grass makes little or no contribution to the overall diet. The systems of housing are generally named after the type of cow confinement (e.g. tethers v. cubicles or free stalls), bed

Table 3.5 Key performance indicators for all year round and seasonal calving dairy herds (Amended from AHDB).

Resource	All year-round	Block/seasonal calving
Fertility	Pregnancy rate (%)	Cows & heifers calved in first 6 weeks (%) Empty rate (%)
Herd replacements	Age at first calving (mo.) Herd replacement rate (%)	Herd replacement rate (%) Live weight at first calving, Mature weight (%)
Feed costs	Purchased feed costs (ppl) Milk from forage (litres)	Milk solids kg and per ha Milk from grass/forage (litres)
Milk yield	Mean lifetime yield (L/day)	Milk solids/cow and/ha
Genetic merit	Production Lifetime Index (£PLI)	Calving Index (CI) (£ACI autumn & £SCI spring CI)
Overheads	Excl. rent & finance (ppl)	Excl. rent & finance (ppl)

type, bedding used and floor type. The choice of housing will reflect the availability of bedding, which affects the manure stacking and slurry/effluent handing system that need to be installed.

In wet climates that have longer winter periods (approx. ≥ 6 mo.), the buildings are more likely to be an 'umbrella' type that covers the milking shed/parlour and cow housing, so that water pollution and the volume of effluent produced can be minimized. The protection of natural water courses, along with ground and surface water is protected by limitations to the type and quality, season and place where efficiency can be applied. In addition, application of manures and effluent will be subject to limitations that are applied according to the calculation of nutrients, particularly nitrogen, that have been applied or become available from green and artificial fertilizers. These limitations are more stringent in nitrate vulnerable zones, field margins, near water courses and lakes, and in organic production systems. The management and comfort of the cows is of great importance to their health and welfare, with greater cow comfort increasing cow lying time, which increases milk yield and lowers the incidence and prevalence of lameness.

3.5.2.1   Free Stall/cubicle Systems

The 'free stall' or 'cubicle' system is the most common system in the EU, mid- and southern USA, China, the UK, Ireland and New Zealand. Cubicles are an efficient use of space and bedding for housing dairy cows but are not suitable for male cattle that urinate in the centre of the cubicle. The main design characteristics of cubicles should be:

- At least 5% more cubicles than animals in the group in the UK, to lower bullying and maximize lying time, but this is often not applied in the USA where larger herds create greater flexibility
- Wide enough to allow animals to lie down and stand up without touching the divisions, with the actual width depend on division design (up to 1.2 m) and animal live weight
- Long enough to accommodate the body and head of the cow and have lunging space at the front (0.7 to 1 m), to allow the cows to move forwards when getting up from a lying position
- Fitted with a brisket board in front of the cow, to help locate the animal so she has space in front of her to get up and lie down. These should be movable to accommodate differing size of cows and stop dunging on the beds
- Made to have a fall of 2 to 3 % from front to back of cubicles, to improve comfort and drainage
- Scraping passage width behind rows of cubicles should be a minimum of 3 m, while feed passages should be at least 4.6 m wide.

The aim should be to maximize cow comfort and welfare, best assessed by lying time, which ideally should be over 10 hours per day. This has been associated with better welfare, disease prevention and improved productivity. There should be at least one cubicle per cow in the UK and the design and size of the cubicle should be in accordance with the live weight and size of the cow (Table 3.6).

The cubicle design, size, bedding material and management are some of the main important components of this system. The design of the divisions is important, with cantilever divisions fixed above ground at the front, that have no leg at the back being more favourable, as these accommodate lying without causing hock damage.

Table 3.6 Area allocation for loose-bedded (UK) and free stall/cubicle bed length (UK and USA) for dairy cattle according to live-weight.

Live-weight (kg)	Deep litter yard area (m²)			Cubicle/free stall bed length (m)			
	Bedded	Loafing	Total	Open front		Closed front	
				UK *	USA	UK	USA
500	6.0	2.5	8.5	2.10	2.05	2.40	2.05
600	6.5	2.5	9.0	2.20	2.15	2.45	2.15
700	7.0	3.0	10.0	2.30	2.30	2.55	2.55
800	8.0	3.0	11.0	2.40	2.40	2.70	2.70

* Double these for stalls that have cows facing each other head to head.

The provision of high levels of comfort and cleanliness are important factors in the management of dairy cows, and the use of sand beds, rubber mats or mattresses, with regularly replaced clean bedding materials, is important in the maintenance of low levels of bacterial contamination, mastitis pathogens and prevent hock damage. Cow comfort and this welfare have increasingly become a subject of cow and system evaluation, using high bed occupation rates, number of cows lying, good lying posture and appropriate animal placement within the bed while standing and lying, along with hock rubbing and knee swelling being and cow cleanliness some of the main 'cow signals' being applied to the success of bed size, suitability of bed type, cleaning out and bedding application. In addition, scoring the cleanness of cow feet, legs and flanks is used to indicate the adequacy of scraping out and bed maintenance, cleanness and bedding material application rates and regularly. This is essential in preventing mastitis and maintaining low milk bacteria scan (Bactoscan) counts.

The proportion/number of cubicles available per cow is subject to differing welfare regulations and farm assurance recommendation being applied in differing countries. The UK welfare regulations and farm assurance schemes state that there must be least 1 cubicle available per animal and there should be 5% additional 'spare' cubicles available for each group of animals. The occurrence of 'overstocking', where there is fewer than 1 cubicle per cow, has been a subject of several surveys in Canada and the USA. In large herds with many thousands of cows, it is claimed that milking takes place continually, followed by which cows tend to spend time eating and drinking, so cows can lie for 10 h/day despite such 'overstocking'.

Cubicles and free stalls are not suitable for housing calving cows and animal welfare regulations in many countries stipulate that cows calving indoors should be isolated in a calving pen or placed in suitably open areas with a clean deep litter bed. These requirements relate not only to the health and safety of the cow and calf, but also to the need to accommodate natural behaviour. Moreover, regular bedding and cleaning of calving facilities is an essential element in lowering the risk of potential contamination of the cow by mastitis causing pathogens and infection of the calf by pathogens that result in enteric disorders such as cryptosporidiosis and respiratory disease.

3.5.2.2 Deep Litter and 'Pack' Bedded Systems

In areas where cereal crops are grown, deep litter bedding systems may be used to house dairy cattle. These systems can provide a good level of cow welfare comfort and are essential for calving cows. More recently, in dry climates, dried manure has been used as a 'pack' bed for dairy cows. In deep litter bedding systems, it is imperative that adequate amounts and regular provision of clean dry bedding material are applied, along with a separate feeding and watering area that can be cleaned in order to reduce the risk of bacterial contamination and mastitis. The main criterion used to design and assess this system is the allocation of enough space per animal. A separate feed alley and area for water troughs be sited to lower wetting and contamination of the bed. In addition, cows that are on heat should be removed to prevent mastitis due to the bed becoming disturbed.

3.5.2.3 Tie Barns

Some countries continue to use tie barns, where cows are tied by the neck. These mostly involve smaller herds both in cooler climates, such as Wisconsin and Canada, and in warmer climates, such as Thailand. In some units, cows are moved from the stalls to the milking parlour, but mostly they are permanently tethered during the winter and milked in the stalls. In both cases it takes a relatively long time to milk the cows, which limits the system to small herds. Moreover, the extreme restriction of cow movement and exercise can lead to hock swellings and lameness associated with abnormally low levels of hoof wear. These systems do tend to keep the cow and claw horn clean and dry, provided the beds are well bedded, well drained and dung is regularly cleared away.

3.5.2.4 Herd Homes

The introduction of herd homes in New Zealand has been increasing in recent years. These are low-cost polythene tunnel-type structures, with fully slatted floors. The impact of the introduction of these on dairy cattle has yet to be determined.

3.5.2.5 Wood Chip, Concrete Feed-pads and 'Stand-off' Areas

The use of low-cost pads or free draining area is common in pasture-based systems of New Zealand and Australia. These are used to feed cows supplements of silage and/or other feeds following milking, during periods of poor pasture growth, but also to hold cows 'off' pasture when wet soil conditions would cause pasture damage. More recently, these have been replaced by housing and or covered by roof structures, mainly due to increasing regulations regarding nitrate leaching and animal welfare. The opportunity for cows to lay down is limited and number of days cows can continuously be kept on these is limited by welfare regulations.

3.5.2.6 Solid Concrete Flooring

Flooring should provide comfortable slip free footing, be firm and durable. Floors should have a fall that facilitates drainage, so that they provide a relatively dry walking surface and maintain lower relative humidity levels, to help enhance animal welfare and prevent mastitis and respiratory diseases. Smooth surfaces increase the risk of slippages and injuries, especially dangerous in high-traffic areas and where cows/heifers may exhibit bulling behaviour. Concrete flooring wears smooth over time and cattle are less confident walking on smooth floors. Tamping and grooving of concrete flooring successfully improves cow comfort and drainage. The grooves should run in the opposite direction to direction cows travel, because this is much less slippery. The parallel grooves should be 35 mm apart and not exceed 10 mm wide and have smooth edges. Concrete that has a rough finish will increase the rate of claw horn wear, by up to 20%, potentially exasperating negative claw horn accumulation rates, that are associated with negative energy balance during early lactation.

3.5.2.7 Slatted Floors

Slatted floors have become more popular in recent years for housing lactating cows mainly to lower bedding material use. The faeces and urine are trodden through or pushed through using a robot, into the tank below. This helps to maintain good animal welfare by preventing lameness by maintain the lower legs, claw horn and digital area in a cleaner and drier state. The comfort of slats can be enhanced by covering them with rubber. The slats should be wide enough (125 mm) and have a gap that prevents the build-up of faeces on the slats (20 and 40 mm wide), while having a gap that is narrow enough to prevent foot injury and avoid excessive pressure on the sole of the claws (18 to 20% of the total area). The overall accommodation should include some solid-floor area or beds with sand, straw or some other suitable bedding material that makes the cows comfortable, especially their udders.

3.5.2.8 Feed Face/barriers

Feed barriers are designed to maximize feed intake, by maintaining a constant supply of clean feed in front of dairy cattle. This is achieved by keeping feed within reach, while minimizing the labour required to pushing feed up and clean out old feed. This is central to minimizing feed wastage. Allocating enough space at the feed face for each animal is a critical component of animal welfare and in maximizing the efficiency of the herd, minimizing bullying, that increases lameness, infertility and herd wastage, while facilitating the opportunity to maximize animal health, growth and milk yield (Table 3.7).

Open horizontal barriers lower feed intake and increase the risk of bullying or animals stealing feed and supplements that are top dressed onto forages. Diagonal barriers reduce these risks, while the expense of head bale gates provides a discrete feeding space for individual animals, which increases feed intake (5 to 7%) and provides a simple way to restrain animals for management purposes. Thus, locking head bale gates have become very popular on dairy units.

The key requirements for a feed face are that the:

- bottom of the feed trough should be no more than 100 mm above the feet of the animal
- surface should be smooth to encourage feeding and make cleaning easier
- trough or brisket boards should be around 500 mm high for adult cattle
- maximum reach is up to 1.0 m for adult cattle, but varies with age and is less for younger animals
- reach is improved by fixing feed rails and diagonal barriers at a forward angle of approx. 20°

Table 3.7 Feed face/barrier width requirement for different weights of cattle.

Animal weight (kg)	Width (mm per animal)	Ad-lib feeding (mm)
200	400	150
300	500	150
400	550	190
500	600	240
600	650	280
700	700	320
800	750	320

- neck rail height should be adjustable, from 1150 to 1250 mm above floor height for adult cattle and 900 to 1100 mm for younger cattle
- neck rails should be high enough so that an animal's neck should rarely touch it while feeding
- signals that indicate the feed barriers are too low and need adjusting include hair being rubbed off or calluses on the back of the neck.

3.5.2.9 Water Troughs

Milk has a high water content and the supply of fresh clean water is especially important for lactating dairy cattle. Welfare regulations sate that water must always be available, unless under veterinary advisement. The water supply needs to be well able to cope with peak demands and the water troughs should be designed and positioned to minimize potential contamination by food and fouling. They should be placed so there is a low risk of freezing in cold weather and where cattle can access them easily and without interference: i.e. not in a dead end. The water trough should be located at the correct height for the animal (850 mm from the floor for adult cattle, lower for younger animals) and the water level should be 50 to 100 mm below the edge of the trough to minimize splashing that increases the humidity and moisture in the building. Water troughs should be cleaned and emptied regularly, and these can be used to clean the floor of crossover passages. It is essential that the water can drain away quickly, avoiding a build-up of moisture that lowers animal welfare by increasing the risk of disease. In deep litter bed systems, water troughs should be placed away from the bed in a separate scrapable feed alley.

3.5.2.10 Ventilation

Good ventilation is essential to achieve good animal welfare by preventing pneumonia in younger animals and mastitis in adult animals. Ventilation removes stale air, lowering the relative humidity of the internal environment, mainly due to respiration. The placement/aspect of cattle buildings should be used to ensure they take advantage of the prevailing wind direction and opportunity to ventilate naturally. In addition to this, the design of the building should maximize the potential for ventilation even on a still day, without exposing livestock to direct drafts on windy days. It is possible for some, but not all buildings to rely on ventilation on still-air days to be achieved via the stack effect, which is natural ventilation that occurs when the design and location of the building allows the heat of the animals to drive the stale air out through a central air outlet in the roof ridge, while wind speeds of more than 1 m/s drive in fresh air at a lower level through gaps in the sidewalls. This can also be used to drive air out of the opposite side of buildings. The main reasons that natural ventilation fails are when there is a solid sidewall and/or an adjacent building or structure that prevents adequate air flow or increases air speed creating draughts on the livestock. The sidewalls of building should be designed to provide air diffused inlets along the maximum length of both sides of the building, which should be above animal height to protect them from direct draughts. Alternatively, buildings that feed livestock outside the wall of a building should have internal structures that protect animals from greater air speed at animal height.

3.5.2.11 Lighting

Lighting control and intensity are important for providing good animal welfare along with an efficient and safe working environment. Lighting also affects the hormone and production levels of dairy cattle (Table 3.8), and each day a period of darkness (less than 30 lux) is essential to ensure optimal endocrine function. Longer day lengths that provide 16 to 18 hours of light > 170 lux, interspersed with six to eight hours of lower lighting/darkness, increase heifer growth rates, advancing the onset of puberty and increase the milk yield from lactating cows.

3.5.3 Milking Management

The efficacy of milk practice is essential to mammary gland health and animal welfare, with the majority of dairy cattle milked in parlours or milking sheds. In large herds these are typically of herringbone or rotary design. Smaller herds in Europe, Canada and developing

Table 3.8 Lighting requirements for different work and locations.

Work	Lux	Control(s)	Types
Exterior areas	20	Timed (with option of passive infrared (PIR) movement sensors)	High-pressure sodium, metal halide lights
General use	50	Timed (with manual override)	-
Lying and feeding areas (non-photoperiod)	50	Timed (with manual override)	High-pressure sodium, metal halide lights or multiple fluorescent fittings
Lying and feeding areas (during photoperiod)	170 to 200	Timed (with light level sensing)	High-pressure sodium, metal halide lights or multiple fluorescent fittings
Animal inspection	300	-	Portable/localized
Office	500	-	-

countries may use abreast or tandem parlours, or even hand milking in some developing countries. Robotic milking continues to become more common due to better technical innovation and lower availability of labour.

The herringbone parlour/shed is the most common type, mainly due to its being one of the most cost-effective ways to milk large numbers of cows. The aim should be to ensure the throughput is sufficient to allow all the cows to be milked within about two hours. Herringbones can be fitted with clusters to milk one side at once or both side to milk all of the cows at once and are described by the number of cows that can be held, followed by the number that can be milked at any one time, e.g. 48 : 48 or 48:24. Rotary sheds are described by the number of stalls or bales that they contain and the reliability and less operator walking time has made these a popular choice for milking larger herds. Tandem milk parlours allow greater access to the cows and allow individual cows to enter and leave the milking parlour or shed, but these have a slower throughput than herring bones and the operator needs to walk much longer distances during milking.

3.5.4   Milking Equipment and Practice

Most cows are milked mechanically, by alternating between vacuum (approximately 38 to 50 kPa depending on the equipment) and non-vacuum (atmospheric pressure) phases, referred to as pulsations. The milk is removed from the cows by mimicking the suckling of the calf, where vacuum is used to reduce the pressure outside the teat end to below the pressure within the mammary gland, thus resulting in the milk flowing out through the teat canal. In terms of animal welfare, the maintenance of an appropriate and consistent amount of vacuum is one of the most important factors that ensure the health of the mammary gland. Regular maintenance and checking of milk equipment, along with appropriate staff training in milking practice, machine and equipment maintenance, is essential to maintain good animal welfare. In addition, a stock of materials for the replacement of friable materials such as short and long milk and vacuum rubber ware is equally essential. The checks required include:

- annual milking machine maintenance by professionally qualified and equipped contractors
- appropriate staff training and experience
- daily checking of the vacuum gauge for the correct vacuum
- daily checking of the vacuum regulator allowing air into the system
- daily checking of all rubber wear and the instant replacement of pipes that have slits or cracks, which would allow air to leak into the system.

The correct vacuum level, along with the correct rate and ratio of pulsations, which prevent the build-up of tissue fluid and oedema within the teat, is important in efficient milking and to prevent teat damage. The final important factor is the effective function of the rubber teat cup liners, which should be changed approximately every 2500 milkings or annually, whichever is the sooner, to ensure the function of these liners in response to the vacuum and/or non-vacuum phases and prevent any cracking or splitting that may cause mastitis and high somatic cell counts.

More recent precision technology has allowed the addition of greater individual animal monitoring during the milking process that can include regularity of milking visits, milk yield, milk composition and/or conductivity, live weight, camera-based body condition scoring and pressure plate-based mobility scoring as examples.

3.5.5 Milking Frequency

3.5.5.1 Twice and Thrice Daily Milking

Most cows are milked mechanically twice daily at relatively evenly spaced (14 and 10 h or 12 and 12 h) intervals. Milk yields can be increased by milking higher-yielding cows (>6,500 L/ year) three times daily, which increases milk yield (15 to 25%) mainly through enhancement of the longevity and function of the milk-secreting epithelial cells in the mammary gland. The removal of milk that acts as a feedback inhibitor gives rise to less myoepithelial cell damage from stretch and compaction. Moreover, a greater frequency of oxytocin secretion and its effect on cell signalling increase milk yield both during and following the period of increased milking frequency. The greater milk yield increases nutrient requirements. Greater milking frequency increases labour and fixed costs associated with milking.

3.5.5.2 Robot Milking and Greater Milking Frequencies

The application of robots in cow milking has become more common and cows choose to be milked between three and six times a day in early lactation, thereby increasing milk yield beyond that of twice daily milking. Cows may need to be trained to use the milking robot following parturition and a small proportion of cows may need to be collected and encourages to go through the robot daily, especially during late lactation, when their motivation to be milked is reduced due to the lack of pressure from milk within the mammary gland.

The placement of the robot and the greater amount of space available at the entrance and exit to the robot will increase the number of times cows will go into the robot voluntarily and this increases milking frequency and milk yield, provided adequate feed and nutrients are made available. Unlike other systems, each robot typically milks mixed stage of lactation cows, up to 50 in a pen, but fewer early-stage lactation cows because these present themselves for milking more frequently and take a little longer to milk. The robot encourages cows to be milked by offering the cows concentrate at each milking, which provides the opportunity to allocate concentrate feed according to milk yield and offer smaller meals more frequently. Robots allocate concentrate feed according to a set feed plan, starting at a low rate of 2 kg, which can be increased using weekly increments to a max of 12 kg/day, which remains constant during early lactation, before declining according to milk yield in mid- and late lactation. Other factors may be built into the system, such as allocating first lactation animals a set amount of concentrate. The main elements of milking robots include individual computerized teat location, laser guided individual teat cleaning, cup application and removal, allowing individual milk flow monitoring and milking, along with accurate post milking teat spray application. In addition, cows can be individually monitored for live weight, activity (heat detection), rumination and rumen pH, and milk conductivity. This allows cows to be automatically selected out into a management pen for observation, treatment or insemination.

3.5.5.3 Once-Daily Milking

Milking cows once daily has become a more popular option for some farm enterprises in recent years. Lower-yielding cows can be milked once daily, or three times in two days, particularly those producing milk of higher solids such as Jersey and Jersey cross cows in pasture-based systems, with a limited reduction in milk yield. Once-daily milking has been used in early lactation to lower peak labour loads in block calving herds. It can be a useful management approach for the maintenance of body condition during drought periods or the management of dairy cattle in marginal areas where feed supplies may be limited. It allows for greater flexibility of working practices, facilitating managers that have second jobs and/or school age children. The lower milk yield associated with long-term once-daily milk herds is offset by lower labour, fixed and supplementary feed costs. It greatly reduces the distance walked by dairy cattle daily and has a relatively limited effect on somatic cell count (SSC) concentrations, but only provided mastitis is well-managed and the dairy herd has low incidence of mastitis and SSC count initially.

3.5.6 Milk Sale, Quality and Testing on Farm and Processing Facility

Samples of milk are taken from farm milk storage vats prior to collection and from the bulk milk tanker on arrival at the factory. The milk samples from the bulk milk tanker are tested for temperature, fat, protein, somatic cell and urea composition using near-infrared spectroscopy (NIR) and the presence of antibiotics before the milk enters factory processing. Milk samples collected from milk producers are subsequently further tested for milk fat, protein, bulk milk cell count, bacterial count and residues such as antibiotics and/or pesticides, along with the existence of unusual taste and smell. There are set standards and grades. Milk that fails any of the tests is unsuitable for producing quality products and the milk will be rejected. Most milk contracts set a milk price that depends on fat, protein (component yield), bacterial count (hygiene), heat resistant bacterial (plant cleaning and silage quality) and somatic cells (mastitis), along with other components that currently have no commercial value such as lactose and urea. It is extremely important that these samples are collected and stored correctly.

3.6 Dairy Cow Nutrition

The nutrition of high-yielding dairy cows is typically managed using nutrition consultants, diet formulation packages and analysis of ensiled forage nutrient composition and pasture availability and quality. Lower-yielding cows are less challenging and can be managed more easily. The feeding management of dairy cows typically involves several factors and feeding opportunities, such as feed storage, diet mixing equipment and feed out equipment/ opportunities. Dairy cows, with the exception of those milked by robots, are generally allocated into groups according to their physiological stage of lactation; early, mid- and late lactation, dry (> 3.5 weeks far off from calving) and 'transition' (3.5 to 2 weeks close up to calving). This facilitates the provision of suitable diets for the efficient use of feed resources to produce milk and to manage the body condition score and health of the cows.

3.6.1 Digestive Anatomy and Function

Dairy cattle are large ruminants. Their digestive system has evolved to enable the microbial fermentation of cellulose and other fibres in forage-based diets and consists of four main compartments – the rumen, reticulum, omasum and abomasum (Figure 3.3), which are followed by the duodenum, small and large intestine, caecum and colon.

3.6.1.1 The Rumen

The rumen is a large organ (capacity 170 to 190 l), which allows large quantities of forages and effective rumen degradable protein (ERDP) to be digested over a period of time. In the rumen there are bacteria, protozoa and fungi that ferment and break down the feeds consumed by the animal. The rumen-based microflora and fauna grow and multiply while the fermentation of carbohydrates from dietary starch and cellulose produces volatile fatty acids (VFA) mainly consisting of acetic, propionic and some butyric acids. The VFA are largely absorbed into the blood through the rumen wall whose surface area is greatly enlarged by tiny finger-like projections, the rumen papillae. The undegraded feed, rumen undegradable protein and microflora and fauna (microbiome) pass out of the rumen to be digested in the abomasum, thus providing a source of protein for the animal. The microbial protein is

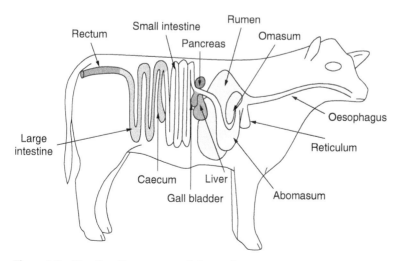

Figure 3.3 The digestive anatomy of the ruminant.

referred to as microbial crude protein (MCP), and these provide ruminant animals essential amino acids in addition to those provided by the feeds consumed. There are also bacteria in the rumen that produce B complex vitamins and some vitamin H or biotin, while Archaea are the species mainly responsible for methane production.

3.6.1.2 Diet Changes

The composition of the rumen microbiome develops in accordance with the composition of the diet offered to the cows, and this occurs over approximately two weeks. In consequence, sudden changes in diet should be avoided. The diet should be changed gradually to avoid potential indigestion and diarrhoea. As the proportions of the microflora and -fauna within the rumen are directly affected by the composition of the diet, so too are the proportions of the differing types of VFA produced. Diets high in structural fibre produce higher proportions of acetic acid to propionic acid, while diets lower in structural fibre produce higher proportions of propionic acid to acetic acid. These VFA proportions directly affect milk composition; high proportions of acetic acid result in a greater milk fat concentrations, while higher proportions of propionic acid favour greater milk protein concentrations. Moreover, the proportions of VFA affect plasma insulin and growth hormone levels and thus affect milk yield and body condition score. The production of high proportions of propionic acid to acetic acid not only tends to reduce milk fat concentration, it potentially reduces milk yield and increases the potential for live weight and body condition gain.

3.6.1.3 Dietary Fibre and Rumination

The rumen and the reticulum respond to the longer fibres that tend to accumulate towards the surface of the rumen liquor and from here they are propelled up through the oesophagus into the mouth to be chewed and re-swallowed during rumination. The cow adds copious quantities of saliva to the ingesta, both on primary consumption and during rumination. Cows can produce up to 100 l of saliva per day, which contains phosphates and bicarbonates that help to maintain the rumen environment at an optimal pH of 6.0 to 6.5. The monitoring of rumen pH using boluses has become more common place, and these can be added to a selection of cows to lower cost.

Dairy cows spend up to 6 to 8 h/d ruminating and the number of times they chew each cud depends on the amount of fibre and 'functionality' (length of fibre) of the diet. The amount of fibre in feeds is measured by chemical analysis (conventionally defined as neutral- or acid-detergent fibre (NDF or ADF). The functionality of the fibre is affected by the levels of chopping or processing. In recent years the physical assessment of fibre content has been applied to dairy cow diets, mainly due to a higher incidence of displaced abomasum (DA) in dairy cows offered mixed rations lacking longer fibre. This involves a set of sieves with decreasing apertures, which allow the lengths of the fibres of the diet to be assessed. Other practical methods for assessing the adequacy of the diet include inspection of the dung to ensure there are very few loose/sloppy faeces, check that the majority of cows lying down are ruminating and to assess that the cows are applying an adequate number of chews to each cud, approximately between 45 and 70. The total of 45 is fairly low and would be common in a low-fibre, pasture-based system, while 50 to 70 chews would be more appropriate for mixed diets.

3.6.1.4   Water Absorption and Gastric Digestion

The omasum can be identified as a small dark structure, relatively hard in structure, which contains many layers of tissue, which gives it an internal appearance similar to the leaves of a book. This organ is mainly responsible for the absorption of water.

The abomasum is relatively small compared to the rumen and has a relatively smooth texture and pale appearance. This is the equivalent of the simple stomach in the non-fermenting species and as such utilizes gastric juices at a low pH to aid digestion.

3.6.1.5   Dairy Cow Nutrition and the Environment

The potential pollution of groundwater, rivers and lakes due to leaching of both nitrates and phosphates from agricultural practices has come under increasing levels of control in most countries. This includes the effective storage and application of manures, including potential restrictions to manure application to prevent damage to water quality and the environment. Moreover, rumen fermentation can produce large amounts of methane which is a particularly powerful 'greenhouse' gas, along with carbon dioxide and nitrogen gasses. The amounts of greenhouse gases produced by ruminants and their global population make them a significant contributor to global emissions. In addition, the transportation of imported of animal feed can increase the carbon footprint of agricultural livestock. These issues may be addressed at the level of both the agricultural system and the individual cow. An example of the former approach is the capture and use of gases from manure using biodigesters. The production of gaseous methane direct from cows can be reduced through manipulation of diet and/or the population of ruminal microbes, mainly to lower archaea numbers in the rumen microbiome and fibre in the diet to increase propionate:acetate ratio in the end-products of fermentation by using maize silage as a partial replacement for grass and pasture. Other products such as garlic, citrus oils and seaweed are useful feed additives that lower methane emissions. In addition, the greater use of home-grown feeds and altering the concentration of dietary nutrient can lower the carbon footprint by lowering overseas import of feeds. Diet formulation and farm practices are evaluated in order to calculate the carbon footprint, compare this with other similar farms and inform mitigation strategies. Finally, the feed efficiency of the dairy industry can be improved by selection and feeding for higher individual yields to offset the feed energy costs of maintenance. Other routes to increased feed efficiency include reduced feed wastage, lowering the number of herd replacements and age at first calving, reducing the number of non-lactating days (50 to 60 d/lactation), increasing longevity and lifetime productivity of dairy cows. All these are key areas where animal management can lower the environmental impact of dairy production.

3.6.2   Feeding the Dairy Cow

As for any animal, the aim of planned feeding is to match the supply of available nutrients to nutrient requirements. In the special case of the lactating dairy cow, nutrient requirement is high, and supply is limited by the capacity of the animal to ingest and digest fibrous feeds that ferment relatively slowly. Thus, the process of dairy cow nutrition is based on two main elements – estimating the feed intake and nutrient requirements of the animal. In this process it is essential to consider the effects of stage of lactation, feed quality and feeding system when planning to provide nutrients in the diet in an adequate concentration to allow the animal to consume these within the constraints of its feed fresh (FMI) and dry matter intake (DMI) potential. Similarly, when planning a diet, it is important not to overestimate the DMI and to ensure that there is sufficient metabolizable energy (ME) (typically overestimate by 5%) in the diet, followed by crude protein (CP) and then minerals and vitamins.

3.6.3 Nutrient Requirements

The nutrient requirements of dairy cattle are generally expressed in terms of ME (MJ/kg or per day) and CP (% per kg DMI or g/d), along with minerals and vitamins. However, lowering the CF has led to more precision in the use of CP in dairy cow, calf and growing heifer nutrition is moving towards the division and application lower CP diets assessed according to effective rumen degradable (ERDP) and rumen undegradable protein (RUP)/and digestible undegradable protein (DUP). The dairy cow requires these nutrients for maintenance and production (i.e. milk production, reproduction and pregnancy, growth and live weight gain). In early lactation the dairy cow will prioritize maintenance and milk production before reproduction, growth or live weight gain. This prioritizing of nutrients towards differing purposes is referred to as nutrient partitioning. Lactating animals also require large quantities of water and substantially more in hot weather/conditions.

3.6.3.1 Energy

Energy is usually considered the first limiting factor in production. Dairy cows require energy for both maintenance and production. Energy is also essential for the function of the microbial population in the rumen. In most countries the energy requirements of dairy cattle are expressed as ME. Due to the importance of supplying energy for the rumen microbes, the ME terminology has been refined to include a measurement of the energy that can be fermented by the microbes in the rumen, which is fermentable metabolizable energy (FME) to ensure that these microbes are supplied with adequate amount of FME to function, degrade feed efficiency and maximize DMI. The USA and some other countries use net energy (NE), which is a measure of the energy directly available to the animal for production. The ME and NE are expressed in ruminant production in megajoules (MJ). The energy content can be calculated from the gross energy (GE) content, which is estimated using a bomb calorimeter, and the energy losses associated with the digestion and metabolism of differing feeds (Figure 3.4), indicating clearly that not all the GE is available to be metabolized by the animal.

3.6.3.2 Protein

The protein requirements of dairy cows are calculated in a similar way as for energy. The most common term presently used to describe proteins for ruminants is CP and metabolizable protein (MP), which is that available for metabolism following digestion and absorption. While the terminology used to describe the protein content of feeds directly reflects the

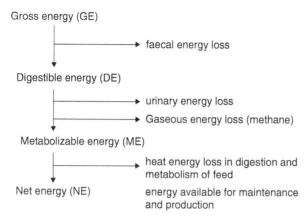

Figure 3.4 Schematic representation of the relationship between gross energy, metabolizable and net energy, and energy losses during digestion.

areas of the digestive system in which it may be digested, this is affected by the natural proportion that may be degraded in the rumen and amount of time the feed spends degrading in the rumen. The overall composition of the diet directly affects the rate that feed passes through the rumen and a larger proportion of rapidly degradable feed competent increases this rate, which lowers the opportunity for ERDP to be fully degraded, thus lowering the proportion of ERDP and increasing the proportion of DUP. Moreover, the proportion of DUP can be enhanced by the application of feed processing technology (typically applied to oil seed meals such as rape/canola, cotton seed, sunflower and soya bean) such as heating, extrusion, encapsulation and other treatments that protect the protein from degradation in the rumen and are used to increase the amount of protein and amino acids supplied to the abomasum.

The final amount of protein that is available to be digested by the dairy cow is that which arrives into the abomasum from two potential sources: DUP and microbial crude protein (MCP) and these are digested in the abomasum to provide MP. The amount of MCP delivered to the abomasum is a function of a combination of ERDP and fermentable metabolizable energy (FME) available to the microbes in the rumen and this ratio is checked to ensure the diet contains an adequate amount of FME. Finally, milk urea concentration can be used to assess the 'balance' between protein supply and utilization and the need to increase or decrease dietary protein supply to potentially increase milk yield when financially viable.

3.6.4 Feed Intake

As a ruminant animal, one of the main factors limiting the performance of the dairy cow is the voluntary feed intake, which is often referred as DMI. The factors that affect DMI can be divided into those that are related to the animal or to the feed.

3.6.4.1 Animal Factors

The main animal factors that affect DMI include weight or physical size, body condition, physiological state and health. In general, larger individuals or breeds tend to have greater DMI. Within a breed, animals with lower body condition (lower fat reserves) tend to have a higher DMI than those with greater body reserves. This is due to blood metabolites regulating intake, through chemostatic signals, and the physical limitation that abdominal fat places on space available for food within the rumen.

Physiological state is an important factor affecting both DMI and nutrient requirement. The main factor for lactating cows is milk yield, which increases DMI substantially. Conversely, DMI becomes limited during the last trimester of pregnancy, due to the increasing size of the foetus reducing the physical space available for the rumen. This reduction in feed intake persists, for up to three to five weeks following parturition. Thus, it is important to take stage of lactation into consideration when estimating DMI. This period of lowered nutrient intake in early lactation coincides with high nutrient demands for milk production. This has been termed the 'energy gap' and over this period that lactating dairy cows tend to mobilize body fat and some protein to meet the nutrients required for milk production. This live weight and body condition loss should be managed by ensuring optimal body condition score (BCS) at parturition (3 to 3.5 on a scale of 1 to 5, or 5.5 on a scale of 1 to 10; see Table 3.9), to allow body reserves to be available, and cows should be offered sufficient nutrients to regain lost live weight prior to mating to optimize reproductive functions, such as regular oestrous cycling, follicle quality, increased oestrous behaviour and detection rates, thus improving conception and pregnancy rates.

3.6.4.2 Feed Factors

The main feed factors that affect DMI include feed availability, type and quality. The DMI of the cow can be reduced when feed availability is limited or pasture availability (height) is low. This has the effect of under-utilizing the DMI capacity of the animal and thus reduces milk

Table 3.9 Body condition scoring of dairy cattle.

5-point scale	10-point scale	Description/target
0	1	
1.0	2	Emaciated/too thin
1.5	3	Too thin
2.0	4	
2.5	5	Target body condition at calving
3.0	6	Target body condition at calving
3.5	7	
4.0	8	Over conditioned
4.5	9	Obese
5.0	10	Obese

yield per cow but may increase milk yield per hectare in grazed animals. The type of the feed affects the DMI mainly through the fibre content (conventionally described by NDF and ADF) and energy concentration (ME) or FME which is the major substrate required by the rumen microflora and -fauna. Thus, the fibre content and energy density of the diet directly affect DMI through the degradation rate of feeds in the rumen. Feeds with higher fibre levels and lower energy concentration, which include straw, tall pasture and late cut silage or hay, tend to degrade more slowly in the rumen, occupy the physical space of the rumen for longer, thus reducing DMI. Conversely feeds that have lower levels of fibre and higher levels of energy concentration, such as young leafy pasture, cereals and some co-products, degrade faster in the rumen and, when offered as an appropriate total diet, result in DMI closer to the animal's maximum potential. The main aim of feeding dairy cattle is to optimize feed intake by offering an appropriate combination of feeds and nutrients on a regular and unrestricted basis.

Other feed factors that affect DMI include the palatability of the feeds and the feeding system employed. A good example of feeds that are likely to have lower intake potentials are pasture with recently applied manure and poor-quality silages. Dairy cows should be offered high-quality silages, which mainly result from mowing pastures before 50% ear emergence, along with good ensiling and silage storage practices that minimize butyric acid production and microbial deterioration. Pasture silages with higher dry matter (DM) content (29 to 32% DM) tend to have a higher intake potential, compared with wetter silages (<25% DM). The management of animal feeding can affect feed intake, and this includes overstocking at the feed face or at pasture and allowing feed quality to deteriorate due to poor clamp face management, feeding-out management and general hygiene.

3.6.5 Feeding and Feeding Systems

The main aims of dairy cow feeding are to optimize feed quality and feed intake through good pasture management, ensiling techniques, feed storage and feeding-out practices. Most lactating dairy cows rely heavily on the consumption of high-quality forages in order to optimize milk yield potential. Dairy cattle can graze fresh grass or be offered conserved grass as silage or hay. These feeds can be complemented with a range of other feeds such as forage maize silage, cereal silages, cereals, co-products and pelleted compound feeds, along with minerals and vitamins. The cost of diet components and diet cost is a very important factor and least costs formulation of lactating cow diets is applied widely through the feed industry, but may have less of a place in early lactation diets were the main goal is the enhancement of fertility and longer-term milk yield. The aim of a total mixed ration (TMR) to provide both a balanced supply of nutrients and the correct substrates for stable fermentation through the day and night results in a more constant rumen pH, increased feed intake and greater milk yields.

3.6.6 Minerals and Vitamins

Dairy cattle require several minerals and vitamins for healthy body function and to prevent deficiency diseases. Macronutrients include calcium (Ca), magnesium (Mg) and phosphorus (P) whose requirement is measured in g/kg feed and Ca in early lactation is added to the diet as low-cost calcium carbonate. Micronutrients required in μg/kg include copper (Cu), cobalt (Co), selenium (Se) and zinc (Zn). The levels of macro-minerals will depend on the forage mineral levels, boluses, etc. and the requirements of the animal according to the physiological stage of lactation/pregnancy and season (see Section 3.6.6.2).

3.6.6.1 Calcium Deficiency (Milk Fever)

The most common problem of dairy cows and the severe form of calcium deficiency is milk fever, which should be prevented to ensure good animal welfare and fertility. This typically presents as extreme muscle weakness in a newly calved cow that can lead to collapse and death within hours, if untreated. Treatment involves administration of calcium salts subcutaneously, or intravenously in advanced cases. However, the risks of milk fever should be prevented by attention to feeding practices during late pregnancy that facilitate early lactation, referred to as the 'transition' period. This involves offering cows diets with low levels of positive potassium and calcium ions, that includes avoiding grazing pastures that have had effluent applied to it and reducing pasture and grass silage intake. This enables cows to begin mobilizing body reserves of calcium from bone just prior to parturition and thus preventing sudden plasma calcium deficiencies (hypocalcaemia) at and directly following calving. This strategy is applied to dry cows that are close to calving (3 to 4 weeks prepartum) and typically involves the addition of a high fire forage to prevent displaced abomasum and addition of negative ion minerals to manipulate the dietary cation:anion balance (DCAB) to induce a mild metabolic acidosis and thereby encourage the mobilization of calcium and phosphorus buffers during late pregnancy (see Section 3.7.4).

3.6.6.2 Magnesium Deficiency (Grass Staggers or Hypomagnesaemia)

Magnesium deficiency in dairy cows is primarily associated with low levels of magnesium (Mg) in spring pasture. This can be exacerbated by the application of artificial fertilizers that can reduce magnesium availability. Early clinical signs of acute magnesium deficiency include hyperexcitability and a 'staggering' gait. The conditions can proceed to death within hours, so prevention is critical. Supplementing the diet or water with magnesium is typically used as a preventive for magnesium deficiencies in spring.

3.6.6.3 Copper Deficiency (Clinical and Subclinical) and Excess

The supplementation of cow diets with copper (Cu) is often required in areas where copper is deficient or high soil molybdenum, sulphur or iron lead to reduced copper availability. This can be prevented by the implantation of long-acting copper boluses into the rumen. This can enhance oestrous behaviour and improve reproductive performance of dairy cattle. However, it is important to combine all sources to prevent excess Cu being supplied and livestock feed should never be offered to sheep.

3.6.6.4 Other Important Micronutrients for Dairy Cattle

The supplementation of zinc and selenium has become more popular, in the belief that these can improve hoof horn quality and immunity and reduce somatic cell count levels (see Section 3.8.3). The vitamin H (biotin) has been seen in recent years to improve hoof horn quality, when offered for prolonged periods of up to 8 to 10 months, and reduce lameness (especially white line disease), and has been associated with increased milk yields. Finally, the availability of more complex (e.g. chelated or bioplex) forms of minerals and application of blouses have become more commonplace on the basis that they may be more bio-available so achieve similar effects on level animal performance at lower levels of inclusion and less risk of environmental pollution. Unfortunately, this may lead to several forms mineral supply, including from diet components, being combined inadvertently and the whole diet mineral supply should be assessed. Unfortunately, the availability of minerals and micro-minerals can interact to reduce their availability, thus suboptimal levels can be created either by a lack in the diet or by reduced availability due to an interaction with another mineral or micronutrient, resulting in suboptimal absorption by the animal. This can lead to a clinical or subclinical deficiency and suboptimal performance. The availability of copper, for example, is profoundly affected by interactions with other elements – sulphur, molybdenum, zinc and iron.

3.6.7 Grazing and Pasture Management

Grazed pasture is one of the cheapest forms of forage that can be offered to dairy cattle. Good management is essential to limit fibre content, encouraging greater DMI and optimizing the nutrient concentration of the pasture. This is achieved using pasture measurement techniques to assess pasture height and available for each day and month, by feed planning (daily, monthly and annually), and by management of grazing frequency, grazing period and stocking rate to control pasture height. Pasture management also includes the incorporation of ensiling during periods of rapid pasture growth. The main aim is to maintain the grass plant in a vegetative stage through regular defoliation. This optimizes the number of tillers and nutrient density by minimizing the opportunity for the plant to enter the reproductive stage, thus limiting the senescent materials and fibre content of the pasture throughout the grazing season.

There are a number of grazing systems available, which allow varying levels of plant management and infrastructure requirements:

- *Paddock grazing*: – the farm is divided into small paddocks according to herd size to allow one, two or three days of grazing. This allows the greatest control of pasture quality, but also has the greatest infrastructure requirements;
- *Set stocking*: – pasture is controlled by the number of animals grazed on a set area;
- *Continuous grazing*: – the area is continually grazed and the stocking rate is adjusted according to pasture availability;
- *Zero grazing*: – pasture is not grazed but cut and carried to the cows;
- *Strip grazing*: – the use of electric fencing to allocate cattle to strips of fresh pasture. This can be used for pasture and forage crops, where there is a high volume of feed.

Finally, ensiling can be used to control plant growth, by cutting down the area to be grazed when pasture growth is rapid during spring, so that silage is available during periods of low pasture growth such as dry summer periods and in winter. More recent precision technology that have been added to pasture management include NIR measurement of pasture height and currently pasture feed quality, including the use of trailed machines and more recently drones. Other developments are location monitoring of cattle and the use of virtual fencing. Greater botanical diversity of pasture species has been introduced recently to support greater wildlife diversity; however, this is are better suited to marginal areas, conservation dairy and beef production systems and specialist dairy product production, rather than intensive dairy production systems.

3.6.7.1 Forage/fodder Crops

In climates where grass and white clover can respond to heavier soil types, adequate quantity and frequency of rainfall, grass silage will be a large component of the diet of dairy cows, due to its good level of crude protein (18% CP) and energy (11.5 MJ/kg ME) concentration. Other forage crops include maize and whole crop cereal silages, which have found to lower methane emissions from ruminants. The most popular of these is forage maize, which is used quite extensively due to the development of faster-maturing varieties that have allowed this crop to be grown in a wider range of environments. Forage maize makes an excellent complement to grass silage, due to its high level of starch, which increases the milk yield of dairy cattle when used at 30 to 75% of the forage in the diet. Other whole-crop cereal silages (e.g. wheat, barley) can be used in combination with grass silage but seem not to be as effective as forage maize in increasing milk yield. In terms of precision technology, the development of portable NIR for more regular assessment of silage quality on farm as an aid to greater precision in monthly diet formulation and precision feeding of dairy cattle. Fodder crops such as fodder beet, turnips and kale can be offered to dairy cattle and are generally strip-grazed to control intake levels to avoid scouring and milk taint. The current need to lower the carbon footprint of dairy systems has led to the use of lower protein diets (from 18 to 15 to 16 % CP), less use of soya and protein resources imported from countries where its growing is related to deforestation and greater use of more locally grown forages and crops, which may include pasture, white clover, chicory and canola/rape seed meal, red clover, peas and beans and other feed resources suited to the local climatic conditions. In addition, this food security has led to a greater focus on ruminants utilizing non-human edible crops and coproducts, along with the need to enhance the feeding value of co-products though feed processing technology. The efficiency of forage use is evaluated by using the milk from forage and the greater the amount of milk from achieving good forage quality, lowers the amount and costs of supplementary feed required to produce milk.

3.6.7.2 Compound Feeds, Cereals and Co-products

These are classified in the feed resource databases into energy and protein sources according to their chemical composition. A range of cereals and protein-rich oil seeds can be used, following some form of processing, for inclusion into dairy cow diets. The compound feeds are a combination of products including, but not exclusively; cereals, oil seeds, minerals and vitamins that are formulated and processed into a pelleted feed containing a combination of energy and protein, with set levels of fat. The feed can be purchased as 'straights', which are single products that can be purchased in bulk loads that require storage, which are combined with silages using mixer wagons. There are an increasing number and range of coproducts from the food, beverage and biofuel industry. These include such products as bread and biscuit meal, vegetables, brewer's and distiller's grains, and maize co-products, to mention just a few. Technological developments include the processing of canola/rape-seed meal to increase the proportion of DUP and thus enhance its ability to supply MP, and the use of technologies to improve the feeding value of coproducts from bioethanol, beverage and the food processing industry, including the use of naturally occurring feed additives such as enzymes, yeast and essential oil that enhance the gastrointestinal tract microbiome, immunity and animal health and welfare, along with the need to lower farm antimicrobial use, carbon footprint and subsequent climate change. The efficiency of milk production is evaluated by the margin over purchased feed, which is measured from amount of milk income produced after the of costs of purchased feed has been deducted.

3.6.8 Feed Storage

Correct and appropriate feed storage is important in ensuring that the quality of the feed is maintained and risks of moulding and production of mycotoxins, which negatively affect animal and human health, are minimized. The addition of mycotoxin binders is expensive, but they are effective when required. It is imperative that feed storage and feeding facilities are designed to ensure that cattle feed and forage cannot be contaminated by bird, pest, rodent, cat or dog urine or faeces and this is an essential part of farm assurance.

3.7 Diet Feeding and Management

3.7.1 Mixed Rations

3.7.1.1 Feeder Wagons and Diet Mixers

The use of total mixed rations (TMR) or complete diets (forages mixed with other concentrated feeds and minerals) has become increasingly popular as dairy cow yield potential has increased. The use of mixer wagons to combine and dispense a pre-mixed diet has become very popular in both indoor and pasture-based systems. This machinery allows the maximum flexibility in the components that can be included in the diet, depending only on the ability of the mixer wagon to render the cow unable to select components from the mixture. These types of diet offer the opportunity to maximize the use of a range of feed resources and the consistency of the type of diet being offered throughout the day and thus optimize DMI and milk yield. This method increases the machinery and labour costs for diet mixing.

A mixed ration is typically formulated to provide enough nutrients for the maintenance requirement of the cow plus a specific level of milk production. These diets are described as 'maintenance plus'. This allows batches of a mixed ration to be made up and offered to groups of dairy cattle according to their milk yield or stage of lactation. The additional nutrients can be offered through feeding systems that dispense feed to groups in the shed or to individuals in the parlour or via computerized dispensers; this has led to the term 'partial mixed ration' (PMR). These mixed rations generally include a combination of forages, protein meals, cereals and other co-products with calcium carbonate and potentially minerals for lactating cows. They may also contain some straw to ensure that the diet contains enough functional fibre ensure adequate salivation and rumination occurs to lower the risk of ruminal acidosis and displaced abomasum.

3.7.1.2   Offering Forages (Silages/cut Forages and TMR/PMR)

Silages and mixed rations can be offered from feed bins, troughs, rings or eaten directly ('self-feed') from the silage bunker. Cows that are required to use self-feed silage bunkers will have a lower DMI compared with cows offered feed freely. It is important to ensure that cows have enough space for all to eat at any one time, which should increase feed intake and milk production and reduce lameness (recommended feed face space is a minimum).

3.7.1.3   Feed Pads

These are common in pasture-based systems and are hard-floored areas or standing areas, often concreted, which are occasionally fitted with a roof structure. Here cows are offered feeds to supplement pasture, usually silage forage-based diets with other available cost-effective feeds such as cereals, co-products and plant-based food waste with diet balancers and minerals. Cows are given access to these feeds following milking, during periods of peak yield or when pasture supply is below that required by the animal (dry periods, cool spring, winter) or when high rainfall leads to wet soils and excessive damage to pasture (pugging or poaching) would be caused by cattle treading the ground.

3.7.2   Supplementing Forage Diets with Concentrated Feed or Compound Feeds

The forage diet of dairy cattle can be supplemented with more concentrated sources of nutrients, thus increasing nutrient intake and subsequent milk yield. Dairy cows respond to a greater extent to these supplements in early lactation and when genetically predisposed to higher milk yields – i.e. when their nutrient demands are greatest. The allocation of concentrated feeds can be achieved on a group or individual cow basis. The feeding rates (kg DM/d) can be managed according to differing approaches:

- lead feeding where cows are fed high rates until peak lactation;
- stepped feeding rates, where differing rates are offered for set periods of the lactation;
- feeding to yield, where cows are offered a feed rate according to the milk yield of the cow, which can be adjusted on a weekly or monthly basis.

The choice of approach will depend on the feeding equipment and resources available. The allocation of concentrated feed to individual cows can be achieved using in-parlour/shed or out-of-parlour/shed automated cow feeders. In more simple systems, cows can be offered feed applied over the top of silage 'top dressed' as a midday supplement or offered liquid feeds from 'lick ball' feeders on an ad *libitum* basis.

3.7.3   Automated Feeding Systems

Automated equipment and electronic tags (or transponders) can be used to operate feeders that distribute feeds to individual cows according to preset levels held on a computer database system. These can be operated in or out of the milking shed/parlour.

3.7.3.1   In-parlour or Shed Feeding

This system, which can be electronic or manually operated, delivers concentrated feeds, usually pelleted or processed cereals, to cows while being milked. It can be used in addition to pasture or silage feeding and as a complement to mixer wagons. It allows individual cows to be offered feed levels according to their individual milk yield. Its limitation is the amount that can be offered at any one time. This should generally be restricted 3 to 5 kg DM at each milking, to avoid the risk of ruminal acidosis caused by consumption of large quantities of rapidly degradable carbohydrates.

3.7.3.2   Out-of-parlour or Shed Feeding

These are electronic systems that deliver concentrated feeds, usually pelleted in nature, to cows throughout the day or night. They reduce the amount of compound feed that is required to be offered at one point in time, thus avoiding fluctuations in rumen pH, and thereby permit higher levels of concentrate feeding with consequent increases in milk yield.

3.7.4   Feeding Management for Dry Cows (Transition or Lead Feeding)

The advent of improved feeding management of dry (non-lactating) dairy cattle has been one of the major advances in dairy cow husbandry. The main aim is to prevent metabolic disorders such as milk fever, ketosis and acidosis, and improve fertility in early-lactation cows. This involves the management of calcium mobilization and body condition score and the introduction of a proportion of the lactation diet before calving to allow the rumen microflora and fauna to adapt to the great increase in nutrient demand at the onset of lactation. To achieve this, specific dry cow supplements, limitations of pasture intake and the provision of fibre (i.e. cereal straw) are key components.

The prevention of milk fever requires the management of calcium and magnesium supplementation before calving. Low positive ions of potassium and calcium, along with the addition of magnesium before calving, will encourage the cow to mobilize body reserves of calcium. Similarly, the management of dietary cation and anion balance (DCAB or DCAD), using negative (chloride) ions added to the diet, induces a mild metabolic acidosis and stimulate the cow to mobilize body calcium and phosphorus salts, which act as buffers. Grass and silage are high in potassium, especially that that has had effluent applied to it, which will increase plasma pH and thus discouraging cows from mobilizing calcium from bone tissue; the levels of grazed grass, grass pasture silage should be restricted in dry cow diets, e.g. by inclusion of cereal silages and fibre into dry cow diets to maintain DMI to satiate the cow and rumen capacity.

3.7.5 Feeding and Management of Cow Body Condition (Body Fat and Protein)

The body condition of dairy cattle is evaluated using visual and/or manual palpation to estimate the level of body fat covering the tail head, ribs and spine. This is expressed using either a 5-point (with half points) or 10-point scale, with the lower numbers indicating lower fat reserves (thinner) and the higher numbers indicating greater levels of fat reserves (fatter, Table 3.9). The main aim is to allow cows to gain weight in late lactation and the dry period. This will allow dairy cattle to calve in adequate body condition (3.5 on a 5-point scale) to enable them to have sufficient reserves to cope with the energy gap in early lactation. The provision of good quality feed and a nutrition plan in early lactation should then ensure that the dairy cow does not lose too much live weight during early lactation and is on a rising plane of nutrition and increasing body condition during the mating period in order to increase the conception rate and thus herd fertility.

3.8 Health

The main focus should be the enhancement of the welfare and longevity of the dairy herd, through disease prevention, recording and the use of a herd health plan that is developed with a veterinary surgeon and good feeding plans developed and applied though your nutrition consultant. The majority of diseases of importance for dairy herds are often multifactorial in nature, with a number of factors that interact together to cause disease. In global terms, the three main health issues that cause cows to be culled from the dairy herd are, in decreasing order:

- infertility;
- mastitis;
- lameness.

These diseases are of great importance in both economic and animal welfare terms and they will be discussed in detail because their control and prevention is central to good dairy herd management. Other major potential animal health issues include hypocalcaemia, hypomagnesaemia, acidosis, displaced abomasum, endometritis, acetonaemia (ketosis) and bloat.

3.8.1 Reproduction and Fertility

On a global basis, poor reproduction or 'infertility' is the most common reason for dairy cows to be culled from the dairy herd. The loss of cows due to infertility and the subsequent need to provide herd replacements is a considerable economic cost, while calving of cows on an approximately annual basis is a key factor in generating high levels of efficient milk production. The efficient management of reproduction is one of the most important factors in dairy herd management. The annual management of reproduction is presented in Figure 3.5. (Further reading can be found in Peters and Ball 2004, *Reproduction in Cattle*.) Close to annual calving or a calving interval (CI) of 365 days is desirable, with seasonal and lower

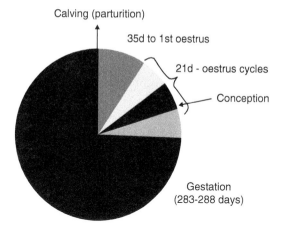

Calving (parturition)

35d to 1st oestrus

21d - oestrus cycles

Conception

Gestation
(283-288 days)

Figure 3.5 An example of the differing components (days) of an annual (365-day calving interval) reproductive cycle of the dairy cow.

milk-yielding herds needing a CI of 365 days to be efficient, while herds that have cows with greater milk yield per cow (> 9,000 l) allowing longer CI's of 380 to 410 days.

3.8.1.1 Gestation

The gestation length of the dairy cow is a relatively fixed period of approximately 283 days, which varies slightly with sex of the calf and breed of the sire. Calves born to sires from the continental beef breeds (e.g. Charolais, Limousin) tend to have longer gestation periods, as do male calves compared to female calves of dairy breeds. In New Zealand the Angus and Angus cross-breeds are favoured as terminal sires compared with the Hereford beef breeds due to the shorter gestation length and ease of calving needed in seasonal calving herds.

3.8.1.2 Puberty and Oestrous Cycles

Dairy heifers reach puberty at around 40% of mature weight and this can be achieved as early as 4 months of age, where the plane of nutrition has been high in early life. The optimal age for heifers to calve is at approximately 2 years of age, at an estimated 85 % mature weight and, as gestation length is relatively fixed, this can be achieved by heifers conceiving at 13 to 15 months of age at 55 % mature weight.

3.8.1.3 Oestrous Cycles and Conception Rate of Lactating Cows

The dairy cow has a natural period of non-ovulation (anoestrus) following calving, which is approximately 35 days long. This period can be minimized by ensuring adequate body condition at calving and providing adequate nutrition following calving. The aims should be to minimize live weight loss following calving and for the cows to be gaining weight by the time of insemination. First oestrus should occur between 20 and 40 days post-partum and this may be recorded in order to determine the return of 'normal' oestrous cycles in readiness for the next oestrous cycle. Dairy cows that have not shown oestrous behaviour following this period may have cystic ovarian disease (COD) and require treatment by a veterinarian. The uterus requires approximately 40 to 50 days following parturition to return to its normal size and function and, as a consequence, conception rate (CR) to inseminations before 50 days post-partum tends to be low. Due to this and the expense of high-quality semen, dairy cows are typically inseminated following standing heats (oestrus) from 50 days post-partum onwards and this may be delayed to 60 days post-partum in higher milk-yielding herds.

The CR to first insemination completed around 50 to 60 days post-partum tends to be lower compared to second and subsequent inseminations. In the assessment of conception rates, first, second and subsequent inseminations should be calculated and monitored separately. The conception rate of Holstein Friesian cows has tended to decline over the last 10 to 15 years. As a consequence, fertility, despite its low heritability, has been included in the breed assessment index for animal selection and breeding purposes.

3.8.1.4 Oestrous Behaviour

The length of the oestrous cycle ranges between 18 and 24 days, averaging around 21 days. The cow is 'on heat' or 'in oestrus' for an average of around 14 hours, but this can vary from 1 hour to 24 hours. Ovulation occurs around 10 to 12 hours following the onset of oestrus, but this timing will clearly be affected by the length of oestrus and the correct animal identification and timing of insemination following oestrus is critical in achieving high conception rates. The amount and duration of oestrous behaviour can vary according to season, ambient temperature, housing environment, breed, body condition, social interaction and plane of nutrition. Oestrous behaviour tends to be lower in warmer climates or periods, during winter (reduced light), in housed conditions and for cows that have lower social status within the herd. The oestrous behaviour is likely to be higher for cows in good body condition, with adequate and appropriate nutrition including mineral supplementation, which are housed or grazed in compliance with the welfare regulations, housing codes of practice and conformance to the relevant farm assurance guidelines.

3.8.2 Factors Affecting Fertility

3.8.2.1 Oestrus Detection

The use of cow observation, which is increasingly aided by tail paint or automation, supported by accurate recording and a good communications system, is an important factor in heat detection. This system relies on observation of cows expressing oestrous activity, identification of the correct animal and timely insemination that follows ovulation. Manual observation requires animals to be observed at regular intervals through the day and in the evening and for this approach to succeed, cows should be observed as many as four times daily for an adequate period time to identify cows that are standing to be mounted or mounting the front of herd mates. In terms of management it is important to be able to correctly identify individual animal, potentially from a distance. The use of freeze branding and electronic tagging is quite common, in addition to the legal requirement for ear tagging.

3.8.2.2 Aids to Oestrus Detection

The trend to larger herds and to all-year-round calving has led to the development of several aids to the detection of oestrus to ensure timely insemination, high levels of conception and pregnancy rates (PR).

3.8.2.3 Tail Paint and Pads

Purpose-specific paint or pads of paint can be applied to the 'tail head' on the spine. Cows that have been 'mounted' by other cows can be observed and recorded at milking time and submitted for insemination.

3.8.2.4 Electronic Monitors

During the oestrous period the activity level of cows on heat tends to increase beyond the normal levels. Meters that measure the number of steps or activity of the cow can be used to assess cow activity and the possible occurrence of oestrus. Similarly, the body temperature of the cow tends to be higher during oestrus, and this can also be monitored and interpreted in a similar way. However, these technologies can give 'false positives' in cows with high activity or body temperature for reasons other than oestrus.

3.8.2.5 Hormone Tests

Kits are available to measure milk progesterone levels on-farm. Progesterone is secreted from the corpus luteum. Thus, it is high during the dioestrous period after ovulation and increases further in pregnancy. In a non-pregnant cow, milk progesterone levels fall sharply about 19 days after the previous oestrus and remain low for about 4 days, then start to rise at the time of ovulation. Analysis of milk samples for progesterone on days 7, 19 and 21 after previous oestrus can either predict optimal time for insemination or give a good early indication of the success of a previous insemination.

3.8.2.6 Vasectomized or 'Teaser' Bulls

The intermittent use of vasectomized or 'teaser' bulls can also increase oestrous behaviour levels. Undoubtedly the most successful way to achieve high fertility is through natural service. However, this is inconsistent with the need for genetic improvement of the herd that can be gained from the access to nationally and internationally ranked sires using artificial insemination.

3.8.2.7 Target Body Condition Score

The health and productivity of dairy cows has been enhanced by the regular application of body condition scoring and adherence to achieving target body condition for dairy cows (Table 3.10). This should maximize fertility and milk yields, and avoid metabolic disorders associated with over condition, such as ketosis. The body condition of the cows is assessed at key points: calving, 60 days pp, 100 days prior to dry off and drying off. The actual body condition of the animal informs us about the success of longer-term animal nutrition, while body condition score change informs us about the adequacy of the shorter-term, current nutrition.

Table 3.10 Target body condition for dairy cows to maximize milk yield and fertility, by avoiding metabolic disorders.

	Body condition			
Stage of lactation	UK (1 to 5)	NZ (1 to 10)	USA (1 to 10)	USA (1 to 5)
Parturition	2.5 to 3.0	5.0 to 5.5	5.0 to 5.5	2.5 to 3
At 60 d pp	2.0 to 3.0	4.5 to 5.0	5.0 to 5.5	2.0 to 3.0
At 100 d prior to drying off	2.5 to 3.0	4.5 to 5.0	5.0 to 5.5	2.5 to 3.0
At drying off	2.5 to 3.0	4.5 to 5.0 *	5.0 to 5.5	2.5 to 3.0

* Lactation lengths are often shorter and dry periods are longer in NZ and gain in BCS can be made during the early dry period depending on milk price.

In terms of body condition score change, loss of body condition should be limited during the first 60 days of lactation (0.5 on a scale of 1 to 5) to avoid infertility; whole body condition score gain should be avoided entirely during the 60 days dry period, more especially during the 3-week transition period prior to calving to avoid calving difficulty and the risk of ketosis post-partum.

In New Zealand lactation length can be shorter, lengthening the dry period of cows managed in seasonally calving herds. Seasonal spring calving results in cows consuming autumn pasture during late lactation, making it notoriously difficult for cows to gain body condition during late lactation. At this point, depending on the need for cows to achieve optimal body condition, cows will be either supplemented if milk price is higher or dried off to gain body condition during the extended dry period.

3.8.3 Mastitis

Mastitis is the second most common reason for culling cows from the dairy herd, affecting approximately 35% of cows annually (the range for 95% of herds being between 5 and 60%). It is caused by a bacterial infection of the mammary gland via the teat canal. The bacteria involved are classified as *contagious* (e.g. *Staphylococcus*, *Streptococcus*) because they are typically transmitted between cows through poor hygiene at milking, and *environmental* (e.g. *Escherichia coli*). Clinical mastitis results in inflammation of the affected quarter and can cause considerable pain and discomfort. Consequently, mastitis represents a considerable challenge to the welfare of the dairy cow. Factors that affect the incidence of mastitis are shown in Figure 3.6.

3.8.3.1 Economic Effect of Mastitis

Mastitis reduces the economic efficiently of the dairy herd by causing losses and increasing costs. The losses associated with mastitis include:

- liquid milk sales (antibiotic milk discarded or offered to calves);
- milk price (lower price for milk with higher somatic cell counts;

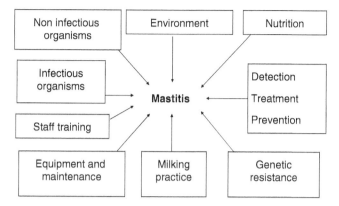

Figure 3.6 Main factors associated with mastitis of dairy cattle.

- milk component levels (reduced due to mastitis);
- milk production (long-term reduction).

Increasing costs associated with mastitis include:

- treatment (antibiotic or other);
- labour (treatment, dry cow therapy, separation from main herd);
- herd replacements (cows culled due to high SCC or clinical mastitis)
- along with the increased risk of antimicrobial resistance (AMR).

3.8.3.2 Management of Mastitis

The level of mastitis in the dairy herd can be monitored using the somatic cell count (SCC) levels in the milk. This is essentially a measure of white blood cells recruited to combat chronic (typically non-clinical) infection with organisms of contagious mastitis (e.g. *Staphylococcus*). The maximum SCC allowed in bulk milk varies considerably in differing countries; within the EU, UK and New Zealand a level of 400,000 (cells/mL) is applied, while in Australia (600 to 700,000 cells/mL) and the USA (750,000 cells/mL) higher levels are applied. Milk that exceeds these levels will not be collected by milk purchasers or will attract demerit points and much reduced milk price (Table 3.11). In practice, there are moves in the USA to reduce the maximum levels to 400,000 cells/mL. In all countries the annual mean SCC levels achieved for milk are well below the maximum levels.

Milk purchasers use milk quality payment schemes to maintain and increase the quality of milk supplied by milk producers, and in some schemes SCC levels below 50, 100 and 150,000 cells/mL can attract additional payment for good milk quality. The bulk milk SCC levels are monitored by milk purchasers and used to calculate milk price in payment schemes, apply demerit points or refuse to collect milk considered not to be suitable. On the farm the management of mastitis is best described as proactive, where a positive approach is used to prevent, rapidly diagnose and treat mastitis in order to maintain low SCC levels. The main

Table 3.11 Examples of bacterial quality and somatic cell count levels used in milk purchase in differing counties (000/mL).

Country	Maximum bacterial count	Maximum somatic cell count
Denmark	100	400
France	100	400
Germany	100	400
UK	100	400
Australia	600	750
New Zealand	500	400
Canada	100	500
USA*	400	700 to 750

* Varies with state.

potential for cows to be infected with mastitis is during mechanical milking. A key issue is the need to maintain low levels of SCC throughout the herd in order to minimize the risk of cross-contamination between cows with mastitis (high SCC > 250,000) and cows without mastitis (low SCC < 250,000). Milking heifers (with low SCC) before cows with higher SCC can prevent herd SCC from increasing, milking individual cows with high SCC following lower SCC cows and the use of pre-milking teat dip and wearing gloves during milking can reduce the risk of spreading the mastitis bacteria. The application of teat dips following milking is a key point at which mastitis-causing bacteria can be prevented from gaining access into the mammary gland, by protecting the teat canal from contamination while the sphincter muscle, that typically closes the teat canal, remains open following milking. The sooner cows with clinical mastitis are diagnosed that will directly reduce the opportunity for other cows to be contaminated (Table 3.12) and lower the potential severity of the disease for the individual animal and whole herd.

3.8.3.3 Mastitis in Organic Dairy Herds

In organic herds, antibiotics are not used as first line of treatment for mastitis, unless withholding this treatment is likely to compromise the welfare of the animal. These greater restrictions to use antibiotics make the prevention of mastitis a key management strategy for organic herds. Organic milk producers emphasize the importance of good milking equipment design and maintenance, and hygienic milking practices, particularly the wearing of gloves for milking. The use of non-antibiotic treatments for the treatment of mastitis is also considered to be important and some of these include vaccination, drenching with vinegar and the use of arnica, peppermint udder creams and cold water applications to minimize mammary inflammation, which is typical to this disease. The efficacy of these is unproven.

Table 3.12 Prevention and treatment of mastitis.

Measure	Action
1. Teat dip or spray	Post-milking teat treatment – always (cheap and effective)
	Check adequacy of application (rate of product use and teat coverage)
	Pre-milking teat treatment – problems with contagious bacteria spread at milking
2. Clinical cases	Prompt diagnosis and treatment
3. Dry cow therapy	Long-acting antibiotics for high SCC cows
	Teat sealant for cows and heifers that have low SCC and those that have not had mastitis
4. Culling	Cows that have high SCC, persistent and recurring cases of mastitis
5. Equipment testing and maintenance	Observation of teats for normality of colour following milking and to ensure no damage of teat sphincters
	Daily check and instant replacement of rubber wear that has cracks and/or splits
	Daily check on vacuum level, pulsator and vacuum function
	Regular replacement of rubber cup liners according to the number of milkings or annually, whichever is the sooner
	Professional annual check of milking machine
6. Staff training	Milking practice, machine maintenance and cow management, along with communication and record keeping
9. Facility management	Maintenance of beds, tracks, area s around gateways and water troughs
8. Animal breeding	Selection of sires with the ability to enhance the mastitis resistance of the herd

3.8.4 Lameness

Lameness is the third most common reason for cows to be culled from the dairy herd, but this it is a serious welfare issue due to the pain involved. The incidence of lameness in dairy cattle is approximately 35% of cows *per annum*, but ranges from as low as 5% to as high as 60% on differing farms. Lameness is a multifactorial disease and the main factors involved in the cause and prevention of lameness include environment, especially housing and cow tracks, animal management and handling, genetic conformation, nutrition and regular hoof trimming and foot bathing.

The more common forms of dairy cows lameness are related to the foot and/or claw horn (Figure 3.7). It can take many forms, but these may broadly be considered within two categories:

- disorders of the sole and hoof horn – these are usually non-infectious in origin and include sole bruising and ulceration, white line disease, toe ulcers and foot rot (as a secondary infection);
- infectious conditions of the skin adjacent to the hoof – e.g. digital and interdigital dermatitis, necrobacillosis ('foul').

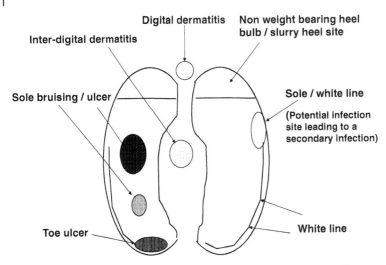

Figure 3.7 Areas of the cow's weight-bearing claws and main types of lameness.

3.8.4.1 Locomotion and Mobility Scoring

Mobility scoring (Table 3.13) and the identification and accurate recording of claw horn disorders (Figure 3.7) and regular foot trimming are essential to the prevention and treatment of lameness. Mobility scoring involves observing cows walking to assess how evenly cows bear weight in each foot, the evenness of the strides they take, the arch of the back and movement of the head. Table 3.13 describe how these are used to score mobility on a four-point scale and used to record the prevalence (number of cows lame on any one day) and severity of lameness. The main aim of mobility scoring is to identify and diagnose individual lame cows (score 1) as soon as possible, so that appropriate treatment can be applied to lower both the

Table 3.13 Mobility score and the description of locomotion (mobility) and lameness.

Score	Mobility	Description
0	Good	Walks with even weight bearing and rhythm on all four feet with flat back. Long, fluid strides
1	Imperfect	Steps uneven rhythm or weight bearing, or strides shortened. Affected limbs not immediately identifiable
2	Impaired	Uneven weight bearing on a limb that is immediately identifiable and/or obviously shortened strides (back might be arched)
3	Severely impaired	Unable to walk as fast as a brisk human pace (cannot keep up with healthy herd) Lame leg easy to identify, might not be weight bearing. Back arched when standing and walking. Very lame

Amended from Whay et al. 2003; AHDB 2010.

number of animals that progress to severe lameness (scores of 2 and 3) and length of time the cows spend lame. |Recent surveys of UK dairy producers showed that farmers did not see the value proposition of this approach. However, some milk purchasers have added regular mobility scoring and the prevalence of lame cows in dairy herds to their farm assurance schemes, with penalties for those who fail to meet their standards.

The correct identification of lesions (e.g. claw horn haemorrhage, digital dermatitis; Figure 3.7) and puncture damage also helps to identify hazards, risks and corrective measures at the herd level. This type of approach reduces the potential for lameness to contribute to other health issues through reduced feed intake, loss of live weight, milk yield and fertility. Early diagnosis also reduces the labour and costs of treating severely affected animals.

3.8.4.2 Types of Lameness

Sole and white line damages account for the majority of lameness in dairy cows. However, the infectious conditions, digital dermatitis (DD) and interdigital dermatitis (IDD), are an increasing problem in the UK, EU and the USA and have become endemic on many farms. DD and IDD are not common in New Zealand and other pasture-based systems.

3.8.4.3 Sole Bruising and Ulceration, and Puncture

This is a common problem and is typically at its greatest level at around 120 days following calving. It results from damage that occurs to the corium when it is trapped between the bone tissues within the hoof. Prolonged standing on concrete and walking on hard surfaces such as cow tracks is a major predisposing factor, as is inadequate (or improper) foot trimming. The resilience of the foot structures is also compromised around the time of calving and early lactation. This can be seen by the greater intensity of bruising and potential ulceration in Figure 3.7. This condition predisposes animals to sole puncture, and handling of cows on tracks and raceways, allowing them to walk that their own pace and avoid rocks and stones, is essential in preventing lameness. The maintenance and repair of concrete yards, and to some extent raceways, play an important role in preventing lameness. Animal signals that indicate a lack of adequate space include them raising their head above the shoulder height, while being handled on tracks or pushed up in a collecting yard.

3.8.4.4 White Line Disease, Disorders and Toe Ulcers

The white line, indicated in Figure 3.7, is where the wall horn is cemented to the sole horn. This is weaker than other parts of the claw. In consequence, this area of the claw horn is more subject to physical damage due to wear and damage from twisting and walking, while bruising in this area also occurs. Problems associated with this area of the claw are referred to as white line disease, disorders, erosion and bruising and ulceration. This area is particularly prone to damage in systems where cows walk long distances. The rotation of the distal pharynx (P3) can similarly trap the horn-producing lamellae at the toe and lead to toe bruising and ulceration. Good handling facilities of adequate size to provide the correct amount of space and careful use of 'backing gates' and movement of dairy cattle are essential in the prevention of lameness. Incorrect handling and lack of adequate space creates twisting forces that separate the anatomically weak structure of the white line. Placement of rubber matting at any point where cows make sharp turns, such as backing out of rotary milking bales, will lower white line damage and the potential for secondary infections of the lamellae.

3.8.4.5 Foot Rot
This seems to be quite common in New Zealand. It is most frequently a secondary infection and is often associated with ingressions of infectious organism through the white line/sole area (Figure 3.7), which is in contrast to infectious lameness seen in other dairy cow systems of management, which usually presents as digital or interdigital dermatitis. It is most apparent during wet conditions and when cows are confined on concrete pads (feed pads) to be offered feed and where cow tracks and lane ways have wet and poorly maintained areas. Feed pads and tracks or lane ways are commonly used in the pasture-based systems of New Zealand and Australia. Good construction and maintenance of tracks and lane ways are imperative in reducing foot rot, and wet conditions in general tend to reduce claw horn strength and resilience to cow housing and management.

3.8.4.6 Digital and Interdigital Dermatitis
The primary cause of this infectious disease is a spirochete, which is very resilient, survives in manure and as such is more common in housed animals. This infection is spread through manure and can be reduced by attention to floor hygiene (e.g. twice-daily scraping and/or flushing with water). It can however be spread by frequent (inadequate) scraping with automated scrapers. Regular use of clean footbaths becomes essential where the disease is endemic. Some farms incorporate foot bathing as a daily routine. Individual cows may need to be treated with a licensed antibiotic spray. Digital dermatitis is not presently a common problem in pasture-based systems.

3.8.5 Environment and Lameness

3.8.5.1 Pasture-based Systems
In pasture-based systems, which are common to New Zealand, Australia and some areas of Europe and the USA, the cows are managed in large herds, often using paddocks which are grazed in rotation and, as a consequence, cows in these systems walk long distances. In these circumstances the most common types of lameness are white line disease and foot rot, which is a secondary infection that has often resulted from an infection of the white line at the heel area of the outer (lateral) claw, which tends to wear faster than the toe in these systems. The other types of lameness include sole bruising and ulceration, interdigital damage and swelling due to high stocking rates (paddock pressure). There is less infectious skin disease (e.g. DD), but this is increasing with an increasing prevalence of housing.

In pasture-based systems the careful handling of dairy cattle and the infrastructure used to convey cattle to and from pasture are key areas of management in the prevention of lameness. The provision and maintenance of good-quality cow tracks, the steady movement of cattle (at their own speed) along tracks, the prevention of manure build-up and occurrence of wet muddy conditions and the accumulation of small stones or the development of rough surfaces where cows are required to walk, are key areas in the prevention of lameness. On tracks drovers should be more than one fence post distance away from the last cow. Ideally cows should make their own way to being milked, which can be facilitated by automatic time-controlled gate opening devices.

3.8.5.2 Housing and Lameness

In many countries, cattle are housed either permanently or, more commonly for four to six months of the year, when pasture growth is low due to cold wet conditions. Dairy cattle confined in housing or feed areas with concrete flooring may have more feet and leg problems. Due to increasing herd sizes the free stall or cubicle housing systems have become the most common. In these systems sole bruising and ulceration, white line disease and digital and interdigital dermatitis are the most common types of lameness. Provision of at least one stall or cubicle available for each cow, preferably with 5% additional (empty) stalls, will increase lying time and reduce sole and white line-related lameness. These stalls or cubicles should be of an appropriate size (Table 3.6) and construction to allow the cow to lie comfortably and have enough 'lunge space' to allow the cows to rise and reduce hock damage. These cubicles/stalls should provide a comfortable bed. Cow mats are common but not ideal. The best material would appear to be sand, which provides comfort when lying at rest and purchase for the feet when the cow is changing position (standing up and lying down).

Loose housing systems should have a bedding area and separate loafing/feeding area, which can be cleaned regularly to minimize bedding use and incidence of mastitis and milk SCC levels (Table 3.11). Tie barn systems, where cows are tethered, are much less common overall, but are still popular in some parts of Europe and Canada, where smaller herds are housed. In these systems, sole bruising along with claw overgrowth and hock swelling are more common types of lameness due to lack of exercise.

The exact details of housing requirements for dairy cattle, such as space allocation and appropriate cubicle/stall dimensions according to animal live weight, can be found in the building standards of each country along with reference to welfare codes of practice and farm assurance guidance notes.

3.8.6 Nutrition, Genetics and Lameness

3.8.6.1 Acidosis and Subacute Rumen Acidosis

Laminitis, which should not be confused with sole haemorrhages arising from mechanical damage to the suspensory apparatus of the foot, arises from disturbances to the blood and oxygen supply to the corium, the area of horn production. The condition, which may affect all four feet, is extremely painful. The skin above the hooves is hot to the touch though the hooves themselves may feel cold. This lameness is associated with nutritional disorders, especially acute (pH < 5.0), or intermittent or chronic subclinical rumen acidosis (pH < 5.5). A reliable indicator of subclinical acidosis is low milk fat composition. This has become more common in recent years. The use of diets with high levels of rapidly digestible carbohydrates or sugars and potentially low levels of dietary fibre and short forage chopping can result in low pH due to higher rate of fatty acid production in the rumen fluid (especially lactic and propionic acids). A low rumen fluid pH can result in the death of some rumen bacterial populations leading to the release of endotoxins that mediate an inflammatory response and cause the constriction of blood, oxygen and nutrient supply to the corium, where the hoof horn-producing lamellae are located. This causes a disturbance to horn formation, which can be sufficiently severe to result in a break or crack appearing on the outer wall of the hoof wall of the outer (lateral) claw, which typically occurs at the heel of the foot.

3.8.6.2 Vitamins and Minerals

The structural integrity of the hoof horn depends on the effectiveness of the keratinization of epidermal cells and this can be affected by diet, e.g. vitamins A, D, E and H (biotin); minerals calcium, phosphorus and magnesium; trace elements zinc and selenium (Table 3.14). Dietary deficiencies of minerals, vitamins and trace elements lead to disturbances in the keratinization process. This can result in decreased horn quality and development of secondary infection. Calcium, phosphorus and manganese are involved in the development and maintenance of bone and collagen formation. The addition of biotin and zinc sulphate has been found to reduce the levels of lameness, especially white line disease, and improve the rate of healing of hoof horn. Copper and cobalt supplementation may also affect hoof and foot health. However, such dietary supplementation will not compensate for poor genetics, environment and/or management.

Table 3.14 Preventing and reducing the incidence of lameness of dairy cattle.

Area	Factors to prevent/reduce lameness
Housing	Adequate space, fee stalls (number, size and design), Clean flooring and maintenance, additional rubber matting
	Good layout, collecting yard (adequate design and size)
	Appropriate collecting yard space and backing gate operation
Handling	Good handling practices of cows in housing, collecting yards and tracks.
	Good housing, yard, collecting yard and track/race size, design and maintenance.
	Don't rush and/or push up cows too tightly on tracks, collecting yards and other handling situations
Hygiene	Regular scraping to reduce occurrence of slurry heel, spread of digital dermatitis
Genetics	Good conformation; foot, leg and hoof angle
Nutrition	Avoid low moisture content silages and rumen acidosis
	Application of rumen stabilizers that lower the effect of low rumen fluid pH
	Adequate macronutrient (Ca, P), micronutrient (Zn, Cu, Se) and vitamin nutrition
	Addition of Biotin (vitamin H and B vitamins) where appropriately high-yielding cows have supplemented diets
Management	Regular professional foot trimming
	Regular application of foot bathing to control DD
	Appropriate cow handling and moving, backing gate operation
	Recording of mobility issues, cause and treatment – inform actions to prevent occurrence

3.8.6.3 Genetic Selection

The selection process favours cows with steeper hoof and mid-range leg angles, which allow the cow to wear the toe of the claws and this has also been related to stronger hoof horn quality. This selection of dairy cows and sires for good 'conformation traits' such as leg and foot angle has been successfully applied to reduce the number of cows with low hoof angles and 'sickle' shaped hocks that tend to develop overgrown claws at the toe area. A slight overgrowth is indicated when the outer (lateral) claw is slightly longer than the inner (medial) claw and this should be corrected by hoof trimming before the cow develops an inability to wear the hoof wall at the toe.

3.8.7 Hoof Trimming

The routine trimming of cows' claws is a common practice for the prevention of lameness in countries such as the UK, the USA and Canada. This is typically carried out at drying off from lactation. This should be carried out by a qualified hoof trimmer, veterinarian or farmer who has completed an accredited hoof-trimming course. While good hoof-trimming is a major contributor to the control of lameness in dairy cattle, poor, overzealous trimming can make matters worse. Therapeutic foot trimming, e.g. in the management of a sole ulcer is normally accompanied by the application of a 'block' to the undamaged to one claw to take the weight off the affected claw while it heals. This also brings about an immediate reduction in pain during locomotion.

3.8.8 Other Potential Health Problems

3.8.8.1 Hypocalcaemia

Lactating dairy cattle produce large amount of milk, which contains calcium. This requires them to mobilize body reserves of calcium from their bones. However, during early lactation the requirement for calcium for milk production can result in a shortage of calcium in the blood plasma (hypocalcaemia). Acute calcium deficiency can result in lack of muscle function that is enough to cause paralysis and rapid death. Affected cows can be treated with calcium borogluconate injections, but the main aim is to prevent the occurrence of this calcium deficiency in the blood (see Section 3.6.6.1).

3.8.8.2 Hypomagnesaemia (Grass Staggers)

During periods of rapid pasture growth, typically in spring or following late autumn applications of nitrogen fertilizer, the magnesium levels of pasture can be low and result in a deficiency of magnesium in the plasma. Magnesium is required for muscle function. In acute deficiency, animals will initially show signs of 'staggers' and this can rapidly proceed to convulsions and death. Prevention involves giving magnesium supplements, which are typically added to water or included in concentrated diets offered at milking time. Since magnesium is unpalatable the most effective method of supplementation is by addition to water troughs. However, this will not succeed if cows have access to an alternative source of fresh water.

3.8.8.3 Acidosis and Subacute Rumen Acidosis

This disease has become more common in recent years and is classified as acidosis with a rumen pH < 5.0 and subacute rumen acidosis (SARA) with a rumen liquor pH < 5.5. These have become common due to the use of high levels of rapidly digestible carbohydrates or sugars and potentially low levels of dietary fibre and forage chopping, which has resulted in low pH due to higher rate of acid production leading to death of protozoa and some bacterial species in the rumen with increased production of lactic acid. The low rumen fluid pH results in low milk fat composition (below 2.9%) and potentially lowered dry matter intake. Attempts to prevent rumen acidosis in cows given diets high in starch and low in NFD and or functional fibre include the dietary inclusion of bicarbonate of soda in the short term, the use of yeast preparations (dead), which utilize lactic acid, in the longer term, or the inclusion of highly digestible fibre (HDF) into the diet, usually as part of the compound feed offered at milking. Other options include the inclusion of some chopped straw in the diet may be an option, since this will stimulate salivation and thus increase the supply of endogenous sodium bicarbonate. However, this may cause an overall reduction in nutrient intake and thus an undesirable reduction in milk yield.

More recently the application of diet separation sieves to check the feed particle length of mixed rations has become more common (Table 3.15) to ensure mixing of the diet leave sufficient amounts of functional fibre. In addition, the assessment of dung consistency to check it's not too loose and checking that the rumen is full (rumen fill), that the majority of cows are ruminating while lying down and that they chew cud each cud bolus between 50 and 60 times before swallowing are cow signals that are used to assess the adequacy of functional fibre in the diet.

3.8.8.4 Bloat

Bloat is caused by the gas from rumen fermentation becoming trapped in a foam of air bubbles. The problem typically arises when cows graze pasture legumes that contain a protein that creates a 'strong' coating on the air bubble, making it resistant to being broken down. This build-up of gas bubbles results in the rumen crushing the lungs and large abdominal blood vessels of the animal, leading to death. This disease can be prevented by treating cows with bloat oil and or piercing of the rumen to let out the froth. However, the use of anti-bloat pasture species is much more practical than dosing animals with oils or other techniques. The main prevention is controlling access by cows to pastures likely to cause bloat, and the use of plant varieties that have low bloat potential.

Table 3.15 Maize/ corn silage, haylage, and TMR particle size recommendations for lactating cows.

Screen	Pore size (mm)	Particle size (mm)	Maize silage	Haylage	P/TMR
Upper Sieve	19.1	19.1	3 to 8	10 to 20	2 to 8
Middle Sieve	7.9	7.9 to 19.1	45 to 65	45 to 75	30 to 50
Lower Sieve	4.1	4.1 to 7.9	20 to 30	30 to 40	10 to 20
Bottom Pan	0	< 4.1	< 10	< 10	30 to 4

3.8.8.5 Acetonaemia (Ketosis)

Ketone bodies are produced as a result of the excessive mobilization and incomplete oxidation of fat, in cows that are too fat at the time of parturition (Table 3.9). The main prevention is to control live weight and condition score through proper nutrition in the transition period and early lactation.

3.9 Heifer Rearing and Transition into the Dairy Herd

3.9.1 Strategies

The overall replacement rate is typically around 20% to 25% of the dairy herd annually. Truthfully the lower the herd culling rate and replacement rate the lower the carbon footprint and cost of milk production. Conversely, this will lower the rate of genetic improvement of the herd. The main thing is to ensure excellent management of heifers to ensure they come into and remain in the herd, so that fewer are lost before first calving and fewer young cows are culled from the herd. Loss of these will be most costly in terms the lack of return on investment and the most damaging to the genetic improvement of the herd. Dairy heifers are typically provided from the dairy herd by selective breeding from the cattle in the herd that are the most productive, fertile and have the desired conformation and mating these to high genetic-merit sires, with desired dairy characteristics. The alternative is to buy heifers, but this introduces increased risk of disease introduction, variability in cost and unsuitability to the dairy system.

In herds where non-sexed semen is used, a 25% replacement rate will require mating a minimum of 50% of the highest-merit cows in the herd, using high genetic-merit semen from artificial insemination or possibly natural breeding in order to provide sufficient herd replacements on an annual basis. Recent changes to farm assurance standards require dairy bull calves to be maintained on the dairy unit or reared by allied units. Consequently, many herds are using sexed semen, which produces few bull calves and they may inseminate cows to produce cross-bed calves for the beef industry. While New Zealand continues to need to concentrate on seasonal calving and has a 'bobby calf' processing chain for young male dairy calves, which may include cross-bred beef calves when market prices are low.

The optimal economic performance of dairy heifers will be achieved by calving dairy heifers at 22 to 24 months of age. While many countries achieve this, all year calving herds in the UK dairy industry have on average been consistently calving heifers around 4 months older. The incidence of pneumonia due to damp, cold and inclement environment and greater reliance on pasture are two potentially contributory factors, along with feed cost. While seasonal calving herds must and the USA manages to calve cows for the first time at 24 months of age, which requires heifers to be served at 13 to 15 months of age. While the USA, the UK, EU and China generally reach the optimal 55 % mature weight at service and 85 % mature weight at first calving, those calving in grazing systems often calve for the first time at lower mature weight. This compromises feed intake and milk yield, but more important fertility and may increase the risk of calving difficulty, infertility and premature culling.

Mature weight is highly heritable and thus can be predicted from the parents and breed of dairy heifer, but farmers must be realistic about the true mature weight of the adult animals as genetic improvement and breed will affect adult weight. The application of higher feeding rates, increased protein intake and thus higher growth rates for dairy heifers between 0 and 3 months of age has been found to increase mammary development and subsequent milk yield, while higher growth rates around puberty (40% mature weight) predispose to fat deposition in mammary tissue and this can negatively affect subsequent milk yield potential. Therefore, the rearing and nutrition of dairy heifers differs from that of beef cattle and will have a direct impact on the yield potential of the dairy herd. The effective provision of dairy herd replacements can be achieved through a specific and planned approach using target maturity for age and achieving appropriate growth rates for each phase of development.

3.9.2 Options for the Provision of Dairy Replacements

There is a range of options for the provision of dairy replacements (Table 3.16), which include rearing calves from the dairy herd on the home farm, rearing calves to milk

Table 3.16 Optional methods of providing dairy herd replacements and the effect on requirements, cost and risk.

	Home rearing	Full contract rearing	Contract grazing to calving	Purchased
Genetic improvement	Full control	Full control	Full control	Very limited control
Growth rate and maturity	Full control	Need contracts and monitoring	Need contracts and monitoring	Very limited control
Feeds	Full control	Limited control	Limited control	No control
Contracts	Not required	Contract required	Contract required	Not required
Infrastructure	Full requirement	Limited needs	Limited needs	None required
Labour	Labour, training and peaks	Limited requirement	Limited requirement	Only required for selection of animals
Finance	Low	Outward flow of cash	Outward flow of cash	Outward flow of cash
Land use	Requirement, but can use land not suited to dairy	Not required	Not required	Not required
Transport	Limited requirements	Required	Required	Required
Biosecurity	Full control	Limited control	Limited control	No control
Cost	Full control	Some control	Some control	No control
Risk	Low	Medium	Medium	High
Flexibility	Low	High	High	High

weaning and later transferring them to a 'contract grazier' or purchasing in calf heifers or freshly calved heifers as replacements. There are advantages and disadvantages to each of these options. If contract rearing is practiced, all contracts should be legally binding documents, drawn up by a suitably qualified and experienced person. These must clearly state targets for growth rates and live weight/maturity according to animal age and penalty clauses if targets are not met. They should include regular monitoring and reporting of heifer development. There should be a health plan and a contingency feeding plan, which should be developed with a veterinarian and nutritionist, documented and monitored.

3.9.3 Dairy Heifer Rearing Programmes

3.9.3.1 Rearing Young Calves

Most dairy calves are removed from their mothers shortly after birth and many are offered pasteurized colostrum to avoid the potential transfer of Johne's disease, followed by which they are reared artificially. Milk is offered by training calves to drink from a pail or suckle from a teat or from a mechanical calf feeding machine. Suckling systems, where calves are suckled on a cow on a restricted basis or where multiple calves suckle a nurse cow, are less common in developed countries, but are used regularly in developing environments. Calves are offered whole milk, milk replacer or colostrum. In addition, calves are offered specialized calf starter feeds and forages to encourage rumen development. The main objectives are to achieve low mortality and produce healthy calves that have few disease problems and grow rapidly (750 to 950 g/d) during the first 3 months. The single most important factor in ensuring good calf-rearing practice is the adequate provision of high-quality (high immunoglobulin concentration) colostrum from the first two milkings post-partum This must be offered within the first 6 to 12 h of birth, in enough quantity (10 to 12 % of live weight) to ensure adequate passive immunity transfer.

3.9.3.2 Whole Milk Feeding

The use of whole milk offered at approx. 4 to 5 litres/day (L/d) (or 10% of live weight) is popular in many countries and will achieve growth rates of 630 to 650 g/d, which are below the growth rates recommended for dairy heifers. Whole milk is deficient in nutrients, vitamins D and E and trace elements – iron, manganese, zinc, copper, iodine, cobalt and selenium. To achieve optimal growth rates for dairy calves, whole milk requires the nutrient concentration (fat, lactose and protein) to be increased along with additional vitamin A. These need to be achieved without substantial increase to feeding volume (L), with the addition of high-quality milk replacer, with additional lactose and high protein level (26 to 28%) or preferably with a specifically designed milk supplement. Increasing the feeding level of whole milk above 5 l/d is not recommended; this will reduce solid feed intake, delay rumen development and weaning from milk, which will increase rearing costs and negatively affects mammary development. Milk from cows being treated with antibiotics is not recommended for feeding to dairy heifers.

3.9.3.3 Colostrum Feeding Systems

Colostrum feeding is more popular in some counties than others, depending on calving pattern and other marketing opportunities for colostrum. Colostrum feeding at 4 to 5 l/d results in high growth rates (700 to 750 g/d) and healthy calves. Continuing to feed colostrum may delay the development of an active immune system in the calf and a period of 'low' immunity, the 'weak' period between passive immunity from colostrum and active immunity in the calf, will occur within 1 to 2 weeks post-weaning or following the removal of colostrum from the diet. Changing the diet to whole milk 3 weeks prior to milk weaning will help avoiding a clash between milk weaning and low immune function.

3.9.3.4 Milk Replacers

Milk replacers are typically either skimmed milk or whey-based milk powder. Skim milk powders and whole milk contain caseins, which coagulate in the abomasum and increase retention time, while whey-based milk powders do not form clots. The available comparisons of skim milk versus whey protein concentrate indicate that calves offered skim milk-based milk replacer do not seem to perform better than those offered whey protein concentrate. Heat damage, which can be estimated by testing the lysine content, can severely affect the digestibility of milk replacers and subsequent calf growth rates. The best performance will be achieved from highly digestible milk replacers that contain fractionated milk proteins (skim base) and natural antibodies, which increase disease resistance in the digestive tract and provide good-quality proteins. Milk replacer powders recommended for dairy heifers contain 20 to 21% fat along with additional lactose and 26 to 28% crude protein. The liquid volume of milk and concentration of replacer in the liquid are important factors, while most milk replacers have been reconstituted at 125 g/l, current practice is to offer 150 g/l in general and for this to be increased on a sliding scale up to 175 g/l when ambient temperatures fall below 5°C. Calves offered milk replacers at 600 g/d they should achieve growth rates around 750 to 900 g/d, depending greatly on management, environment, nutrition and health. The need to lower antimicrobial use has more natural additives being included in milk powder and starter diets. These enhance the microbiome of the intestinal tract and immunity of the animal using prebiotics such as saccharides and yeast cell walls and probiotics such as yeast and lactobacilli spp., along with other natural substances such as essential oils.

3.9.3.5 Ad Libitum Milk Feeding

Ad libitum feeding of milk is not recommended for dairy heifers, due to this practice resulting in slow rumen development and inadequate balance of nutrients in milk.

3.9.3.6 Cow Calf Systems

Cow calf systems have become increasing popular due to the direct impact of milk purchasers and the poor perception of consumers regarding cow-calf separation. Some farmers have nurse cows and operate multiple suckling systems which involve running a number of calves with one or more 'nurse' cows. This system can be effective provided that calves receive sufficient milk (10 to 13 % birth weight) to achieve adequate growth rates. Farmers sometimes use high somatic cell count cows for this purpose to prevent damage to milk quality supplied to the milk product manufacturer.

3.9.4 Restricted Suckling

The use of restricted suckling of dairy calves in developing countries where the infrastructure to ensure hygiene and support factors are limited can be more successful than artificial rearing and feeding calves from buckets, pails or artificial teats. These systems allow the calf to suckle the dairy cow before milking to encourage milk letdown and again after milking (by hand or mechanically) to remove the residual milk remaining. Depending on the milk yield of the cows, the calf may be allowed one or two full quarters or the residual milk of all quarters. The main factor is to ensure that the calf is allowed sufficient milk to ensure adequate growth, health and development. Calves are typically offered milk up until 10 to 12 weeks of age, up to a maximum of 4 to 5 L/d.

The advantages of restricted suckling systems are the lack of potential infection (enteric disorders or scours) of the calf due to poor feeding, utensil hygiene, prolonged passive immunity for the calf and satiation of suckling behaviour. The cow will produce a greater quantity of milk and be less likely to have mastitis. The disadvantages are the potential to prolong the anoestrous period in the dam with twice daily suckling of the calf, which can be alleviated by reducing the suckling frequency to once daily to initiate ovarian activity.

3.9.5 Weaning from Milk

Early weaning systems allow calves to be weaned from milk at five to six weeks of age when intake of the dry, cereal-based starter feed is 1.5 to 2 kg/d for three consecutive days prior to weaning. However, this system restricts milk intake to approx. 10% of birth weight, which restricts growth rate to around 450 to 500 g/d. Dairy heifers and larger dairy beef breeds are typically offered milk at around 13% birth weight and weaned around eight weeks of age. In pasture-based systems calves are typically offered milk for longer, until 8 to 12 weeks of age. In New Zealand calves are generally weaned according to live weight, which is related to breed – approximately 80 kg for Jersey, 85 kg for Friesian Jersey cross and 90 kg for Friesian calves, which is achieved between 8 and 10 weeks of age. This equates to approx. double birth weight plus 5 to 10%. The UK and the USA wean dairy heifers at double their birth weight. However, calves are not weighed on many farms, so age and adequacy of growth/health are more typical characteristics. Delaying the weaning of calves that have had health issues and made inadequate development is the better potential approach, rather than weaning strictly according to age.

3.9.6 Organic Dairy Systems

Organic systems have specific requirements for calf rearing and at present most specify feeding of whole milk until 12 weeks of age. Milk feeding level will be a minimum of 10% birth weight, but maximum milk feeding level will depend on the cost of organic calf starter diets and forage quality and availability. In these cases, individual country and milk company guidelines should be followed.

3.9.7 Solid Feeds and Feeding

3.9.7.1 Calf 'Starter' Feeds

Young calves should be offered calf starter and will consume small amounts (200 g per head per day) of palatable cereal-based feeds within the second week of life. These cereal-based feeds are key to the development of the rumen and ruminal papillae, which respond well to volatile fatty acids produced from rumen fermentation. Specialist calf supplement feeds and meals need to be highly palatable, should be offered in small amounts initially and replaced daily, to encourage early and increasing consumption levels. Any leftovers can be collected and given directly to older (weaned) calves.

Good-quality calf supplements for dairy calves should be made from highly digestible components, 22% crude protein (CP) with a good amino acid profile (e.g. soya bean meal). However, due to the need to strive towards carbon neutrality, the importation of soya into the EU and UK is likely to be replaced by locally gown peas, beans and canola (rape seed meal). Dairy heifer growth and mammary development are increased by higher levels of utilizable proteins (amino acids) in the diet. The levels of sugar (50 g/kg and fat (35 g/kg) need to be limited in barley-based diets, as calves have a limited capacity to digest these.

3.9.7.2 Calf Starter and Feeding Levels

Calf starter feeds should be offered *ad libitum* prior to the time of weaning from milk but restricted thereafter according to the availability and quality of pasture or forage. The body condition of heifers can fluctuate, low body condition can be used to indicate the need to increase feeding levels, while short-term increases in body condition should not be a reason to decrease feeding levels.

3.9.7.3 Forages

Ad libitum access to clean, dust-free fibrous feeds, preferably chopped straw, should be offered to satisfy the investigative need of young calves for oral activity from approx. the beginning of the third week of life Insufficient access (level offered or feeding space) to forage will result in calves sucking and chewing other objects in their surroundings, such as each other, buildings, fences and anything they can reach, included string used to fix up gates or fences. Grazing calves will be consuming some pasture but will benefit from being offered straw or hay with a high stem component, which need to be kept dry and covered from rain, to prevent subsequent mould and aflatoxin development. The consumption of these forages will aid rumen development, although the main contributor to this is the consumption of cereal-based calf starter diets.

3.9.7.4 Water

All livestock should have access to clean fresh water at all times. Calves should be offered good-quality, fresh clean water that should be changed twice daily. The exception is a small proportion of calves that drink water as if it was milk, and these should have their access limited to feeding periods twice daily for the first week or so. Care should be taken to ensure that watering facilities can be cleaned scrupulously, as it can harbour pathogens such as cryptobiosis.

3.9.7.5 Bedding

Housed calves, unless housed on slatted floors, will require bedding materials. Calves will eat bedding and will eat this to a much greater extent when cereal straws or stalk hay is not provided separately. Wood shavings, sawdust, straw, wood chip and sand all make suitable bedding materials and can be used in combination. Calves prefer the softer, more comfortable, bedding types, and straw has the added advantage of developing layers, increasing the opportunity for the top layer to remain dry for longer. Bedding choice generally will depend on availability. The cost needs to be considered according to ability to keep the bedding dry and subsequent amount required, and suitability to maintain the relative humidity in the building below 75% (see Section 3.9.8.3); however, in damp climates this humidly can be greater during winter. Bedding is important in providing physical and thermal conform for calves, along with its role in maintaining air quality in general and at calf height especially.

3.9.8 Calf Housing/management Systems

3.9.8.1 Pasture-based Management

In pasture-based systems, such as found in New Zealand, calves can be housed but are frequently reared at pasture in groups (mobs) of 20 to 40. They are housed briefly and, once they have learned to suck from an artificial teat, are offered milk at pasture from either from a machine or a 'calfeteria' (mobile milk vat with many teats, at least one per calf), which delivers colostrum, whole milk or milk replacer at approximately 4 to 5 L per head, each day. Unfortunately, drinking speed varies greatly between calves and unless the system can regulate milk on an individual calf basis this will result in calves drinking very differing levels of milk.

3.9.8.2 Housed Calves

The main aims should be to provide a warm clean environment and prevent the development of pneumonia (Table 3.17). This can be achieved by the provision of buildings with adequate air space and natural ventilation. Calf buildings should be built to allow the prevailing wind to pass directly through the top portion of the building to remove moist air, while avoiding

Table 3.17 Minimum space requirements for calves in group housing.

Calf weight (kg)	Space requirements per calf (m^2)
50 to 84	1.5
85 to 140	1.8
140 to 200	2.4

any direct draught onto the animals. Conditions of high relative humidity in the building can be avoided through attention to good ventilation, regular (daily) addition of bedding and minimizing accumulation of water, through daily cleaning of any water, good drainage and limited addition of water through washing down.

In between groups or batches of calves, the buildings should be cleaned out, washed down thoroughly and rested (1 month) or disinfected between each batch of calves. This includes water troughs and bowls, as these harbour disease organisms. This is referred to as an 'all in, all out system' and can be applied to sections of buildings if required, as in pasture-based systems, where multiple groups of calves may use the building for short periods of time.

3.9.8.3 Calf Hutches and Tethering
Calf hutches, wherein calves can be kept outdoors in physical isolation but in social contact, have become popular in recent years. The main reason is to restrict the spread of respiratory infections. In some countries, calves can be tethered without a hutch (not within the EU). Hutches should be moved onto new areas for each new calf to prevent disease build-up. Hutches should be placed on well-drained areas, cleaned using a similar approach that described above (Section 3.9.7.2). These systems are labour intensive.

3.9.8.4 Individual Pens and Group Housing
An individual pen for calves allows individual monitoring of feed intake and is favoured in early weaning systems. The calf should have sight of and contact with other calves. These systems are labour intensive and as a result group rearing has become more popular as herd sizes increase. Cleaning is essential using a similar approach to that described above (Section 3.9.7.2).

3.9.8.5 Mechanical Feeding
Due to shortages of skilled labour and increased herd sizes, the use of machines for feeding dairy heifer calves is becoming more popular. The level of control and information provided varies greatly between machines. They can be used at pasture or in housing systems. They do require a skilled operator, but they remove much of the work involved in calf feeding.

3.9.9 Disease Prevention and Minimizing Mortality

One of the main factors in preventing disease and mortality is the adequate provision of good-quality colostrum, soon after calves are born. The main diseases that calves are likely to suffer include enteric disease (scours), clostridial diseases (see Sections 3.9.3.3), joint ill and pneumonia. A disease prevention and treatment plan for dairy calves should be put in place with the advice of a veterinarian.

3.9.9.1 Joint Ill
Joint ill is a serious disease that can be fatal. Prevention is the key and as soon as possible after birth, the umbilical cord should be treated with a suitable iodine-based solution, in the

calving paddock or calving box. Further applications of iodine-based liquid until the cord has dried, and regular checking for a navel swelling, will allow the opportunity to identify and treat any infections quickly using suitable antibiotic therapy as advised by the veterinarian. The regular cleaning and replacement of bedding of calving boxes and calf transport equipment will help prevent infection, in addition to navel treatment. This should be added to the farm's herd health plan.

3.9.9.2 Enteric Disease (Scours)

Enteric diseases should be prevented through high levels of building management ('all in, all out' system for pens, with resting or disinfection), personnel and equipment cleaning and hygiene. This includes effective biosecurity measures that prevent visitors bringing disease onto the calf unit and into contact with the calves. On units where Rotavirus has been a problem, cows may be vaccinated before calving, so that they provide colostrum with specific antibodies against this organism. The prevention of pathogen challenge is essential, grouping calves of similar ages (less than three weeks' difference), application of all in-all out approaches, cleaning out and disinfection of all materials, pens and buildings. Twice daily assessment and scoring (1- to 4-point scale) of faeces and the prompt treatment of calves with poor faecal consistency (≥ 3). The treatment of scouring calves should include the prompt administration of electrolyte solutions to prevent dehydration. The identification of the pathogen involved, and suitable treatment can be identified through faecal sampling. Scouring calves should be isolated from unaffected calves to prevent disease transfer and kept warm (possibly using heat lamps) and dry to maximize their opportunity for survival. Pens that have held sick calves should be thoroughly cleaned and disinfected before further use. On the reintroduction of food, colostrum can be useful to enhance immunity at the mucosal surface of the gut wall.

A planned approach to calf health management is essential. All calves should be closely observed twice daily for signs of health or incipient disease. The unit should have a store of electrolyte preparations and suitable calf scour treatment products. Colostrum can be stored frozen for emergency use, and should be thawed in hot water, not in the microwave. There should be a herd health plan for the calf unit, which may incorporate (e.g.) a cow vaccination programme when Rotavirus is endemic.

3.9.9.3 Bovine Respiratory Disease, Pneumonia and *Mycoplasma bovis*

Bovine respiratory disease (BRD) and pneumonia is most likely to occur in housed calves and is best prevented by attention to building design and management (avoid overstocking, provide adequate air space and good ventilation; see Section 3.9.7.2). This is more prevalent in damp, cold and changeable winter weather in the UK. Any calves, whether housed or kept at pasture, that develop coughing, which can equally be scored on a 4-point scale, along with nose and eye discharge, should be examined by the veterinarian, a suitable diagnosis and treatment should be sought immediately, the cause identified, and prevention strategies put in place. These may include improvements to colostrum feeding, building ventilation, bedding strategy and eventually vaccination in addition. Older heifers should not be housed within the same air space as younger calves, to prevent the transfer of pneumonia. Recently, *Mycoplasma bovis* (M. Bovis) has become more common on dairy farms that typically presents itself as pneumonia, but can manifest as a middle ear infection, which can be identified and will need to be treated using antibiotics that are effective against M. Bovis.

3.9.10 Stock Tasks

The main stock tasks will include animal identification, de-horning, supernumerary (extra) teat removal and vaccination.

3.9.10.1 Animal Identification

Accurate identification of dairy heifers is essential, not only for traceability, but also for herd improvement and practical management of dairy cattle. Legislation requires the accurate identification of individual animals, and this is achieved through ear-tagging with an individual animal and herd number. These tags will be placed into the ears soon after birth. In many countries this is linked to a national animal identification scheme and animal passport system.

3.9.10.2 De-horning and Supernumerary Teat Removal

Dairy calves will require de-horning and possibly the removal of any supernumerary teats at approximately five to six weeks of age. It is important that local anaesthetic be used during the disbudding/dehorning processes to ensure animal welfare, minimize growth checks and comply with local legislation. It is essential that these tasks are not carried out at the same time as any other changes such as vaccination, weaning or changes in housing.

3.9.10.3 Vaccination

Vaccination against pneumonia, clostridial infections and/or lungworm may be necessary where dairy calves are likely to be infected by these. An appropriate herd vaccination programme should be applied according to the recommendations of the veterinarian and added to the farm's herd health plan.

3.9.11 Growing Dairy Heifers

Following the calf rearing point, dairy heifers will be managed at pasture and potentially housed during winter periods in countries where weather conditions are inclement or may be fully housed. During period of grazing the control of parasitic infections will be required. In addition the provision of adequate forage and supplementary feeds, and regular monitoring of health and growth rate are the main tasks required to ensure that heifers are well grown and ready for service at 13 to 15 months to create a pregnancy and transfer to the dairy herd (Table 3.18).

3.9.11.1 De-worming

At pasture, young animals are particularly susceptible to parasitic worms of the intestine and potentially the lungs. Control measures will depend on the age of the animal, access to pasture and the infection that exists on the pasture. Pasture used by older animals may be

Table 3.18 Energy and protein requirement and targets for live weight gain and wither height in growing Holstein Friesian heifers.

Age (months)	Weight gain (g/d)	Live weight (kg)	Wither height (cm)	Metabolizable energy (MJ/kg)	Crude protein (%/kg)
2	900	95	86	12	18
3	900	123	90	12	18
6	850	200	104	11	16
14	800	392	128	10	14
20	750	527	135	10	14
22	750	572	139	11	15
23	750	595	140	11	15

infected with parasites and necessitate the more frequent control of parasitic infections in younger animals. Parasite infection can be controlled by the use of clean pastures that have not been infected by older animals and reducing the potential infection by mixed grazing with other animal species not susceptible to the same species of parasites. The control of parasites may need to be backed up with regular use anthelmintic treatments while at pasture and housing to eliminate adult worms, followed by a second treatment following housing to prevent re-infestation from the developing larvae.

3.9.11.2   Service (Insemination)

The natural service or insemination of dairy heifer needs to take place at 13 to 15 months of age and the heifer will need to be 55 % mature weight. This first service should be with a sire that has an 'easy' calving or 'low calving difficulty' rating for first-calving heifers. This rating can be taken from the 'sire' details for bull semen. Alternatively, one can use an easy calving breed such as Jersey or Angus for AI or natural service. Many dairy heifers are synchronized using intrauterine devices and then inseminated to ensure they come into the dairy herd at 22 to 24 months at 85 % mature weight. The body condition of heifers should not be a problem, but calving condition scores of 3 to 3.5 (on a 1 to 5 scale) and 5 to 5.5 (on a 1 to 10) New Zealand scale are recommended. There is a range, because breed and genetic merit within breed tends to affect actual condition scores for dairy cattle.

3.9.12   Transition of the Heifer into the Dairy Herd

Increasing the longevity of the dairy cow through careful heifer management will reduce the cost of rearing replacements. This will maximize herd genetic merit and productivity, thus increasing the profitability of the dairy herd. The introduction of heifers into the dry cows and the milking shed/parlour or shed before calving will reduce the number of stresses experienced by heifers around calving.

3.9.12.1 Heifer (First Lactation Cow) Fertility

Infertility can be a major problem for first-lactation dairy cattle. First calving should be at 85 % mature weight to prevent problems such as competition for feed and aggression from older cows that may lead to weight loss, decreased conception rates rate and potential culling. It should also reduce the risk of a range of post-partum disorders, such as ketosis, displaced abomasum and infertility. Alternatively, larger herds have the opportunity to maintaining first lactation cows in a group separate from adult cows, during the initial- to mid-part of first lactation.

3.9.12.2 Lameness

Heifers are particularly susceptible to developing sole bruising around first parturition, which can develop into lameness during first and subsequent lactations. Thus careful transition and management of first lactation cows can reduce the incidence of lameness throughout the whole herd.

3.9.12.3 Mastitis

The management of heifers in separate groups, and milking heifers before adult cows, will reduce the risk of transmission of infectious mastitis from adult cows. Teat sealants may also be carefully administered to dairy heifers before first calving to reduce the risk of mastitis-causing pathogens entering the mammary gland during late pregnancy and causing mastitis during first lactation.

3.10 Precision Farming

The development and lower cost of electronic devices, cameras, accelerometers, satellite and localized monitoring of animal location, pH boluses, rumination monitoring, drones, virtual fencing and digital image analysis offer considerable potential for precision management of housed and grazed dairy systems. Some of these technologies are being used as a routine, while others are less developed. The main constraints on their use are the production and interpretation of the information into a useful format as a basis for decision-making, especially the lack of a common platform for managers to be able to access, integrate and interpret data more easily from different systems. The main advantages are greater animal monitoring, which has the potential to enhance animal welfare and productivity.

References and Further Reading

Agricultural and Horticultural Development Board (AHDB). (2021). dairy https://ahdb.org.uk/dairy.

BS5502: Part 40. (2005). Buildings and Structures for Agriculture. Code of practice for design and construction of cattle buildings. British Standards Institution.

Dairy Australia. (2021). https://www.dairyaustralia.com.au.

Dairy, N.Z. (2021). https://www.dairynz.co.nz.

Defra. (2002). Code of Recommendations for the Welfare of Livestock, Cattle, Defra Publications, Admail 6000 London, SW1A 2XX.

Eurostat. (2021). https://ec.europa.eu/eurostat/statistics-explained/index.php?title=Milk_and_milk_product_statistics.

Gordon, I. (1996). *Controlled Reproduction in Cattle and Buffaloes*. Wallingford: CABI Publishing.

Holmes, C.W., Brookes, I.M., Garrick, D.J., MacKenzie, D.D.S., Parkinson, T.J., and Wilson, G.F. (1998). *Milk Production from Pasture*. Wellington, NZ: Butterworth-Heinemann.

Mcdonald, P., Edwards, R.A., and Greenhalgh, J.F.D. (2002). *Animal Nutrition*, 6e. Harlow, UK: Prentice Hall.

Peters, A.R. and Ball, P.J.H. (2004). *Reproduction in Cattle*, 3e. Oxford: Wiley-Blackwell.

Phillips, C.J.C. (2002). *Cattle Behaviour and Welfare*, 2e. Oxford: Wiley-Blackwell.

Pond, W.G., Church, D.C., Pond, K.R., and Schoknecht, P.A. (2004). *Basic Animal Nutrition and Feeding*, 5e. Hoboken, NJ: Wiley.

Roy, J.H.B. (1990). *The Calf: Management of Health*, 5e. London: Butterworth.

Statista. (2021). Production of cow milk in the EU 2013-2020 | Statista. https://www.statista.com.

Wathes, C.M. and Charles, D.R. (1994). *Livestock Housing*. Wallingford: CABI Publishing.

4

Beef Cattle and Veal Calves

Bernadette Earley

KEY CONCEPTS

Management and Welfare of Farm Animals: The UFAW Farm Handbook, Sixth Edition.
Edited by John Webster and Jean Margerison.
© Universities Federation for Animal Welfare 2022. Published 2022 by John Wiley & Sons Ltd.

4.1 The Beef Industry

4.1.1 Livestock Population

Worldwide, beef production is the third largest meat industry (~65 million t globally), behind swine and poultry. In 2015, the major beef producing countries included the United States (US) (11.4 million t), Brazil (9.6 million t), the 28 member countries of the European Union (EU) (7.5 million t), China (6.7 million t) and India (4.5 million t), with the global beef cattle population exceeding 1 billion (Cameron and McAllister 2018). In 2016, Spain, Germany, France, the United Kingdom and Italy held the largest populations of livestock in the EU-28. The highest numbers of bovines were recorded in France (19.0 million head). The livestock population in the EU-28, grew by 1.4% from 2010 to 2016.

'Veal' refers to the slaughtering of bovine animals younger than one year of age (calves and young cattle), and 'beef' reflects slaughtering of older bovine animals. Beef is mainly produced from cattle breeds grown specifically for their meat but can also come from dairy cattle. Male calves from dairy mothers are of no use for producing milk, and their growth potential for producing beef meat is inferior. Thus, many of them are used for veal production. Most notably, the end of UK milk quotas on 31 March 2015 led to increased number of cows being slaughtered (4.0%), reflecting the abandonment of dairy production by some of the smallest farms. The size of the cow herd also grew as a result of favourable feed prices and demand for high-quality beef meat. However, although the production of beef continued to rise in 2016, the total number of bovine animals in the EU-28 remained relatively stable. Almost half (45.2%) of the total EU-28 beef production was accounted for by France (18.7%), Germany (14.7%) and the United Kingdom (11.7%). In each of these countries, production was greater in 2016 than it was a year earlier (Table 4.1). The growth in beef production between 2015 and 2016 was greatest in Cyprus (53.0%), followed by Romania (29.4%) and Bulgaria (25.9%), which were distinctly above the EU-28 growth rate of 2.9%. However, the beef production in Cyprus and Bulgaria remained among the lowest

Table 4.1 EU bovine population: cattle numbers in thousand head (per category) and totals (No.) for the six most populous countries contributing 75% of the total population.

	Total	Age, years			Cows		
		<1	1 to 2	>2	Cows	Dairy	Other
France	19124	5070	3611	10443	7921	3759	4163
Germany	12609	3950	2950	5709	4789	4064	725
Ireland	5902	1633	1311	2957	2205	1088	1117
Italy	6577	1929	1436	2918	2280	1839	441
Poland	5406	1344	1053	3008	2739	2677	61
Spain	6410	2402	767	3240	2862	903	1959
UK	10078	2846	2455	4777	3643	1978	1665
Others	22646	6955	4159	11502	9996	7846	2183
Totals	**88751**	**26130**	**17742**	**44554**	**36435**	**24154**	**12314**

Source: Eurostat.

in the EU-28. Close to two thirds of the bovine meat produced in the EU-28 in 2016 was derived from either bulls or cows (31.4% for each category) (Table 3), which were even greater in other EU Member States. While in the United Kingdom and Ireland the majority of the beef produced in 2016 (68.0% and 66.1% respectively) came from heifers (> 1-year-old females that never calved) and bullocks (> 1-year-old castrated males). The EU cattle price index fell by 3.2% from 2015 to 2016, following a stabilization in 2015 after a fall in 2014. Nevertheless, the price index increased by 7.0% over the period 2010 to 2016 (Figure 4).

4.1.2   Suckler Cow Herds

Suckler beef cows constitute a very important farming sector in the grassland areas of Europe. Suckler beef production is a sustainable system producing high-quality meat, with low feed and labour inputs. In suckler herds, calves remain with the dam at pasture until they are 5 to 9 months of age, when they are weaned and separated from the dam, with many of the weaned animals being transported away from the suckler farms to fattening units. This industry, suckler farms and fattening units, produces very high-quality meat. In Europe suckler herds (cow-calf farms) are located in three main areas, which are the:

- Grasslands of Britain, Ireland, France and northern Europe (27%).
- Mediterranean areas of Italy, Spain, Greece and Portugal (20%).
- Mountain areas of France, Spain and Eastern Europe (16%).

An estimated 65,000 cow-calf producers finish the majority of the progeny as suckler calves, bulls, heifers or steers on their farms. The herd size and acreage managed by cow-calf producers is greater than by pure bred cow-calf beef farms, which manage land more intensively and produce forage crops, with 23% operating at a stocking rate higher than 1.8 livestock units / ha. This system represents 7% of the farms and 8% of the European bovine herd, but the contribution to the beef finishing is important, especially for bull and steer production. They are mainly located in the grasslands of Ireland and UK, and in the forage crops areas of France and northern Europe.

4.1.3   Beef from Dairy Farms

Within the European Union, 123,800 enterprises are simultaneously involved in dairy and beef production, which represent one-quarter of the beef producers and use 17% of the beef farming land. In most cases, beef production has been developed on farms with small milk quotas to contribute 20% of the overall EU beef production. This involves differing types of beef production system, which develop according to land and labour availabilities, and include the fattening of dairy bull calves on the French and/or German farms, and steer and heifer production on pastures in Great Britain and/or Ireland (Table 4.1).

The supply of beef animals in the EU is largely sourced from the dairy herd, except for Ireland, with two-thirds of the cows in the EU being dairy cows. The size of the EU dairy herd is itself is in decline, due to the constraints enforced on milk production by milk quotas and increased milk yield per cow, which has led to a reduction in EU beef production. There has also been a decline of approximately 3% in the EU suckler cow herd between 2000 and 2008 (Figure 4.1). The EU beef and veal sector, which is predominantly beef breeds, has a total production of about 8 million tonnes. This contributes 10% to the total value of agricultural production within the EU, which is the second biggest contributor after the dairy sector, representing approx. 13% of the total production of beef and veal in the world. Since the 1990s beef production in the EU has been gradually declining, falling by 7.6% in the 10-year period 1993 to 2003. In the same period, global beef production increased by 6.3 million tonnes (16.8%) due to the substantial increase in production from other continents, particularly South America which had an increase of 2.6 million tonnes or 26%.

There are over 1,389 million cattle in the world in 2007, which was an increase of 0.6% (7.8 million) compared with 2006. Over 58% of the total world cattle population were held by just 10 countries in 2007, with Brazil holding the majority – 207.2 million cattle. The USA, which is the largest milk-producing country in the world, held 7.0% of world cattle in 2007. The US cattle population has increased 0.3% (301,500) between 2006 and 2007 to over 97 million cattle. In 2007, Brazil held 207.2 million cattle, an increase of 0.6% when compared to 2006, and now accounts for 14.9% of the world cattle population. Other countries saw cattle population fall between 2006 and 2007 with India and China seeing falls of 0.5% and 2.0% respectively. In 2007 India held 12.8% of the world cattle population, while China accounted for 8.4%.

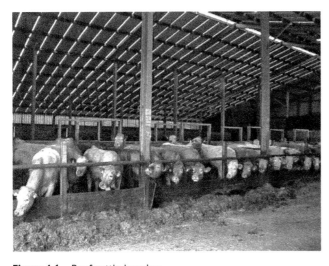

Figure 4.1 Beef cattle housing.

4.1.4 Trends in the UK Beef Industry

In the 1990s in the UK there was a bovine spongiform encephalopathy (BSE) outbreak, and during the associated closure of the export market, a high proportion of dairy and dairy-cross calves were disposed of on-farm in the light of the poor returns achievable (particularly true of pure dairy male calves). Another consequence of BSE was a ban on the consumption of beef from animals aged over 30 months referred to as the Over-Thirty Month Scheme (OTMS), which took more potential cattle for beef production out of the human supply chain. In the UK in 1999 around 902,000 cows and 72,000 head of prime cattle entered the OTMS. By 2001 these figures had reduced to 56,000 cows and 62,000 head of UK prime cattle and the OTMS was finally withdrawn in January 2006. Following a change to the OTM rule, OTM cattle born after July 1996 were allowed into the food chain, subject to BSE testing. With effect from 23 January 2006, the Older Cattle Disposal Scheme (OCDS) replaced the OTMS for pre-August 1996 cattle. The OCDS disposed of older bovine animals, which were permanently excluded from the food chain, and provided farmers with compensation for their stock for a limited period. The OCDS was a voluntary scheme which lasted until 31 December 2008. In contrast, suckler cow numbers almost trebled in Ireland during the past 25 years and they now comprise approximately half of the national cow population of 2.2 million. In the UK, the decline in beef and veal production in 2008 was a direct result of a reduction in prime cattle slaughterings of 130,000 head to 2 million head in 2008 from 2.2 million head in 2007 (6% fall). While prime cattle slaughterings declined, there was a 25% increase in cow slaughterings to nearly 560,000 head. Throughout the UK, cow beef accounted for 20% of total beef and veal production in 2008 compared with 16% in 2007. In Northern Ireland, a similar pattern exists with cows accounting for 19% of total cattle slaughtered in 2008, but only 14% in 2007.

4.2 Quality Beef Production

Success in beef production is dependent on:

1) Breeding from high-quality animals
2) Achieving high animal performance
3) Achieving optimal carcass conformation and fatness at slaughter
4) Clearly defined grassland management programme
5) Low production costs
6) Detailed records of breeding, performance and health

4.2.1 The Product

Carcass quality is a major determinant of price. Conformation and fatness determine the value of a beef carcass. Conformation describes the shape of the carcass in terms of muscle to bone ratio and the proportion of meat in the expensive cuts. The value of a cut of beef depends on attributes of meat quality such as taste, tenderness and juiciness, which are determined by the age of the animal at slaughter, position of the meat on the carcass (e.g. rump, shoulder) and fat concentration within the meat. Generally, meat from cows contains more mature connective tissue (gristle) than meat from prime beef carcasses and is therefore tougher. Prime cuts such as fillet, sirloin and rump fetch higher prices because they contain little or no gristle or visible strips of intermuscular fat.

The proportion of meat in the hindquarter is highest for the progeny of Limousin cows (Table 4.2). Progeny of Limousin (L) and Charolais (C) cows have a similar proportion of fat in the hindquarter, lower than Limousin × Friesian (LF), Limousin × Holstein-Friesian (LLF) and Simmental × (Limousin × Holstein-Friesian) (SLF). The proportion of bone in the hindquarter is highest for progeny of Charolais cows and lowest for Limousin progeny. The meat to bone ratio is highest for progeny of Limousin cows. Under the EU beef carcass classification (EUROP) scheme, each carcass is assessed and classified at the weighing point on the slaughter line.

4.2.1.1 EU Beef Carcass Classification Scheme

The aim of the beef carcass classification scheme was created to ensure a common classification standard throughout the EU. This enables the EU to operate a standardized beef price reporting system and from late 2004. The criteria for classifying beef cattle are based on conformation, fat cover and sex of the animal. The classification scheme uses the following classifications: the conformation, which is the shape and development of the carcass, is denoted by the letters E, U, R, O, P, with E being the best and P the poorest. The degree of fat cover is denoted by the numbers 1, 2, 3, 4, 5, which represent the order of increasing fatness, while the sex of the animal is categorized by letters as follows; A: young bull, B: bull, C: steer, D: cow and E: heifer.

The carcass classification information is returned to the supplier by the slaughter plant. Over 90% of carcasses are classified by machine, which makes use of Video Image Analysis to carry out various measurements of the carcass. As the determination of classification in this

Table 4.2 Carcass composition Limousin (Lim), Charolais and Limousin Simmental (Sim) and Holstein Friesian (HF) cross bred beef cattle.

	Cow breed types				
	Limousin	Charolais	Lim × HF	Lim × (Lim × HF)	Sim × (Lim × HF)
Hindquarter (%)	50	50.1	49	49.7	48.8
Carcass meat (%)	76.5	74.6	74.3	74.4	74.2
Carcass fat (%)	5.9	6.3	7.2	7.4	7.6
Carcass bone (%)	17.5	19.1	18.5	18.4	18.2
Meat: bone ratio	4.4	3.9	4	4.1	4.1

Source: Drennan and McGee (2009).

case is objective, no appeal is possible. In smaller plants, classification is carried out by factory employees who have been licensed by the Department of Agriculture, Fisheries and Food. In these cases, the supplier can appeal the decision of the classifier to the slaughter plant.

The five conformation classes, represented by the letters E, U, R, O and P, define an incremental scale ranging from P (poor), which denotes the worst conformation, to E (excellent), denoting the best. European Union regulations allow for three subdivisions of each conformation and fat class. In Ireland, conformation class P is subdivided into P +, P, and P–, describing declining conformation. The carcass fat classes describe the amount of fat on the outside of the carcass and in the thoracic cavity. The five fat classes are defined, represented by the numbers 1 to 5 where 1 denotes the least fat and 5 the most. Fat class 4 may be further subdivided into low (4 L) and high fat (4 H) (Table 4.3).

Beef carcass classification data in Ireland for 2007 (Table 4.3) show that 87% of steers and 91% of heifers fall into the combined conformation classes of O and R. A better differentiation would be achieved by classifying carcasses on a 15-point scale (e.g. R–, R, R +) rather than on a 5-point scale (Drennan and McGee 2009). It would be more informative, for the same reason, to have carcass fat class equally classified on a 15-point scale as 87% of steers and 85% of heifers were in fat class 3 and 4 in 2007. The mechanical carcass classification system currently in operation at Irish meat processing plants facilitates this expanded system (Drennan and McGee 2009).

The decision when to slaughter a prime beef animal depends on its conformation and fatness. In practice, this occurs when the fat concentration in the carcass is 15 to 20%. A butcher will trim off about half this fat before the beef reaches the consumer and, while this appears wasteful, it is because quality beef requires enough quantity of intramuscular fat ('marbling') to achieve better meat quality. This only occurs when the animal has deposited substantial amounts of 'waste' fat in the subcutaneous tissues and within the abdomen i.e. kidney, knob and channel fat (KKCF). However, one objective of selective breeding in all meat animals is to reduce the deposition of unsaleable subcutaneous and intra-abdominal fat while preserving

Table 4.3 Percentage of beef carcasses in the different conformation (EUROP) classes and fat classes (1, 2, 3, 4 and 5) in 2007.

Animal	Carcass										
	Conformation class					Weight (kg)	Fat class				
	E	U	R	O	P		1	2	3	4	5
Steers	-	7	45	42	7	358	1	11	53	34	1
Young bulls	1	43	42	13	1	368	4	40	51	5	-
Heifers	-	6	55	36	3	291	2	9	41	44	5
Cows	-	1	11	44	44	305	9	13	33	36	10

Source: Department of Agriculture, Fisheries & Food (DAFF 2004, Ireland).

an amount of marbling fat that creates 'tasty' meat. In general, young bulls are leaner than steers at slaughter and a greater proportion are grade E or U (24.2% compared with 10.1%). Heifers are usually fatter than steers at the same conformation class. Cows culled from a herd, especially the dairy breeds, have poorer conformation than steers, but carry more intra-abdominal KKCF at slaughter.

A few key points may be identified in relation to the feeding and breeding of cattle for quality beef production. Feeding cattle *ad libitum* or increasing the metabolizable energy (ME) concentration of the feed (e.g. by feeding cereal concentrates) will increase both growth rate and the relative rate at which they fatten. Early maturing breeds (Hereford, Aberdeen Angus) animals will be fatter than late maturing animals (Charolais, Simmental) when fed the same ration and slaughtered at the same carcass weight. Feeding diets of grass silage or grazed grass produces yellower fat than concentrate feeds and the fatty acid composition of intramuscular fat can be influenced by diet, e.g. the feeding of maize silage.

4.2.2 Eating Quality

Eating quality is a very subjective term in the meat industry. Consumer studies show that tenderness and flavour are the most important characteristics determining the acceptability of meat. Juiciness, smell, colour and texture are next in importance, while leanness and absence of gristle tend to be least important. In the United States and Asian markets, 'marbling' (deposition of fat within the muscle bundles) is highly valued. In contrast, beef for EU markets is required to have little visible marbling. In recent years red meat has been perceived to be 'less healthy' relative to competing white meat products and other foods. This perception has contributed to red meat losing market share. Perceived 'healthiness' of beef is a significant long-term issue for the beef industry.

4.2.3 Beef Consumption and Human Health

Beef fat contains a high proportion of saturated fatty acids which, when eaten to excess, are known to be a risk to health. However, it also contains a proportion of fat molecules that may have beneficial effects (Lolli et al. 2020). These include monounsaturated fatty acids, some long-chain polyunsaturated fatty acids, with the first double bond at the omega-3 position, such as those found in oily fish, and conjugated linoleic acid. It is of major importance to determine how on-farm factors such as diet may affect the fatty acid profile of beef and so influence its positive and negative health attributes. Recent observations have shown, for example, that the inclusion of grass in the finishing diet can enhance key 'health attributes' of beef by increasing conjugated linoleic acid (CLA) concentration and increasing the ratio of polyunsaturated fatty acids (PUFA) to saturated fatty acid (SFA). Beef from grass silage had a 'healthier' fatty acid profile than beef from maize silage. The concentration of CLA and PUFA can be increased by manipulating the finishing diet, e.g. by inclusion of sunflower oil. Muscle from cattle finished on a grass or clover sward had higher PUFA but lower CLA concentrations than animals finished on grass (Moloney et al. 2018).

4.3 Beef Production Systems

Grazed suckler herds are mainly spring-calving, to coincide with the seasonal grass growth profile. In suckler beef production systems, spring-born calves have continuous access to their dams at pasture until the end of the grazing season in autumn, when they are weaned and housed indoors (Drennan and McGee 2009). In dairy calf to beef production systems calves are artificially reared, usually indoors, on milk replacer and concentrates for eight weeks and then turned out to pasture for their first grazing season following which, they are housed indoors. Irrespective of the system used, cattle reared for beef production in cool/temperate maritime climates will spend a significant proportion of their lifetime indoors; therefore, the housing system will influence their overall performance and welfare. The most common systems used for finishing beef cattle in Ireland are shown in Table 4.4.

4.3.1 Beef from the Suckler Herd

Beef suckler cows are kept in a wide range of grazing habitats. These range from herds kept at high stocking densities on improved pastures with high inputs of nitrogenous (N) fertilizer to herds raised extensively in habitats ranging from the European Alps to the great plains of North and South America. Calves born to beef cows stay with their mothers until weaning in late summer or autumn. In Europe, producers sell them into yards for winter feeding before they are finished out of yards in the spring or at pasture the following summer. In North America, weaned calves are typically finished (reared to slaughter weight) in large feedlots.

In Europe, calving is usually concentrated either in early spring, normally before turnout to grass, or at pasture in autumn. When calves are born in the spring, the peak period for

Table 4.4 Finishing systems used on Irish farms and months (mo.) of housing required during the lifetime of dairy bred calves up to finishing.

System	Housing (mo.)	Reference
Under 16M Bull Beef	8	Drennan and McGee (2009)
19M Bull Beef	12	McGee (2005)
19M Heifer Beef	11	Kelly et al. (2010)
20M Heifer Beef (Suckler Bred)	7	Moloney and Drennan (2013)
23M Steer Beef	10	Keane (1999)
24M Heifer Beef (Suckler)	10	Moloney et al. (2013)
24M Steer Beef (Suckler)	10	Drennan and McGee (2009)
24M Friesian Steer Beef [1]	11	Keane (1999)
25M Steer Beef	12	McGee (2005)
29M Steer Beef (Suckler)	10	Keane and Allen (1999)

lactation in the cows coincides with the peak period for production of grass. This reduces the cost of feeding concentrates to cow and calf. It is common practice to house autumn-born calves with their mothers and provide them with access to a special creep area. Such an area provides a place where they may rest and receive concentrate feed without competition from the adult cows. Farmers then turn them out to pasture in spring and wean calves in midsummer at 9 to 10 months of age and weights of 250 to 350 kg (depending on breed). The Meat and Livestock Commission (http://www.mlc.org.uk) publishes annual summaries of the physical and economic performance of recorded beef herds.

The cow herd uses approximately 0.85 and 0.66 of the total energy requirement in calf-to-weanling and calf-to-beef systems, respectively, with about two-thirds and one half, respectively, of the total energy consumed going towards maintaining the cow herd (Montano-Bermudez et al. 1990). Feed is the main variable cost on suckler beef farms and cow winter feed costs are a major proportion of feed costs. In systems that sell calves at weaning, approximately two-thirds of total feed energy goes towards maintaining the cow herd. In systems that rear calves to slaughter, feed energy costs are split approximately 50:50.

4.3.2 Beef from the Dairy Herd

Dairy beef production systems typically involve crossbreeding between dairy cows and semen from beef bulls. Male dairy/beef crosses (e.g. Charolais x Holstein) will all be reared for prime beef. In the UK and Ireland, a substantial proportion of the crossbred females will be retained for use as dams in suckler beef systems. In Brazil, females from local adapted breeds are commonly mated to temperate, high genetic-merit dairy breed males to generate adapted, yet productive F1 females for the dairy herd and the males are reared for beef. The F1 females generally become either terminal females (defined as females whose immediate progeny are slaughtered) or are backcrossed to dairy breed males to generate terminal females.

Farmers producing prime beef from calves born to dairy cows remove them shortly after birth and rear them artificially. This involves providing them with a liquid milk replacer diet until they are eating sufficient digestible dry food to support maintenance and growth. This usually occurs at about 35 to 42 days old. The rearing system employed thereafter will be determined by a variety of factors such as phenotype, the cost and availability of feed, season of birth and seasonal variations in selling price.

The recent conclusion of a Brexit trade deal removes a major threat to food exports and wider trade. However, new non-tariff barriers apply to UK/EU trade since January 1st, 2021. At market level, the current outlook due to Covid-19 and Brexit is difficult to predict. The medium-term market outlook to 2027 is for global food demand to grow in line with population. For most agricultural commodities, prices adjusted for inflation are not expected to grow due to the growth in global supply. Volatility in output and input prices will continue to be a challenge.

The provisional political agreement reached in June 2021 by the European Parliament and Council on the new Common Agricultural Policy (CAP) introduces a fairer, greener, more animal friendly and flexible CAP. Higher environmental and climate ambitions, aligned with Green Deal objectives, are to be implemented from January 2023. The new CAP will also ensure a fairer distribution of CAP support, especially to small and medium-sized family farms and young farmers.

4.3.2.1 Semi-intensive Beef Systems

The expression 'semi-intensive' describes systems in which young cattle live out at grass for one or two summers. There are two options (Table 4.5), where farmers finish cattle either in yards during their second winter or at pasture after a second summer at 20 to 24 months of age. Beef producers normally castrate and rear male calves as steers.

4.3.2.2 Finishing in Yards

Finishing in yards is the most common system for calves born from September to December. Despite financial incentives for earlier (summer) calving, this is still the peak calving period for dairy cows. The calves can grow at 0.7 to 0.9 kg/day over the first winter so that they weigh 200 to 220 kg when the spring comes, and they go out to grass. At this stage of growth, the ruminant digestive system is sufficiently mature to enable them to thrive on a diet of grass alone (without milk or cereals). Such calves achieve weight gains close to 1 kg/day and reach 340 to 360 kg by October or November when they return to the yard. If they are to finish before the following spring, they will then need to receive a highly digestible diet *ad libitum*.

Table 4.5 Outline of semi-intensive beef production from Hereford (He), Friesian (Fr), Holstein (Hol) and Charolais (Ch) calves from the dairy herd finished in yards or at pasture in year 2.

	Finishing			
	Yards			Pasture
	He × Fr	Ch × Fr	Hol	Ch × Fr
Live bodyweight (kg)				
Weaning (5 weeks)	65	70	65	70
Turnout (Year 1)	200	220	220	200
Yarding	340	360	340	360
Turnout (Year 2)	-	-	-	480
Slaughter	420	520	510	600
Age at slaughter (mo.)	12 to 14	14 to 16	18 to 24	20 to 24
Carcass weight (kg)	205	277	260	318
Killing out (%)	51.0	53.2	51.3	53.0
Saleable meat: bone ratio	3.8	4.0	3.4	4.0

This is primarily a mixture of forage (grass or maize silage) with a cereal-based concentrate ration supplement if necessary. An early maturing Hereford × Friesian steer may finish by January at a slaughter weight of 420 kg Heifers will finish even younger and lighter. A Charolais × Friesian steer will grow faster but finish a little later at a much greater weight. A Holstein-type male calf may achieve a similar slaughter weight to the Charolais × Friesian but will take much longer to finish.

4.3.2.3 Summer Finishing

Traditionally farmers used the summer finishing system for calves that were born in mid- to late winter. This is because such animals are sufficiently mature to obtain the maximum benefit from grass during their first summer. Farmers also summer-finish calves from big, late maturing bulls, like the Charolais, that are difficult to fatten in yards over their second winter. If there is no intention of finishing cattle out of yards during their second winter, producers will put them through a 'store' period. During this time the animals receive only silage and supplements of essential minerals and vitamins. They may continue to gain weight at 0.5 to 0.8 kg/day but lose body fat, so that they end the winter bigger but leaner than when they entered it. When such lean and hungry animals return to pasture for their second summer, their appetite for good grass is initially high because they sense that they are thin (or underweight for age). In these circumstances they can achieve growth rates in excess of 1 kg/day on low-cost summer pasture. However, cattle in good to fat condition, moving to spring grass, initially lose weight which they may not recover for several weeks. For the same reason, it is important not to turn out cattle that are nearly finished at the end of winter on to grass; they will need feeding on in yards until they are ready for slaughter. In June 2003, EU farm ministers adopted a fundamental reform of the common agricultural policy (CAP). The reform completely changed the way the EU supports its farm sector. These new 'single farm payments' are linked to respect for environmental, food safety and animal welfare standards.

4.3.3 Intensive Systems for Beef and Veal

Intensive calf-rearing systems are those that involve rearing calves from the dairy herd in confinement from birth to slaughter. This is expensive in terms of housing, machinery, labour and, especially, feed which can account for up to 80% of total costs. Intensive high-input, high-output systems depend on achieving high daily gains. As cattle approach their natural mature weight, the rate of fat deposition increases and since each kg of fat takes about 2.25 times the energy of each kg of muscle (lean meat), feed efficiency declines. It is now recommended that cattle should be slaughtered at fat score 3 rather than 4 L Indeed, this is a trend that has occurred over the past few years. Almost 55% of steers were slaughtered at fat score 3.

It is most common to rear male dairy-type (Holstein-Friesian) calves that have a poorer conformation, so are cheaper to buy than beef × dairy calves, in intensive systems. The strategy in these systems is to offer the highest quality feed available at an economic price and finish the calves as quickly as possible. Inevitably this reduces both the age and weight, and therefore the price, of the animal at slaughter. For a good Charolais × Friesian calf, worth double, it pays to rear it semi-intensively to a greater slaughter weight even though it takes longer. The main feeding options for intensive beef are based on grass silage plus concentrates, maize silage plus (less) concentrates of 'barley beef' (Table 4.6). In the barley beef system, the main feed is cereal with small amounts of protein, minerals and vitamins plus a little straw to encourage rumination. Since barley is more energy-rich than grass or maize silage, this system finishes calves most quickly. It is, however, less profitable than silage-based systems, except where the barley is home-grown and more likely to provoke digestive disorders.

Intensive beef production systems require the confinement of animals throughout their lives at a high stocking density. This increases the risk of infectious diseases, such as pneumonia, relative to systems that permit the animals to spend half the year at pasture. These problems are particularly acute for calves in the first three months of life. In the early days of intensive beef systems, calves were moved to the rearing accommodation and were exposed to carriers of infection directly after weaning at five to six weeks of age. This created serious losses from respiratory disease. Specialist contract-rearing units have developed which provide 12-week-old calves at a weight of 110 to 130 kg and, ideally, an acquired immunity to the major respiratory pathogens of intensive beef units.

4.3.3.1 Cereal and Baby Beef
Cereal-based diets are often used for bull beef production. Beef cattle that are finished indoors are offered concentrate feedstuffs at rates that range from modest inputs through to *ad libitum* access. Such concentrates frequently contain high levels of cereals such as

Table 4.6 Guidelines for intensive beef and veal production systems for Holstein/Friesian bull calves from the dairy herd.

	Grass silage concentrates	Maize silage concentrates	Barley beef	Veal	
				White	Pink
Live weight gain (kg/d)	1.00	1.15	1.30	1.60	1.40
Slaughter weight (kg)	510	490	460	220	300
Slaughter age (mo.)	16	14	11	4	7
Concentrates feed (t)	1.3	0.8	1.8	-	0.8
Milk powder (t)	-	-	-	1.2	0.4
Gross margin (£/head)	160	140	115	30	70
Carcass price (p/kg)	209	204	214	380	240

Source: Meat and Livestock Commission 1994.

barley or wheat. In addition to this, it is essential to provide sufficient roughage in the diet to prevent metabolic disorders from hindering production and causing distress. This is often supplied in the form of cereal straw; this should be fed in the form of 'long fibre'(>10 cm) in order to stimulate healthy rumination and salivation. Straw that is rolled and processed into pellets carries an increased risk of digestive disorders such as rumen acidosis.

Farmers thinking of using 'high-moisture grain' techniques for preserving and processing cereal grains destined for feeding to beef cattle need to know how the yield, conservation efficiency and feeding value of such grains compares with grains conserved using more conventional techniques. The animals on this system achieve a live-weight gain of 1.25 kg per day from 3 months of age and are slaughtered at 450 kg live weight.

4.3.3.2 Veal

Veal is the pale meat (white veal) of calves maintained at the pre-ruminant stage on a liquid diet of milk or milk replacer. Formerly the diet was fed entirely in liquid form. However, it is now compulsory within the European Union to feed some solid feed in the form of digestible fibre to promote rumen development. Traditionally veal was produced by calves of dual-purpose breeds that were fed whole milk after milking, and by suckling calves of multipurpose or beef (e.g. Limousin) breeds. With the introduction of milk substitutes in the early 1960s the production of veal expanded. The carcass weight of veal calves may range from 105 to 140 kg

Veal production is mainly prevalent in the EU, where it was highly stimulated by subsidized milk powder used for calf rearing (as one of the ways of using up the huge milk surpluses in the EU). Veal calves were exclusively given milk or milk substitutes in order to keep them at the pre-ruminant stage, thus avoiding the development of the forestomachs. Slaughtered at 2 to 5 months of age, at a live-weight varying from 100 to 250 kg, they grow rapidly (over 1 kg per day) and provide a high dressing percentage (about 60%), well-conformed and sufficiently fat covered carcass with pale pinkish meat. This last-mentioned characteristic is very important from a commercial point of view (high premiums are paid by consumers for this type of meat) and can only be obtained from pre-ruminant animals on an iron deficient diet. The two main types of veal production can be distinguished.

4.3.3.3 Nursed Veal Calves

This system is limited to two areas in France and includes less than 12% of veal calves slaughtered in France. The calves are mainly offspring of French beef breeds and crosses with dairy cattle. Almost all calves are born on the farm where they are reared, but sometimes a few additional calves are bought. The price of this top-quality product is high (around 18% higher than calves reared on milk substitutes). This system is decreasing because it gives a lower income than suckling calves at pasture which are sold at weaning for further fattening and red meat production.

4.3.3.4 Veal Calves Reared on Milk Substitutes

The production of milk substitute-fed veal calves is mainly localized in western and southwestern France, northern Italy and central Netherlands. Friesians with an increasing proportion of Holstein blood predominate. Most of the calves are born outside the farms where they are reared. They are usually bought from various sources at one to three weeks of age; Italy imports calves for rearing from the Netherlands and France. A significant number is imported into mainland Europe from the UK. Over 85% of the production is organized under contract by dairy and non-dairy companies manufacturing milk substitutes as well as slaughterhouse companies.

4.3.3.5 Feeding and Growth

Milk substitute fed to veal calves mainly contains milk ingredients (milk and whey powder; 70 to 90% of total). Starch derivates, fat substitutes (e.g. tallow, lard and saturated vegetable oils), minerals and vitamins are added in various proportions. Growth rates of an average 1.2 kg per day are common (0.7 to 0.8 kg during the first month, increasing to 1.4 to 1.6 kg during the last part of the fattening period) with an average daily consumption of 1.8 to 2.0 kg milk substitute powder.

4.3.3.6 Alternative Husbandry Systems for Veal Calves

Several alternative husbandry systems for veal calves have been explored to discover one that is more humane and also economically competitive with the intensive method. The aims of these systems are to ensure good welfare by keeping calves in groups with access to straw or other bedding and to provide enough fibrous feed to promote good health and normal behaviour in consequence of normal rumen development. Liquid milk replacer still forms a major part of the diet in order to promote rapid growth and produce quality 'pink' veal that attracts a high price. Veal is perceived as a luxury meat by those prepared to eat it and shunned by others as unacceptable on welfare grounds. It should follow, therefore, that high welfare standards become a major selling point for those seeking to produce high-premium veal for the luxury market. A few honourable entrepreneurs have sought to exploit this market with approval from bodies such as RSPCA Freedom Foods. However, the economic returns to date are not encouraging.

4.4 Beef Breeding and Genetics

The beef herds in the UK and Ireland consist of some pure-bred breeds, e.g. Angus, Hereford, French breeds, but more crossbred cows (British breeds × dairy breeds) mated to the late-maturing beef breeds. The beef breeds in extensive grazing areas such as in France and Spain are predominantly local (rustic) breeds. The ideal characteristics for a suckler cow are as follows:

- Fertility: Calve at 2 years (early puberty), then a calf per year. Herd fertility 90%
- Conformation: Produce a top-grade carcass (EUR) when bred to a good-quality sire

- Milk yield: Sufficient to grow one calf well (but not excessive)
- Ease of calving: To reduce calving difficulty and management
- Docility: Cow should be manageable and safe to work with
- Feed efficiency: Low maintenance requirement
- Cull value: Replacement cost is lower where cull value is higher
- Uniformity: The herd should be reasonably uniform in type so that the progeny will be likewise.

4.4.1 Holstein/Friesian Dams

In areas such as the UK, where most beef comes from the dairy herd, most beef calves have Holstein/Friesian mothers. Until recently the Holstein and British Friesian were two different breeds in the UK but the two breed societies have now amalgamated. There remains, however, a profound difference in the conformation. The typical British Friesian has a superior muscle to bone ratio and proportion of meat in the expensive cuts relative to the long-legged, bony American Holstein. There is steady, and probably unstoppable, trend towards the extreme Holstein type of dairy cow that gives more milk but has a considerably inferior beef shape. One of the reasons for the UK increasing the number of calves it exports into white veal units in continental Europe was the rise in the number of poor-quality Holstein-type male calves. These calves are unsatisfactory for beef production but are so cheap that it is profitable to rear them quickly for veal.

4.4.2 Beef Breeds

The most desirable traits for a beef bull are rapid growth rate, especially lean tissue; excellent carcass conformation, without excess subcutaneous and KKC fat; and good appetite, especially for grass and forages to achieve early finishing. These traits are somewhat incompatible and the relative importance of each depends on the nutrition and environment within the rearing system. Table 4.7 shows the variation in growth rate and fatness of different breeds of pedigree bulls (i.e. weights and backfat thickness at 400 days of age). There is no such thing as one perfect breed, because different types suit different circumstances.

4.4.2.1 Hereford

The Hereford was, for many years, the most popular sire for beef production from the dairy herd. It is a relatively small animal, with an average 400-day weight of approximately 470 kg and a mature weight of 900 kg. The breed has an excellent conformation and finishes quickly due to a large appetite for forages relative to its energy requirement for maintenance. The bulls carry a low risk of dystocia (Table 4.8). The gene for a white face is dominant and therefore the beef producer, seeing a white-faced calf at market, knows that it was sired by a Hereford bull. The bulls are relatively gentle natured. For all these reasons they remain a popular breeding animal for dairy farmers to keep and run with their heifers. They also remain excellent sires of crossbred suckler cows. However, Charolais and Simmental have largely overtaken their role as a first-choice sire of prime beef calves. The beef trade has for

Table 4.7 Performance of principal beef breeds according to pedigree recordings.

	No.	Bull 400 day weights (kg)			Back fat (mm)	
		Range	Mean	1975 to 1990	Range	Mean
Aberdeen Angus	1134	434 to 670	417	+ 86	1.6 to 8.5	4.6
Belgian Blue	508	511 to 655	519	-	-	-
Charolais	3315	453 to 831	617	+49	1.5 to 4.1	2.6
Hereford	1683	361 to 635	469	+ 35	1.3 to 9.3	4.2
Limousin	3404	410 to 669	525	+ 94	1.0 to 5.3	2.6
Simmental	3560	445 to 810	600	+ 73	1.5 to 5.2	3.3
South Devon	1228	424 to 730	546	+ 21	1.5 to 5.5	3.1

Table 4.8 Carcass composition of calves from sire breeds crossed with Friesian/Holstein cows.

	Sire breeds			
	Angus	Charolais	Hereford	Limousin
Weight at slaughter (kg)	393.0	494.0	410.0	454.0
Feed efficiency (g gain/kg feed)	86.0	82.0	88.0	85.0
Killing out (%)	52.5	54.8	52.3	54.7
Carcass:				
Saleable meat (%)	72.5	72.7	71.9	73.3
Saleable expensive cuts (%)	44.1	44.8	44.1	45.4
Fat trim (%)	9.6	9.0	9.7	9.2

Source: Southgate in More O'Ferrall 1982.

many years favoured larger carcasses, although the largest carcasses are now about as big as people and current machinery can reasonably handle. Also, the quality of feed for beef cattle has generally improved. The facility of the Hereford to finish early on poor forage has become something of a disadvantage. When forage quality is good, Herefords fatten too soon.

4.4.2.2 Aberdeen Angus

Aberdeen Angus cattle are black and polled and both these characteristics are dominant. Breeders developed the Angus to produce high-quality beef, with conspicuous marbling, on good land but in the short growing season of northeast Scotland. The traditional Angus is a small, early finishing animal suitable as a mate for heifers but fattens too quickly. There has been a move to increase size in this breed, mainly through importation of bulls from North

America. The average 400-day live weights for Angus bulls are now higher than for Herefords (Table 4.6) and the top of the range is as heavy as any breed other than Charolais and Simmental.

4.4.2.3 Limousin

The Limousin is a red-coloured breed originating from central France. It is, on average, intermediate in weight between the British beef breeds and the very large Charolais and Simmental. It is lean and has excellent carcass conformation with a high killing-out percentage, and a high proportion of meat in the expensive cuts (Table 4.7). This makes it very popular with butchers. Calving problems are lower than for Charolais and Simmental; this makes it a suitable bull for mating with dairy cows to produce beef. Selection for leanness and high killing-out percentage (which implies a small gut) inevitably tends to select against appetite, especially for highly fibrous forages. Limousin crosses are therefore difficult to finish without expensive concentrate feeds. Intensive systems, which house animals in yards and slaughter them by 18 months of age, are most suitable for Limousins. Limousin × Friesian male calves in these systems are usually entire and can be difficult to handle.

4.4.2.4 Charolais and Simmental

It is possible to consider these popular large breeds together with other, less numerous large breeds, such as the Blonde d'Aquitaine and the South Devon. Pure-bred Charolais and Blonde d'Aquitaine have rather similar cream-coloured coats. The Simmental is very like the Hereford in colour. At best, these bulls and their calves grow fast and have the ability to reach a large size and excellent carcass conformation without getting too fat. Since the prime factor determining the price of a beef animal is its slaughter weight, these breeds, especially the Charolais, have become increasingly popular as sires for both dairy cows and suckler beef cows. The dairy farmer who sells male calves at 10 days of age can get more money for a Charolais cross that may finish at 580 kg than for a Hereford cross that may finish at 450 kg However, the dairy farmer cannot afford obstetric problems since they compromise the prime source of income, namely subsequent lactation performance. The suckler beef industry can only generate income from the sale of calves (and ultimately the cow) so, inevitably therefore, they often use very large bulls and carry the greater risk of dystocia (Table 4.8). To maximize slaughter weights, calves from these large bulls, whether out of dairy or beef cows, are best suited to 20- to 24-month systems. Most calves have the capacity to finish well (if slowly) off grass. The Charolais and Simmental breeds are continuing to increase in size and growth rate to 400 days (Table 4.9). The rate of improvement in these traits has been less impressive in the native red South Devon breed.

4.4.2.5 Belgian Blue

Breeders have developed the modern Belgian Blue from a breed similar in appearance to the traditional blue-roan beef shorthorn. They have selected for 'double muscling' (i.e. heavy muscling), especially in the hindquarters. This leads to a very high muscle to bone ratio but abnormalities of skeletal development, especially a reduction in pelvic dimensions. Cows carrying the double muscling trait in the homozygous form are seldom able to give birth normally and will need a caesarean section. The homozygous double-muscled animal also does

Table 4.9 Effects of sire breed on calving difficulties and calf mortality in suckler cows, dairy cows and heifers.

| | Suckler cows | | Holstein /Friesian | | | |
| | | | Cows | | Heifers | |
Breed of sire	**Dystocia (%)**	**Mortality (%)**	**Dystocia (%)**	**Mortality (%)**	**Dystocia (%)**	**Mortality (%)**
Aberdeen Angus	3.1	1.3	-	-	2.3	5.8
Hereford	3.8	1.6	1.2	2.9	3.1	6.2
Friesian	-	-	2.5	5.0	7.4	7.9
Limousin	7.2	4.4	3.2	6.1	8.1	9.7
Charolais	9.6	4.8	4.2	5.2	-	-
Simmental	9.3	4.2	3.1	5.6	-	-
South Devon	7.4	4.1	2.4	5.6	-	-
Belgian Blue	-	-	4.3	5.4	-	-
Average	**6.7**	**3.4**	**3.0**	**5.1**	**5.2**	**7.4**

Source: Allen 1990.

not thrive, partly because of a poor appetite and partly because of a predisposition to infectious diseases, especially pneumonia. In the natural state, this trait is a lethal recessive. However, F1 hybrid calves from a double-muscled bull do grow rapidly (although they are difficult to finish) and have a good carcass quality. The incidence of dystocia when using a Belgian Blue bull on a Holstein/Friesian cow is no worse than for a Charolais bull. There are no special welfare problems in the crossbred calves. However, the breeder who elects to use Belgian Blue semen must accept the welfare problems involved in producing the pure-bred double-muscled bulls.

4.4.3 Suckler Cow Breeds

The beef herds in the UK and Ireland consist of some pure bred breeds, e.g. Angus, Hereford, French breeds but more crossbred cows (British breeds × dairy breeds) which are then mated to the late-maturing beef breeds to produce the generation of calves for slaughter as prime beef. Most suckler cows in the UK are not pure-bred but first crosses between two pure breeds. This is partly because genetic traits relating to maternal behaviour and calf survival are more likely to improve by heterosis (hybrid vigour) rather than by selection within breeds. It is also partly because dairy farms are regularly producing and selling suitable half-bred heifers for the suckler herd, such as Hereford × Friesian or Limousin × Friesian. Such animals, which have been reared artificially, with little or no contact with their own mothers, manage the responsibilities of motherhood very well.

Over the last 200 years the Hereford has become the most popular breed of suckler cow in the world outside the hottest areas of the tropics. The ability of the breed to thrive and fatten on poor-quality grasses and forage may now be a disadvantage in a bull intended as a sire of calves destined for slaughter as prime beef. It is, however, an excellent trait for a bull siring hardy beef cows able to subsist and regularly produce calves, at least cost, on range in the USA, Australia or on the hills of the UK. Other traditional hardy British beef breeds include the Aberdeen Angus, Beef Shorthorn, Galloway and Welsh Black.

4.5 Behaviour

4.5.1 Social Behaviour

Cattle in the wild form large, stable herds whose size appears to be limited only by the availability of pasture. Being part of a herd contributes to a sense of security since it reduces the risk of capture for a large animal that cannot hide. On open range and given plenty of space, cattle form stable subgroups. A dominance hierarchy is established, whereby each cow knows its place. Cattle perceive a predator as a threat but not as a source of real alarm if they can maintain a satisfactory flight zone and can see (or think they can see) an escape route. It is possible to build these principles into handling systems for range cattle. Removing an individual from a herd will cause it distress. One exception is the cow about to calve, who will isolate herself from the herd to give birth. Having licked her calf clean and suckled it she will then leave it to lie hidden and go back to the herd. She will only return to feed her calf 4 to 6 times during the first few days until it is strong enough to run with the herd.

4.5.2 Reproductive Behaviour

The cow normally has one calf per year, after a pregnancy of nine months. There are small genetic differences in the duration of pregnancy that are largely due to the genotype of the calf. A Holstein/Friesian cow carrying a calf to a bull of her own breed has a gestation period of 281 days. If (to use an extreme example) the sire had been a Limousin bull, gestation would take 287 days. Table 4.8 gives values for the incidence of dystocia (calving difficulties) and calf mortality in suckler cows and dairy cows (Holstein/Friesians) artificially inseminated to bulls from different breeds. The traditional British beef breeds, Hereford and Aberdeen Angus, carry a lower incidence of dystocia, which is one reason why farmers traditionally use them to inseminate heifers. Their relatively small size and equable temperament is another reason why they are suitable to have running with heifers.

The incidence of dystocia in Holstein/Friesian cows is less than in suckler cows although, for calf mortality within the first two days of life, the reverse is true. The incidence of dystocia is higher for the cows mated with very large beef bulls, Charolais and Simmental. However, the risk of dystocia is due at least as much to the pelvic dimensions of the cow as the size of the bull. Left to themselves, beef cows are more likely than dairy cows to ensure that their calf stays alive (Table 4.8). Breeders have selected Belgian Blues for very heavy muscling, to the extent that many pure-bred cows are unable to calve normally; such cows require repeated, premeditated caesarean section and this constitutes a major welfare problem. However, the incidence of dystocia in Holstein/Friesian cows mated to Belgian Blue bulls is no greater than for the Charolais. Artificial insemination (AI) studs, for dairy and beef cows, keep records of the performance and progeny tests of their individual bulls. These include records of calving difficulty. When selecting a bull for AI it is possible to take this into account, to avoid, for example, mating a bull that carries a high risk of dystocia to a cow with a history of calving difficulties.

Cattle have no discrete breeding season. A non-pregnant sexually mature female will show oestrus at intervals of about 21 days throughout the year. When beef cows are on pasture or open range, natural service by a bull running with the herd is practically obligatory. When cows are confined, it is possible to induce and synchronize oestrus and ovulation using hormone treatments. There are two approaches, both of which rely on controlling the end of dioestrus, which initiates the period of rapid follicular development. This involves either injection in dioestrus of prostaglandin to destroy the corpus luteum, or insertion and timed withdrawal of progesterone-releasing intravaginal devices (PRIDs). The probability of fertilization following synchronization of oestrus followed by AI is unlikely to exceed 65%, so most beef farmers need a 'sweeper' bull to serve those cows that do not conceive to AI. However, AI does make it possible to use bulls of much higher genetic merit than one is likely to find on the average commercial beef farm.

4.6 Nutrition and Feeding

4.6.1 Digestion

When a cow grazes at pasture, all plant material enters the large paunch, or reticulorumen, where it is mixed, diluted with saliva and subjected to microbial fermentation. The end-products of microbial fermentation of plant carbohydrates (sugars, starch, cellulose and hemicellulose) are absorbed, largely across the rumen wall, as the volatile fatty acids; acetic, propionic and butyric acid, which form the major source of dietary energy for ruminants. The digesta that leave the reticulo-rumen and pass into the abomasum (which corresponds to the true stomach in humans) contain large amounts of microbial proteins. These are subjected to further digestion and form the ruminant's principal supply of amino acids. The adult ruminant derives most of its nutrients from reactions in the rumen. The small intestine (duodenum, jejunum) is the major source for absorption of amino acids and minerals. The large intestine (caecum and colon) acts as a second fermentation chamber, but normally contributes less than 8% to nutrient uptake.

4.6.2 Metabolizable Energy

By far the greatest quantity of nutrients absorbed from the gut is used as a source of energy (i.e. metabolizable energy; ME) to fuel the work of maintenance, activity and production. The

ME requirement is expressed in megajoules per day (MJ/day) and the ME concentration in the feed is expressed in MJ ME/kg dry matter (DM), which abbreviates to M/D. The DM intake of a ruminant is stimulated by its requirements for nutrients, especially energy, but restricted by the rate it can digest the food it eats, principally the amount of unfermented matter it can carry within the rumen. A growing calf or lactating cow will have a greater hunger for nutrients per unit of body weight than an adult, non-pregnant, non-lactating animal. However, the less digestible the food (i.e. the lower the M/D) the more difficult it becomes to meet its energy requirements within the constraints of gut fill. The M/D of pasture grass and the best silages should be greater than 10 MJ/kg DM and can sustain weight gains of 1 kg/day or more. Cereals, with an M/D close to 13 MJ/kg, can provide enough ME to sustain maximum weight gains. However, they are deficient in protein and other essential minerals and vitamins. Moreover, a diet based almost entirely on cereals will not provide enough long fibre to stimulate rumination and can lead to problems such as bloat and rumen acidosis.

4.6.3 Protein

Ruminants, like all animals, require amino acids as essential building blocks for growth, reproduction and lactation and as constituents of all the enzymes that drive the processes of metabolism. Most of the amino acid requirements of beef cattle are provided by acid digestion in the abomasum of proteins synthesized within the rumen. This may be termed effective rumen degradable protein (ERDP). Rumen microbes synthesize their own proteins, partly from true protein in the diet and partly from simple sources of non-protein nitrogen (NPN), such as urea. In the natural state this urea arises from the recycling of blood urea, via the saliva or by direct absorption across the rumen wall. Blood urea is an end-product of protein catabolism within the body and, in simple-stomached animals, almost entirely excreted in the urine. The ability of ruminants to recycle urea is an elegant adaptation to seasonal shortages of protein and water, e.g. during the dry season in the tropics. In areas (e.g. the USA) where cattle are finished in feedlots on high-cereal diets, it is possible to meet amino acid requirements in part by providing a dietary source of NPN. In some high-producing ruminants (e.g. dairy cattle) it is not possible to meet amino acid requirement from the 'natural' mixture of microbial and undegraded dietary protein (UDN) that enters the abomasum (see Chapter 3). In these circumstances the diet can be supplemented with a protein source that is resistant to microbial degradation. However, there are probably no circumstances where it would be cost-effective to provide supplementary UDN for beef animals.

4.6.4 Minerals and Vitamins

Diets based wholly on fresh or conserved grass are likely to provide enough calcium, but phosphorus and magnesium may be marginal. In certain cases, the diet may be deficient in copper, cobalt or selenium and all these deficiencies may stunt growth. It is possible to feed exact amounts of minerals by incorporating them into the concentrate ration. It is also possible to offer cattle free choice in mineral licks. However, intake is erratic and does not relate to requirement. Moreover, selenium (and possibly copper) is toxic in excess. Some cattle may therefore consume too little and some too much. One of the most popular ways of delivering copper, cobalt and selenium to beef cattle is within a bolus that lodges in the rumen and releases these minerals at a steady rate; this is usually effective, but sometimes the bolus is lost.

Cattle have no dietary requirement for vitamin C and can acquire B vitamins and vitamin K (biotin) as end-products of microbial synthesis in the rumen. Green grass and silage are good sources of carotenes, the precursors of vitamin A. Sun-cured hay is a good source of vitamin D, and whole cereals good sources of vitamin E. Generally, adult cattle are unlikely to suffer from deficiencies of the fat-soluble vitamins A, D and E, but body reserves of these drop during the winter. Calves are born with almost no fat-soluble vitamins in their body and normally acquire them by drinking colostrum. The colostrum of beef and dairy cows in late winter may contain very low concentrations of fat-soluble vitamins. This gives the calves a poor start and makes them particularly vulnerable to infectious diseases of epithelial surfaces, such as diarrhoea and pneumonia.

4.6.5 Water

The *Codes of Recommendations for the Welfare of Livestock: Cattle* (DEFRA 2003) state that 'cattle should have access to sufficient fresh, clean water at least twice daily.' This is necessary to maintain the water content of the body tissues while sustaining inevitable and regulatory losses. Cattle also require water for milk production and to sustain the continuous culture of microbes in the rumen. Published figures for the water intake of cattle range between 50 and 150 g/kg bodyweight per day. It is greater during lactation and hot weather and less when the food is very wet (e.g. fresh grass or grass silage). The first response of cattle to a water shortage is usually to reduce food intake. Ideally, cattle should have access to clean water almost continually. If only allowed access to water twice daily they should be free to drink for as long as they want on each occasion.

4.6.6 Feedstuffs

4.6.6.1 Grass

Grass is almost the perfect food for beef cattle. The most nutritious part of the plant is the young leaf, so its digestibility (and M/D) is greatest before the emergence of the seed heads. Grazing management should aim to ensure that the grass is long enough (at least 7 cm) to ensure that the cattle can consume enough during daylight hours, but not so long that it becomes stemmy and fibrous. Well-managed grassland provides enough ME and protein for maintenance and lactation in beef cows and for maintenance and growth in calves receiving milk from their mothers. It also provides enough ERDP. It cannot, however, sustain economically acceptable weight gains in calves from the dairy herd that are receiving neither concentrates nor milk from their mothers before they reach 200 kg in the case of British breeds or 300 kg for the larger continental breeds. This is because of the constraints of gut fill in the immature rumen. Cattle that receive all or nearly all their food from fresh and conserved grass may, in certain areas, suffer debilitating deficiencies of copper, cobalt, selenium or phosphorus. Such animals may be more susceptible to an acutely fatal attack of hypomagnesaemia or grass staggers. Increasing grass crop yields by application of inorganic fertilizer (N, P and K) inevitably reduces concentrations in grass of the trace elements (Cu, Co and Se). The claim of organic farmers that their cattle are far less prone to mineral deficiency diseases has a basis in that they do not reduce the concentrations of trace elements because they grow less per hectare.

4.6.6.2 Conserved Forages

It is possible to sun- or air-dry grass crops and conserve them as hay or compact them into an air-tight clamp or big, covered bale, and conserve them anaerobically as silage. Well-made grass silage has a greater nutritive value than hay because the crop is cut at an earlier, leafier stage. When making grass silage for dairy cows, it is important to cut the grass very young to maximize M/D. For beef cows, it is usual to leave the crop a little longer to achieve a greater yield but lower M/D (*c.* 10 MJ/kg). The anaerobic fermentation of grass sugars (ideally by lactobacilli) in the silage clamp increases the acidity of the crop and inhibits further microbial breakdown. In effect, the crop is pickled. However, appetite for grass silage when it is fed on its own can be disappointing, partly because it digests slowly in the rumen and partly because it can contain a relative excess of ERDP. Both fermentation rate and appetite can be improved by the addition of a more rapidly fermentable feed with a relative excess of ME. Such ingredients include cereals, a root crop (turnips or fodder beet) or maize silage.

Well-made hay is less nutritious than silage but extremely palatable. Soft meadow hay made from a range of grass species is particularly suitable for encouraging young calves to develop an appetite for roughages. Barley straw has little nutritional value but is a good dietary supplement for cattle eating large quantities of cereals. The long, hard, relatively indigestible fibre dilutes the quickly fermentable starchy cereals and provides the necessary stimulation for increased rumination and therefore more salivation. Both these factors reduce the risk of ruminal acidosis. It is possible to improve the nutritive value of straw by treating with alkali – sodium hydroxide or ammonia. Alkali causes the cell walls to open up and release more fermentable cellulose from its bonds to unfermentable lignin. Alkali-treated straws have an M/D close to that of hay. In any year, economics strictly determine the case for alkali treatment of straw; if the grass crop (hay or silage) is poor (in a wet summer) or in short supply (in a dry summer) then it pays to treat the straw crop.

4.6.6.3 Maize Silage

Maize (corn) silage is an excellent feed for all beef cattle in areas where the crop can be grown successfully. Yields of ME per hectare can be very impressive. The M/D is excellent, but it is slightly deficient in ERDP. Properly supplemented, maize silage can sustain growth rates in excess of 1.0 kg/day. It is particularly effective when fed in combination with grass silage, not least because DM intakes are usually better for maize silage than when feeding grass silage alone. A mixture of 75 parts maize silage and 25 parts grass silage on the forage wagon is ideal for finishing cattle.

4.6.6.4 Cereals

The main nutrient in barley, oats and wheat is starch, which makes these cereals highly concentrated forms of ME for cattle. They are marginal or slightly deficient in protein, both as ERDP for the rumen micro-organisms and as a source of essential amino acids for growing or lactating cattle. When they constitute a major part of the ration (e.g. in a barley beef system) they may promote very rapid growth, but this will cause early-maturing breeds (e.g. offspring of Hereford and Angus bulls) to fatten too soon. All cereals may predispose to ruminal acidosis through too-rapid fermentation, unless diluted with long fibre. Oats is the safest cereal in this respect, being the most fibrous, but it is more expensive per unit of ME than barley or wheat.

4.6.6.5 Root Crops

Root crops such as fodder beet, swedes and turnips have a DM content of less than 200 g/kg but are rich in sugars and very palatable. They are deficient in protein and minerals. A small quantity of a root crop such as fodder beet (e.g. 5 kg/day) can make an excellent supplement to grass silage. In the north and east of England and Scotland it is possible to grow roots as the main energy feed for wintering beef cattle. However, such a diet will need supplementing with protein, minerals and fat-soluble vitamins.

4.6.6.6 By-Products and Crop Residues

Most pelleted compound rations for cattle contain large proportions of by-products or residues from crops grown primarily for direct human consumption. The most common by-products that farmers feed their cattle are the protein-rich residues from plants such as soya bean, rapeseed or groundnuts. These are grown primarily as sources of vegetable oil for human consumption. Others include sugar beet pulp, a highly palatable source of digestible fibre, and maize gluten, the crop residue after extraction of most of the starch from maize. Both sugar beet and maize gluten are reasonably well balanced in the ratio of ERDP to ME and it is possible to feed them directly to cattle as straights. In areas where it permitted, feed manufacturers may also incorporate small quantities of fishmeal into compound feeds as an excellent source of undegradable amino acids, minerals and vitamins. In the past, manufacturers used meat and bone meal from abattoirs. However, since the epidemic of BSE it is illegal, in Europe, to include feed of animal origin in diets for cattle. The total ban on the use of meat and bone meal was introduced in 2001. The BSE crisis led to the European Union banning exports of British beef with effect from March 1996; the ban lasted for 10 years before it was finally lifted on 1 May 2006.

4.7 Environment and Housing

The UK Department for the Environment, Food and Rural Affairs Welfare Codes outline legislation and provide guidelines based on the principles of the 'five freedoms' (Chapter 1). These animal welfare guidelines are the application of sensible animal husbandry practices to the livestock present on the farm. Moreover, the five freedoms provide a structure for the evaluation of the welfare of an animal or group of animals in various environments (Chapter 18). The overall welfare of cattle is defined by their physiological and behavioural state as they seek to reconcile exogenous influences with their natural endogenous state. Exogenous factors include the physical environment (temperature, humidity, wind, photoperiod and so on) and social environment (feeding, housing, stocking rate, area per animal). Endogenous state is influenced by (e.g.) breed, age, sex, weight and temperament and impacts on social order (competition, aggression, dominance order, leadership and so on).

4.7.1 Housing Design

Beef cattle are normally outdoors at pasture for a 7 to 8-month period each year. Housing of cattle is designed to provide shelter from winter climatic conditions and protect pastures from undue damage (poaching) in wet conditions, particularly in the months of December and January when grass is in short supply. Housing provides structured management (feeding, drinking, health check) under controlled conditions. It also aids effective slurry and effluent control. Slatted floor and loose-bedded systems are two main house types used for accommodating beef animals. In many instances, hybrid house types have developed which are constructed using combinations of the above, particularly in the situation where facilities have evolved over time, e.g. the addition of a slatted feed passage to a loose straw-bedded house. Many of these houses utilize liquid manure storage systems. The move away from the traditional design layouts of open yards with self-feed silage has also been driven by the management problems associated with the high volumes of dirty water produced with these designs due to the high levels of annual rainfall.

Slatted floor housing is the most relevant housing system in areas such as Ireland where the availability of straw is low and the cost prohibitive. Alternatively, and preferably, each pen may be divided into a well bedded area and a concrete area behind the feed fence at either side of the central feeding passage. Each pen is separated from the next by a gate which can be swung across daily to enclose the cattle in the bedding area and permit the concrete standing area behind the feed fence to be scraped down using a tractor. The building should be designed to permit the maximum amount of air movement without incurring draughts. This is best achieved by installing space boarding to a depth of at least 1 m and preferably 2 m below the eaves, and an open ridge, with flashing upstands to either side over the central feed passage. The air, which has been warmed by the cattle, and which leaves the building by this open ridge, will prevent the entry of rain or snow in all but the most severe conditions. In addition, over the winter, the ridge will probably let out about 100 times more moisture (from the cattle) than it will let in.

4.7.1.1 Essential Elements of Good Building Design

Essential elements of good building design include the following:

- All houses should be adequately ventilated, allowing for an adequate supply of fresh air, thus facilitating heat dissipation and preventing the build-up of carbon dioxide, ammonia or slurry gases.

- Floor surfaces should be even and non-slip. All buildings should be adequately ventilated with enough air exchange to meet the animals' requirements.
- The accommodation should contain enough natural or artificial light so as not to cause discomfort to the animals. Artificial light should also be provided to enable adequate inspection of the animals, especially cows in late pregnancy and of young calves.
- Each building accommodation should have a suitable smoke or fire alarm system installed in order to detect fire or smoke at an early stage.

Special requirements for slatted floor housing include the following:

- Housed stock should have freedom of movement and ample floor space for lying, grooming and normal animal-to-animal interactions.
- A well-designed, properly constructed and fully maintained slatted floor unit for cattle provides the necessary comfort with minimum distress or injury to the cattle.
- Escapes/creeps should be provided, if young calves are housed with adults, i.e. sucklers.

4.7.1.2 Feed Barriers

Design of the feed barrier should include the following:

- There should be enough space for all animals to feed comfortably at the same time.
- The feed trough should be sufficiently large so that animals always have adequate access to food.
- Avoid any sharp edges or projections on the feed barrier or on the pen divisions, which could cause injury to cattle.
- The feed should be kept within reach of the animal.

4.7.2 Bedding Area

The goal of a reasonably clean, dry comfortable bed is easier to define than to achieve. Cattle are undoubtedly very comfortable when lying in deep, clean straw. However, straw is probably too expensive unless a farm produces its own straw, and prohibitively so in some areas of good beef country such as Ireland. The main problem is that cattle urinate and defecate indiscriminately. This makes it more difficult to maintain the bedding reasonably dry and clean even when the feed is dry (e.g. barley and straw) and practically impossible when the main feed is low dry matter grass silage. It is possible to house adult, non-lactating beef cows and growing cattle over six months of age on slatted concrete floors. These are far from ideal as a mattress to lie on, but they can be kept clean and dry if the gaps between the slats are 40 mm wide and the cattle are stocked densely enough to tread the dung between the slats. However, young calves less than six months of age should not be kept on slatted floors because 40 mm gaps are too wide for their feet and the stocking density necessary to ensure that the slats stay clean increases the risk of provoking pneumonia in these young animals. It follows that while pregnant beef cows may be housed on slatted floors, it is no place for a beef cow to rear her calf, still less give birth.

Beef cows and fattening heifers can be accommodated in cubicles. They are obviously unsuitable for males, who urinate into the middle of the cubicle bed. The dimensions of the cubicle should be determined by the size of the largest animal that they are likely to accommodate. Each animal should be able to lie down entirely within the cubicle without interference from its neighbours (e.g. being trampled upon), change position (stand up and lie down) without difficulty, yet, so far as possible, urinate and defecate in the dunging passage. A cubicle for a Hereford × Friesian suckler cow should be at least 2 m by 1 m. Fine tuning of the standing position can be achieved by adjusting the neck rail or brisket board at the front of the cubicle.

4.7.3 Space Allowance

The recommended space allowances for beef cattle (Table 4.10) show that the minimum space allowances for cattle used in livestock production are those for animals housed in slatted-floor pens. This is because more traditional, bedded systems require more space per animal to maintain the integrity of the bedding (Table 4.10) and because slatted-floored systems require a certain stocking density in order to tread the dung between the slats and stop it building up inside the pen. It is essential that cows or fattening cattle that are given restricted amounts of concentrate feed animals can all feed at the same time. The recommended trough spaces for cows are 0.6 to 0.8 m and for growing cattle are 0.4 to 0.6 m, depending on age and cattle breed. A group of 10 yearling cattle on slats with 0.4 m trough space per head and a floor area of 1.6 m^2 per head would require a square pen 4 m wide by 4 m deep. While the recommended minimum air space is 12 m^3 per head and so for pens 4 m by 4 m either side of a 4 m wide feeding passage, the average height of the building would need to be 5 m. Examples of housing designs accommodating these basic environmental requirements are given later.

The housing of adult cattle raises concerns regarding space and flooring. There is inadequate evidence regarding the effects of concrete slatted floors on animal wellbeing, although the preferences exhibited by cattle for softer surfaces may prompt the development of systems that combine the waste-control advantages of slats with a softer coating. The provision of adequate housing space allowances is critical to the welfare status of cattle. Insufficient space allowance may induce a state of chronic stress, prevent animals from performing their natural behaviour and may impair immune function and performance. Figure 4.1 provides an example of beef cattle housing.

Table 4.10 Space requirements for beef cattle.

	Calves (weeks of age)		Fattening cattle > 1 year	Beef cows
	0 to 6	6 to 12		
Floor space (m^2)				
Straw bedded	2	2	3 to 4	4
Slatted floor	-	-	1.4 to 2.2	3.0 to 3.7
Air space (m^3)	6	10	12	12

Source: DEFRA 2007.

4.7.4 Housing Suckler Cows and Calves

Housing for suckler cattle should provide clean, comfortable, well-ventilated, draught-free accommodation for calves with suitable accommodation for cows. Housing should permit the accommodation of cows and calves in small groups according to calf age, to minimize the spread of disease from older to younger calves. A straw-bedded creep should always be provided for autumn/winter/early spring calves.

There are three types of housing for cows with suckling calves:

1) Slatted housing with creep area;
2) Cubicle housing with creep area;
3) Loose housing with creep area.

The above systems can be combined and the most usual combination is slatted and loose housing, where cows are easy-fed along slatted passages. A kerb height of 200 mm to 250 mm and a width of 200 mm is required to retain bedding material between the slatted and bedded areas. The floor area required per cow and calves is the same as that required for loose housing of cattle.

Calving boxes should be provided for calving cows indoors. In slatted units where the creep area is at the back of slats, part of the creep area may be partitioned off to provide a suitable calving box. In larger herds a further box may be provided to keep cows with calves for a few days following calving and the floor area should not be less than 14.5 m². Calving boxes may be provided in an adjoining building. It is recommended that there should be a crush gate, set out 600 mm from the wall to facilitate handling of suckler cows within the calving box, and Figures 4.3 and 4.4 show some suggested layouts for housing sucklers.

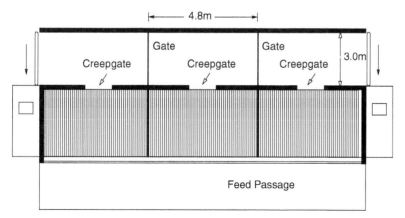

Figure 4.2 Slatted house and creep area (*Source:* Department of Agriculture, Fisheries & Food, 2007, Ireland).

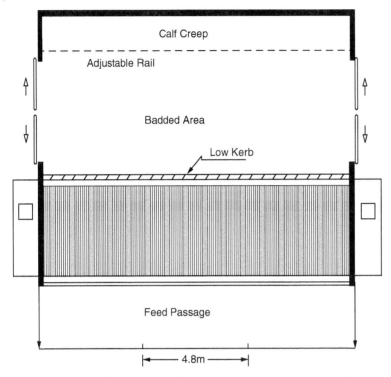

Figure 4.3 Bedded/slatted house (*Source:* Department of Agriculture, Fisheries & Food, 2007, Ireland).

4.7.5 Design of Creep Area

A creep area of at least 1 m^2 per calf should be provided for spring-born calves and up to 1.75 m^2 per calf for autumn-born calves. A solid floor is preferred, with a fall of at least 1 in 30 (recommended 1 in 20) towards a drainage channel, which discharges liquid into an underground tank. Slatted floor pens that are normally used to house cattle may be used as creep pens, by covering the slats with straw and a suitable material to prevent straw bedding entering the slurry tank is recommended. In this situation, underfloor draughts should be excluded as far as possible.

The location of the creep area depends on:

- The preferred management system: autumn, winter, early spring or late spring calving. No creep area is required for late spring calving.
- Where part of the herd is early calving it is recommended that the creep area be located at the end of the house with calved cows accommodated in the adjoining pen.
- Where most of the herd is housed after calving the preferred location of the creep is at the back of the slatted area. The recommended minimum width is 3 m.

It is recommended that there is a separate external access to the internal divisions of the creep area, particularly in autumn and winter calving herds, to facilitate concentrate feeding and calf inspection. It is recommended that the barrier between the cow area and the creep is a tubular steel gate framed with 50 mm tubular steel, which has a creep gate incorporated. Cows should be able to see the calves, using a wall that is 1.1 m to 1.2 m high, which has a horizontal top rail that is set at 1.5 m over floor level. There should be one creep gate per pen provided.

4.7.6 Handling Facilities

Cattle that are brought into an indoor yard system, having been out at grass all summer, are well adapted to a fibrous diet and reasonably immune to the endemic viral and bacterial organisms that cause infectious pneumonia. Management, therefore, presents few problems. The objective is to feed the cattle so as to achieve pre-set targets for weight gain at the least possible cost. The most useful aid to management is, therefore, a good set of weigh scales and an efficient arrangement for moving cattle in and out of their pens and over this weighbridge at intervals of about four weeks. Cattle may be driven fairly easily in groups into a collecting pen large enough to contain all the cattle from one pen in the beef rearing unit. They may then be driven down a race with solid sides and a curved approach to a weighbridge and a crush, where individuals may be restrained for routine treatment or administration of preventive medicine. The high, solid sides to the race prevent the cattle from being distracted or startled by the presence of handlers or other alarming objects in front of them, and the curve in the race encourages them to follow their leaders until it is too late to try to escape.

4.8 Management of the Suckler Herd

4.8.1 Breed Selection

The ideal characteristics for a suckler cow (e.g. fertility, conformation, docility) were listed in the section on breeding and genetics. Strategies to achieve these targets include:

1) Continue to buy in some replacements as dairy cross heifers and breed from these to produce second cross (75% continental) replacements. The amount of dairy breed in the cow herd can be reduced to 30% to 35% on average, meaning that the majority of progeny will have minimal dairy genes.
2) Breed toward 100% continental beef cows, using careful selection and breeding programmes to maintain adequate milk output, and backcrossing two different continental breeds to secure hybrid vigour. In all but the very largest herds this system will involve the use of artificial insemination for replacement breeding.

Pure-breeding is seldom recommended for commercial herds, principally because the loss in hybrid vigour is too great, probably up to 22% less weaned calf live weight per cow bred. If replacement heifers are being bred from within the herd it is recommended that an AI sire be used; otherwise, the stock bull will have to be replaced every two to three years to avoid inbreeding. Where second and third cross replacement heifers are being brought into a herd, it is recommended that sires with proven maternal traits be used to produce these heifers.

4.8.2 Management of Fertility

Fertility targets for a suckler herd are:

- Calving interval: 365 days;
- Calving block: 90% of the herd calves within 10 weeks;
- Fertility: 5% or less of the herd is culled for infertility.

The two major factors affecting reproductive efficiency in suckler herds using natural mating are the interval from calving to first heat (postpartum interval) and conception rate. Heat detection efficiency is a further significant factor when AI is the method used for breeding. One of the major causes of poor reproductive efficiency in beef cows is an extended interval from calving to first ovulation, or postpartum (pp) interval. This interval is considerably longer in beef than in dairy cows and is influenced by several factors including pre and post-partum nutrition, suckling frequency, age of cow, season and the presence of a bull. Moreover, the time from calving to first pp heat is very dependent on body condition. Thus, body condition scoring on a scale of 0 (very thin and emaciated) to 5 (grossly over-fat) is a practical aid in assessing and ensuring the provision of adequate nutrition at this important time. Spring calving cows on good pasture are on a high plane of nutrition during the breeding season and a body condition score of 2 is satisfactory when breeding commences. The high nutrient intake from grass, assuming adequate leafy pasture is provided, offsets the adverse effects of low body condition on fertility. In contrast, autumn-calving cows offered silage are on a lower plane of nutrition during the breeding season and should have a body condition score of 2.5 at the start of breeding.

Fertility can be a problem in autumn calving cows, with cows bred indoors it is essential to provide adequate nutrition during the breeding period, either as good-quality silage or a moderate quality silage with the addition of about 2 kg of concentrates daily. Autumn calving cows achieve greater weight gains during the summer at pasture and regularly achieve body condition scores of 3 or better at calving. In fact, there is a danger that cows become over fat, and pasture restriction may be necessary prior to calving. Nutrition is not as important following successful breeding and a body condition score of 2 is adequate at turnout in spring.

4.8.3 Breeding Seasons

The season of calving influences both the breeding management and the yearly feeding program. The winter feed requirements of a cow rearing one calf are about 1.5 times those for a pregnant cow. Thus, autumn-calving cows lactating throughout the winter require about 1.8 tonnes more silage over a 5-month winter period than spring-calving cows. In the spring-calving suckling system there may be two target calving periods:

- **Early spring** calving (January and February) where the intention is to produce a strong calf at turnout to grass, especially in the early grass growing areas, and a heavy weanling by the autumn;
- **Late spring** calving (mid-February to mid-April) targeted at turnout to grass from mid- to late March.

4.8.4 Artificial Insemination

The success of any AI program depends on two main factors:

- **Heat (oestrus) detection** rate, shown to be 75% in good dairy herds;
- **Conception** rate to AI, with success rate to natural service shown to be 60%.

Heat detection in suckler herds is more difficult than in dairy herds. The intensity of heat is not as strong and does not last as long. The cow in heat is the one that stands to be mounted. However, cows that are most active at mounting are usually those cows which have either been recently in heat themselves or are about to come into heat shortly. Detecting the highest possible number of cows in heat each day during the breeding season presents a major challenge for suckler herd owners. In dairy herds it has been shown that early morning and late evening are the best times for observing the highest proportion of cows in heat. These data also indicate that three further checks at about 3–4 hours apart are required to detect 90% of cows in heat. Therefore, to achieve the highest possible number of cows in heat each day of the breeding season requires five regulated daily inspections.

4.8.5 Oestrus Synchronization

Oestrus (heat) synchronization is a management practice that can help beef producers improve production efficiency and economic returns. It can help shorten the breeding and calving seasons and help increase calf weaning weights. Its purpose is to control oestrus and ovulation in cycling females, so that breeding can be completed in a short period of time. Instead of females being bred over a 21-day period, synchronization can shorten the breeding period to less than 5 days, depending on the programme selected. The use of synchronization has great potential for improving beef production, but it requires good management for success. Producers should understand the advantages of, as well as the requirements for, a successful oestrus synchronization programme. They should also know how the different oestrus synchronization products and programmes work, and the expected results and costs involved before initiating the practice.

4.8.5.1 Requirements for Oestrus Synchronization

1) A well-planned and implemented programme for successful results.
2) Fertile heifers and cows on an adequate nutrition programme.
3) Quality semen for AI, and experienced inseminators.
4) Healthy, aggressive, fertile bulls for synchronized natural breeding.
5) Sufficient labour input at breeding and calving times.
6) If possible, facilities for bad weather during concentrated breeding and calving periods.

4.8.6 Management around Calving

Management of the suckler cow in the final two months of pregnancy can have a major influence on cow health, calf survival and calf diseases. The increased use of highly muscled bulls has inevitably increased the risk of obstetric problems. However, this can be offset by attention to body condition of the cow and feeding during the final two months of pregnancy. The ideal condition score (CS) at calving is 2.50 to 3.25. Above a CS of 3.5 there is an increase in calving difficulty. Cows with a body condition score higher than 3 should be on a restricted diet and given as much exercise as possible.

Cows whose CS is below 2 should be separated and given extra feed but care should be taken in the final month as the calf is now putting on about 0.5 kg per day. The weight gain of the calf over the final 4 to 6 weeks has a big influence on calving problems. The overall 'fitness' of the cow also has a bearing on calving process, so exercise is important too. The interval from calving to first ovulation in beef cows is highly dependent on body condition. This is another reason to optimize body condition at calving. Increasing the level of postpartum nutrition for a thin cow, even to very high levels, has a negligible effect on the interval to first ovulation.

4.8.7 Management of Cows and Calves

Ideally, spring-calving herds should be turned out to grass before calving but, because of the fickle nature of the spring and the shortness of the summer in classic beef country, this is usually impracticable. This means indoor calving, which carries severe risks of infection. The main problems of infectious disease for the newborn calf in a suckler herd are septicaemia, usually caused by *Escherichia coli*, and enteritis caused by viruses such as Rotavirus. Both organisms are inevitable inhabitants of winter accommodation for adult cattle. Calves born into such an environment can be infected with *E. coli* at birth and the resultant septicaemia may (at worst) kill them within two to three days. Rotavirus and other enteroviruses usually induce diarrhoea beginning in the second week of life, which can also be fatal or may severely stunt the calf's development.

Turnout to grass should take place as soon as possible. The main risk for the cows at this time is hypomagnesaemia, and magnesium supplements are essential. If the cows are not getting a concentrate ration, these minerals can be incorporated into a block, added to the water supply or delivered from an intra-ruminal bolus. The bulls are introduced to the cows in June, when the weather is good, and the cows are on a high plane of nutrition and gaining condition. In these circumstances, fertility should be high.

4.8.8 Weaning Suckled Calves

Within seasonal, grassland-based suckler beef production systems in Ireland, the majority of calves are spring-born and reared with their dam at pasture for approximately eight months until the end of the grazing season in autumn when they are weaned. In addition to removal from the dam, the weaning procedure may be compounded by other stressors, e.g. change of diet (grass and milk to conserved feed with or without concentrates), change of environment (outdoors to indoors), transport/marketing, de-horning and castration. Weaning therefore is a multifactorial stressor, in which nutritional, social, physical and psychological stress are combined. Psychological stress is present in the form of maternal separation and social disruption, whereas physical and nutritional stressors are often present in the introduction and adaptation to a novel diet and novel environment. At or shortly after weaning, calves are housed indoors over the winter period and offered grass silage, which is generally supplemented with concentrates. Concentrate supplementation of suckling, grazing beef calves prior to weaning is commonly referred to as 'creep feeding', and serves to compensate for decreasing milk yield and forage, and to improve calf weaning weights (Lynch et al. 2019). Additionally, this practice is often advocated as a means of reducing weaning stress in calves through the familiarization to a palatable feed, such as concentrates and has been reported to decrease morbidity in feedlots (www.agriculture.gov.i.e./schemes/Suckler Scheme).

Calves that are weaned abruptly in the autumn, housed and introduced to silage and concentrates have a low feed intake initially. All calves should be provided with a concentrate creep feed prior to weaning. While suckled calves may be slow to adapt to creep feeding, the stress that normally occurs following weaning will be reduced considerably if calves are consuming 1 kg of creep feed daily prior to weaning. The preferred option is to keep the herd in a properly fenced field with a good grass supply or with silage (or hay) fed and the cows removed gradually (up to one-quarter on any one occasion) to a location away from the calves. As the calves remain in the same herd, with adequate feed supplies, the upset caused is reduced considerably. During this period the concentrate creep can be increased gradually to about 1 kg per calf daily. Where calves are intended for castrated, it is preferable that they are castrated at least four weeks prior to weaning date, or at least two weeks after the calf has been weaned (see Section 4.11.1). In Ireland cattle can be castrated, other than by a veterinary practitioner, before it attains six months of age using a Burdizzo or before it attains eight days of age using a rubber ring (DAFM (2014) S.I. 127 of 2014), in both cases without the use of anaesthesia and analgesia (S.I. 107 of 2014). Over these age limits, local anaesthesia, using a prescription only medicine (POM), must be administered by a veterinary practitioner to animals intended for castration. It is illegal to castrate an animal over six months of age without veterinary involvement. In Ireland the Suckler Herds Welfare Scheme was introduced in 2008 in order to improve the standards of animal welfare and the breeding quality of animals in suckler herds. Details are given in Box 4.1 (www.agriculture.gov.i.e./schemes/Suckler Scheme).

4.8.9   Health and Welfare Problems

In general, the spring calving suckler cow is given very little concentrate and therefore has no opportunity to obtain supplementary minerals in the regular diet. The energy and protein requirements of most suckler cows in late pregnancy can be supplied by silage. Normally, grass and good-quality silage are reasonably well balanced in terms of major minerals, but deficiencies of trace elements can occur. The most common trace mineral deficiencies in cattle consuming forage are copper, iodine, selenium and cobalt. Deficiencies can cause a range of health problems that affect growth, performance, disease resistance and reproduction. Some of the chemical symptoms of deficiencies in copper, iodine and selenium are common to each other. These are stillbirths, abortions, lowered immunity to diseases such as calf scours, pneumonia, mastitis and below normal survival rates in calves around the time of birth.

A definitive diagnosis of trace mineral deficiencies can be tedious to obtain. Doing a large range of tests and/or giving a large selection of mineral supplements can be costly. Sometimes a blood test could show a deficiency but if there are no clinical signs and performance is satisfactory there is unlikely to be a response to extra mineral supplementation. Blood samples and feed analysis do not give a full diagnosis and are best used to support a clinical diagnosis by a veterinarian. Suckler cows in late pregnancy can be offered powdered mineral supplements at 100 g/day, which can be sprinkled on the silage or minerals can be offered in mineral blocks or licks. Cows offered poor quality hay or straw should receive mineral supplementation including calcium, phosphorus, sodium and magnesium. However, offering pre-calving cows excessive amounts of calcium combined with low amounts of magnesium can result in milk fever immediately following calving. Therefore, pre-calver minerals should contain little or no calcium (depend on the forage) but up to 15% magnesium in the mineral mix.

4.8.9.1 Acute Hypomagnesaemia (Grass Tetany)

Acute hypomagnesaemia, or grass tetany, is still the biggest killer of suckler cows each year. Cows need to be supplemented with 20 g of magnesium per day during the months of April and May. Mineral feeding options are:

- high magnesium bucket licks – not very expensive but some cows' intake can be very low
- pasture dusting – again, not very expensive and is very effective but can be time consuming to apply
- high magnesium compound feeds – effective but expensive
- water medication – is effective and some products are relatively inexpensive but cows may not drink a lot in wet weather or if fresh water is available from streams
- magnesium bolus – expensive compared to other methods but does provide reasonable control.

4.8.9.2 Mastitis

Of the several causes of mastitis, only microbial infections are important. Although bacteria, fungi, yeasts and possibly virus can all cause udder infection, the main agents are bacteria. The most common pathogens are *Staphylococcus aureus*, *Streptococcus agalactiae*, *Str. dysgalactiae*, *Str. uberis* and *Escherichia coli*, though other pathogens can cause occasional herd outbreaks. Mastitis occurs when the teats of cows are exposed to pathogens which penetrate the teat duct and establish an infection in one or more quarters within the udder. The course of an infection varies; most commonly it persists for weeks or months in a mild form which is not detected by the stockperson (i.e. subclinical mastitis). With some pathogens, typically *E. coli*, the infection is frequently more acute and there is a general endotoxaemia with raised body temperature, loss of appetite and the cow may die unless supportive therapy is given. When clinical mastitis occurs, the effective therapy is a course of antibiotic infusions through the teat duct.

The necessary steps to eliminate infections are:

- treat all quarters of all cows at drying off with antibiotic products specifically designed for dry cow therapy
- cull chronically infected cows.

4.8.9.2.1 *Control of Environmental Mastitis*

The key to controlling environmental mastitis is prevention, by reducing the number of bacteria to which the teat end is exposed.

Attention should be paid to the cows' environment:

- The cow environment should be as clean and dry as possible.
- Cows should not have access to manure, mud, or pools of stagnant water.
- The dry cow's environment is as important as the lactating cow's environment.
- The calving area must be clean.
- Stalls should be properly designed and maintained.

The following factors are important in considering cow bedding:

- The number of bacteria in bedding depends on available nutrients, amount of contamination, moisture and temperature.
- Inorganic materials (such as crushed limestone or sand) are low in nutrients and moisture, and thus low in bacteria.
- Finely chopped organic bedding (such as sawdust, shavings, recycled manure, pelleted corn cobs, various seed hulls, chopped straw) is frequently high in bacteria numbers.

The facts about teat dipping include:

- Post milking teat dipping with a germicidal (germ-killing) dip is recommended.
- Dipping controls the spread of contagious mastitis.
- Teat dipping exerts no control over coliform infections.
- Barrier dips are reported to reduce new coliform infections; however, they do not appear to be as effective against environmental streptococci and the contagious pathogens.
- Attempts to control environmental mastitis during the dry period, using either germicidal or barrier dips, have been unsuccessful.

4.8.9.2.2 *Summer Mastitis*

Autumn-calving cows immediately after weaning and during the six to eight weeks of the dry period are at high risk of summer mastitis. Other high-risk groups are the fattening cull cows and in-calf heifers. Summer mastitis is an acute, painful, bacterial infection of the udder that occurs mainly during the months of July, August and September. Research in the UK indicates that almost 70% of cases occur in August, with 25% split between July and September and the remainder at other times of the year including the winter months. It is believed that flies play a major role in the spread of the disease, first by causing damage to the teat orifice and second by transmitting the bacteria from infected udders to healthy ones. However, the evidence for this is mostly circumstantial, with the highest incidence of the disease coinciding with the month of highest fly populations. While most cases occur in dry cows, in-calf heifers and milking cows are also susceptible. The disease has also been found in maiden heifers and even in male cattle, though this is rare.

4.8.9.3 Parasitic Diseases

The two most important species of parasitic roundworms affecting grazing cattle are *Ostertagia*, which causes gastritis, and *Dictyocaulus*, which causes pneumonia. Both species overwinter on pasture and, therefore, can affect calves shortly after turnout. If, as is likely, the pasture was grazed by cattle the previous year, it pays to delay turning out young calves until early May, by which time most of the over-wintered *Ostertagia* larvae will have died. If calves do become infested and excrete eggs on to the pasture, there is a second build-up of larvae on the pasture by the middle of July. Ostertagiasis in cattle can be controlled effectively by pasture management, but many beef farmers consider it necessary to dose young calves with anthelmintic drugs in their first summer at grass. Cows and yearling cattle that have previously been exposed to a low level of parasitic challenge develop an effective immunity.

The lungworm, *Dictyocaulus*, is a much more dangerous parasite which causes husk or hoose, a severe, incapacitating parasitic pneumonia. Affected animals have difficulty in breathing, develop a characteristic deep, husking cough and lose condition extremely fast. The most elegant way to control husk is to vaccinate the calves with two oral doses of irradiated (and thus attenuated) larvae before turnout. It is, however, often cheaper to control the condition with appropriate anthelmintics.

4.9 Calf Rearing

4.9.1 Birth and Calving Pens

Unless cows are calving outdoors, they should be confined in a spotlessly clean and disinfected calving box and well bedded down with fresh straw to minimize the risk of infection to cow or calf at the time of parturition. Assuming a normal delivery, the first tasks for the stockperson are to ensure that the calf can breathe properly, and then disinfect the navel with iodine or with an antibiotic spray. The next essential is to ensure that the calf drinks an adequate amount of the cow's first milk (colostrum) in the first 12 hours. Colostrum provides not only food but also maternal antibodies to protect the young calf against the common infections that it is likely to encounter in early life (see Section 4.12).

The teats of mature Holstein/Friesian cows may hang far below the abdominal wall and may be difficult for the young calf to locate. If the calf is left with its mother, the stockperson should ensure that it is feeding satisfactorily. Many good stock-people like to remove the calf from its mother as soon as possible, before the maternal bond has developed, to minimize distress for both cow and calf. If so, the cow should be milked out and the calf offered three to four feeds of colostrum during the first day of life. For calves born to Holstein/Friesian cows, each of these first feeds should be of 1.5 litres. Having started rearing the calf individually, it is a matter of choice whether to rear it up to weaning in an individual pen on restricted amounts of milk replacer fed from a bucket twice (or, later once) daily or to rear it in a group with free or controlled access to milk replacer sucked through a teat.

4.9.2 Management of Artificially Reared Calves

This section deals with the artificial rearing of calves born to dairy cows, for the first six months of life, whether destined as dairy replacements or for beef.

Box 4.2 presents a brief summary of the most important aspects of the European Communities (Welfare of Calves) Regulation 1995 and 1998 amendments, which apply to calves less than 6 months of age (see DEFRA 2009a, for legislation relating to farmed cattle). Many of them have relevance to calves reared to produce white veal and were designed to prevent the worst abuses of welfare involved in the practice of rearing these animals on all-liquid diets and in individual pens without bedding. Nevertheless, the principles apply to all calves.

4.9.2.1 Welfare of Calves up to 6 months

According to the European Communities (Welfare of Calves) Regulations 1995 and 1998 amendments (ECWCRA 1995, 1998), calves shall not be kept permanently in darkness and to meet their behavioural and physiological needs, the accommodation shall be well lit, by natural or artificial light, for at least eight hours a day. All housed calves shall be inspected by the owner or the person responsible for the animals at least twice daily and calves kept outside shall be inspected at least once daily. Any calf which appears to be ill or injured shall be treated appropriately without delay and veterinary advice shall be obtained as soon as possible for any calf which is not responding to the stock-keeper's care. Where necessary, sick or injured calves shall be isolated in adequate accommodation with dry, comfortable bedding. Calf accommodation must be constructed in such a way as to allow each calf to lie down, rest, stand up and groom itself without difficulty. No calf shall be confined in an individual pen after the age of eight weeks, unless a veterinarian certifies that its health or behaviour requires it to be isolated in order to receive treatment.

Calves that are kept in groups should have access to an unrestricted space allowance for each calf, which should be at least equal to 1.5 m^2 for calves of less than 150 kg, at least 1.7 m^2 for calves from 150 to 220 kg and at least 1.8 m^2 for calves weighing 220 kg or more. The floor should be smooth, but not slippery to prevent injury to the calves. This floor shall be suitable for the size and weight of the calves and form a rigid, even and stable surface. The lying area shall be comfortable, clean and adequately drained and shall not adversely affect the calves, and appropriate bedding shall be provided for all calves less than two weeks of age (ECWCRA 1995, 1998).

All calves shall be provided with an appropriate diet adapted to their age, weight and behavioural and physiological needs, to promote good health and welfare. To this end, their food shall contain sufficient iron to ensure an average blood haemoglobin level of at least 4.5 mmol/L and a minimum daily ration of fibrous food shall be provided for each calf over

2 weeks of age, the quantity being raised from 50 g to 250 g per day for calves from 8 to 20 weeks old. Calves that are housed in groups and not fed *ad libitum* or by automatic feeding system, should have access to the food at the same time as the others in the group. All calves over 2 weeks of age shall have access to enough quantity of fresh water or be able to satisfy their fluid intake needs by drinking other liquids. However, in hot weather conditions or for calves which are ill, fresh drinking water shall always be available. Finally, calves shall not be muzzled and all calves shall be fed at least twice a day and calves should not be tethered, except for group-housed calves which may be tethered for periods of not more than 1 hour at the time of feeding milk or milk substitute (ECWCRA 1995, 1998).

4.9.3 Systems for Feeding Artificially Reared Calves up to Weaning

4.9.3.1 Bucket Feeding: Twice Daily
During the first week calves should be offered 2 × 1.5 litres/day of milk replacer, reconstituted at 125 g powder/litre (375 g powder/day), which should be offered at blood heat (40°C). During the second week, milk replacer should be increased to 2.0 to 2.5 litres/feed at 125 g powder/litre (500 to 625 g powder/day) and a dry calf starter ration (e.g. based on cereals) and roughage in the form of hay or barley straw should be introduced. Weaning can take place when the intake of calf starter is more than 1 kg/day, on three consecutive days, which occurs at approximately five weeks of age. At this point each calf will have consumed approximately 20 kg of milk powder.

4.9.3.2 Bucket Feeding: Once Daily
During the first and second weeks of life milk replacer should be offered twice daily (see bucket feeding twice daily) and at the third week of age calves can be offered milk replacer at 2.0 to 2.5 litres/day in a single feed that contains 450 to 500 g powder. While starter feed and roughage should be offered, and calves weaned as calves offered milk replacer twice daily (see bucket feeding twice daily). Intake of milk replacer prior to weaning will be approximately 16 kg.

It is essential to provide access to fresh clean water for all calves.

4.9.3.3 Teat Feeding
- Calves may simply be fed once or twice daily from buckets with teats attached. This is natural and healthy.
- Dispensers that deliver freshly mixed milk replacer at blood heat:

1) *Ad libitum* **milk dispensers:** Most calves thrive on this system but intakes of milk powder to 5 weeks of age are likely to exceed 30 kg per calf, which substantially increases feed costs relative to bucket feeding. Moreover, calves that have had *ad libitum* access to milk powder may be eating much less than 1 kg/day of calf starter ration at this time. One strategy to encourage intake of dry feed is to restrict time of access to the teat for the last week

before weaning or make it more difficult for the calves to drink by progressively constricting the milk supply line.

2) **Computerized milk dispensers** which recognize individual calves, wearing transponders, dispense controlled rations (e.g. 400 g/day of milk powder) and provide records of any calf which fails to drink its full ration.

3) **Acidified milk dispensers**: These can deliver acidified milk replacer at room temperature. Acidification helps both to preserve the feed in the dispenser and to reduce the risk of diarrhoea by maintaining a low pH in the abomasum.

4.9.4 The Bought-in Calf

The artificial rearing of calves on their farm of birth can usually be accomplished without mishap. Unfortunately, most beef calves from the dairy herd are moved off their farm of origin at about one to two weeks of age into specialist rearing units. This may involve trips through two or more markets, and transport, sometimes for the full length of the country. Such animals are deprived of normal food, water and physical comfort, and are confused, exhausted and exposed to a wide range of infectious organisms, of which the most important are the *Salmonella* bacteria. By the time they reach their rearing unit, they are likely to be infected, dehydrated and stressed, and need special care if they are to survive.

On arrival, bought-in calves should be rested in comfort in deep straw. In very cold weather, they may benefit from a little supplementary heating for the first two to three days. Water should be available, but they should be offered no milk replacer for at least 2 h after arrival. If they arrive in the evening, they can be left until the following morning. Some people feed 1.5 L of milk powder at 125 g powder/L for the first feed. It is probably wiser to give two 1.5 L feeds of a proprietary glucose/electrolyte solution (or one tablespoonful of glucose and one teaspoonful of common salt in 1.5 L of water) to rehydrate the calves and provide a minimal supply of energy but keep the gut empty of nutrients until the calves have been able to eliminate most of the enteric bacteria acquired in transit. Thereafter, feeding can be as described above. An injection of fat-soluble vitamins A, D and E is also advisable, especially for calves purchased in the late winter. A preferable alternative to this remedial action is for specialist calf rearers to negotiate contracts with dealers who can guarantee to supply calves from their farm of origin to the rearing unit on the same day and with the minimum of disturbance and mixing.

4.9.5 Feeding after Weaning

After weaning, calves are fed a concentrate ration plus hay, straw or silage *ad libitum*. The amount of concentrate being offered and its protein concentration are governed by how fast the calf is expected to grow. If it is to be turned out to grass in the spring and reared for slaughter at 18 to 24 months, it should get no more than 3 kg/day of concentrate with a protein concentration of 180 g/kg plus hay or silage *ad libitum*. Calves in contract-rearing units, which need to achieve as much weight gain as possible by 12 weeks, and barley beef calves, will probably be given unrestricted access to concentrates and consume more than 4 kg/day.

In this case the protein concentration in the post-weaning concentrate diet should be no more than 160 g/kg, and it may pay to feed roughage in the form of straw rather than hay or silage. Since calves are likely to eat less barley straw than hay or silage it follows that they will tend to eat more concentrates when straw is the only source of roughage. If the calves are to be reared intensively on a high concentrate ration and slaughtered at 12 to 16 months of age, it pays to adapt them to a high concentrate ration as quickly as possible. If the mainstay of their subsequent diet is to be grass or maize silage then, equally, it makes sense to introduce these feeds as soon as possible.

4.9.6 Housing Young Calves

The basic requirements of calf housing are that it should be constructed so it can provide clean, dry, draught-free accommodation without risk of injury to the health of animals and workers. The building design needs to allow feeding, cleaning, disinfection and general hygiene along with the thorough inspection of calves and easy stock management. The accommodation needs to have adequate air space and ventilation and there should be space for the isolation of sick calves.

Calves may be kept in single pens, in groups, or in a combination of both. When group penned, the minimum permissible pen floor space per calf of less than 150 kg is 1.5 m^2 but 1.7 m^2 is recommended. Calves between 150 kg and 220 kg have a minimum space requirement of 1.7 m^2 per calf and calves over 220 kg require 1.8 m^2. However, as a general guide a total floor area of 2.3 m^2 per calf with a cubic air capacity of about 7 mm^3 per calf should be provided. For larger herds a double range of pens with a central feeding passage is suitable. The passage shall not be less than 1.2 m wide. Movable pen divisions may be used to facilitate different space requirements and cleaning systems. Individual pens shall be a minimum of 1.0 m wide by 1.5 m in length, but 1.7 m length is recommended, especially for isolation pens.

4.9.6.1 Pens

European Union Regulations state that individual pens for calves except those for isolating sick calves should not have solid walls but shall have perforated walls which allow the calves to have direct visual and tactile contact. Calves more than eight weeks old may not be kept in individual pens unless a registered veterinary surgeon certifies that its health or behaviour requires it to be isolated in order to receive treatment. The greatest threats to the health and welfare of the young calf are infections which may cause septicaemia, enteritis (leading to diarrhoea or scours) and pneumonia (see Section 4.12). The organisms responsible for these conditions are widespread and young calves, especially those which are moved through markets, are practically certain to be exposed to some degree of infection. The prime specification for a calf house is, therefore, that it should be as hygienic as possible, not only on the surfaces of the walls, floor and feeding utensils, but also in the air itself. It should be power washed with hot water or steam and disinfected before the first calves of the season arrive, and this process should be repeated between successive batches. Whenever possible, the rearer of bought-in calves should practice an 'all in, all out' policy and avoid introducing new baby calves into an already infected building. Hygiene and humidity are also controlled by ensuring effective and appropriate drainage under the individual group pens.

Air hygiene is determined mainly by air space per calf and, to a much lesser extent, by ventilation. This is because the animals are the prime source of pathogenic organisms, but ventilation only removes a small proportion of these organisms from the air in the building; most die *in situ* (for further explanation, see Webster 1985). Preweaning calves require 6 m^3 air space per calf to ensure reasonable air hygiene, and post-weaning calves 10 m^3. In temperate climates, effective air movement (a minimum of four air changes per hour) can be achieved by natural ventilation through strategically placed inlets and outlets. Whether reared in groups or individual pens prior to weaning, calves are normally grouped after weaning and reared in follow-on pens. The simultaneous stresses of mixing and weaning can increase the risk of disease at this time, especially pneumonia. One advantage of rearing batches of calves in groups and feeding them from a teat is that they can be kept in the same group and in the same accommodation from the time of arrival until turnout. Calves are initially restrained in the back of the pen by straw bales, which are taken down at weaning and used as bedding. The small increase in feed costs prior to weaning may be more than offset by reductions in the cost of housing and of disease.

4.9.7 Rearing Calves for Veal

The intensive production of veal in Europe and North America in the latter part of the twentieth century involved the confinement of calves for life in individual wooden crates and the feeding of a liquid milk replacer diet, deficient in iron, to ensure white meat. The European Communities (Welfare of Calves) Regulation (1995, 1998; see above) have now prohibited the worst welfare excesses of this system. Calves over eight weeks of age must not be penned individually and the food for all calves shall contain enough iron and a minimum daily ration of fibrous food. Nevertheless, the system continues to present many welfare problems. Group housing is typically on slatted floors, which can become very slippery, especially given the liquid, projectile nature of faeces from calves on liquid diets. This problem is exacerbated when entire bull calves, reared to heavier weights, approach sexual maturity and attempt to mount one another.

4.10   Routine Management Procedures

This section describes routine procedures in husbandry and preventive medicine common to most beef farms. The skills that enable the stockperson or veterinary surgeon to carry out painful procedures like castration and de-horning with speed, safety and humanity are not to be learnt solely from textbooks but by direct, practical instruction from trained operators.

4.10.1 Castration

Castration is performed on calves because it reduces management problems associated with aggressive and sexual behaviour. The production of beef from castrated male cattle is still preferred in Ireland, and in numerous other countries such as the UK, the USA, Australia and New Zealand. Castration is a husbandry procedure, which can cause pain and discomfort, and, if done incorrectly, may result in subsequent health problems.

The legal requirement for the use of anaesthesia for castration in cattle varies considerably between different countries depending on the method involved and the age of animals. In Ireland, use of anaesthesia is required for surgical/Burdizzo castration of cattle over six months of age. In contrast, castration of calves without use of anaesthesia must be done before they reach two months of age in the UK. In Ireland and the UK, rubber ring castration (or use of other devices for constricting the flow of blood to the scrotum) without use of anaesthesia can only be performed in calves less than seven days of age. In New Zealand, cattle over nine months of age must be castrated using an effective anaesthetic. In Germany, castration of cattle without use of anaesthesia is allowed only in animals less than four weeks of age. By contrast, there is no legal requirement for the use of anaesthesia for castration in the USA. In all of the countries where the administration of anaesthesia is required for castration, the procedure must be done either by a veterinarian or under veterinary supervision. This technicality is based on the fact that anaesthesia constitutes an act of veterinary surgery. So far as the welfare of the calf is concerned, anaesthesia would bring relief from pain at any age.

4.10.1.1 Castration Methods

Burdizzo castration is based on the principle that crushing destroys the spermatic cord carrying blood to the testicles, leaving the skin of the scrotum intact. A Burdizzo emasculatome (or clamp) is used to crush the spermatic cord, but blood supply to the scrotum is preserved. Each spermatic cord is crushed twice (second crush below the first) for 10 seconds each along the neck of the scrotum with the Burdizzo clamp to ensure completeness of the castration procedure. With this technique, the testicle is left to atrophy in the scrotum, and because of the lack of an open wound the potential for haemorrhage or infection is minimized.

Banding castration involves use of a specially designed elastic band with the aid of an applicator around the neck of the scrotum, proximal to the testicles. This will cause ischaemic necrosis of the testicles, eventually leading to testicular atrophy and sloughing of the scrotum.

Surgical castration techniques for male cattle involve opening the scrotum with a scalpel or sharp castration knife, to expose the testicles. Traction is then applied manually to the exposed testes and spermatic vasculature to allow complete removal of the testicles. Manual traction usually provides adequate haemostasis for small calves. However, the use of an emasculator in place for 30 seconds that crushes and cuts the spermatic vessels is recommended for all ages to improve haemostasis. Proper surgical hygiene must be observed during the castration procedure to avoid any unnecessary cross-contamination, infections or sepsis. Concurrent clostridial immunization is recommended.

Everybody who rears male calves for beef should ask himself the question 'Is castration necessary?' If the cattle can reach slaughter weight in 18 months or less, the answer is almost certainly no. Entire male cattle grow lean tissue faster than steers or heifers, and the population advantages of bulls have increased in importance since the ban on the use of anabolic steroids as growth promoters for beef cattle.

4.10.2 Disbudding

Disbudding and dehorning are husbandry management procedures, which as a principle are deemed undesirable by society, but permitted in law because there are perceived benefits to human and animal safety. The primary reasons stated for removal of horns or horn buds is to make the handling of cattle easier and to reduce the risk of injuries (in cattle, other animals and human handlers) associated with horned cattle. Disbudding involves the destruction of the cells of the horn bud and is defined as the removal of horns in calves up to two months (mo) of age. Dehorning refers to the removal of the horn after attachment of the horn bud to the skull, occurring at approximately two mo of age. Farmers as well as veterinarians, in many countries, consider removal of the horn buds a painful procedure for calves. Disbudding and dehorning procedures are therefore regulated by animal welfare laws. Within the European Union (EU), the disbudding procedure is regulated by European Council Directive 98/58/EC based on the Recommendation Concerning Cattle. In addition, cautery disbudding is recommended by the European Food Safety Authority, and is the only method allowed in Ireland under S.I. 127 of the Animal Health and Welfare (DAFM 2014), which permits disbudding of calves up to four weeks of age by thermal cauterization (Marquette et al. 2021). Cornual nerve block with local anaesthetic is currently the accepted technique to anaesthetize the horn bud prior to its removal. Under Irish legislation, calves can be disbudded under two weeks of age without use of local anaesthesia or analgesia. Administration of a local anaesthetic as a prescription only medicine (POM) by a non-veterinarian stockperson is permitted under Irish legislation for the disbudding of calves from two weeks to four weeks of age. For calves older than four weeks, administration of a local anaesthetic prior to disbudding under veterinary supervision is mandatory.

4.10.3 Emergency Slaughter

The most humane procedure for slaughtering casualty cattle is for either a veterinary surgeon or a licensed slaughter person to kill the animal on the spot using an approved procedure such as shooting it with a captive bolt and then cutting the throat. If, however, the animal can be transported to an abattoir, it is more likely to be killed and butchered in such a way as to render the meat fit for human consumption. Within the EU the welfare of the animal is now largely covered by the EU Council Regulation (EC) No. 1 of 2005. On 5 January 2007 new EU rule (Council Regulation (EC) 1 of 2005 on the protection of animals during transport and related operations) on the protection of animals during transport came into operation. The Council Regulation has been given legal effect in Ireland by the European Communities

(Animal Transport and Control Post) Regulations 2006 (S.I. No. 675 of 2006; UK legislation see DEFRA 2009b.) The general rule is that unfit animals may only be transported if the intended journey is not likely to cause them unnecessary additional suffering.

Sick or injured animals may be considered fit for transport if they are:

- slightly injured or ill, and transport would not cause additional suffering; in cases of doubt, veterinary advice shall be sought;
- transported under veterinary supervision for or following veterinary treatment or diagnosis. However, such transport shall be permitted only where no unnecessary suffering or ill treatment is caused to the animals concerned.

(Complete list see Annex 1, Chapter 1 of Council Regulation (EC) No 1/2005.)

Transport of weak, sick or injured cattle to a slaughterhouse will clearly cause unnecessary suffering if the animal is in severe pain which is exacerbated by movement; a broken leg is an obvious example. A calf that is too weak to move could reasonably be transported to a slaughterhouse if it is carefully carried on to (and off) the lorry. The larger animal, such as the downer cow that collapses and develops paralysis post-calving, presents a more difficult problem. She may be reasonably comfortable where she lies and equally so if on deep bedding in a lorry. Any procedure that involved dragging the live recumbent cow over the ground to enter and exit the lorry would constitute unnecessary suffering and the owner should arrange for the animal to be killed on the spot. The whole issue of the moving of casualty animals is complex. For advice see the *Fitness to travel: guidance note* (DEFRA 2009b) and EU Council Regulation (EC) No. 1 of 2005. The method of disposal of carcasses should be in accordance with the requirements for the disposal of waste as laid down in Council Regulation 2002/1774/EC (as applicable) (see Annex 1, chapter 21, Disposal of carcasses).

4.11 Calf Health and Welfare

The objective of a well-designed herd health programme is to address multiple areas of management in order to reduce the likelihood of disease outbreaks occurring in calves and adult animals and is a necessary step if economic returns are to be realized. The aim of successful calf rearing is to produce a healthy calf which is capable of optimum performance throughout its life from birth through to finishing. A suitable calf-rearing system has good animal performance with minimal disease and morbidity and optimal growth rates, low cost and labour input. The survival of the calf involves all of those factors, plus a suitable post-birth environment, management and nutrition.

4.11.1 Colostrum

The first and most important feed given a newborn dairy calf is colostrum. Maternal colostrum provides the main source of immunoglobulins for the newborn calf. Immunoglobulins help to maintain the animal's health and reduce mortality rates by helping to eliminate foreign agents in the body such as bacteria and viruses. In the bovine species, immunoglobulins do not cross the placenta in utero, and the newborn calf is, therefore, dependent on antibodies obtained through ingestion of colostrum. The two main classes of immunoglobulin are IgG class (approximately 80%) and IgA (8–10%). IgG protective antibodies operate within the general circulation; IgA provides protection at mucosal surfaces, especially the gut wall. It is of vital importance that all calves are fed two litres of colostrum within one hour of birth and receive a second two-litre feed four to six hours later to ensure that enough IgG is absorbed across the gut wall.

Colostrum feeding should continue as long as possible after birth. While immunoglobulins are not absorbed after 24 hours they continue to provide local protection in the intestinal tract. The timing of colostrum feeding is important due to the loss of absorptive sites in the intestine over the first 24 hours and competition from bacteria in the intestine. Calves that receive inadequate colostrum are more susceptible to neonatal infections. This problem can be particularly severe in calves that that have been moved off their farm of origin and through markets. In these circumstances, there is greater risk of exposure to infection. Circulating IgG levels may be lower due to inadequate colostrum feeding on the farm of origin and less effective when challenged by pathogens from a different source.

4.11.2 Calf Mortality

Calf mortality can best be subdivided into four main categories; abortions (foetal loss at less than or equal to 270 days' gestation), perinatal mortality (foetal loss at greater than 270 days' gestation and mortality during the first 24 hours of life); neonatal mortality (death between 24 hours and 28 days) and older calf mortality (death between 29 and 84 days).

Morbidity and mortality of the young calf represent a major cause of economic concern for beef producers. Septicaemia and enteric disorders caused by strains of *E. coli*, Rotavirus, *Neospora*, Coronavirus, *Cryptosporidium* or by *Salmonella* species are the main cause of neonatal mortality. Older calf mortality is mainly dominated by respiratory infections and salmonellosis. Disease is not a simple matter of exposure of a susceptible animal to an infectious agent such as a bacterium, virus or fungus. Calves are exposed to infectious organisms from the moment of birth, and natural defence mechanisms usually prevent the establishment of disease. Animals develop disease because of a complex relationship between the host (animal), the infectious agent and the environment. Control of the agent is largely based on prevention of exposure, immunity and chemotherapeutic agents (drugs). Diagnosis and correction of health problems usually involves clinical, immunological, haematological and therapeutic approaches. In recent years there has been major emphasis on reducing the reliance on antibiotics in animal production, which demands nutritional management procedures aimed at elevating passive immunity in calves.

4.11.3 Calf Diarrhoea

Outbreaks of diarrhoea in calves are associated with the interaction of potentially pathogenic enteric micro-organisms with the calf's immunity, nutritional state and environment. An outbreak may be triggered by a single infectious agent but is mainly due to mixed infections. The most common organisms involved are *E. coli*, *Salmonella* species, rotavirus, coronavirus and *Cryptosporidium*. Dehydration, acidosis, impaired growth rate and death are the major consequences. A number of preventive measures have been adopted to control calf diarrhoea. Control of *E. coli* infection may be achieved by hyperimmunization of the dam with an *E. coli* antigen, thereby providing passive immunity to the calf (via ingested colostrum) during the first two to three weeks of life, before it can produce its own antibodies.

4.11.3.1   Salmonellosis

Salmonellosis in calves is mainly caused by the organisms *Salmonella dublin* or *S. typhimurium*. *S. typhimurium* DT104 is highly pathogenic to calves, resulting in a high incidence of mortality. Furthermore, it has a wide range of antibiotic resistance and is capable of rapidly developing new resistance patterns. It is also an important cause of human food poisoning. In acute cases of calf salmonellosis, a septicaemia may occur, accompanied by blood-stained diarrhoea. Calves that are affected more severely have an elevated body temperature (greater than 40°C), are debilitated and have reduced feed intake. The calf may become infected as early as the second day of life, with highest incidences occurring at one to five weeks of age. Outbreaks of *S. typhimurium* are usually associated with purchased calves. Salmonellosis superimposed on calves with pre-existing pneumonia leads to an exacerbation of clinical signs and pulmonary damage. Thus, purchased calves should be carefully examined on arrival so that any infection may be quickly diagnosed. Prevention is again highly dependent on ensuring that the calf receives adequate colostrum after birth.

4.11.4   Respiratory Disease

The underlying cause of bovine respiratory disease (BRD) is extremely complex, with the involvement of viruses, bacteria and *Mycoplasma*. The incidence of infection (morbidity) is usually high, but the mortality rate is variable. Viruses that have been predominantly isolated from outbreaks of calf pneumonia are infective bovine rhinotracheitis (IBR), respiratory syncytial virus (RSV), parainfluenza-3 virus (PI-3 virus) and bovine virus diarrhoea–mucosal disease (BVD-MD virus). Predisposing factors are those that affect the magnitude of the infectious challenge (e.g. overstocking, poor hygiene, inadequate ventilation) and those which affect immuno-competence (ability to fight infection). These include stress, draughts and fluctuating temperatures, poor nutrition and/or concurrent disease. In most cases it would appear that the primary infective agent is viral, producing respiratory tract damage that is subsequently extended by *Mycoplasma* and secondary bacterial infections. Viruses are unaffected by antibiotics; however, antibiotic treatment is usually administered to treat secondary bacterial infections. *Mycoplasma* species are resistant to antibiotics which act on the cell wall, and an antibiotic specific to the cell nucleus is required to inactivate it. In order to direct the appropriate treatment strategy, nasal swabs should be submitted to the appropriate regional veterinary laboratory for accurate identification of the pathogen(s) involved. In addition, *Mycoplasma* species are known to suppress the calf's immunity to disease. Of these, *M. bovis* is the most pathogenic and can act in unison with *Pasteurella* species to produce a very severe form of pneumonia. Following suppression of immunity the animal's ability to withstand an attack from *Pasteurella* and other organisms is reduced. *P. haemolytica* is an important secondary agent in respiratory disease. Pathological changes occur in the lung tissue, leading to consolidation and respiratory distress. Negative consequences for the welfare of animals that survive a respiratory disease attack are that they may end up as 'respiratory cripples' with permanent lung damage.

Bovine respiratory disease, which can terminate fatally, affects both the dairy and beef industry and is the most important disease affecting calves in terms of animal welfare and agricultural economics. In an Irish survey in a slatted unit containing 6399 beef cattle, over a six-month period respiratory disease was the most frequently recorded cause of morbidity and mortality, and this observation agrees with reports from large feedlots in the USA.

Outbreaks of respiratory disease occur throughout the year but are particularly common in late autumn and early winter when young animals are brought indoors. Disease occurrence is most common in herds of two- to six-month-old animals; in severe outbreaks most calves in a herd are affected. Environmental factors and adverse animal management practices can also predispose animals to disease. Environmental factors include draughts, inadequate ventilation and poor air hygiene which facilitate the spread of infectious agents within the herd. The importance of sound animal management cannot be overlooked and factors such as adequate colostrum intake in early life, prevention of co-mingling of different age groups and avoidance of stressful procedures (e.g. weaning, castration, de-horning) during high-risk periods for disease cannot be overemphasized.

Numerous vaccines provide a range of combinations of live and/or killed antigens, active against IBR, RSV and PI-3 virus, *Pasteurella* spp. and *Haemophilus somnus*. Intramuscular modified-live virus vaccines quickly induce long-lasting immunity. Intranasal modified-live virus vaccines induce immunity at the mucosal surface. However, response to these vaccines is only evident in calves over one month of age when their own immune system is active. It is difficult to successfully vaccinate young calves against these diseases because protective colostral antibodies block the vaccine, resulting in maternal antibody interference with vaccination. Development of vaccines effective against the *Pasteurella* organisms and other bacteria that cause pneumonia has been difficult, and success cannot be guaranteed.

Detection methods for respiratory distress are mainly based on visual inspection; however, this method has proven to have limited sensitivity (62%) for detecting BRD. Currently, the detection of microbial agents associated with the BRD is slow, difficult and expensive. Accurate detection of BRD is crucial for effective treatment; however, detection is difficult as cattle do not show clinical signs of the disease until the later stages of the disease process. Furthermore, some of the symptoms associated with BRD such as depression, loss of appetite and increased rectal temperature are not specific to BRD. Early detection of BRD can be achieved by blood tests studying the acute phase proteins and serum haptoglobin can signal if an animal is infected with BRD.

More recently, there have been advances in technology that can aid with the detection of BRD. The Whisper® Veterinary Stethoscope System (Whisper, Geissler Corporation, MN,

USA) is a computer-aided lung auscultation system that classifies acoustic patterns in lung sounds that has been developed to diagnose BRD. The Whisper system contains a stethoscope that measures lung sounds, and a software package that analyses these sounds and assigns an objective score between 1 and 5 (1 = normal, 5 = chronic) to each animal. The Whisper stethoscope score, coupled with measuring rectal temperature, has proven successful in the early detection of BRD.

4.11.4.1 Bioacoustics for Early Detection of Bovine Respiratory Disease in Calves

In recent years, monitoring techniques have been developed to discriminate cough sounds, along with an algorithm for automatic detection of coughing sounds. These monitoring bioacoustics using microphones show good precision and sensitivity. They can monitor many individuals. They are non-invasive and non-contact so do not influence the animals in their normal behaviour and have no need for light to do accurate measurements.

4.11.4.2 Prevention of Pneumonia in Calves

The following are important factors in prevention of pneumonia.

- Many vaccines provide a variety of combinations of live and/or killed antigens. However, experience indicates that responses to these vaccines were only evident in calves > 2 months of age, when their own immune system was active.
- Good housing, good nutrition (including mineral and vitamin supplements) and good management, while not preventing an outbreak of respiratory disease in calves, undoubtedly minimize the long-term negative effect of the disease. They allow a more rapid recovery, thereby preventing the development of chronic cases.
- Rear calves in groups of similar age in well-ventilated draught-free buildings.
- Work in close association with the veterinary surgeon. Collection of nasal mucus samples or swabs for laboratory diagnosis will direct the administration of the appropriate antibiotic treatment.
- Regular temperature checking is useful to guide both diagnosis and observation of treatment effect.
- Minimize exposure of the calf to the infectious agent. This may be achieved using closed herds, screened replacements and positive herd immunity.
- Oral rehydration is particularly beneficial under practical conditions, as loss of body fluid is often associated with pneumonia.
- Vaccination may help to attain optimum livestock productivity through disease prevention. However, vaccination is effective only against specific organisms.
- Note the overall role of pre- and postnatal nutrition, including trace elements and vitamin supply.
- In those herds that are known to have trace element deficiencies, or to have a high tetany risk, young calves may need supplementary magnesium and trace elements for optimal health and immune status.

4.12 Finishing Beef Cattle

This section describes the management of cattle reared for prime beef from weaning, in the case of suckled calves, or six months of age, for artificially reared calves, to the time of slaughter.

4.12.1 Winter Feeding

Two classes of beef animals will require winter feeding in yards:

1) Weanlings from the suckler herds and store animals from dairy/beef systems animals entering their first winter and at least a year from slaughter
2) Finishers – animals being finished for slaughter over the winter.

The main difference, from a feeding viewpoint, between the two types is that weanlings have time after the winter to exhibit compensatory growth whereas the finishers do not. However, weanlings are still immature and relatively underdeveloped, so a minimum rate of gain is necessary to ensure essential bone and muscle growth. For dairy calf-to-beef production systems this minimum has been set at about 0.5 kg/day.

Grass silage is an integral part of most beef production farming systems in northern and north-western Europe. Besides silage being an important feedstuff for cattle, especially when they are housed indoors, silage production can be integrated into farming systems in a manner that makes an essential positive contribution to both effective grassland management and internal parasite control with grazing animals. Furthermore, nutrients collected from housed livestock can be best recycled by spreading the manures on the grassland used for producing silage. Generally, the level of concentrates fed to weanlings and store cattle in winter is low. Reducing or eliminating concentrate feeding towards the end of winter is sometimes practiced. Within the EU, beef production has been influenced by legislative requirements, such as age limits for the application of premiums and the ban on the sale of animals over 30 months of age (to control the threat of BSE). Such requirements have been gradually removed and animals are likely to be finished at an age that best suits market demands.

Most beef finishing systems use a confinement system based on conserved forages (e.g. grass or maize silage) and concentrates composed mainly of grains (e.g. barley), protein sources (e.g. soya bean meal) by-products (e.g. non-forage fibre sources), minerals and vitamins. Concentrates are a major cost element in feeding beef cattle in winter, particularly finishing cattle. The optimal feeding system is one that considers daily live-weight gain, feed efficiency, seasonal variations in market prices and regional variations in perception of beef quality. When forages are supplemented with concentrates, forage intake declines. This is known as substitution. The present economic level of concentrate supplementation for finishing steers offered silage *ad libitum* is in the range 4 to 7 kg per head daily depending on factors such as concentrate costs; type of animal being finished and anticipated carcass price. Concentrates are normally fed at a flat rate throughout the finishing period either as one or two discrete meals per day or as part of a mixed ration. In recent years, mainly because of the need to hold cattle until specific dates to collect premiums, the practice of varying the level of concentrates throughout the finishing period has developed. Feeding a lower level early on prevents animals being finished before their eligible premium dates, and then if they are not finished as the eligible premium date approaches, the level of concentrates is increased to permit rapid disposal after the retention date has passed. Manipulating growth rates in the finishing period can have an adverse effect on meat quality as there is evidence that a declining rate of gain before slaughter predisposes to poorer-quality meat. Furthermore, Mediterranean markets require carcasses with muscle which is light red in colour and fat which is white in colour. These colour traits are more likely when animals are fed a high level of concentrates towards the end of the finishing period.

4.12.2 Housing and Welfare

Housing protects animals from adverse weather conditions and provides structured management (feeding, drinking, health check, etc.) under controlled conditions. In many Irish beef production systems, animals are generally housed in a concrete slatted-floored facility for a four- to five-month winter period at 2.2 m^2 per head for 500 kg animals (Dodd 1985) and fed *ad libitum* grass silage with concentrate supplementation. Provision of adequate space allowances during the housing period for cattle determines their welfare status. High stocking densities of less than 2.0 m^2 per head have been shown to adversely affect the frequency and duration of lying and levels of aggression within groups. Animal behavioural studies indicate that intensive stocking rates on slatted floors can present a significant challenge to the successful adaptation of cattle to confinement. Cattle are social animals and establish social bonds and hierarchy among themselves. In large groups (>100 animals) with minimum space allowances, individual animals appear to have difficulty in memorizing the social status of all peers, which increases the incidences of social aggressiveness and oral stereotypies in cattle. The abrupt breakage of the social bond or hierarchy through regrouping and relocating may lead to social stress and an animal may respond with abnormal behaviour and impaired performance. European beef production systems generally consist of a grazing season followed by a four to five-month winter housing period. Recently, there have been growing concerns regarding the welfare of beef cattle accommodated indoors, particularly in relation to floor type and space allowance. A review (22 papers) and research studies completed at Teagasc showed housing beef cattle on concrete slatted floors, with and without overlaid with rubber had no effect on feed conversion efficiency, gain or carcass weight but resulted in a greater number of hoof horn lesions. In terms of space allowance on concrete slats (2.0, 3.0, 4.5 and 6.0 m^2 per head) and on straw with 6.0 m^2 per head, found that heifers given 4.5 m^2 per head had a greater gain and lying time than those with 3.0 and 6.0 m^2; however, space allowance had no effect on carcass weight and while 3.0 m^2 per animal was enough space for housing finishing heifers, while 2.0 m^2 per animal was too low. However, as animal grow space requirement increases and the equation $y = 0.033w^{0.667}$ was enough to estimate the space requirements of finishing beef cattle on concrete slatted floors (Keane et al. 2018a, 2018b).

4.12.3   Summer Grazing and Pasture Management

The allocation of summer pasture for all animals should be enough to meet their feed requirements. A supply of clean fresh water should always be available, and the pasture area should be free of hazards that may cause injury to the animals. An adequate supply of good-quality pasture for suckler cows in spring and early summer ensures rapid weight recovery, good milk production and good reproductive activity. Paddock grazing or the use of a buffer area allows better budgeting of the grass available, thereby matching the demand of the animals with grass supply. A flexible approach to grassland management is essential to control within- and between-year variation in grass growth.

Overstocking that results in cows losing weight is not acceptable and it may be necessary to reduce the stocking rate in autumn or during dry summers in order to maintain adequate feed supply. Overstocking in the autumn lowers calf growth and the cow will not establish adequate body condition to sustain her during the winter period. Moreover, delays in weaning on scarce autumn pasture can also result in rapid loss of body condition in suckler cows.

4.13   Handling, Transport and Slaughter

4.13.1   Handling

Although cattle are a domesticated species, the handling of cattle by humans can result in increased stress, agitated behaviour and even injury or death, especially if the animals are not used to being handled or are handled in an inappropriate manner. The following recommendations are designed to ensure good welfare during the handling and movement of cattle.

- Animals should be treated and handled in a manner which avoids injury and stress. Goads or electric prodders should not be used.
- The movement of animals from one paddock to another, or to penning facilities, should be done without recourse to excessive force. Beating the animals, or the presence of an untrained aggressive dog which causes the animals to panic, is not acceptable.
- At the time of movement, check for any abnormal behaviour, lameness, reluctance to move or isolation from the remainder of herd.
- Cattle need to see where they are expected to move to, i.e. if going indoors or into a truck make sure that lights are on and corridors are clear.

Grandin (2007) has pioneered the design and management of high-welfare handling systems for cattle. One essential feature of these is proper attention to the principle of the flight zone (Figure 4.4). The flight zone is described as the area around an animal, which if penetrated by the handler, will be re-established by the animal by moving away. Flight zones can vary widely depending on whether an animal has been raised in extensive or confined conditions and its level of tameness or wildness. To avoid undue agitation of the animal, the handler should work at the edge of the flight zone. If the handler penetrates the flight zone too deeply, the animal may try to run back past the handler, or if it is in a race, rear up and attempt to escape (Grandin 1992).

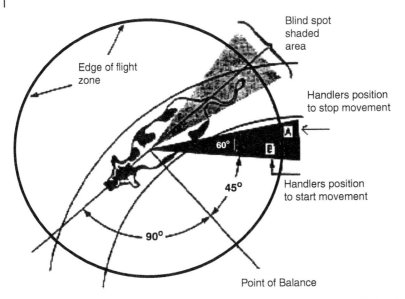

Figure 4.4 The flight zone. *Source*: (Grandin 2007). Reproduced with permission from Professor Temple Grandin.

4.13.2 Transport

The transport of livestock can have major implications for their welfare, and there is strong public interest and scientific endeavour aimed at ensuring that the welfare of transported animals is optimal. Physical factors such as noise or vibrations; psychological/emotional factors, such as unfamiliar environment or social regrouping; and climatic factors, such as temperature and humidity, are also involved in the transport process. Alterations in immune function resulting from transport stress are particularly relevant to younger animals, and illness in young cattle following road haulage is not uncommon. The handling and marketing of animals prior to the journey to the abattoir must not involve extended periods of feed withdrawal as, in addition to the welfare consequences, this will result in bodyweight loss and reduction in meat quality. Feed withdrawal will also increase the impact on animal welfare, through hunger and metabolic stress.

While it is well established that transportation of cattle is a stressor that causes a quantifiable response measured, for example, by a significant increase in blood cortisol, stress during transport resulting in physiological or pathological changes can be reduced with good management practices. The age of the cattle transported can have a great effect as instances of morbidity and mortality are greater in transported calves younger than three weeks of age, which may be compounded by the stress incurred by simultaneous weaning. One of the most prevalent examples of transport stress is 'shipping fever' in transported cattle. The disease may have first appeared as early as the late 1800s to early 1900s when cattle were first transported by railroad. The aetiology of shipping fever is complex. However, the simple definition, 'the occurrence of pulmonary infections during or after transit,' is accurate enough.

4.13.3   Stunning and Slaughter

The purpose of stunning an animal before slaughter is to render it unconscious and hence insensible to pain, before death occurs due to exsanguination. Conventionally, cattle have been stunned mechanically, such as by captive bolt, although there is some commercial use of electrical stunning, e.g. in New Zealand and the UK. The captive bolt, when used correctly, has been shown to be an extremely effective method of stunning. Halal (Islamic) or Shechita (Jewish) ritual slaughter often involves the throat-cutting of cattle which have not been stunned. Since 1995 animal welfare legislation around slaughter has been covered by Council Directive 93/119/EEC covering a wide range of animals and slaughter circumstances. The European Commission has revised the legislation to reflect new knowledge and advanced scientific evidence and the new Regulation (Council Regulation 1099/2009) was published in 2010. Information on humane killing and slaughter methods, together with the relevant legislation, is provided by the Humane Slaughter Association (https://www.hsa.org.uk). Methods of restraint causing avoidable suffering must not be used in conscious animals because they cause severe pain and stress:

- Suspending or hoisting animals (other than poultry) by the feet or legs;
- Indiscriminate and inappropriate use of stunning equipment;
- Mechanical clamping of the legs or feet of the animals (other than shackles used in poultry and ostriches) as the sole method of restraint;
- Breaking legs, cutting leg tendons, or blinding an animal to immobilize them; severing the spinal cord;
- The dragging of disabled animals and other animals unable to move while conscious is prohibited; stunned animals may, however, be dragged.
- Conscious animals should not be dragged, dropped or thrown (OIE, 2008, Animal welfare code https://www.oie.int/en/home).

4.14   Animal Welfare and the Beef Industry

The scientific consideration of farm animal welfare is important, due to the ethical obligation to maximize health and well-being and eliminate suffering in animals that are under human stewardship, and the need to fulfil the requirements and demands of the general community and to improve the efficiency of animal agriculture by optimizing animal health and productivity. In addition, within the European Union, the OIE, community-wide legislation is continually being changed/drafted and implemented with a view to safeguarding farm animal welfare, and it is important that such laws be based on objective, evidence-based scientifically derived information. In 2017 the EU commissioned an expert group 'Platform on Animal Welfare' and this European Commission is responsible for:

- providing appropriate information and where necessary training on EU legislative requirements
- ensuring that EU legislation is properly implemented and enforced
- in extreme cases ta action against EU countries that have failed to implement legal requirements

How this is achieved:

- inspections and controls undertaken by the Food and Veterinary Office to check that competent authorities in EU countries apply EU legislation in an effective and uniform way
- the Standing Committee on the Food Chain and Animal Health provides a platform for representatives of the Member States to discuss issues of public or animal health or animal welfare and when necessary approve urgent measures
- For scientific opinions reference is made to EFSA (European Food Safety Authority)

Welfare quality assessment has been developed, which scores animal feeding, housing, health and behaviour (Table 4.11) to calculate an overall cumulate comprehensive score, which suitable for research, but needs to be simplified for commercial use or farmers. This indicates a drive to include positive states in welfare assessments and this is highlighted in the Five Domains model (Table 4.12).

In Ireland and Belgium beef producers use an animal welfare index (AWI), which incorporates elements of the Austrian Tiergerechtheitindex (TGI) animal needs index, which use methods that assess the housing system and the management of a farm through selected indicators (Mazurek et al. 2010; Lawrence et al. 2014).

4.14.1 Factors Affecting Animal Welfare

Many factors contribute to the overall welfare of domestic farm animals and beef cattle. These factors may be endogenous or exogenous, directly and indirectly influencing

Table 4.11 Principles and criteria for good welfare.

Principles	Welfare criteria
Good feeding	1) Absence of prolonged hunger
	2) Absence of prolonged thirst
Good housing	3) Comfort around resting
	4) Thermal comfort
	5) Ease of movement
Good health	6) Absence of injuries
	7) Absence of disease
	8) Absence of pain induced by management procedures
Appropriate behaviour	9) Expression of social behaviours behaviour
	10) Expression of other behaviours
	11) Good human-animal relationship
	12) Positive emotional state

Source: (Blokhuis et al. 2010).

Table 4.12 Animal welfare perspectives of the five freedoms, domains and welfare principles of the welfare quality project.

Five Freedoms [1]	Welfare principles [2]	Five domains [3]
Hunger and thirst	Good feeding	Food and water deprivation
Discomfort	Good housing	Environmental challenge
Pain, injury and disease	Good health	Disease and injury
Fear and stress	Appropriate behaviour	Behavioural restriction
Normal behaviour		
		Mental state

[1] UK Farm Animal Welfare Council (1993, 2009).

[2] Welfare quality project (WQP) Blokhuis et al. (2010).

[3] Mellor and Beausoleil (2015).

Table 4.13 Endogenous ad exogenous factors affecting farm animal welfare.

Endogenous		Exogenous	
Genetic or physical conditions	Social conditions	Physical environment	Social environment
Breed	Competition	Temperature	Housing
Sex	Aggression	Humidity	Feeding
Age	Leadership	Wind	Age
Weight	Dominance behaviour	Photoperiod	Stocking rate/ space allowance
Temperament			

Source: (Grandin 2000; Moberg and Mench 2000).

subsequent responses in the animal and are summarized in Table 4.13. The genetic components of beef cattle and physical conditions they are maintained in are included in the endogenous factors, while the exogenous factors refer to the external environmental and social factors.

4.14.1.1 Animal Health

An animal that is diseased, injured or otherwise in poor health is assumed to have reduced welfare, as basic concepts of animal welfare imply health and well-being. The Brambell Committee Report (Brambell 1965) argued that disease is a principal cause of suffering in

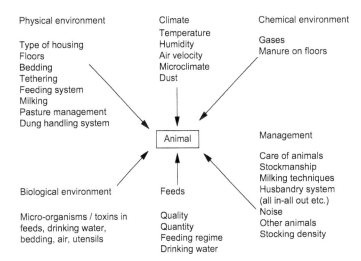

Physical environment

Type of housing
Floors
Bedding
Tethering
Feeding system
Milking
Pasture management
Dung handling system

Climate
Temperature
Humidity
Air velocity
Microclimate
Dust

Chemical environment

Gases
Manure on floors

Animal

Biological environment

Micro-organisms / toxins in
feeds, drinking water,
bedding, air, utensils

Feeds

Quality
Quantity
Feeding regime
Drinking water

Management

Care of animals
Stockmanship
Milking techniques
Husbandry system
(all in-all out etc.)
Noise
Other animals
Stocking density

Figure 4.5 Essential environmental factors affecting animal health.

animals and that measurement of disease or disease risk is of major importance in evaluating the overall welfare of animals. An animal may become diseased or injured through impaired functioning of its immune system, the build-up in its environment of noxious agents or organisms, physical trauma from its surroundings or other animals or inappropriate feeding and management (Webster 1994, 2011). Genetic factors may predispose animals to ill-health, such as the selection for muscle growth or excessive body condition resulting in dystocia. In addition, environmental constraints placed upon animals may lead to the development of pathology, such as horn quality and growth. The type of disease condition recorded, and the way that it is measured will depend on the type of animal, its environment and the management system, while most environmentally induced problems for animal health are multifactorial in nature (Figure 4.5).

4.14.1.2 Application of Production Measurements to the Evaluation of Welfare

Animal production measurements can be a useful component of welfare assessment as they provide a medium to long-term measure of animal responses and can be quite sensitive to adverse husbandry situations and procedures, such as rates of dystocia, carcase scores, morbidity and mortality rates. Where 'welfare-friendly' systems are being developed, measurements of animal production also ensure that such systems are commercially practicable. Measurements of animal production alone, especially if evaluated on a system, rather than on an individual animal, basis, are usually not sufficient to determine animal wellbeing, as the most efficient systems in terms of production may not satisfy individual animal requirements, such as the freedom to express normal behaviour.

4.15   Precision Livestock Farming

More precision livestock farming (PLF) applications are being used in the beef industry and these are based upon using monitoring systems (through image and sound analysis techniques, sensors and ICT) to monitor animals' health status and welfare and detect diseases and disorders at an early stage. Farmers can, by automating the process, receive real-time information about their livestock and optimize animal health and welfare in a timely and accurate way. These include computer-controlled feeders, which recognize individual animals, are increasingly being used on dairy and beef farms and can automatically record aspects of feeding behaviour, that may help detect animals that are sick through changes in feeding behaviour.

Other areas include a category of automation consists of devices that can be attached temporarily to the animals specifically for monitoring their behaviour. These are most commonly accelerometers, but other devices such as pedometers, simple tilt switch devices or GPS devices have also been used. Several relatively cheap, small and accurate electronic devices are now available that can be used to measure the time animals spend standing and lying. Accelerometers attached to various body parts have been used to automatically detect the occurrence of other behaviour patterns such as sleep patterns in dairy calves, while other devices have also been used to automatically record animals' location.

Ready availability digital imagery along with the development of computer programmes that can 'read' such images, has resulted in the possibility of using automated image analysis ('computer vision') to take measures of animal behaviour and computer programmes have been used to detect behaviour changes caused by lameness. In recent years considerable improvements in experimental outcomes with computer vision-based technologies have come about due to advancements in the field of algorithms called convolutional deep neural networks. Applications include the estimation of live weight from images of beef cattle.

References

Blokhuis, H.J., Veissier, I., Miele, M., and Jones, B. (2010). The Welfare Quality® project and beyond: safeguarding farm animal well-being. *Acta Agriculturae Scandinavica: Section A, Animal Science* 60(3): 129–140.

Brambell, R. (1965). *Report of the Technical Committee to Enquire into the Welfare of Animals Kept under Intensive Livestock Husbandry Systems*. London: Her Majesty's Stationary Office.

ECWCRA. (1995). Statutory Instrument (S.I.) No. 90 of 1995 - European Communities (Welfare of Calves) Regulations, 1995. https://www.irishstatutebook.ie/eli/1995/si/90/made/en/print (accessed 14 December 2021).

ECWCRA. (1998). Statutory Instrument (S.I.) No. 138/1998 - European Communities (Welfare of Calves) Regulations, 1998. https://www.irishstatutebook.ie/eli/1998/si/138/made/en/print (accessed 14 December 2021).

Farm Animal Welfare Council (FAWC). (1993). *Second Report on Priorities for Research and Development in Farm Animal Welfare*. Tolworth, UK: MAFF.

Farm Animal Welfare Council (FAWC). (2009). *Farm Animal Welfare in Great Britain: Past, Present and Future*. London, UK: Farm Animal Welfare Council

Grandin, T. (2000). *Livestock Handling and Transport*. 2e. Wallingford, UK: CABI.

Keane, M.G. and Allen, P. (1999). Effects of pasture fertiliser N level on herbage composition, animal performance and on carcass and meat quality traits. *Livestock Production Science* 61: 233–244.

Keane, M.P., McGee, M., O'Riordan, E.G., Kelly, A.P., and Earley, B. (2018a). Effect of floor type and space allowance on performance and welfare of finishing beef cattle: a meta-analysis. *Livestock Science* 212: 57–60.

Keane, M.P., McGee, M., O'Riordan, E.G., Kelly, A.P., and Earley, B. (2018b). Performance and welfare of steers housed on concrete slatted floors at fixed and dynamic (allometric based) space allowances. *Journal of Animal Science* 3: 880–889.

Kelly, A.K., McGee, M., Crews, Jr., D.H., Fahey, A.G., Wylie, A.R. and Kenny, D.A. (2010). Effect of divergence in residual feed intake on feeding behavior, blood metabolic variables and body composition traits in growing beef heifers. *Journal of Animal Science* 88: 109–123.

Lawrence, P., McGee, M., and Earley, B. (2014). Animal welfare index (AWI): an on-farm welfare evaluation of beef farms in Ireland and Belgium. Irish Journal of Agricultural and Food Research. In: Proceedings of the Agricultural Research Forum, Tullamore, Co. Offaly, Ireland: 10th March 2014, P17 (peer reviewed).

Mazurek, M., Prendiville, D., Crowe, M.A., Veissier, I., and Earley, B. (2010). An on-farm investigation of beef suckler herds using an animal welfare Index (AWI). *BMC Veterinary Research* 6: 55.

McGee, M. (2005). Recent developments in feeding beef cattle on grass silage-based diets. In: *Silage Production and Utilisation. Proceedings of the XIVth International Conference (a Satellite Workshop of the XXth, International Grassland Congress), July 2005, Belfast, Northern Ireland* (ed. R.S. Park and M.D. Stronge), 51–64. Wageningen Academic Publishers.

Mellor, D.J. and Beausoleil, N.J. (2015). Extending the 'Five Domains' model for animal welfare assessment to incorporate positive welfare states. *Animal Welfare* 2015 (24): 241–253.

Moberg, G.P. and Mench, J.A. (2000). *The Biology of Animal Stress: Basic Principles and Applications for Animal Welfare*. Ed. Wallingford, Oxon, UK. CABI Publishing.

Moloney, A.P. and Drennan, M.J. (2013). Characteristics of fat and muscle from beef heifers offered a grass silage or concentrate-based finishing ration. *Livestock Science* 152: 147–153.

Webster, J. (1994). *Animal Welfare. A Cool Eye Towards Eden*. Oxford, UK: Blackwell Science Ltd.

Webster, J. (2011). Zoomorphism and anthropomorphism: fruitful fallacies? *Animal Welfare* 20: 29–36.

References and Further Reading

Allen, D. (1990). *Planned Beef Production and Marketing*. Oxford: Blackwell Scientific Publications.

Cameron, A. and McAllister, T.A. (2018). Antimicrobial usage and resistance in beef production. *Journal of Animal Science and Biotechnology* (2016) 7: 68

DAFF. (2004). *Expenditure Review of Beef Carcase Classification Scheme*. Dublin, Ireland: Department of Agriculture, Fisheries and Food.

DAFM. (2014). Statutory Instrument (S.I) 127 of 2014. (http://www.irishstatutebook.ie/eli/2014/si/127/made/en/pdf) and S.I. 107 of 2014 (http://www.irishstatutebook.ie/eli/2014/si/107/made/en/print#).

DEFRA. (2003). *Codes of Recommendations for the Welfare of Livestock: Cattle*. London: Department for Environment, Food and Rural Affairs. http://www.defra.gov.uk.

DEFRA. (2009a). *On Farm Animal Welfare Legislation*. London. Department for Environment, Food and Rural Affairs. http://www.defra.gov.uk.

DEFRA. (2009b). *Fitness to Travel: Guidance Note*. London: Department for Environment, Food and Rural Affairs. http://www.defra.gov.uk.

Dodd, V.A. (1985). Housing for a beef unit. Veterinary Update, April, 6–13.

Drennan, M.J. and McGee, M. (2004). Effect of suckler cow genotype and nutrition level during the winter on voluntary intake and performance and on the growth and slaughter characteristics of their progeny. *Irish Journal of Agricultural and Food Research* 43: 185–199.

Drennan, M.J. and McGee, M. (2009). *Producing High Quality Carcasses from Grass-based Suckler Beef Systems*. Occasional report, Teagasc.

Earley, B., McGee, M., and Fallon, R.J. (2000). Serum immunoglobulin concentrations in suckled calves and dairy-herd calves. *Irish Journal of Agriculture and Food Research* 39 (3): 401–407.

Farm Animal Welfare Council. (1986). *Report on the Welfare of Livestock at Markets*. RB 265. London: HMSO.

Grandin, T. (1980). Observations of cattle behavior applied to the design of cattle handling facilities. *Applied Animal Ethology* 6: 19.

Grandin, T. (1992). Handling and transport of agricultural animals used in research. In: *The Well-being of Agricultural Animals in Biomedical and Agricultural Research* (ed. J.A. Mench, S.J. Mayer, and L. Krulisch), 74. Greenbelt, MD: Scientists Center for Animal Welfare.

Grandin, T. (ed.) (2007). *Livestock Handling and Transport*, 3e. Wallingford: CABI Publishing.

Humane Slaughter Association. (2000). Electrical stunning of red met animals. http://www.hsa.org.uk (accessed 14 December 2021).

Humane Slaughter Association. (2001). Captive bolt stunning of livestock. http://www.hsa.org.uk (accessed 14 December 2021).

Humane Slaughter Association. (2004). Emergency killing (video). http://www.hsa.org.uk (accessed 14 December 2021).

Keane, M.G. (1999). Comparison of carcass grades of steers in the Republic of Ireland, Northern Ireland and Great Britain. *Farm and Food* 9: 6–9.

Keane, M.G., O'Riordan, E.G., and O'Kiely, P. (2009). Dairy calf-to-beef production systems. Teagasc, Report.

Lolli, V., Zanardi, E., Moloney, A.P., and Caligiani, A. (2020). An overview on cyclic fatty acids as biomarkers of quality and authenticity in the meat sector. *Foods* 27: 9. (12):1756.

Lynch, E., McGee, M., and Earley, B. (2019). Review: weaning management of beef calves with implications for animal health and welfare. *Journal of Applied Animal Research* 47: 167–175.

Marquette, G.A., McGee, M., Stanger, K., Fisher, A.D., and Earley, B. (2021). Horn bud size of dairy-bred and suckler-bred calves at time of disbudding. *Irish Veterinary Journal* 74: 17.

Ministry of Agriculture, Fisheries and Food. (1983). *Codes of Recommendations for the Welfare of Livestock: Cattle*. London: MAFF Publications.

Ministry of Agriculture, Fisheries and Food. (1984a). *Energy Allowances and Feeding Systems for Ruminants, RB 433*. London: HMSO.

Ministry of Agriculture, Fisheries and Food. (1984b). *Cattle Handling, B 2495*. London: HMSO.

Ministry of Agriculture, Fisheries and Food. (1986). *Annual Reviews of Agriculture*. London: HMSO.

Ministry of Agriculture, Fisheries and Food. (1995a). *Agriculture in the United Kingdom 1994*. London: HMSO.

Ministry of Agriculture, Fisheries and Food. (1995b). *Summary of the Law Relating to Farm Animal Welfare* (reprinted 1998) PB 2531. London: MAFF Publications.

Meat and Livestock Commission. (1994). *Beef Yearbook*. Milton Keynes, UK: MLC.

Molony, A.P. (1999). R & H Hall Technical Bulletin. Issue No. 4.

Moloney, A., O'Riordan, E., Schmidt, O., and Monahan, F. (2018). The fatty acid profile and stable isotope ratios of C and N of muscle from cattle that grazed grass or grass/clover pastures before slaughter and their discriminatory potential. *Irish Journal of Agricultural and Food Research* 57: 84–94.

Montano-Bermudez, M., Nielsen, M.K., and Deutscher, G.H. (1990). Energy requirements for maintenance of crossbred cattle with different genetic potential for milk. *Journal of Animal Science* 68: 2279–2288.

More O'Ferrall, G.J. (ed.) (1982). *Beef Production from Different Dairy Breeds and Dairy Crosses*. The Hague: Martinus Nijhoff.

Murphy, B.M., Drennan, M.J., O'Mara, F.P., and McGee, M. (2008). Performance and feed intake of five beef suckler cow genotypes and pre-weaning growth of their progeny. *Irish Journal of Agricultural and Food Research* 47: 13–25.

Petit, M. and Lienard, G. (1988). Performance characteristics and efficiencies of various types of beef cows in French production systems. *Proceedings of 3rd World Congress on Sheep and Beef Cattle Breeding*, 19–25 June 1988, INRA, Paris, 2: 25–51.

Sarzeaud, P., Becherel, F., and Perot, C. (2008). A classification of European beef farming systems, EAAP Technical series No. 9. in EU beef farming systems and CAP regulations 2008. 23–31.

SCAHAW. (2001). The welfare of cattle kept for beef production. Publication of the European Commission, Health and Consumer Protection Directorate-General by the Scientific Committee on Animal Health and Animal Welfare (SCAHAW) SANCO.C.2/AH/R22/2000. Adopted 25 April 2001. http://europa.eu.int/comm/food/fs/sc/scah/out54_en.pdf (accessed 14 December 2021).

Weary, D.M., Jasper, J., and Hötzel, M.J. (2008). Understanding weaning distress. *Applied Animal Behaviour Science* 110: 24–41.

Webster, A.J.F. (1985). *Calf Husbandry, Health and Welfare*, 2e. London: Collins.

Webster, A.J.F. (1995). *Animal Welfare: A Cool Eye Towards Eden*. Oxford: Blackwell Scientific Publications.

Webster, A.J.F., Saville, C., and Welchman, D.B. (1986). *Alternative Husbandry Systems for Veal Calves*. Bristol: University of Bristol Press.

Williamson, M. (1998). Straw in Europe. Chalcombe Publications, ISBN 0 Q48617411.

5

Sheep

Cathy Dwyer and Pete Goddard

KEY CONCEPTS

Management and Welfare of Farm Animals: The UFAW Farm Handbook, Sixth Edition.
Edited by John Webster and Jean Margerison.

5.1   Introduction

In the past, the focus for animal welfare was on intensive, indoor agriculture, particularly of pigs and poultry, and sheep were not considered to have many real welfare issues, probably because they are usually farmed outdoors with naturalness seen to be important. With much more emphasis now being placed on quality of life aspects, which affect all managed animals, there is a responsibility to consider how livestock management can deliver the greatest welfare benefit to sheep. By using welfare frameworks, such as those provided by the Five Freedoms (Farm Animal Welfare Council 2011) or the Five Domains model (Mellor et al. 2020), and the increased use of proactive farm health plans and risk avoidance strategies, there is the opportunity to consider management actions (or omissions) from the individual sheep's perspective. Production requirements or environmental constraints create welfare challenges, which management needs to mitigate. These challenges include lameness, perinatal lamb loss, undernutrition, internal and external parasitism (and the development of anthelmintic resistance), predation, effects of climatic variability and the impact of specific management practices: castration, tail docking, shearing, transport and slaughter.

The impact of these on sheep welfare can be minimized or eliminated through knowledgeable shepherding and veterinary advice.

This chapter builds on previous editions, providing updated information on developments, thinking and new opportunities for the welfare management of sheep. The chapter provides information about many common sheep management systems and practices, both within the UK and more globally, and emphasizes those human actions that have the greatest potential to affect sheep welfare and considers how the success of these actions can be evaluated.

Since previous editions of this chapter, there have been developments in methods to assess sheep welfare, and to evaluate how well a producer is achieving good welfare. These will be discussed. The fact that the public already believes sheep systems to have an inherently high level of welfare, due primarily to the high degree of naturalness and lack of intensification, may have resulted in less focus on welfare assessment in this sector. Consequently, there is less consumer pressure to encourage sheep producers to adopt higher standards through the sale of welfare-premium products. However, there have been developments, for example, in commitments to tackle issues such as lameness or neonatal mortality, that are having an impact on sheep welfare.

5.2 The Sheep Industry Worldwide

5.2.1 Development and Structure of the Industry

There are well over a billion sheep worldwide, living in widely different environments and managed in diverse ways, from nomadic subsistence systems to the intensive lowland production of fat lambs or dairy sheep. Sheep are well adapted to harsh environments, and can exploit environments that other livestock, such as cattle, cannot. In some countries, such as many parts of Asia and sub-Saharan Africa, sheep (and goats or other livestock) represent a family's financial reserve or 'bank', to be sold in times of need but otherwise representing the family's status. This can lead to the number of animals being more important than their condition. In many subsistence systems, knowing when to sell or slaughter livestock in the face of feed or water shortage is key to sustainability or even survival.

The country with the largest sheep population (around 150 million animals) is China, and large sheep populations are also found in Iran, Australia, India, Nigeria and Sudan. Australia and New Zealand are dominant in many aspects of sheep production, particularly with a focus on wool and meat, respectively, for export. In sub-Saharan Africa and Asian countries, sheep play an important part in the rural economy. Ruminant numbers are increasing to provide protein for the rapidly growing human population, though within this general picture, the trend in sheep numbers is variable and in some countries the number is declining in favour of cattle. As a result of increasing ruminant numbers, there are concerns about rangeland degradation; many rangelands are already under severe pressure, a critical concern in countries where livestock production is paramount. A vicious cycle can ensue if carrying capacity is exceeded and overall animal production declines. In such areas, innovative management systems can provide solutions; greater use of crop residues/green by-products (e.g. -rice straw) and mixed ruminant animal/plantation enterprises has been shown to be very effective at a local level. Climate change impacts will also play a part in the suitability or otherwise of areas for ruminant production; drought conditions have been a factor in the decline in sheep numbers in New Zealand, for example. Sheep production, along with other types of farming, may be subsidized in some countries and this may also have an impact on the profitability of sheep farming and thus sheep numbers.

Sheep are amongst the earliest domesticated ruminants, probably arising from the Mouflon around 11,000 years ago in the region around Iran and Iraq. Sheep produce a range of commodities useful to humans including meat, milk, fleece and hides, dung for fertilizer and fuel, and even portage in some regions. The relative importance of these features varies with the breed and system of management (Table 5.1). There are around 1000 breeds, composites and crossbreeds in commercial production (about 80 of these are found in the UK), each generally well suited to their environment and management conditions. These management conditions range from those which can deliver individual animal care, such as dairy sheep production, to large extensively managed or ranched flocks for meat or wool. Sheep may also still be 'shepherded' in many countries where animals are taken to and from pasture and are under constant human supervision for all or part of the day. Under very extensive conditions, sheep may rarely encounter humans and may be gathered only periodically for selection for breeding or slaughter, or for shearing. It is essential under these conditions that sheep are well adapted to their environment and possess suitable fitness traits, as individualized care is largely absent, and sheep must rely on their own adaptive abilities to cope and survive. Within such systems, although there is great capacity for behavioural freedoms, there is considerable opportunity for poor welfare to arise; as animals are inspected only infrequently, injury and disease will go undetected. These systems may still be highly managed, but the management occurs at the level of the flock, often based on the response of the average animal, and not at the requirements of

Table 5.1 Examples of sheep breeds and their main uses.

Type of sheep	Primary use	Example types
Hill/upland	Producing store lambs for finishing, replacements and draft ewes	Scottish Blackface, Swaledale, Welsh Mountain, Cheviot
Fat-tailed breeds (found mostly in arid regions)	Milk (pelts from Karakul lambs used for traditional fur coats)	Awassi, Karakul, Chios, Small-tailed Han, Red Maasai
Fine-wool	Wool	Merino types, Rambouillet
Mutton/terminal sire	Meat	Suffolk, Texel, Down breeds, Border Leicester, Dorper
Dual purpose	Meat & wool	Polworth, Corriedale
Milking	Milk production	British Milksheep, East Friesian, Lacaune, Laxta, Sarda
Hair sheep	Meat	Soay, Persian, Peliquey, Barbados Blackbelly

individual sheep. Key management decisions in these systems relate to selection of the correct breed and breeding of individuals with desirable characteristics: good mothering abilities, resistance to parasitic disease and lameness, and a low incidence of lambing difficulty.

While there is a worldwide trade in sheep products, the movement of live animals for slaughter has declined over recent years as a result of good chilling and freezing technologies to preserve meat, and through public concern over live exports of stock for slaughter. However, there are still some movements of live animals between countries, such as large shipments of lamb from Australia and Romania to the Middle East to meet cultural or other requirements. Biosecurity requirements now often restrict the movement of genetic material to semen and embryos rather than live animals.

5.2.2 Sheep in the United Kingdom

Sheep production in the UK has embraced many recent technical advances, such as ultra-sound scanning for pregnancy determination, and electronic identification for precision management. However, sheep farming is still largely governed by the geographical conditions where production takes place. Sheep can be found in areas ranging from lowland pastoral and arable areas, which can be readily cultivated, and where different enterprises can be more cost-effective than sheep farming, to upland and hill areas where conditions are potentially much more severe, with a predominately unimproved rough grazing. In these latter areas, which account for around one-third of the available agricultural land in the UK, there are few other options for converting the available biomass into food owing to the severity of the climate, difficulty of terrain and low soil fertility. Over the course of centuries, several sheep breeds have been developed to maximize the potential of the environment and nutritional resources available. (A brief description and pictures of UK breeds, can be found here: https://www.nationalsheep.org.uk/uk-sheep-industry/sheep-in-the-uk/sheep-breeds.) This is coupled with the development of integrated management systems to allow movement of sheep when natural resources become scarce. In addition to producers of meat and wool, sheep are agents for managing the countryside in hill and upland areas.

There are around 35 million sheep in the UK, but numbers fluctuate depending on market forces. Flock sizes vary widely from small hobby farmers with tens of ewes to large commercial flocks with several thousand ewes. The principal output of the UK sheep industry is prime lamb (the top-quality finished meat product) and mutton from older animals. Prime lamb is produced from the offspring of terminal sires and hardy pure-bred or prolific crossbred ewes. The UK is more than 100% self-sufficient in lamb production, but seasonality, and demand for specific cuts, also provides a market for imported lamb, particularly from New Zealand and Ireland. Other than in a small number of specialist flocks, wool accounts for virtually no income for the sheep farm; shearing costs are often not covered and wool removal is considered primarily as a welfare action. The low value of wool, and the cost of its removal, have led to an upsurge in interest in 'wool-shedding' breeds in some flocks, where the fleece is lost naturally in the summer and the animals do not require shearing. In the UK only a small number of sheep are involved in milk production, which is much more commonly seen elsewhere in Europe (particularly Spain, Italy and Greece), the Middle East and Asia. Sheep may also be produced for their skins.

In the UK, sheep production traditionally falls into two main categories: hill and upland systems, and lowland systems. These are dependent on each other, but the distinction capitalizes on different environmental resources and the capabilities of different breeds and their crosses (Figure 5.1). This results in a stratified breeding and production system across the UK. Recent developments, for example, with composite breeds, or drives to increase productivity, have reduced the reliance on stratification in sheep breeding.

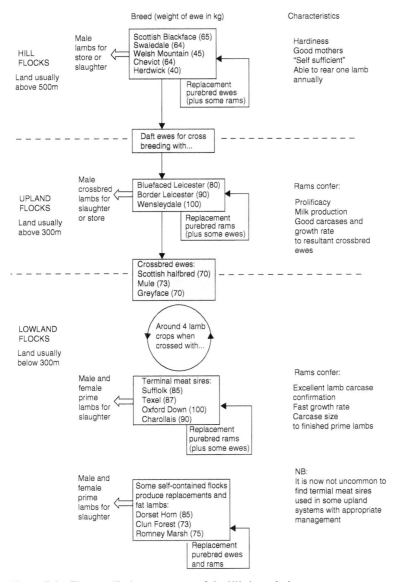

Figure 5.1 The stratified arrangement of the UK sheep industry.

5.2.2.1 Hill and Upland Production

About half the national flock is found in hill and upland areas where ewes represent the main reservoir of the breeding stock. A primary output of this system is the crossbred ewe (developed by crossing hill breed ewes with long wool rams), which forms around 80% of the lowland breeding stock. Other animals sold include older pure-bred ewes, which are unable to sustain further lamb production in the harsh upland environment (usually after three crops of lambs), ewe lambs (to be retained for breeding in the hill and upland systems) and male lambs (often castrated 'wether' lambs) as store animals for fattening (finishing) with preferential feeding. The process of movement down the hill of these older ewes is called 'drafting'.

Traditional breeds are still commonly used as hill animals, which have been used for generations on the same land, and are sometimes referred to as 'hefted', where the sheep are familiar with the landscape and location of resources. Hill breeds of ewe require characteristics of hardiness and good mothering ability and are generally more 'self-sufficient' than lowland breeds but have lower prolificacy with fewer lambs per litter. However, several composite or 'new' breeds are also being developed: to increase survival characteristics in 'Easy Care' breeds of sheep, or litter size and growth rates. The Easy Care sheep combine hardy survival characteristics with health traits (e.g. resistance to foot rot and parasitism). Some have been selected to be wool shedding to avoid the labour and cost of shearing low-value fleeces. In hill and upland systems stocking rates may be as low as one sheep per hectare overall, yet often there will be some improved grazing, usually close to the farm buildings ('in-bye') where stock can benefit from preferential nutrition at key times of the production cycle, e.g. at lambing, as these animals are never housed. The extent of the in-bye available may determine the carrying capacity of the enterprise. These areas may also allow conservation crops, such as silage or hay to be made.

Upland farms, which usually have a more favourable environment for sheep, take the draft ewes from hill farms and cross them with a long wool breed, such as a Border or Blue-faced Leicester. Crossing hill ewes with larger long wool breeds retains the good maternal traits of hill breeds in a larger framed ewe which can produce more and larger lambs per litter. The resultant female lambs move to lowground farms to cross with terminal sires, and males may go directly for slaughter from the farm. These farms also make better use of a two-pasture system whereby there is a relatively small area of improved pasture and a relatively large area of unimproved hill integrated into a complete management approach. The improved pasture can be utilized primarily during lactation and lamb growth. If a rest period can occur from mid-August (when grass can regrow) the area can be used again to provide a flush of improved nutrition during the pre-mating and mating periods.

5.2.2.2 Lowland Production

The crossbred ewes from the upland system move to lower ground and are bred to terminal sires of meat breeds to produce lambs with excellent carcass characteristics for the prime lamb market. Crossbred ewes have traits of increased body and litter size and the ability to produce sufficient milk for twin lambs – lambing at typically upwards of 160%. The potential for the crossing of a large number of breeds allows the industry to respond rapidly to changes in market demand, by selecting sires that can provide desirable traits for the market. Stocking densities are much greater (around 12 ewes per hectare) and there is considerable scope for active pasture management. This can involve use of rotation grazing, where ewes are moved from one relatively small pasture to the next, sometimes every few days or weeks, to gain the maximum benefit from the grazing area available. In addition, there is a use of mixed swards, which can contain novel plant mixtures, including chicory, plantain and other plants. These can provide variety and interest to the ewe, may encourage a greater intake and can contain medicinal components, such as tannins, that can reduce worm burdens.

5.2.3 Dairy Sheep Production in Europe

Sheep dairying is common in parts of Mediterranean Europe, and can be combined with meat production, often of light or suckled lambs, in a dual-purpose system. Milk is usually processed into cheese, and the system is less intensive compared to dairy cattle, based around grazing. Dairy sheep can be hardy breeds, producing one or two lambs each year, which are suckled by the ewe for up to six weeks. Lambs are then weaned and sold for the light lamb market, and ewes are milked for the remainder of the lactation period. Although milk yields are lower, the systems provide two products, milk and lamb, and the milk it used to generate a higher-value product in cheese, such as Feta (Greece), Roquefort (France), Manchego (Spain) and Pecorino Romano (Italy).

5.2.4 Wool Sheep Production in Australia

Australia is the largest producer of fine apparel wool in the world, although this may be combined with meat production in some areas. The backbone of the wool industry is the Merino breed, originally imported from Spain, but selected to have a very wrinkled skin, generating more wool per area of skin, and for very fine wool characteristics. Sheep bred for wool are often run in very large flocks of several thousands of animals on some of the most extensive grazing lands in the world. Unlike other forms of production, where animals may have human interactions on a frequent basis, wool is taken from sheep relatively infrequently, once or twice a year, and can be harvested from male and female sheep.

Australian sheep farmers are responsive to the market signals they receive and may invest in crossbred lambs when the market is favourable for meat production, or for purebred Merino lambs when the wool price is good. Shearing is usually carried out by contractors ('roustabouts'), who travel around the country to shear, trim and process fleeces. As these contractors are often paid by the number of animals sheared, often speed is seen as more important than the welfare of the animal, and animals may sustain a significant number of shearing cuts and injuries.

5.2.5 Sheep Production in Low- and Middle-Income Countries

Unlike the more industrial production of meat, milk and wool seen in European countries or Australia, many of the world's sheep are found in low- and middle-income countries, where they may be managed to produce a range of products, and are usually managed under various forms of pastoralism. This can be nomadic, where sheep, shepherds and the families that depend on them may move continually to access feed for their animals, following the patterns of grass growth. Alternatively, animals may be taken out to graze daily, but return to the same location at night. Generally, the land on which animals graze is not owned by the herders, and may be common grazing land, where each family flock may mix with other flocks.

These forms of pastoralism allow shepherds to respond to the availability of grazing or watering points. However, the lack of land ownership can mean that shepherds may be denied access to land. There is little opportunity for improvement of the flock beyond seeking other places to graze, and contact with other flocks can cause problems of biosecurity and the spread of disease. With the impact of global warming on weather patterns, these farmers and their flocks can be vulnerable to sudden drought, or changes in forage availability.

5.3 Selection and Improvement

Traditional sheep markets and agricultural shows are places where breeders of livestock displayed their best animals, yet superficial phenotypic characteristics are not necessarily correlated with important market or health requirements, e.g. for ewes to experience trouble-free parturition. Even the experienced stockperson's eye, while able to ensure animals remain of a particular type, is less able to evaluate the genetic potential of breeding stock. However, standardized classification methods, for example, for overall fatness and conformation of crossbred animals, can have a place in pure-bred selection programmes. Much of the sheep breeding in the world has no coordinated improvement strategy but, in some countries, genetic improvement programmes identify animals with advantageous characteristics and disseminate this genetic superiority. As yet the use of genetic improvement in the sheep sector has not been fully exploited. The earliest examples related primarily to production traits and the recent focus has included health issues such as parasite tolerance/resistance and resistance to foot rot. With a move to more easy-care systems of sheep production, maternal traits and lamb survival are also key selection criteria. Some traits can be evaluated in contemporary comparison trials (either within- or between-flock comparisons) as part of a sire reference scheme, which requires recording of a range of criteria to indicate the genetic merit/superiority or breeding value of stock. In systems where feeding and disease are managed to a high standard, improved breeds can exploit these conditions. Molecular techniques particularly genome sequencing, are starting to be used to identify animals of high genetic merit. There are also known gene-specific characteristics (e.g. Boorroola sheep with increased fecundity, and greater muscle mass in Texel sheep). Accurate measurement of certain carcass characteristics *in vivo* has been achieved using ultrasound scanning of muscle and fat depth at key sites. The use of computed tomography (CT) carcass analysis has allowed an even greater precision and identification of the most superior meat sires and so more rapid genetic progress can be made. Video image analysis systems have been developed to objectively evaluate carcasses. Genetic algorithms are used to separate genetic and environmental effects on performance to generate estimated breeding values (EBVs) within sire reference schemes and maximize the speed of genetic progress. Such schemes have the potential to focus increasingly on health and welfare criteria, but these aspects have yet to be fully exploited.

5.4   Natural History and Behaviour

Wild sheep species can still be found in Europe (the mouflon: *Ovis orientalis*), Asia (the argali: *Ovis ammon*) and in North America (Mountain Bighorn: *Ovis canadensis* and Dall's sheep: *Ovis dalli*), as well as feral sheep, such as the Soay sheep found on the Soay Island and St. Kilda in Scotland. Sheep have been able to exploit a range of different habitats, including deserts, mountains, islands and lowlands, and have adapted to feed on a range of plant species from cactus to seaweed.

Factors that encouraged the early domestication of sheep included their gregarious, flocking nature, and their size, which made for easy control and individual handling. Sheep also have a promiscuous mating pattern, show good maternal care and give birth to mature, mobile offspring, all characteristics that contributed to domestication. Sheep are not aggressive towards humans and, as ruminants, do not compete directly for the same food resources. Over the intervening years, animals with desirable behavioural and production traits have been selected (directly or indirectly) to adapt to particular systems and environments.

Sheep are sexually dimorphic, with larger size in males, and may be horned in both sexes, in males only or polled depending on the breed. In horned breeds males have larger and more elaborate or curving horns than females, as horns are used as symbols of strength and dominance in inter-male aggression. In temperate regions, sheep are seasonal breeders, with the ewes coming into oestrus in the autumn, lambing in the spring and lactating in the summer reflecting availability of forage. In the tropics, sheep are less seasonal, and some breeds can be managed to produce three litters of lambs in two years, rather than one litter per year. Litter sizes are generally between one and three lambs, although four or five lambs is possible. Sheep can live to up to 20 years, although farmed sheep are usually considerably younger when they reach the end of their productive life (generally less than 10 years).

5.4.1   Social Organization

Sheep are strongly social, and will become distressed, agitated and vocal when socially isolated or separated from flockmates. In wild sheep, the social group is a very important component of anti-predator defences, and this response is maintained in domesticated sheep. Sheep also show allo-mimetic responses, where they follow one another, and synchronise their behaviour with other sheep. Originally these behaviours helped the wild ancestors of sheep to evade detection and capture by predators but can facilitate shepherding and moving sheep becomes easier once the sheep at the head of the movement understands where to go. Sheep social behaviour can be broadly described as gregarious, with strong flight reactions when alarmed, following, a very strong bond between ewes and their lambs, and learning responses, such as features of the environment, passed from older adults to younger animals through allo-mimetic behaviour. Sheep-friendly handling systems minimize isolation and encourage sheep to move of their own volition, by utilizing the strong desire of sheep to follow others.

While grazing, sheep will disperse across a given area, with different individuals displaying varying degrees of sociability. Lowland breeds show stronger tendencies to remain together, whereas hill ewes will disperse more widely. During lactation ewes are less gregarious, and a ewe and her lamb may move much further from the flock during spring and summer than during the winter.

5.4.2 Inter-sheep Behaviour

Sheep flocks display a complex social structure. Sheep have the capacity to recognize and remember a considerable number of other individuals (and humans), retaining this information for at least two years. Recognition is based on visual cues, and olfactory information when at close quarters. Sheep respond to the emotional content in faces, avoiding human and sheep faces that show signs of anger or stress, and approaching calm and relaxed faces. Although overt aggression is rare, sheep maintain a social hierarchy through gaze, pushing or foreleg kicking and displacements from feeding or resting areas. This can mean that subordinate animals are usually the last to feed, excluded from the shaded or sheltered resting areas and at the back of any movements. Marked instances of aggression are shown between males during the breeding season, who will fight for access to females by butting and chasing. Significant injuries can occur at this time, particularly in horned breeds, although males can live together amicably in male flocks when oestrus ewes are not present. Competition for feed resources will occur in both sexes when limited supplementary feed is available or when sheep are housed at high stocking density, or recently mixed, seen as butting or barging behaviour. Mixing sheep of the same breeds induces some aggressive interactions and avoidance of one another initially, although the flock will become integrated in time. Mixing sheep of different breeds often results in persistent maintenance of two sub-flocks that do not integrate.

The strong mother–young bond is the most marked inter-animal behaviour displayed, and in some systems the female lambs will remain with the matrilineal flocks for many years, although young ewes cease to associate with their mothers over time. Mother ewes form an exclusive attachment with their own lambs soon after birth, based on initially on olfactory (odour) memory and discrimination of their own offspring. An early and effective ewe–lamb bond is critical in terms of lamb survival, and management practices should facilitate its establishment. Moves to establish easy-care sheep flocks rely on the selection of individual ewes that demonstrate (among other qualities) particularly strong maternal behaviour.

Sheep are not particularly vocal animals but maintain social relationships through postural and behavioural cues. They are strongly visual with good visual acuity and approximately 270-degree vision, so have a wide field of view. Grazing sheep will frequently stop grazing and look around, with vigilance behaviour increasing in smaller groups. Sheep alert their immediate neighbours to perceived danger by standing alert and upright, with the head held above the height of the shoulders or moving off with a stiff-legged gait. When alarmed, sheep will sometimes congregate at a vantage point, which gives them a panoramic view of their surroundings, and turn to face the disturbance. Sheep show little mutually affiliative behaviour, such as grooming, but do appear to have preferred grazing partners.

If isolated, sheep will vocalize to regain neighbour contact, and mother ewes will bleat to call their lambs to them, often accompanied by a raised head gesture. Vocalization patterns between the ewe and her newborn lamb are a significant and specialized aspect of the ewe–lamb bond, with a preponderance of low-pitched bleats.

5.4.3 Reproductive Behaviour

Ewes, in the absence of a ram, show little overt behavioural change when in oestrus. In the presence of a ram, ewes in oestrus sometimes seek out the ram and may show a tail waggling or fanning behaviour before standing to be mounted, though it is usually the ram that does most of the seeking. Prior to mating, the ram will explore the perineal area of the ewe and display one or more of a number of specific behaviours: raising the head, stretching the neck and curling the upper lip, called 'flehmen'. He may also vocalize and paw the ground. Some of these actions may be seen a short distance from the ewe. This pre-mating phase in the ram is generally short. The ram will then mount the ewe from behind and perform one or sometimes a small number of ejaculatory thrusts before dismounting. After dismounting the ram will often stand alongside the ewe with head lowered and after a few minutes the ram will go off to seek another oestrous ewe. If several rams are kept together in the pre-mating period, an increasing level of competitive encounters is seen, with rams challenging each other in head-to-head combat. This can result in serious injury. If several rams are used together, competitive encounters can occur if there are too few ewes relative to the number of rams, which may reduce the overall mating efficiency.

5.4.3.1 Behaviour at Parturition

Lambing is a critical period in the shepherding calendar. Neonatal lamb mortality is a significant welfare concern, and a loss of production for the farmer. Most lamb losses occur on the day of birth, or within the first week of life, and thus a successful lambing period can set the success of the business for the coming year.

If ewes lamb outdoors, the first sign of parturition is likely to be the ewe isolating herself from the remainder of the flock and seeking a desirable location to give birth. Thereafter, in both housed and outdoor situations, the ewe will become increasingly restless, often alternating short periods of standing and lying, scraping the ground and turning around. The first stage of labour is indicated by evidence of abdominal straining and may last up to six hours, during which the cervix dilates, and uterine contractions begin. Disturbance at this point may interrupt the process. The start of second stage labour is often marked by a rush of foetal fluid as the allanto-chorionic sac (the first 'water bag') ruptures and the amniotic sac appears intact at the vulva in around 50% of births. Part of the foetus becomes visible within the amniotic membranes. During this period, the ewe may alternate standing and lying but she usually lies down as the lamb's head passes through the vulva. Further abdominal contractions are seen and the foetus is expelled, connected by the umbilical cord. Many lambs are born within the amniotic sac. The amniotic membranes are usually broken by either vigorous movements of the lamb or when the ewe turns around to lick her lamb. If this behaviour fails to clear these membranes from around the lamb's nose it can prevent respiration, unless cleared by the shepherd. Generally, lambs are born headfirst (anterior presentation), with the forelegs extended into the birth canal. However, lambs may be presented with one or both legs retracted, back legs first or breech. These presentations are riskier for lamb mortality, and ewe death, and may require obstetric assistance to correct presentations. Dystocia, a difficult or prolonged labour, is a significant contributor to lamb mortality, thus ewes that can lamb easily without help are an important selection goal, particularly for easy care or maternal sheep breeds. Most ewes with normally presented lambs complete the second stage of labour in around an hour. Third stage labour involves expulsion of the placenta (afterbirth). Most ewes pass the remaining foetal membranes within two to three hours.

The birth of the lamb stimulates great interest in the foetal fluids and then the fluids in the lamb's birth coat from the ewe, which triggers intensive licking responses and frequent low-pitched bleats. These characteristic low-pitched bleats or 'rumbles' from the ewe are made with the mouth closed (compared to the open-mouthed, high-pitched bleats such as made by distressed sheep) and are made exclusively to the lamb associated with care-giving. Licking and bleating behaviours are a crucial part of the bonding process as this is when the ewe learns the smell of her own lamb and develops exclusivity in her attachment to her own lambs, which can occur within 30 minutes of birth. Thereafter the ewe will discriminate between her own and other lambs, only allowing her own lamb to suck, and rejecting all other lambs. If ewes are prevented from interacting with their lambs during this period, by shepherding actions or interference by other ewes, then the time window to form a bond with the lamb will pass and the ewe may reject her own lamb.

Immediately after birth, the lamb raises and shakes its head, rapidly develops more coordinated movements and attempts to stand. The neonatal lamb typically stands between 5 and 20 minutes after birth. Once standing, the lamb will attempt to locate the teats and begin to suck (usually within 30 minutes of birth and most lambs will suck within the first hour). Sucking by the lambs provides the lamb with colostrum, or the first milk, which is high in fat and contains antibodies. Lambs are born with limited energy supplies and utilize energy to metabolize brown fat and generate heat so need to obtain sufficient colostrum to stay warm. Antibodies do not pass over the placenta from the ewe. The lamb is thus born immunologically naïve and needs to gain protection from colostrum. For the first six hours after birth the neonatal lamb gut is permeable to immunoglobulins from colostrum to pass into the lamb's bloodstream so early sucking can protect the lamb from infection. Successful sucking also plays a role in the lamb learning to recognize the ewe, which is crucial for effective bonding. Successful sucking is shown by the vigorous waggling of the lamb's tail, nosing by the ewe of the lamb's rump, and may be accompanied by the lamb butting the udder, especially in older lambs. These actions may be hindered by the delivery of a further lamb, the over-zealous actions of the ewe or the inappropriate actions of a maiden ewe.

Disturbance during lambing can lead to rejection or desertion of the lamb by the ewe or subsequent mismothering (where other ewes attempt to 'steal' the newborn lamb). Sensitive and careful shepherding is required to provide obstetric care when needed, but also to allow ewes the time and space to establish strong bonds with their lambs. Lambs that are quick to stand and suck after birth have a higher probability of surviving and develop a better bond with the ewe. The lamb will feed initially from the ewe about 3 or 4 times per hour. As the lamb matures, the frequency of feeding will decline, though intake increases over the early weeks of lactation. Ewes of some breeds are notoriously poor mothers, showing less licking or grooming behaviour, fewer low-pitched bleats and a higher frequency of aggressive or disinterested responses towards their own lambs. In any breed, abnormal behaviour during the lambing period (which may be due to fatigue after a long lambing or a long period between multiple births, disturbance, overcrowding in the lambing shed, or inexperience) can result in rejection or desertion of the lamb, or mismothering. Undernourished ewes may also show poor maternal behaviour, and have higher lamb mortality, compounded by smaller weaker lambs, less colostrum and less milk.

5.4.4 Daily Activity Pattern

Sheep show a diurnal rhythm of behaviour, usually spending the night on higher ground, if available, and then descending and grazing during the morning. During the day, the main activities of sheep are alternating bouts of foraging and grazing (20 to 90 minutes) and resting (45 to 90 minutes), before animals move back up the hill to camp in the evening. Depending on the quality of grazing (or supplementary dietary components) sheep will feed for around 8 hours per day but can increase this period to up to 12 hours if food is scarce. While resting, sheep ruminate for much of the time. They will also sleep for short periods, interspersed with short grazing bouts at night.

5.4.5 Abnormal Behaviour Patterns

Abnormal behaviour patterns, sometimes suggesting environmental deficit in other species, are not commonly seen in sheep, perhaps because sheep are rarely managed in intensive conditions that can lead to stereotyped behaviour. Most reported abnormal behaviours are shown by sheep in individual pens and some instances of repeated rearing, route-tracing and star gazing have been described. Wool-pulling of the fleeces of other pen mates can also be seen under some conditions and may suggest that the social or nutritional environment is not optimal. Occasionally, early rearing conditions can affect lamb behaviour resulting in pica (eating non-food items) and altered social behaviour such as inappropriate male mating behaviour.

5.4.6 Human–animal Interactions: The Stockperson

Different management systems inevitably result in different amounts of human contact: ranging from shepherded systems, where sheep have frequent daily contact with humans, to very extensive systems where only a few contacts occur per year. The quality of any interactions between the stockperson and sheep is crucial in maximizing the value of positive experiences (supplementary feeding, for example) and minimizing potential negative impacts of handling. Often sheep are gathered, moved, exposed to loud noises, pushed through raceways and experience stressful or unpleasant events (such as dosing, injections, restraint and shearing) as their main interactions with humans. Although each of these interventions is intended to improve sheep health and welfare, they are associated with fear, pain and discomfort in the sheep, which associate handling with these negative experiences, which makes future sheep movements more stressful. Sheep are very capable at learning and can be encouraged to move through raceways and other handling systems by exploiting their desire to follow one another, and move towards lit areas, often in a circular motion, rather than relying on forcing sheep by the use of fear-inducing stimuli. Once sheep are familiar with the routes and farm routines they can be moved and handled more readily, to the benefit of both sheep and shepherd.

In some traditional transhumance[1] systems, which have been practised for centuries, the continual presence of the carer results in the sheep becoming habituated to him or her, and sheep may even seek out the company of their shepherd. In these systems sheep are often led by the shepherd, whereas in systems in the UK, Australia or New Zealand it is more common for sheep to be driven with the shepherd behind the flock. In large, extensively managed flocks where the individual contact between the stockperson and sheep is limited and handling infrequent, there is limited scope for any positive human–animal interaction to reduce the negative impact of any interactions, and humans are largely viewed with fear by sheep. When large mobs of sheep are handled it is very difficult to deliver individual care. Well-handled sheep show less avoidance of humans but in some extensive systems opportunities to provide 'gentling' experiences do not exist. It is not known whether providing a positive experience (e.g. supplementary feed) in relation to aversive procedures may attenuate the negative effects. Some farmers argue that having sheep that will approach humans is not desirable in very extensive flocks, particularly if walkers and dogs may enter the pasture. However, sheep that exhibit strong flight reactions at the presence of the stockperson should also be avoided as this can prevent routine inspection and identification of problems. Stockperson knowledge and behaviour in interacting with the flock is particularly important to ensure that sheep will tolerate inspections at a close enough distance to allow health and welfare assessments. Sheep should be cared for by enough personnel with adequate knowledge of sheep and the particular husbandry system adopted, and stockpersons should be able to recognize problems at an early stage. The stockperson should be able to recognize any shortcomings of the system and attempt to compensate for these. The Farm Animal Welfare Council (FAWC) suggested that for one stockperson, an upper limit of 1000 sheep (with additional help at times such as lambing) was reasonable, but suitably qualified, trained and motivated stockpeople can be in short supply.

---

1 Seasonal movement of people with their livestock, typically to higher pastures in summer and to lower valleys in winter.

5.4.7 Behavioural Interactions: Dogs

Dogs are perceived as predators by sheep and, while dogs are used to move or gather sheep over extensive terrain, close proximity to dogs is aversive to sheep. The natural behaviour of sheep towards herding dogs is flight or distancing, often to the edge of the sheep's flight zone. If dogs chase sheep in an uncontrolled way, sheep may injure themselves and, on sheep farms adjacent to urban areas, dog worrying is becoming an increasing concern. Disturbance by dogs of sheep prior to lambing can lead to abortion. Sheepdogs used for herding should not be used in closely confined handling areas where sheep cannot display distancing behaviour, and their presence can cause panic, which makes handling more difficult. Dogs should be trained not to bite or grip sheep. While herding dogs need appropriate training, some breeds, such as the Border Collie or Australian Kelpie have been selected to maximize innate herding traits. At lambing time, ewes may become aggressive towards dogs and will often face towards dogs and stamp to protect their offspring. For this reason, use of dogs when moving ewes with lambs at foot can be ineffective as ewes will not move away without their lambs.

In contrast, dogs of certain breeds, such as the Maremma and Anatolian Shepherd, can be used for sheep protection, mostly in high altitude areas, where large predators, such as wolves or bears, can be a problem accounting for a significant number of losses. These dogs are very passive around stock and sheep appear to bond with the guarding animals from a young age. The use of guarding dogs appears to be increasing on a world scale.

5.5 Reproductive Biology

All British breeds of sheep, except the Dorset horn, are seasonally polyoestrous (and even Dorset horn sheep may show an anoestrous period) and short-day breeders, commencing cyclic activity as daylength decreases in late summer. Typically, ewes start to come into oestrus in late summer, in a series of approximately 24-hour cycles of ovulation every 16–17 days. In ewe lambs, puberty is reached at around 8 months of age if nutrition has been adequate and they have reached 50% of adult weight. Thus, well-grown lambs could be ready to breed at the end of their first summer. While photoperiod and diet are influential in promoting the organized release of sex hormones, the introduction of the ram may trigger the onset of reproductive activity in suitable prepubertal lambs. In these lambs, ovulation occurs at least once before the first behavioural oestrus. Ram lambs may also reach puberty and be fertile in their first autumn, often at a lower percentage of mature weight than ewe lambs, but maximum fertility is not reached until around two years of age. The potential for such lambs to breed can pose a significant management challenge, for which castration is the often-adopted solution, unless male lambs can be fattened for sale at an early stage or managed apart from female lambs.

In temperate latitudes, the onset of seasonal breeding activity is dependent on decreasing daylength; nearer the equator the breeding season may be extended over the whole year, though temperature, rainfall and nutrition exert some control. The hormone melatonin, produced by the pineal gland during the hours of darkness, has a pivotal role in relaying photoperiodic information to the hypothalamus; a shorter period of secretion increases the sensitivity of the hypothalamus to oestradiol and reproductive activity is suppressed. As daylength shortens, a longer period of melatonin secretion reduces the sensitivity of the hypothalamus and seasonal reproductive changes are seen. (Administration of melatonin produces a similar effect and can be used to advance the breeding season.) Ewes in very poor body condition may not display oestrus. Rams are also influenced by similar seasonal effects, again mediated by melatonin (though in many breeds, mating is possible all year round). As a result, in practice fewer ewes are allocated to each ram at either extreme end of the breeding season. Testis size, semen quantity and quality and sexual activity are all affected by seasonal influences and the libido of ram peaks with short daylength.

The introduction of males into a group of females at the start of the breeding season causes the majority to ovulate within a week, providing there has been no male exposure prior to this. This 'ram effect' is primarily pheromonal. Since the first oestrus of the season is 'silent' (not accompanied by behavioural signs), it will be 18 to 20 days before overt oestrus is displayed in most animals. Ovulation rate, which is highest in the early part of the season, controls litter size. Following mating, spermatozoa must reach the site of fertilization (the midpoint of the uterine (Fallopian) tube) within 12 to 24 hours of ovulation (24 to 30 hours after the onset of sexual receptivity – i.e. around the end of oestrus). In hill flocks, around 40 to 50 ewes are run per ram, around 50 to 60 in lowland flocks. Maternal recognition of the embryo commences at around day 12 and embryo invasion into the uterine mucosa occurs at around 16 to 18 days, with attachment to the maternal endometrium completed by around day 30. Twin foetuses are almost always dizygotic (non-identical) and are generally found in opposite uterine horns. Sheep develop a cotyledonary placenta with specialized attachment zones at the uterine caruncles.

Well-managed mating periods can achieve greater than 90% fertility of ewes joined with the ram. The main causes of foetal loss once implantation has occurred are serious feeding mismanagement and infection. Ewes typically produce between one and three lambs per pregnancy, following a pregnancy lasting 142–150 days. Hill ewes and ewe lambs have smaller average litter sizes than older or lowland ewes. Ewes with a large litter size may need additional support at lambing time and, in hill flocks, ewes producing twins are often at a significant nutritional disadvantage.

5.5.1 Manipulation of Reproduction

Reproduction may be manipulated to achieve a higher lambing percentage, to encourage early lambing (or out-of-season lambing) or to facilitate a compact lambing period. Lambing percentage should be set to best match the farm's resources. Early lambing or the assisted increase in litter size also dictates that, to ensure lamb survival and welfare, facilities, labour and feeding management must be appropriate. For example, early lambing may require the provision of enhanced shelter. No manipulative methods should be a substitute for poor management and indeed they will work best where overall flock management is of high quality. In some flocks simply improving ewe condition at mating can have the biggest positive effect.

The main reproductive methods employed commercially include the use of intravaginal progesterone-impregnated sponges or devices which suppress the release of pituitary hormones and hence normal oestrous activity. On removal, oestrus commences from around 24 hours later. Artificial insemination (AI) in sheep is more difficult than in other species, usually requiring a veterinary procedure (laparoscopy), and is not common in commercial sheep production. However, synchronization of oestrus allows a compact lambing period in naturally mated flocks, which improves management efficiency at lambing. Where synchronization has been used, one ram is needed per 10 to 15 ewes.

Exposure to vasectomized males can advance the breeding season in certain breeds. In some flocks, melatonin implants are used to simulate short daylength and thus advance the breeding season to produce early lambs. In some systems, although uncommon in the UK, an accelerated lambing regime may be used, where ewes give birth more frequently than once per year (for example, 3 litters in 2 years, or 4 litters in 3 years). These can be very productive systems, but require skilled and careful nutritional and health management, and can take their toll on the ewes, and indeed the stockpeople.

Artificial insemination and embryo transfer (ET) are established techniques to accelerate genetic improvement in a flock (primarily through higher selection intensity) or to introduce a new genotype. AI is also used in situations where biosecurity requirements prevent the movement of rams and thus can be particularly important in an international context, though some diseases (such as foot and mouth disease) can still be transmitted. Compared to AI, ET allows more selection pressure to be exerted on the female and requires multiple ovulations to be produced in donor ewes in a multiple ovulation and embryo transfer (MOET) programme. These are invasive manipulations, and carry welfare risks for the ewe, and the potential to produce animals ill-suited to their environment.

The production of transgenic animals (those with additional, extraspecific DNA incorporated into their genome) or cloned animals, such as Dolly the sheep, while the subject of some public welfare concerns, is not a common practice and consideration is beyond the scope of this chapter.

5.6   Management

5.6.1   The Range of Management Systems

In general terms, the way a flock is managed depends on the target end-product. This could be anything from prime lamb or a top-quality breeding ram to a supply of milk. The aim is to deliver this based on the natural resources and facilities available through stockpersonship and appropriate breed selection. The timing of key activities in the shepherding year is predicated by the seasonal ability of a ewe to lamb and successfully rear her lamb(s) when grass growth sustains maximal lactation. Economic production requires the best available grass, supplemented by conserved forage and cereal crops. Given the annual production cycle and the fact that young females will not usually be recruited into the breeding flock until one or two years of age, it is not possible to make rapid changes to systems, and in the more challenging environments where sheep are kept there is minimal scope for alternative systems to develop. In these harsher, wetter areas of the UK, systems are primarily dependent on grass, with sheep gaining body condition over the summer and relying on body reserves (in the form of fat deposits) over the winter.

In the stratified system of sheep production in the UK (Figure 5.1), ageing ewes move from hill flocks to more equitable lowland conditions, allowing one or possibly two more crops of lambs. Store lambs also move down the hill and some hill sheep are moved to less harsh conditions each autumn. Central to the decision of when to move ewes is the capability of the ewe to sustain herself through natural grazing, as determined principally by incisor tooth presence and condition; once prehension is compromised the ewe's ability to survive on a grass-based diet declines. Sheep with missing permanent incisors are described as 'broken mouthed'. While incisor teeth provide a benchmark for decision-making, the condition of cheek teeth (premolars and molars) is also important as they can be in poor condition, yet these are not easily (and so are rarely) examined.

5.6.2 Management of Rams

5.6.2.1 Examination of Rams

Rams should be examined about 10 weeks prior to use, in order that corrective actions can be effective before the breeding season; rams need to be in a fit and active condition, able to seek out ewes and mate successfully. The inspection should include body condition, teeth condition and lameness. All young rams should be closely examined to exclude the possibility of transmitting hereditary problems to their offspring (e.g. entropion). Rams should also be inspected for evidence of superficial abscesses and, if found, the presence of caseous lymphadenitis (CLA, caused by *Corynebacterium pseudotuberculosis*) must be excluded. Palpation of the testes and accessory organs will reveal any obvious abnormalities or injuries, in which case veterinary advice should be sought.

In many flocks several rams are used in large groups of ewes, so underperformance by a single ram may go undetected, or a small overall reduction in flock fertility may be seen. When only one or two rams are used in a smaller group, the effect of underperforming individuals can be much more dramatic. Estimates of infertility and subfertility range from 3% to 10% in the UK. To ensure that the ram can produce adequate good-quality semen, samples are sometimes collected using either an artificial vagina (AV) or electro-ejaculation (EE), which involves electrical stimulation of the nerve plexus near the pelvic genitalia with a lubricated rectal probe. In the UK, this latter technique is restricted to veterinary clinical use on welfare grounds as it is a potentially stressful and painful procedure. The only real indicator of a ram's ability is the subsequent pregnancy rate, a combination of libido (keenness to mate ewes) and fertility.

5.6.2.2 Feeding of Rams

Rams are, for most of the year, usually maintained outdoors in bachelor groups on a grass diet. While it is important to maintain their condition, rams should not get too fat. Body condition score (BCS) should be monitored and should be around 2.5–3 during this

Table 5.2 Sheep body condition scoring (BCS).

Score	Descriptor
0	Extremely emaciated and on the point of death. It is not possible to detect any muscular or fatty tissue between the skin and bone.
1	The spinous processes are felt to be prominent and sharp. The transverse processes are also sharp, the fingers pass easily under the ends and it is possible to feel between each process. The eye muscle areas are shallow with no fat cover.
2	The spinous processes still feel prominent, but smooth, and individual processes can only be felt as fine corrugations. The transverse processes are smooth and rounded, and it is possible to pass the fingers under the ends with a little pressure. The eye muscle areas are of moderate depth, but have little fat cover.
3	The spinous processes are detected only as small elevations; they are smooth and rounded, and individual bones can be felt only with pressure. The transverse processes are smooth and well covered, and firm pressure is required to feel over the ends. The eye muscle areas are full, and have a moderate degree of fat cover.
4	The spinous processes can just be detected, with pressure, as a hard line between the fat-covered eye muscle area. The ends of the transverse processes cannot be felt. The eye muscle areas are full, and have a thick covering of fat.
5	The spinous processes cannot be detected even with firm pressure, and there is a depression between the layers of fat in the position where the spinous processes would normally be felt. The transverse processes cannot be detected. The eye muscle areas are very full with very thick fat cover. There may be large deposits of fat over the rump and tail.

Source: **AHDB 2015.**

maintenance period (see Table 5.2). Rams should be included in vaccination programmes, parasite control measures and lameness care. Prior to the breeding season, rams should be placed on a rising plane of nutrition to achieve, in lowground flocks, a BCS of around 3.5–4 on introduction to the ewes. Accustoming the rams to supplementary feeding facilitates continued feeding during the mating period, as at this time their natural grazing inclinations are significantly reduced and failure to maintain sufficient condition will reduce their reproductive success; rams can lose up to 15% bodyweight during a six-week tupping period. Individual feeding also leads to rams being easier to catch for the purpose of undertaking routine tasks. When tupping has ended, rams are removed, inspected and placed on a maintenance diet.

The technique is designed to produce a highly reproducible system and is based on the assessment of the prominence of the spinous and transverse processes of the lumbar vertebrae, the degree of fat cover of the latter and the presence of muscle and fat below the transverse processes. The fullness of the eye muscle (longissimus) is also assessed.

5.6.2.3   Introduction of Rams to the Breeding Flock

Depending on the mating strategy, entry of the rams may be preceded by the use of a teaser (vasectomized) ram, up to a month before the rams are joined, to encourage the ewes to commence cyclic behaviour or to synchronize their oestrous cycles (when introduced to already cyclic females). It is common to use a colour marker (raddle), applied directly to the brisket of the ram or via a keel harness, to colour the rump of the ewe, indicating that mounting has occurred. The colour is usually changed after 14 days to allow successive oestrous cycles (or the work of individual rams) to be monitored. A lack of evidence of mounting or a succession of colour marks indicates a problem with either ram or ewe, such as infertility or embryo loss, and prompt veterinary advice should be sought, especially if more than 15% of ewes return to first service. Recording of colour marks is the main route by which some flocks predict lambing if ultrasonography is not employed. When rams are used in teams, it is important to closely observe the rams for signs of excessive competition. This is a particular problem if rams are used in pairs. Vasectomized rams, turned into the flock three to four weeks after mating, can be used to identify non-pregnant ewes, which will continue to cycle.

5.6.3 Management of Breeding Females

Ewes should enter the breeding period in optimum condition. This may be difficult to achieve, given that most will have been lactating the previous summer. Particularly in hill flocks, the ewe will also need to be assessed for her ability to survive over the coming winter and allow her in utero lamb(s) to develop at the same time. The two months before tupping is a vital period if annual flock performance is to be maximized. Much research has been conducted into the feeding and management of ewes before and after mating, and up-to-date advice on the optimal nutritional management of the ewes can be found from AHDB, Quality Meat Scotland and Beef and Lamb NZ Beef, amongst others (see further reading section). A full description of ewe nutrition is beyond the scope of this Chapter, but maintaining ewes in good nutrition throughout the reproductive period is recommended, such that ewes enter the key 30-day period around mating at BCS 3-3.5, with good nutrition and low stress maintained to promote ovulation and prevent embryo losses.

Legs and feet must be in good order, and, for hill sheep, the presence of a full set of incisor teeth is vital. Hill ewes whose tooth condition means that they are unlikely to be able to graze effectively should be drafted to lowground flocks where conditions are more favourable. Palpation of the udder in ewes which have reared a lamb will indicate whether subsequent lactation might be affected, e.g. if there are swellings, lumps or evidence of abscessation. These can indicate previous mastitis and a possible compromise to subsequent lactation and consequent lamb growth. These considerations should be applied to stock animals, home-bred replacements and bought-in animals, for which biosecurity considerations also apply (Section 5.13.2). Culling criteria thus include poor teeth, unresolved lameness, mastitis, previous reproductive problems that may prejudice normal fertility and easy birth, and failure to achieve, on lowground flocks, a BCS of 3 by one month after weaning. If required, ewes should receive vaccinations against diseases such as enzootic abortion and toxoplasmosis in advance of the breeding season. Certain vaccines should not be given concurrently, and adequate time must be allowed. This is a good point in the year to review the flock's health plan with the unit's veterinarian, who may examine a selection of animals.

5.6.4 Pregnancy

Once the rams are removed, ewes should be maintained on a good plane of nutrition with no abrupt changes, to support embryo implantation, which is complete by day 55 after joining. While most embryo loss is thought to occur at this time, in hill flocks it may be difficult to avoid some weight loss, unless sufficient quality in-bye grazing remains available. Younger animals (ewe lambs but also two-tooth ewes (aged 12–18 months) which have just entered the breeding pool should continue to receive a high-quality diet to allow their own growth to continue.

From around 40 days post-mating it is possible to examine ewes using ultrasonography to determine pregnancy and foetal numbers. However, the most accurate diagnosis is made at around day 80, when foetal aging may also be possible. The main value in scanning ewes is to allow nutrition in the last third of pregnancy to be tailored to maternal needs, based on foetal load. For most flocks, nutrition in mid-pregnancy (2 to 3 months) should aim to maintain weight and condition; only individual sheep may need supplementary feeding. Ewe lambs and two-tooth ewes will need attention and access to the best available grazing. For early-lambing flocks, abundant natural vegetation may still be available and lead to some sheep becoming too fat. Over-fat ewes can have difficulties at parturition and during mid- and late pregnancy may suffer from the metabolic condition, pregnancy toxaemia, particularly if subjected to sudden food restriction. They may also produce small lambs. Undernourished ewes are at greater risk of diseases, which may prejudice their own and their offspring's survival.

From around six to eight weeks prior to expected lambing, at a time when naturally available feed is low, around 70% of growth of the foetus occurs, with consequent demands on the mother. It is usual to place ewes on an increasing plane of nutrition and to provide food in a form that they can consume, given that the enlarging uterus reduces available space for the rumen. For hill sheep bearing single lambs there is reliance on natural resources and body reserves to meet the doubling in feed requirement of even a single-bearing ewe. Ultrasound scanning allows the separation of ewes with multiple foetuses for increased feeding over this period. Supplementary feeding can also accustom ewes to the type of feed that will be available if they are housed for lambing and, for hill ewes which remain outdoors, it accustoms them to emergency feeding as may be required in storm conditions.

Better nutrition during pregnancy has significantly reduced ewe and lamb mortality since the 1940s. As well as avoiding metabolic problems around the time of parturition, correct nutrition promotes the birth of vigorous lambs of good birthweight, with sufficient brown fat reserves for thermoregulation and adequate nutrient reserves to allow them to stand and suck within a short period, crucially important for survival in cold and wet conditions. Good nutrition in late pregnancy also facilitates optimal expression of maternal behaviour, and a good supply of colostrum and milk.

During the last third of pregnancy, ewes may receive booster vaccinations to maintain their protection and increase the amount of colostral antibody available to their lambs. Potentially stressful procedures should be avoided immediately prior to expected lambing. For the same reason, if ewes are to be housed, they should be moved to sheds well in advance of lambing.

5.6.5 Lambing Management

5.6.5.1 Preparation for Lambing

Lambing represents one of the most important, and stressful, periods in the sheep year. The first 24 to 48 hours after birth are the most critical in terms of lamb survival and present a significant window of opportunity for stockpersons to provide support. Preparations for lambing will depend on the system and must address the likely events that could lead to significant welfare problems. Where more close supervision is available, key issues relate to assisting (at the right time) during parturition, resuscitation, dealing with hypothermia, ensuring early sucking and the consumption of adequate colostrum, the adequacy of the ewe–lamb bond, and fostering or artificial rearing if required. For hill and upland sheep lambing outdoors, it is not possible to deliver the same quantity of care and thus it is critically important that self-sufficiency traits are present in the flock. In addition, ewes should be in the target body condition and be on familiar land, hefted to where they can find shelter if required or artificial shelter provided. In these systems, with possibly one stockperson for over 1000 ewes, individual care will generally not be provided to the same extent as in low-ground flocks.

Particularly for indoor lambing, and where mating was synchronized, adequate experienced surveillance is required. Everyone involved should know when to intervene in case of a protracted birth (sometimes becoming involved too early is counterproductive), which manual methods can be employed to resolve dystocia, and when to seek help. Stockpersons should know how to attempt resuscitation, how to ensure adequate colostrum has been taken by the lamb (and what to do if not) and the importance of hygiene measures, such as dipping the navel to dry and seal the umbilical stump to prevent infection. There needs to be good access to pens (and ways to move sheep around easily), provision of individual penning, adequate lighting, facilities to care for sick ewes and those which abort, facilities to treat hypothermia in lambs (heat lambs and hot boxes), and arrangements for the collection of placental material, dead lambs and dirty bedding. A marking and recording system is required to ensure correct bonding when ewes and lambs join communal groups.

It is usual to prepare a lambing toolkit that contains commonly required items in a single place (Box 5.1).

5.6.5.2 Ewe Behaviour at Lambing

It is important to be able to recognize the signs of labour (Section 5.6.5.4) and know when to provide assistance to ensure the welfare of both the ewe and lamb(s). However, hill sheep and other more self-sufficient or 'easy-care' breeds will usually lamb unaided. Although most ewes can deliver without intervention, for those that do have difficulty the welfare consequences, for ewe and lamb, can be very severe if not assisted. Stockpersons observing ewes in difficulty are only likely to be able to assist a proportion of ewes, thus easy lambing traits are vital for these flocks. Additionally, although a strong ewe–lamb bond exists in hill ewes, human disturbance at the birth site may cause the ewe to abandon the new lamb. However, it is still possible to provide some pens for ewes and lambs and protection from the worst of the weather by building shelters from large straw bales.

Box 5.1 Contents of a good lambing toolkit

General
- Record book/pencils, marker sprays/crayons, torch and spare batteries
- Water, buckets, soap, disinfectant solution, hand towels
- Rubber rings and applicator
- Disinfectant for lambing pens

Assistance at lambing
- Obstetrical lubricant, disposable gloves
- Strong iodine solution for dipping navels (and suitable dip cup)
- Digital thermometer (works quickly and no chance of broken glass)
- Lambing ropes/tapes/aid for repositioning lamb's head
- Scissors

Support for lambs
- Towels for drying lambs, heat lamp/hairdryer
- Warming box for hypothermic lambs
- 20% glucose solution (10 mL/kg), 50 mL syringe/19 G 3 cm needles/antiseptic swabs
- Respiratory stimulant (e.g. doxapram drops)
- Oral rehydration solution

Support for ewes
- Calcium borogluconate solution for injection (and means for administration)
- Magnesium sulphate solution for injection
- Propylene glycol for oral administration
- Prolapse retainer/harness
- Antibiotics (as prescribed by vet)
- Pain relief (e.g. non-steroidal anti-inflammatory drugs) in case of difficult lambing
Needles and syringes

Artificial feeding
- Stored (frozen) colostrum or artificial colostrum powder
- Stomach tubes, large syringes/feeding bottle
- Graduated plastic jugs
- Bottles, teats and disinfectant
- Ewe milk replacement powder
- Hypochlorite solution for disinfection

For housed sheep, triplet-bearing ewes or those with poorer maternal traits, individual attention will be more helpful. Hygiene of the indoor lambing environment needs considerable effort if infectious disease is not to become a problem. Pre-lambing shearing, for ewes housed for part of the winter, may be used to reduce heat stress in later pregnancy, and can make it easier to see what is happening at lambing time.

Once lambed, the housed ewe must be observed for signs of acceptance of her lambs and her willingness to let them suck. Other events that can lead to lamb morbidity include ewes failing to groom lambs or rejection of lambs, attempted stealing of lambs by ewes yet to lamb and aggression towards lambs. Ewes lambing for the first time are more likely to show behavioural disturbances and can be slower to allow the lamb to suck and obtain a good supply of colostrum. Colostrum contains a high level of energy, minerals and vitamins, and provides immunoglobulins (antibodies against specific diseases), which must be ingested since no antibodies pass to the lamb across the placenta. This helps the lamb to resist diseases endemic in the lambing environment (e.g. watery mouth, which is seen when lambs ingest environmental organisms such as *E. coli*). It also confers non-specific immunity and is a direct source of heat to a cold lamb. Colostrum also contains growth factors, which help mature the neonatal gut, and play a role in the lamb learning to distinguish its own mother from other ewes.

Ewes housed for lambing are often kept with their lambs in individual pens for around 24 to 48 hours. Placental material (afterbirth) is collected for hygienic disposal and pens are cleared of contaminated bedding, disinfected and re-bedded prior to reuse. Alternatively, lambing ewes are housed to lamb in indoor groups. Depending on the weather conditions, they are then turned out in small groups to sheltered paddocks which allow ready observation in case of mismothering, poor maternal behaviour or ill health. If ewes with young lambs remain for too long in the relatively confined conditions of housing, they risk mismothering and infection rates increase.

5.6.5.3 Newborn Lambs

To ensure its survival, the newborn lamb must rapidly become dry, stand, consume an adequate amount of colostrum and develop a bond with its mother. Lamb birthweight varies with breed and litter size: single Blackface lambs weigh between 3.5 and 5 kg; twins will each weigh around 0.5 kg less, whereas single Suffolk lambs weigh 4.5–7 kg During periods of poor weather, particularly when wet and windy conditions combine, the core body temperature of wet or even partially dry lambs can fall quickly, leading to hypothermia. Lamb mortality, in all major sheep producing countries, is estimated between 15 and 25%, although significant between-farm variation can occur, with dystocia, hypothermia, starvation and mismothering the main contributors to lamb losses outside. Lamb survival is enhanced if they stand and suck quickly to replenish energy reserves; lambs slow to stand have greater difficulty in maintaining body temperature. Sucking can be delayed in low birth-weight lambs, triplet lambs, lambs that have experienced a difficult or prolonged labour and in ewes lambing for the first time. These lambs may be more likely to require extra care and attention to ensure that they can suck from their mothers and may need additional heat or feeding in the first day after birth. Other causes of lamb death include stillbirth and infectious disease (particularly in indoor lambing flocks), with a small percentage due to congenital abnormalities and predation in outdoor flocks. From a welfare perspective it is important to recognize that a large proportion of these losses is avoidable.

It is imperative that lambs receive adequate colostrum as soon as possible (ideally within 2 hours) and certainly within 6 hours of birth before 'closure' of the gut wall to immunoglobulin passage. Ingestion of colostrum (and later milk) into the abomasum (the true, glandular stomach) can be assumed in lambs whose abdomens have a full appearance on palpation behind the last ribs. Extra colostrum can be collected from ewes with large volumes, stored and fed to orphaned or weak lambs and be deep frozen in advance of the next year's need. Colostrum has laxative properties which help the lamb to pass contents from the foetal gut (meconium). Moving ewes to new locations to give birth can mean that there is an absence of colostral antibody to 'local' disease organisms. The colostrum from suitably immunized cows or goats can also be used but bovine colostrum can lead to anaemia in lambs. Artificial powdered colostrum is also available, when other sources are not possible, although there is some evidence this provides lower concentrations of immunoglobulins in lamb blood.

5.6.5.4 Assisting during Parturition

Manual delivery of the lamb(s) must be undertaken with care and rigorous attention to hygiene. This is to avoid injuring the ewe and/or lambs, and to prevent inter-animal transmission of disease and to protect the stockpersons. Several organisms present in some lambing ewes can cause serious disease in humans (i.e. they are zoonotic) and, even if all appears normal, their absence cannot be assumed. *Chlamydophila abortus* is among the organisms of particular concern to pregnant women, leading to the recommendation that pregnant women should not work with sheep (since these may abort if infected) and particularly lambing ewes, the products of lambing (or abortion) and lambs needing artificial rearing. Flocks with specific disease problems or those buying in young females or receiving pregnant ewes should seek veterinary advice about the risks and control measures that can be adopted. For more details, see Sargison et al. (2018).

Stockpersons must be able to recognize the stages of parturition, act appropriately when a ewe needs assistance and be able to correct malpresentation of lambs. If a ewe has been straining hard for 15 minutes or more and there is no sign of progress she should be examined to determine the cause: principal reasons include inadequate dilation of the cervix, abnormal presentation or dystocia due to the disproportionate size of the foetus. Birth injuries sustained during a difficult or prolonged birth (either natural or with overzealous human assistance) can result in stillbirth, failure to thrive or morbidity in the lamb. This may be because of physical injury, cerebral haemorrhage or anoxia in lambs deprived of oxygen from placental exchange before respiration commences. Dystocia is responsible for many ewe deaths and is a significant welfare concern.

It is good practice to dip the navels of housed lambs (Figure 5.2a) in a strong iodine solution at birth and ideally four to six hours later as part of the disease control strategy. It is important that the solution covers the navel right up to the abdomen. Iodine speeds desiccation of the remaining umbilical cord (Figure 5.2b) and reduces the chance of infectious organisms causing navel ill or subsequent joint ill.

5.6.5.5 Resuscitation

Some newborn lambs need encouragement to start breathing, especially if the birth process has been long or difficult. For lambs with a heartbeat (which can be easily felt at the

Figure 5.2 Use of iodine for navel dipping: (a) applying strong iodine solution soon after birth; (b) a dry navel and withered umbilical cord. Photographs by permission of Kay Aitchison.

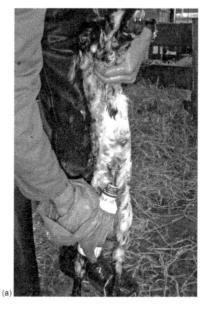

(a)

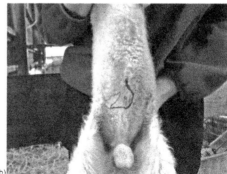

(b)

front of the chest just behind the forelimb) but no obvious respiration, several simple actions are often sufficient. The nose and mouth should be cleared of foetal membranes and the lamb should be vigorously stimulated, for example, by rubbing with clean straw. The nose can be tickled with straw, which often stimulates sneezing followed by breathing. Gently swinging the lamb by the hind legs can prompt respiration and facilitates drainage of foetal fluids from the chest and airways. Respiratory stimulants can be applied to the underside of the tongue. While artificial respiration could be attempted using a purpose-made device, direct 'mouth-to-mouth' methods should not be practised due to the zoonotic disease risk.

5.6.5.6 Dealing with Hypothermia

Hypothermia can be a common issue in newborn lambs, especially those born outside in wet and windy weather, when the lamb's brown fat and energy reserves for thermoregulation can be quickly exhausted. Even if lambs are healthy and in a good nutritional state, weather conditions at lambing time, particularly in hill and upland areas, may be such that they are unable to dry, stand and suck sufficient colostrum quickly enough, and the ewe may not have selected a sufficiently sheltered birth site. Hypothermia dulls cognitive experience and consciousness; thus it is possible that noxious experiences of hypothermic lambs are reduced and so it is difficult to assess the overall welfare impact of this state. The body temperature of lambs that have not dried or stood up within a short period can fall rapidly. Any lamb showing signs of dullness, lethargy or failing to follow or suck from its mother should be assessed by taking its temperature: the normal temperature of a lamb is 39–40°C and lambs at risk can have temperatures of 37–39°C. In individual cases, drying the lamb and either stomach tubing (see Section 5.6.5.7) with warm colostrum or intraperitoneal injection of a warm glucose solution may be effective. Lambs with temperatures below 37°C require urgent attention if they are to survive. For lambs more than 4–6 hours old, which will have exhausted their built-in brown fat reserves, the sequence of events should be to dry, then provide energy (by intraperitoneal glucose injection if it is weak and unable to support its own head), then warm the lamb. If a hypothermic lamb is warmed abruptly in the absence of an energy supply, it can develop a hypoglycaemic coma and die. A further aid to reduce the incidence of hypothermia is the temporary use of jackets for newborn lambs.

5.6.5.7 Stomach Tubing

Stomach tubing is a method for providing supplementary milk or colostrum, where the expectation is that lamb will continue to feed from its mother, and the additional feed is to help warm a lamb and prevent starvation. Milk or colostrum can be delivered directly to the stomach via a catheter tube with a smooth, rounded end with an offset opening. With the lamb sat across the stockperson's lap, the lamb's head is raised, and the lubricated tube gently introduced over the back of the tongue. The tube can be easily advanced as the lamb swallows and force is not required. Its advancement down the oesophagus (gullet) can then be observed externally as it passes down the left side of the lower neck in the jugular groove. It is crucial that the tube is not located in the trachea. This is unusual, but fluids introduced into the lungs of a debilitated lamb will likely lead to death. To prevent this occurring stomach tubing should only be carried out with lambs that are able to swallow and not with weak or unconscious lambs. If the tube is in the trachea its advancement down the neck will not be seen or felt and in some cases the lamb may cough and exhibit signs of discomfort. The tube is advanced until around 20–25 cm is in the lamb, when the tip should be in the stomach. A graduated feed bottle or syringe is attached to the external end of the tube and warm (body temperature) colostrum or milk, as appropriate, is delivered under gravity or gentle positive pressure. The tube is then gently withdrawn with the bottle still attached. The equipment should then be cleaned for subsequent use (e.g. using hypochlorite solution) and a record made of the time and amount given to the lamb.

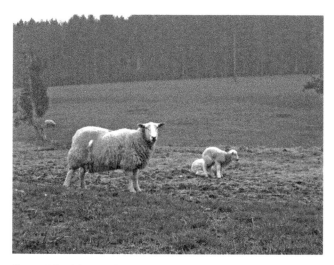

Figure 5.3 A hungry lamb showing a characteristic stance. The lamb should be fed milk and the ewe checked for mastitis. Younger lambs adopting this stance may also be hypothermic. Photograph by permission of Paul Roger.

5.6.5.8 Early Sucking: Provision of Colostrum

It is important that stockpersons can recognize hungry lambs (Figure 5.3) and take appropriate action. Hungry lambs have an arched back, tucked abdomen and it will not be possible to palpate a full stomach. Using a rule of thumb of 50 mL/kg, a 5 kg lamb will require 250 mL colostrum (and later milk) per feed, four times a day. Weak lambs may need initial feeding by stomach tube.

5.6.5.9 Artificial Feeding, Fostering and Adoption

Intervention will be required if ewes die, fail to lactate sufficiently well to feed their lambs, or in some systems when ewes give birth to more than two lambs. Lambs that exhibit a strong suck reflex, even those which have yet to take colostrum, can be fed via a bottle. As with tube feeding, it is important to ensure that feeding implements are scrupulously clean and milk substitutes correctly formulated. While lambs may need individual attention to teach them to suck, they can very easily be moved to automatic milk-feeding systems that can provide ad libitum milk access for lambs. From the stockperson's perspective, this is vital if a large number of orphans are expected. More simple systems such as buckets with teats attached are also effective. From about three weeks a palatable creep feed in pelleted form and high-quality hay should be given as well. It is then possible to consider weaning lambs at around six to eight weeks of age if solid feed intake is adequate.

Vigorous lambs can be fostered on to suitable ewes using several different methods. As ewes form a bond with a lamb via odour, the most successful methods involve masking or altering the smell of the foster lamb to one that the ewe will accept. Best results can be obtained by a 'wet-foster' where the foster lamb is coated with birth fluids from the recipient ewe or using the skin of the ewe's dead lamb to mask its own individual smell. It is helpful if the weight of the lamb to be fostered matches that of the ewe's own lamb. Sometimes cross-fostering can be done immediately at lambing and as the ewe is establishing a bond with its own offspring (usually within 30 minutes of birth). This method is used to move one lamb from triplet-bearing ewes to a ewe with a singleton. If there has been a delay in the fostering process the acceptance rate can be improved by manually mimicking the cervical sensation of the lamb passing through the birth canal if carried out within about 12 hours of the ewe having given birth. Alternatively, ewes are retained in a yoke system where they have no choice but to allow the foster lamb to suck. This latter method may take up to 3 days and is considerably less successful than wet foster or other odour masking approaches that mimic the natural way a bond is formed by the ewe. Often the welfare of the ewe is overlooked in these systems: there must be ready access to feed and water, scrupulous hygiene (as the ewe cannot move and mastitis may occur if the pen is not cleaned) and a minimal period of restraint.

5.6.6 Lactation

The udder of the ewe should have been checked prior to tupping, but if lambs fail to thrive the ewe must be examined again for evidence of adequate milk production. In the first six weeks, the 'pre-ruminant' lamb's growth is dependent primarily on the ewe. Thereafter, milk remains a crucial component of the lamb's diet as it begins to eat herbage, the rumen develops and until this can adequately compensate for the nutrients supplied by milk. For the ewe to produce sufficient milk, the diet must be adequate, and she must remain healthy. The ewe's nutritional needs are greatest in early lactation and in most systems, this is planned to coincide with available spring grass. Ewes with a high lactation potential (up to around 2.5 L per day) require voluntary food intake or feed offered to be sufficient to meet demands and further weight may be lost (up to 5% of bodyweight) as fat reserves are utilized. This is not usually a problem if ewes are in the target condition at lambing time and if there is enough protein in the diet. There may be an advantage in the separate feeding of ewes rearing multiple lambs (which produce up to 40% more milk) to provide them with a higher plane of nutrition (or providing supplementary 'creep' feed to lambs). It is common to continue the pre-lambing feeding regime of a diet with high digestibility. The periparturient increase in shedding of roundworm eggs by the ewe (resulting from perinatal immunosuppression) may affect maternal condition and thus milk production. Maximum milk yield is seen around the third lactation and vigorous lambs have a positive effect on milk production.

5.6.7 Weaning

Weaning is usually undertaken when lambs are 12 to 16 weeks old, although natural weaning is closer to 6 months of age, but the timing is dependent on the system. Weaning is usually done abruptly across the whole group, although fence line or gradual weaning can also be carried out. By this time, lambs are not primarily reliant on ewes for nutrition, although still suckling, but significant psychological bonds still exist. Weaning causes transient distress in both ewe and lamb, and a short check in lamb growth, and any concurrent other stressors for the lamb (such as moving to new paddocks, mixing, vaccination) should be avoided. Early weaning of lambs in dairy breeds (which may occur at 6 weeks of age) or frequent lambing systems require the young lambs to be provided with appropriate concentrate diets. If lambs are weaned onto grass too early, they will fail to thrive or reach their growth potential. However, early weaning may be part of a farm strategy to control intestinal parasites by moving lambs, following anthelmintic treatment, to pasture with a predicted low level of infectivity (e.g. previously ungrazed by sheep that year or used for conservation crops).

5.6.8 Autumn Lambing

A small number of flocks based on the Dorset Horn or Poll Dorset breeds, with their less pronounced reproductive seasonality, can be managed for autumn lambing to target Easter markets, which are otherwise short of fresh lamb. However, this system requires a high standard of management and the availability of freely draining land if the ewe flock is to be outwintered during the lactation period. Alternatively, ewes and lambs are kept indoors with early weaning of lambs at around 6 to 8 weeks with the move to high-quality creep feed available *ad libitum* and the provision of good-quality hay. Lambs can reach a market weight of 40 kg by 16 weeks of age. In some southern counties of the UK it is common to fold (move across) ewes and lambs on winter roots and brassicae, e.g. direct-drilled kale, rape and turnips.

5.7 Management of Hill Sheep

Within the stratified system of UK sheep production (Figure 5.1) hill sheep represent the starting point. Reliance is primarily on nutrition from uncultivated natural hill vegetation with inherently low nutrient value, and supplementary feeding when required. Sheep can tolerate low environmental temperatures, providing they are well fed, have good fleece cover and are dry. Hill sheep have been selected to utilize body reserves efficiently over the winter (i.e. during pregnancy and early lactation), for ease of lambing and the development of local knowledge (hefting), allowing them to take advantage of protective natural landscape features. Pure-bred sheep are generally found in these systems, which are often closed flocks with male and female replacements bred on farm.

Key management activities are focused on late pregnancy and early lactation when body reserves can become depleted and ewe deaths due to inanition (particularly if ewes entered the winter in low body condition) are a real possibility. Supplementary feed can be supplied through conserved forage, root vegetables or feed blocks, based on ewe BCS and weather conditions. Some ewes are routinely moved to areas of improved or more sheltered grazing such as in-bye land or areas of improved hill grazing, and potentially supplementary feeding of concentrates and minerals if required. Additional planning in these systems include consideration of supplying emergency rations in case of storm or heavy snowfall or moving sheep to shelter if adverse weather is forecast.

5.8 Management of Lowland Flocks

The main advantages for lowland flocks compared to hill systems are the more favourable weather conditions, the longer grass-growing season and seasonal housing. These combine to allow a more flexible management programme to be developed. Rotational grazing may also be used, with grazing at higher stocking rates, but frequent movement to a new pasture, to improve the utilization of forage, and ewe nutritional management.

Shelter, or more permanent housing, is provided primarily to protect ewes and lambs at lambing time or more generally over the late winter and early spring when weather conditions, combined with an increased nutritional demand on pregnant ewes, are most challenging. Simple shelters (either adjacent to the farm buildings or on protected pastures) can be erected for use by lambing ewes. An advantage of these temporary shelters is the avoidance of a long-term build-up of infectious disease agents. Corrals of large straw bales can also be used at pasture to provide additional shelter to groups of ewes and lambs once turned out to grass.

5.8.1 Winter Housing

Housing sheep for all or part of the winter is common practice in some areas. Supplementary heat is not required, but it is important that the effect of the wind and draughts at sheep height is reduced, for example, using space boarding or suitable netting. Adequate ventilation and air movement are essential to avoid hot and humid conditions that predispose sheep to respiratory disease (Figure 5.4). Conditions underfoot must remain dry and sheep need to lie

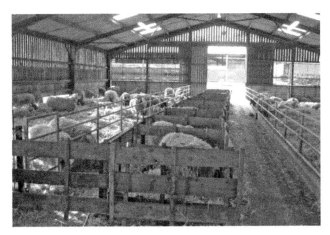

Figure 5.4 A well-ventilated lambing shed with individual pens for ewes and lambs. Photograph by permission of Kay Aitchison.

on a dry bed. While slatted floors are sometimes used, more generally sheep housing have solid floors bedded with straw or wood shavings. These require regular maintenance to avoid dampness and resultant foot problems, such as foot rot. Poor quality or incorrectly spaced slats result in foot and leg injury and have high maintenance costs. Slatted floors should not be used for lambing ewes or young lambs. Sufficient lighting must be available such that sheep can be inspected at any time.

Winter housing reduces energy needed to maintain growth and production when weather is poor, can ease management of sheep with the ability to stock at high density and rests available pasture. In some countries at Northern latitudes, sheep are housed for up to six months to avoid the winter weather. Disadvantages include the potential higher prevalence of infection, particularly respiratory disease and neonatal infection, and the need for greater attention to foot care. Sheep are housed in groups (ideally less than 30 animals per pen); larger groups do not allow stable social structures and make it more difficult for stockpersons to deliver individual care.

Space per animal, feed and watering arrangements need to be enough to avoid competition and aggression or displacements, and sheep should have constant access to forage (Figure 5.5). There should be enough trough space to allow all sheep access to concentrate feed at the same time (Table 5.3).

After lambing, ewes and their lambs are often temporarily housed in individual pens to ensure a good ewe-lamb bond. Individual pens can be constructed using wooden or metal hurdles (Figure 5.4), with provision for temporary feed and water supply. There should be at least one pen per eight ewes, but more pens may be needed for synchronized flocks. Pens should be cleaned and disinfected between lambing ewes, to prevent disease spread. There also need to be facilities for fostering lambs and for orphan lambs. Orphan and sick individuals need additional heat, usually provided by a suspended infrared lamp.

Table 5.3 Recommended minimum space allowances (m^2) and trough space per animal for housed, unshorn sheep (source: Codes of Recommendations for the Welfare of Sheep, UK).

Type of sheep	Space allowance (m^2)	Feeder space (cm)
Large ewe in lamb (60–90 g)	1.2 to 1.4	45
Large ewe with lambs (up to 6 weeks)	2.0 to 2.2	45
Small ewe in lamb (45–60 kg)	1.0 to 1.2	30
Small ewe with lambs (up to 6 weeks)	1.8 to 2.0	30
Lambs up to 12 weeks old	0.5 to 0.6	-
Lambs and sheep 12 weeks to 12 months old	0.75 to 0.9	30
Rams	1.5 to 2.0	50

*Shorn sheep will require around 10% less space.

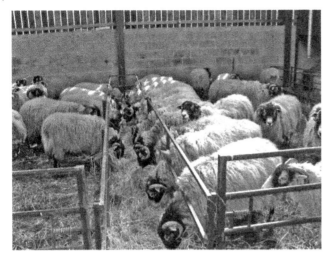

Figure 5.5 Housed sheep being fed from a gangway between pens, facilitating the stockperson's work. Photograph by permission of Paul Roger.

5.9 Management of Fatstock

The end product of prime lamb production is the fat lamb (Figure 5.1). Lambs are generally sold at 40 kg live weight, around 50% of their mature weight, with a killing out percentage of up to 50%. Lambs can be sold off the ewe (i.e. before weaning) and if the ewe has been well fed, lambs can be sold from 10 weeks of age when they weigh around 20 kg Beyond this age, provision of high-quality pasture and control of intestinal parasites are important if lambs are to be marketed early and feeding costs controlled. Most lambs are sold at some point after weaning, finished on late summer grass and sold as dictated by the prevailing market conditions.

European markets exist for 'light' or suckling lambs of a particular weight at certain traditional times of the year, which can be an additional product from the dairy industry (Section 5.2.3). In the UK, lambs that are not sold off grass at the end of the summer are usually sold on for fattening for sale in the autumn or winter (store lambs). As grass growth declines, additional foodstuffs are substituted to maintain growth rates, including root crops, grass or arable by-products. Concentrates may also be used if there is a need to target a specific market window of opportunity. If sheep are closely confined outdoors on poorly draining ground in wet winter weather, poaching can be a serious problem, resulting in foot problems and disease, especially if there is no dry lying area. In some countries, feedlots are used for finishing lambs, where lambs are held in yards, usually outdoors, in large groups and rapidly finished on grains. To avoid ruminal acidosis, sheep also need access to a suitable source of forage to maintain rumen function.

5.10   Organic Sheep Production

Organic principles require a whole-system approach that precludes the use of synthetic inorganic fertilizers, pesticides, growth regulators, preventative antibiotic use, livestock feed additives and genetically modified foodstuffs. Livestock must be fed on organically produced foods. For sheep farming, organic systems rely primarily on efficient grassland management, crop rotations (where the land allows cultivation) and animal manure to maintain soil fertility, with minimal inputs from outside the system. For hill sheep systems this does not have a major impact and so, for some producers, conversion in relation to feed inputs, is relatively straightforward. Organic regulations place restrictions on husbandry procedures, such as routine tail docking, and permits castration only under some conditions.

There is a compulsory requirement to develop a plan to promote health and introduce disease control measures that lead to progressively less dependence on conventional medicines. Thus, organic systems focus on health and welfare promotion, in tune with flock health planning (Section 5.13.1). Requirements of organic standards restrict the use of anthelmintics on a routine basis, favouring pasture management to avoid exposure of susceptible stock (principally lambs in their first grazing season) to infection. This may not always be entirely satisfactory. For example, significant gut damage can be caused by some worms (e.g. *Nematodirus* species) before there is evidence of parasite eggs through faecal counts. Even with exemplary management some use of anthelmintics is almost always essential to ensure effective control of internal parasites. The restricted use of some preventive medicine strategies is, to some, less acceptable from an animal welfare perspective than providing a comprehensive disease reduction and prevention programme incorporating conventional medicines. Some of the reported reductions in health problems on organic farms may be the result of reduced stocking density.

5.11   General Nutrition and Feed Management

The key to economic sheep production is to maximize the contribution of home-produced resources, primarily grazed grassland (including silage aftermaths) during the summer months and conserved fodder over the winter months. This usually allows the feeding of concentrates to be reserved for ewes in the last few weeks of pregnancy or in early lactation if enough spring grass growth has not yet occurred (especially in early-lambing flocks).

5.11.1   Pasture Management and Conservation

Since grass supplies around 90 to 95% of the overall energy requirement, good grassland management is vital. Elevation and climatic conditions influence grass growth. On lowland farms grass use is concentrated on the summer growing season and maximized through high stocking densities. Assessment of pasture growth and availability (kg of dry matter per hectare) can be assessed by sward sticks or plate meters to aid decisions on stocking densities. Grazing at high sheep densities does, however, encourage the build-up of gastrointestinal parasites. In contrast, sheep on extensive or upland/hill farms rely on poor quality natural (rough) grazing. These sheep will usually need supplementary feeding, particularly towards the end of pregnancy, often through the provision of hay or feed blocks.

Once grass growth declines or ceases, sheep in lowland systems rely on conserved feeds, primarily hay or silage. Silage must be of adequate quality that is maximized at a low moisture content (dry matter above 25%) where an adequate level of acidity has been achieved through efficient manufacture and storage. The making of field-cured hay is very sensitive to the weather and in the UK the balance in production has shifted to a major extent to silage. Commercial assessment of both hay and silage is available. Correct storage is also important if the nutritional value is to be preserved.

5.11.2   Root and Forage Crops

Once natural grass growth declines, supplementary food is needed through feeding a range of green fodder crops, such as kale or rape, root crops such as turnips, or arable by-products. Store lambs may be moved to graze arable areas where surpluses exist. These crops subsequently form an important part of the early winter diet, often fed in combination with conserved grass (usually hay) to avoid digestive problems. Root crops can also be harvested to be fed later in the winter and around lambing time. If free access is required through the autumn and winter, the land must be suitable to carry the sheep if conditions become very wet; poaching of the ground and inadequate dry lying areas can lead to significant health and welfare concerns. Some of these crops have a low dry matter content (e.g. DM of swedes is 12% compared to grass silage 25% and hay 85%). Access is usually through strip grazing controlled by electric fencing; however, electric net fencing should not be used if horned sheep are present. Broken-mouthed sheep or those with erupting incisors ('four tooth', in their second winter) may be unable to eat root crops sufficiently and can lose condition rapidly.

A regional supply of crop by-products, undersown cereal crops and aftermaths can be utilized in the autumn, providing adequate note is taken of their nutritional contribution. In many lowland areas, good supplies of sugarbeet tops can be obtained. (It is necessary to allow adequate wilting of sugarbeet tops to avoid oxalate toxicity and digestive problems.) This feed is highly attractive to ewes, which can become over-fat during pregnancy, and if fed as a high proportion of the diet will need supplementing from 8 weeks before lambing.

5.11.3   Concentrate and Compound Feeds

Concentrates are cereal-based and rapid ingestion can lead to ruminal acidosis. For this reason, concentrates are usually introduced gradually, with amounts built up over a few days. This may be more difficult to regulate in large groups of sheep where some consume more than others. Compound feeds are usually pelleted, or cubed feedstuffs made to a specific protein, energy, mineral and vitamin composition. Compound feeds are generally expensive and reserved for feeding to match the nutritional needs of ewes in the last six to eight weeks of pregnancy and early lactation. Such compound diets alone do not provide sufficient fibrous roughage for sheep; therefore, good-quality straw may also be provided *ad libitum*. A further method is the feeding of a complete diet to housed sheep, generally based on pelleted dried grass with vitamin and mineral additions

Feed blocks are also used as a dietary supplement, especially for sheep wintered outdoors. These have a high energy density and can contain urea (as a non-protein nitrogen source) and balancing minerals. Blocks are particularly useful in areas where access is difficult. They resist weathering and last a considerable time but can be expensive and not all sheep will use them to the same extent, particularly if unfamiliar with supplementary feed. Putting replacement blocks at different locations around the hill may encourage more even feeding and prevent the ground being excessively trampled around feed blocks.

5.11.4 Minerals and Vitamins

Two main factors affect the adequate supply of minerals and vitamins in the diet: the local soil type and the content of any supplementary feedstuffs. Some areas of the UK are recognized as being deficient in key minerals or trace elements, principally copper, cobalt and selenium. Subclinical effects of deficiency can affect productivity through reduced growth rates or suboptimal reproductive performance. Provision of mineralized feed blocks or appropriately supplemented concentrate feed are ways to compensate for deficiencies. Supplements can be given on an individual basis, often through oral dosing of slow-release boluses, which lodge in the rumen, or depot injections. Copper supplementation, though often necessary, should be used carefully as it is relatively easy to provide a toxic overdose. Magnesium supplementation may be needed in spring as rapidly growing grass has a low concentration. When required, vitamins are usually provided in compound feedstuffs. In emergency cases, some vitamins and trace elements can be given by injection.

5.11.5 Water

A supply of clean water should always be available, even though non-lactating sheep eating high moisture-content grass may not drink regularly. In extensive conditions, water is often provided from natural sources. Where water is provided artificially, the supply must be checked and cleaned regularly. Indoor watering arrangements must minimize the chance of faecal or food contamination. If sheep are gathered around a water trough this suggests that either the supply has failed, or it has become contaminated. Sheep unfamiliar with automatic watering devices, such as at markets or slaughterhouse lairages, may be reluctant to drink. Transported sheep often choose to eat rather than drink following unloading from a vehicle.

5.12   Nutritional Disorders

5.12.1 Pregnancy Toxaemia/'twin Lamb' Disease

Occurring in late pregnancy and around parturition, this condition is due to an imbalance of energy supply and utilization with low maternal glucose availability due to foetal demand, coupled with a reduction in rumen volume. Twin-bearing ewes are most at risk. Over-rapid mobilization of body fat reserves results in the appearance of ketones in the blood, causing depression, unawareness and loss of appetite and, if not rapidly corrected, leads to coma and death. If signs appear shortly before parturition, the birth of lambs can be hastened, for example, by steroid injection or a caesarean operation. In some cases, ewes may spontaneously abort. Feeding of high-quality hay and concentrates and administering oral glucose or propylene glycol over several days can also be effective, if diagnosis has been prompt. In many cases treatment is futile, and euthanasia of the ewe may be necessary. The condition is best avoided through correct ewe nutrition based on foetal load. Blood sampling a selection of ewes 4 weeks before lambing can indicate diet adequacy by measuring betahydroxybutyrate.

5.12.2   Urolithiasis

Urolithiasis is a disease seen primarily in castrated (wether) lambs receiving a highly concentrated diet. There is a blockage of the urethra, usually as it curves sharply over the ischium, by mineral sediments and proteins which precipitate in the urine. Clinical signs are primarily abdominal discomfort, straining, sometimes kicking at the abdomen, possibly accompanied by urine dribbling. A number of surgical approaches can be attempted but usually the long-term prognosis is poor, and efforts should be made to correct the nutrition of at-risk stock.

5.12.3   Copper Deficiency and Toxicity

Many soils of the UK, and consequently the grass growing in these areas, are unable to provide enough dietary copper for sheep. The availability of copper is reduced in the presence of competitive elements, principally molybdenum and sulphur. Concentrate feeds for sheep usually contain adequate amounts of copper. Copper is an essential trace element needed, for example, for red blood cell formation. A true assessment of the copper status can only be achieved through liver analysis, though blood samples are often taken to provide a general guide. The classical sign of copper deficiency (hypocuprosis) is congenital swayback in newborn lambs where a defect in the nervous system (demyelination) leads to lambs being unable to coordinate their hindlimbs or even stand. In these cases, it is difficult to effect a cure and euthanasia must be considered for welfare reasons. In growing lambs that appear normal at birth, signs of swayback (enzootic ataxia) include failure to thrive and the fleece may develop a characteristic appearance of dullness, dryness and lack of crimp in the wool. Adult ewes experiencing copper deficiency may show ill thrift. An adequate copper status in the ewe may not necessarily prevent symptoms occurring in her lambs. The margin for copper excess over adequacy is relatively small and there is a real danger of overdosing sheep; copper toxicity is the most commonly diagnosed cause of poisoning in sheep. Providing copper supplements by way of intra-ruminal slow-release boluses should not be undertaken in sheep receiving a diet which is supplemented with even a small amount of copper (e.g. compound feeds, mineral blocks or mineral powders with added copper). Copper poisoning results in haemolysis, jaundice and kidney failure and is usually the acute result of chronic copper accumulation. It is occasionally seen in sheep gaining access to cattle feed which has a greater copper content.

5.12.4 Cobalt Deficiency

As with copper, many areas are deficient in cobalt, which is a constituent of vitamin B12 (cobalamin). Thus, sheep that rely mostly on grazing are more likely to suffer and rapidly growing animals are more at risk and can even die. The onset of cobalt deficiency is usually insidious, with sheep failing to thrive. Signs include poor appetite, loss of weight, anaemia and a poor coat. Diagnosis is through blood sampling. Remedial action on an individual basis may involve vitamin B12 injection or the use of an intra-ruminal slow-release bolus if sheep are of an adequate size to accept the bolus. Treating ewes will facilitate the passage of increased amounts of vitamin B12 in their milk. For long-term control, pasture dressing with cobalt may be considered, but this is very expensive. Toxicity through overdosing is unlikely.

5.12.5 Selenium Deficiency

Nutritional muscular dystrophy, known colloquially as white muscle disease or stiff-lamb disease, is due to either selenium or vitamin E deficiency. Young lambs (often under 4 weeks old) appear stiff or unable to stand. Emergency treatment requires individual supplementation (usually via injection) of affected lambs. Both selenium and vitamin E can be included in diets for ewes in late pregnancy or in lamb creep feed if problems are expected in a particular locality. Excessive selenium can lead to toxicity.

5.12.6 Hypomagnesaemia (Grass Tetany/staggers)

Though not common, hypomagnesaemia is sometimes encountered in early lactation, during periods of rapid grass growth. The low concentration of magnesium available in rapidly growing spring grass, coupled with maximum milk production, places a large demand on body magnesium reserves. In acute cases, ewes may be found dead. Affected ewes appear nervous, excited or apprehensive with muscle trembling, particularly around the face. Clinical signs may be precipitated by strenuous events (e.g. gathering or transport). This is an emergency condition and treatment involves intravenous administration of a suitable electrolyte and mineral solution (which may contain calcium since hypocalcaemia often occurs concurrently). Recovery can be very rapid. Flock management should ensure adequate magnesium in the complete diet or the provision of a suitable mineral mix or feed block where concentrates are not fed at pasture.

5.12.7 Hypocalcaemia

This condition usually occurs around the time of lambing, though can occasionally occur prior to lambing if feed intake is interrupted (e.g. by snowfall). It occurs because of disturbed calcium metabolism and the inability of the ewe to maintain circulating calcium concentrations. Over-provision of calcium in the diet prior to lambing may precipitate the condition as the ewe will not develop an efficient calcium regulation mechanism geared to responding to peak demand. Clinical signs include muscle tremors, incoordination, rapid breathing and recumbency. Untreated ewes become paralysed and coma follows quickly. Treatment by intravenous calcium borogluconate (usually followed by a subcutaneous 'depot' injection to prevent a relapse) leads to rapid recovery.

5.12.8   Listeriosis

Listeriosis is primarily seen as a rapidly deteriorating encephalitis in adult sheep, which initially appear disorientated and may collapse on their front legs. They may also circle and drool saliva, with food impacted in their mouths. It is associated with feeding silage (usually big bale silage) which has been contaminated with large numbers of *Listeria monocytogenes*. This organism is relatively common in the soil and herbage. However, bacteria present can multiply in silage which has become spoiled through not achieving sufficient acidity and pose a threat to sheep. If individual cases are seen, a thorough investigation of the feed source should be made to restrict the number of further cases.

5.13   Health and Disease

5.13.1   Risk-based Health Planning and Preventive Strategies

Flock health planning is fundamental to all sheep enterprises and a requirement of farm assurance schemes. It provides a structured way to evaluate the disease and welfare risks to the flock, based on previous experience and local knowledge, and to develop a strategy to minimize or eliminate these risks. For example, health plans may set the timetable for condition scoring, vaccination, parasite and lameness control (see Table 5.4 for an example), and actions for biosecurity. Drawing up and amending a calendar in the light of actual or possible disease threats is a key part of the health planning review. Reactive 'fire brigade' measures to deal with day-to-day problems are inefficient for the farmer and are likely to have a negative impact on the sheep (e.g. the need to gather sheep more frequently to apply treatments). Health planning is also a way to incorporate best practice in disease control (e.g. the strategic use of vaccination) and welfare standards through advice from the farm's veterinary adviser. Depending on the sophistication of data recording, it also provides the opportunity for benchmarking health and production against previous performance and/or that of similar local enterprises. There is opportunity to incorporate a number of targets which can range from essential or aspirational (e.g. reducing lamb losses or the reliance on anthelmintics). Being a risk-based activity, it provides an opportunity to focus on diseases that have the greatest effect on the health and welfare of the sheep.

For any health and welfare programme to succeed, stockpersons must be able to identify signs of illness, yet these initial signs can be subtle and often non-specific. Generally, behavioural signs appear first, e.g. a sheep may spend more time lying down, be slow to rise when approached or hang back behind the rest of the flock. Sheep may be listless and adopt abnormal postures. Of more diagnostic help are symptoms such as coughing or rubbing up against solid objects. The state of the fleece can be a useful guide to general condition, especially

Table 5.4 An example of indicative timing for some basic preventive actions in a northern hemisphere, spring-lambing flock.

Month and key events	Preventive action
October – mating	
November	
December	Bluetongue vaccination within the vector-free period
January	Check for fluke eggs
February	Booster vaccination for pregnant sheep: costridial disease/pasteurellosis
March – lambing	Worming of ewes before moving to clean pasture
April	Check for fluke eggs
May – shearing	Dip or spray ewes Regular dosing of lambs for gut parasites if indicated – begin worm egg counts, depending on
June	Ectoparasite control grazing
July – weaning	
August	Spraying/dipping/pour on against ectoparasites. Active foot care for all stock. Vaccination against abortion agents. Pre-breeding inspections begin feet, teeth, udders
September	Start replacement stock on clostridial/pneumonia vaccination programme. Booster vaccination for rams 4–6 weeks before mating

when compared to the remainder of the flock. Any sheep giving cause for concern must be subject to more detailed examination.

In tick areas, additional control measures will be needed. Liver fluke treatment to be added depending on risk factors and forecast. Strategic sampling will be required depending on specific disease risks e.g. internal parasites. Trace element monitoring may be indicated.

5.13.2 Flock Biosecurity

In general terms, biosecurity concerns the prevention of introduction of new diseases to the farm and the spread of disease on the farm. This can be achieved principally through regulation of the arrival of replacement stock or contact with neighbouring sheep through fences, but also through the movement of humans (e.g. stockpersons attending gatherings where sheep are present). For flocks sharing common grazing or where animal contact commonly occurs, it is sensible for adjoining properties to have broadly similar policies for mutual benefit. Disease can also arrive via other routes: for example, wind-born spread of foot-and-mouth disease virus. Biosecurity may be practised within the farm with different groups of sheep of different disease status or at increased risk of disease. Biosecurity also concerns the export of disease agents from the farm to neighbouring properties and the control of zoonoses.

It is vital that new arrivals undergo a quarantine period to allow surveillance for diseases in incubation, performance of any screening checks and application of treatments such as vaccination, foot treatment or parasite control to bring new arrivals up to the same health status as resident animals. It is particularly important that anthelmintic-resistant worms and drug-resistant liver fluke are not introduced, through correct treatment during the quarantine period. Quarantine should be for at least three weeks, preferably four. If possible, bought-in pregnant ewes should lamb separately from the main flock. The disease risk imposed by the arrival of new stock can be reduced through purchasing replacements from flocks of known disease status and which may be assured or monitored through several national schemes (e.g. enzootic abortion; Maedi-Visna; caseous lymphadenitis). However, for some diseases such as Johne's disease, it is impossible to be sure that incoming sheep are clear. Veterinary advice should be sought to maximize the value of the quarantine period. If quarantine arrangements are to be truly effective, stockpersons must adopt a high standard of cleanliness between handling incoming and resident animals, the latter usually being handled first in the working day. For many 'closed' flocks it is often only rams that are brought in so the effort of applying a quarantine period is reduced.

A high standard of general hygiene will minimize the opportunity for newly introduced diseases to spread around the farm. It is particularly important to adopt a high standard of hygiene at lambing time when abortion agents are spread by foetuses and discharges from infected ewes. Thorough cleaning and disinfection are required also after de-stocking of buildings, including fixtures and fittings. Specific cleaning and disinfection regimes are required in cases of notifiable disease.

Hygienic practices should extend to keeping equipment clean, disinfected or sterilized and in good condition both during and after use, e.g. dosing guns and foot trimming shears. Vaccination equipment must be kept as clean as possible and needles changed at the recommended frequency as they can act as a route for disease spread and lead to abscess formation. Blunt needles are likely to damage the sheep and will cause unnecessary pain.

5.13.3 Vaccination

Vaccination to provide protection against a range of serious diseases should be part of each flock's health plan. On organic units, specific approval for prophylactic vaccination will be required unless control is required as part of a statutory programme (e.g. bluetongue). The timing of primary and repeat vaccination needs to precede the peak risk periods, and for lambing ewes, booster vaccinations are given two to four weeks before lambing to maximize the antibody content of colostrum. It is important that ewes are handled calmly to avoid stress at this time. Some vaccines should not be given concurrently, and advice should always be obtained as part of the flock health planning process.

5.13.4 Diseases with a Significant Impact on Sheep Welfare

While the presence of any disease will reduce the welfare status of an individual sheep, several specific diseases are of major importance in the UK and around the world.

5.13.4.1 Lameness

Lameness in sheep can be due to a range of infectious and physical causes, though scald, classic foot rot (infection with the bacteria *Dichelobacter nodosus*) and contagious ovine digital dermatitis (CODD) are most often responsible. Non-infectious causes include injuries, foreign bodies, laminitis, interdigital fibromas and congenital abnormalities (e.g. corkscrew-shaped claws). Sometimes poor general body conformation may place abnormal load on the limbs. Exposure to a very high plane of nutrition such as a particularly lush pasture can result in laminitis, a painful inflammation of the sensitive laminae of the foot; affected animals can be lame in all four feet and rendered immobile due to the pain associated with this condition. Laminitis usually resolves once the plane of nutrition is lowered. Post-dipping lameness has sometimes been observed due to the build-up of *Erysipelothrix rhusiopathiae* organisms in the dipping solution.

Along with perinatal mortality, lameness probably represents the most important welfare problem for sheep, both in terms of the impact on individual sheep of the painful condition and the sometimes-high proportion of affected sheep in a flock. It is also an economic problem, affecting growth, lactation and reproductive behaviour. In the UK, the bacterium causing scald and footrot is present on 97% of farms. Infections are spread most easily in warm and moist conditions, which can be year-round with the changing climate, and generally from sheep to sheep as they move through well-used areas such as gateways, races and handling areas. Lameness can also be passed from ewes to their lambs in spring and summer.

To control the disease it is important that it is treated as soon as it is observed, to reduce the spread between animals, by giving long-acting antibiotic injections (in consultation with the vet), and applying antibiotic spray to the affected foot. Separation of affected animals from the rest of the flock can also help reduce animal to animal spread. Foot-trimming and bathing are no longer advised as they are ineffective and can actively contribute to the spread of the disease between animals.

Reducing the risk of outbreaks requires good flock management, such as the Five Point Plan advocated by AHDB (https://ahdb.org.uk/knowledge-library/lameness-in-sheep-the-five-point-plan). This is based on the five principles of:

1) Culling animals that have persistent cases of lameness to build resilience
2) Treating even mildly lame sheep as soon as possible to reduce spread
3) Reduce the disease challenge by treating and separating affected animals
4) Quarantining incoming animals for 28 days with regular foot inspections
5) Vaccination if levels of lameness are high and before high-risk periods such as housing.

5.13.4.2 Internal Parasites

Strategies to control parasites in the intestinal tract and liver should be one of the major components of flock health planning. There is not space here to explore fully the various factors that should form part of a control programme. The most important elements are: sound pasture management in relation to nematode parasite epidemiology; the use of faecal egg counts (to assess worm burdens) which can be conducted on-farm using proprietary kits; selection for breeding of animals with greatest genetic resistance; and, lastly, the strategic use of

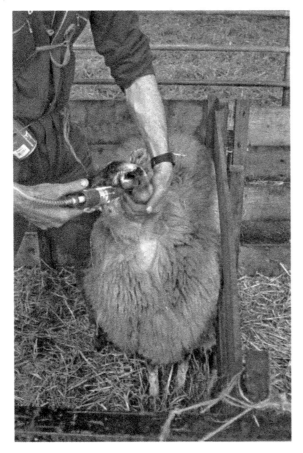

Figure 5.6 Administration of an anthelmintic drench to a ewe using a properly calibrated dosing gun. Photograph by permission of Kay Aitchison.

anthelmintic treatments. The use of rams with resistance to worms can be achieved through estimated breeding values for faecal egg counts. While oral dosing of sheep (Figure 5.6) with liquid anthelmintics is a straightforward task, it does need to be done carefully to avoid damaging the pharyngeal area of the mouth.

Lambs in their first grazing season are at greatest risk of nematode infection. Not only will disease lead to health and welfare concerns but lambs with a high worm burden will not thrive. Strategic worming of ewes is also needed as they show a periparturient rise in worm egg output, which contaminates early grazing. Maximizing the use of clean grazing (land not used for sheep since the last season or used previously for hay or silage crops) or rotational grazing with cattle is possible on some lowland farms. However, some parasites can remain a threat from year to year, particularly *Nematodirus* species which are a threat to 6- to 10-week-old lambs eating increasing amounts of grass. Changing climatic patterns have resulted in a northerly extension in the range of parasites such as *Haemonchus contortus*. Tapeworms are generally controlled by adherence to regimes for nematodes and regularly worming farm dogs. The protozoon parasites, *Coccidia* spp., can cause problems in lambs of 4 to 6 weeks of age where there is a rapid increase in infectious organisms from older to younger lambs, particularly if the lambing period is extended, before natural immunity develops. *Cryptosporidium parvum* affects younger lambs and is a zoonosis.

Sheep with soiled perineal areas, primarily due to worm-induced diarrhoea, are more prone to blowfly attack and fly strike (cutaneous myiasis). The necessity for tail-docking of lambs may be reduced if worm control strategies lead to reduced faecal soiling. Given the seriousness of poorly controlled parasitic disease, several initiatives have been developed to provide targeted advice on control strategies. For example, the Sustainable Control of Parasites in Sheep (SCOPS) programme aims to provide an overall control strategy with less reliance on anthelmintics. This is particularly important as there is widespread resistance to many of the currently available wormers. Resistance is more likely to develop if sheep receive a suboptimal dose: when treating a group of sheep, always adjust the dosing gun in relation to the weight of the heaviest sheep in the group and ensure that the dosing gun itself has been calibrated accurately. Anthelmintics can be grouped into five main families based on their active principles. On veterinary advice, products from these families can be used together or on an annual rotation but on some properties multiple resistance means that none of these is entirely effective.

5.13.4.3 Ectoparasites

One of the major ectoparasitic diseases affecting sheep welfare is sheep scab, caused by the mite, *Psoroptes ovis*. The presence of the mite on the skin surface causes an allergic reaction in the sheep to mite faeces, resulting in a serous exudate on which the mites feed. The allergic response is accompanied by intense irritation, causing the sheep to rub, scratch and bite, leading to self-inflicted injury. Thus, one of the first signs of scab is patchy fleece loss and very frequent scratching and rubbing against fixed objects. Mites are easily spread from sheep to sheep, and can also be passed on through environmental contamination, as mites can live off the host for up to 17 days. Mites prefer warm and moist conditions and disease is most prevalent in the autumn and winter on fully fleeced animals. There is a legal requirement to treat sheep with scab in the UK, and it is a notifiable disease in Scotland. Sheep scab can be treated by plunge dipping in organophosphate dips (although with associated human and sheep health and welfare risks), or by injection of macrocyclic lactones (such as ivermectin). Prevention of sheep scab infestation through effective quarantine of bought in stock or maintaining a closed flock, boundary control and biosecurity is required.

A range of other ectoparasites affect sheep and cause stress, pain and discomfort, and can transmit important diseases: e.g. the sheep tick (*Ixodes ricinus*) which transmits louping ill virus, lice, keds and mange mites. The greenbottle (*Lucilia sericata*) and bluebottle (*Calliphora* spp.), which are the major cause of flystrike/cutaneous myiasis, are the most reported ectoparasite problem in many flocks. Regular inspection of sheep around periods of fly activity is crucial to identify affected sheep for immediate treatment. Blowfly eggs are laid on moist, faecally contaminated wool, usually around the tail area. When these eggs hatch the larvae (maggots) burrow into the sheep leading to large ulcerated areas, subject to secondary infection. Flystrike is more common in warm, wet areas and when sheep are more tightly stocked. It is a life-threatening condition and can lead to significant losses. Prevention requires regular inspection, shearing and removal of soiled material around the tail and anus, and other management to reduce the build-up of faecal material, such as effective internal parasite control to reduce diarrhoea. Pour-on or plunge dipping products can also be used, although young lambs should not be dipped. Dipping to control ectoparasites is stressful and should not take place if sheep are hot, thirsty, wet, tired or fully fed.

5.13.4.4 Mastitis

Mastitis (inflammation of the mammary gland) in meat sheep often goes undiagnosed, and untreated, until a pre-breeding inspection. Since mastitis occurs mainly in the first month of lactation, it should be suspected if lambs fail to thrive as milk production will be affected, and ewes are reluctant to allow lambs to suck due to the pain associated with the condition. Ewes with clinical mastitis can become systemically ill and require prompt treatment to reduce inflammation and restore lactation. On inspection, the udder will be swollen, hardened, hot and inflamed, often with superficial purple discolouration, and only watery fluid may be drawn from the teat. This is a severe condition and even some treated ewes may die or ultimately lose, through sloughing, the affected part of the udder resulting in permanent damage of the udder. Since the organisms responsible are spread in the environment, for housed ewes in particular a high standard of hygiene must be employed and ewes with mastitis should be segregated from other sheep.

5.13.4.5 Zoonoses

Zoonotic diseases are those capable of being transmitted from animals to humans. Sheep can carry several zoonotic infections, many of which are prevalent at around lambing time, when pregnant women are particularly at risk from diseases causing abortion in sheep. Risks are associated with foetal fluids, placenta and the lambs themselves (both live and dead), and potentially with ewes sometime before lambing, so it is recommended that pregnant women do not work with sheep, or come into contact with anything that may be contaminated.

Enzootic abortion of ewes (EAE), caused by *Chlamydophila abortus*, is the most diagnosed type of abortion in sheep, and is spread from infected to susceptible sheep at lambing time through the products of an infected birth. Sheep infected for the first time will abort at the next lambing. Abortion 'storms' can occur when infection is introduced and spread in a naïve flock. Thereafter around a third of ewes could abort annually. Vaccination, maintaining a closed flock or purchasing replacement females from certified EAE-free sources is one way to avoid abortion through this cause.

Toxoplasmosis, caused by *Toxoplasma gondii*, a protozoan parasite, is another common cause of abortion in sheep. Toxoplasma has a complex life cycle involving a final host, usually cats, and a range of intermediate hosts that includes sheep. Between sheep transmission is not thought to occur but the disease can be spread by having infected cats able to access sheep feed or sheds. Vaccination against this cause of abortion is available. *Salmonella* spp.,

Campylobacter spp. and several other organisms can cause abortion or enteritis in sheep and result in zoonotic disease.

Orf (contagious pustular dermatitis) is a viral disease-causing skin lesions, and lesions at junctions of the skin and mucous membranes, for example, around the mouth of lambs. This results in transmission to the ewe's teats and udder. Orf can also affect the lower limbs and genitalia and can lead to ill thrift. In cases of severe infection, a live vaccine should be considered. Humans can experience, sometimes, quite severe lesions following exposure to both field cases and the vaccine and so should be careful to wear protective gloves when handling affected sheep or administering vaccines. The virus can remain viable in the environment for a considerable period.

5.13.4.6 Notifiable Diseases

Several diseases of ruminants are defined as 'notifiable', requiring notification the competent authorities who will instigate an investigation. Notifiable diseases of relevance to sheep in the UK are foot and mouth disease, bluetongue, anthrax, scrapie and sheep scab in Scotland.

5.14 Routine Husbandry Procedures Affecting Sheep Welfare

Several procedures or practices are carried out in the management of sheep, which may reduce sheep welfare in the short term, even if the longer-term goal may improve welfare. Some procedures are, however, generally negative for sheep welfare, although they may make management easier.

5.14.1 General Handling

Interaction between individual sheep and the stockperson can be infrequent, especially on hill farms, but will be required on occasions for various health and welfare procedures, such as vaccinating, shearing, worming and foot care. The infrequency of these direct interactions can make these stressful for the sheep, and skill and care to minimize pain or fear in these interactions is required.

Individual sheep can be caught in the field with a crook to hook the sheep above the hock. If sheep are too flighty to approach, they will need to be herded into a small handling pen, or into housing. Sheep can then be caught by gradually reducing the range of movement in the pen until the animal can be caught and restrained against the handler's legs or gently held against the side of the pen, usually by holding the chin with one hand, and pressing a knee against the lumbar vertebrae in front of the stifle. Animals should not be caught by the fleece, horns, ears or tails, which can cause pain, bruising and, in the case of horns, may break off and cause considerable bleeding.

A sheep can also be cast (tipped over to rest with its hindquarters on the ground and its back against the stockperson) to facilitate some activities. In this position, most sheep tend not to struggle and procedures such as foot trimming and removing soiled wool from around the breech (dagging) can be accomplished single-handed. Although this position usually means the animal stays still, time spent in this position should be minimized, and avoided for late pregnant ewes. Sheep can be cast by turning the head horizontally, towards the tail, with mild to moderate force, and applying downwards pressure on the rump.

5.14.1.1 Gathering and Moving Sheep

One common need in any sheep system is to move animals between grazing areas or to collect them together for selection or other husbandry treatments. For hill flocks, gathering is a major exercise sometime involving the collaborative efforts of local farms whose sheep share the same open hill. Sheep are traditionally gathered on foot, with herding dogs, although the use of quadbikes has made this easier for the shepherds. Gathering can be a stressful process for the sheep and people involved, and it is important to be aware of fatigue in the flock if gathering is over a long distance or of a long duration (often many hours). The start of the gather is when the first sheep are grouped together, and not when the last sheep is collected when the drive phase begins. Sheep gathered early in the day may experience significantly more stress than those gathered at the end of the process. Gathers on hot days are often avoided but, if necessary, must be conducted in such a way that sheep do not become fatigued and dehydrated, by slowing the pace of the movement, and allowing animals to recover along the way. Similarly, dogs should not be allowed to harass straggling individuals or those at the back of a large mob whose forward movement is restricted by stationary sheep. Sheep should be given the opportunity to demonstrate their innate following ability, which is thwarted if they are rushed. In large, extensive flocks, gathering may limited to only a few occasions each year, typically five gathers per year at key management times, whereas this may occur more frequently in lowland flocks. If ewes with lambs at foot are to be gathered, additional time must be allowed; if the lamb cannot keep up with the ewe she will usually turn back and make the overall process more difficult. In some situations, supplementary feed can be used, and ewes and lambs will be attracted by the sight and sound of a rustled feed sack or rattled bucket.

5.14.1.2 Handling Facility Design

In order to handle and treat large numbers of sheep handling systems of pens and races are required, which can be permanent, where the animals are moved to the facilities, or temporary, where pens can be built in the corner of fields. Well-designed systems work with the behaviour of the sheep to encourage the sheep to want to move in the desired direction, such as towards an opening or back to the field. Curved raceways, which allow the sheep always to be following a sheep in front, and to see a way forward, are far more effective in achieving a flow of animals than races with tight corners. Since sheep find isolation aversive, the pens should allow as much visual contact as possible and the working methods should minimize the times when sheep are isolated. In yards and buildings, sheep are easily disturbed by shadows and loud noises (see also Grandin 2019, for more details on handling livestock). Individual handling is also stressful to the sheep and most common practices such as dosing, vaccination or condition scoring do not require individual isolation and can be conducted in small pens or raceways with the stockperson working alongside.

Handling systems should include a gathering pen, of sufficient size to accommodate the largest mob, a way of easily encouraging sheep into smaller pens (such as some form of crowding gate), a raceway system by which sheep can be moved from these smaller pens and a working area where, for example, husbandry treatments are applied. Newer systems that incorporate swinging gates, which can be lifted over the backs of sheep, electronic shedding gates, and hydraulic systems can improve the ease of working with large numbers of sheep by a single stockperson and can improve sheep (and handler) welfare through reducing human frustration and fatigue. Ideally, as much of the area as possible should be covered to allow work to be conducted in the dry and to prevent sheep becoming overheated in the summer under the direct sun.

5.14.2 Identification

Sheep can be marked permanently by tattooing, horn branding, electronic identification (EID), ear tags (metal or plastic) or ear notching, and temporarily by marker sprays and crayon colour marking. However, ear notching is not recommended as more useful and less painful alternatives are available. Within the EU and the UK it is a requirement that all sheep destined for the food chain are marked with EID. In the UK requirements sheep must be tagged within six months of birth (if housed indoors), or before they are moved from the farm, using tags that provide official identification of the animal to improve traceability in case of disease outbreaks.

There is a variation in the retention rate and the damage to the ear on insertion of tags, which should be placed in the lower ear margin, avoiding major blood vessels or cartilaginous ridges. Poor tagging practice can lead to tags being caught and torn out, causing pain and ear damage. It is best practice to apply tags in cooler weather, using clean equipment, to avoid fly nuisance or possible flystrike and infection.

Although farmers can choose to tag animals only as they leave the farm, making use of EID information can improve health and welfare management of sheep. Electronic tags can be read by use of a hand-held reader or automatically by devices which can be incorporated into the weighing crate of a handling system. This allows information to be collected automatically for downloading to a farm's management database.

5.14.3 Transport

Sheep are transported regularly for management and trade purposes. It is generally accepted that transport, even under optimal conditions, is stressful to the sheep and thus should be minimized. Sheep transport can vary from one or more ewes and lambs in a trailer towed around the farm by a four-wheel-drive motorbike to large numbers of market-weight sheep transported in pens in the holds of ships between Australia and the Middle East. The main risks to welfare, which increase with longer journeys, are fitness to travel, exposure to novel environments, movement restrictions due to confinement, vibrations and sudden noise, mixing with other animals, temperature and humidity, and feed and water restriction.

There is wide support for the proposal that the long-distance transport of slaughter sheep should cease in favour of moving frozen or chilled products, although this can present problems for countries without a secure cold chain. Within Europe, there are considerable movements of live sheep to satisfy seasonal demands. However, long-distance transport can cause many problems for sheep, particularly sea transport, and is unequivocally to the detriment of sheep welfare. Welfare considerations should include several pre-shipment practices: gathering, shearing and collection in feedlots to accustom them to transport conditions, including feeding from troughs. These alone can introduce a range of environmental and psychological stressors. During the sea journey, mortality can be high, though has declined over recent years following the introduction of improved veterinary standards. The main problems leading to mortality are failure to eat, salmonellosis and heat stress. Heat stress occurs when poorly adapted, densely stocked sheep fail to cope with a high heat load, despite panting and other short-term heat-reducing physiological changes. Inter-country or inter-region transport of any livestock has the potential to introduce exotic disease and to make individual transported animals more susceptible to disease through the negative effect of stress on the immune system. In addition, the increased contact between unfamiliar animals increases the opportunity for disease to spread. In many countries, there has been considerable public pressure to end live animal export and to slaughter animals as close to the point of production as possible.

Within the EU, there are comprehensive rules relating to distances, journey duration and transport conditions, but enforcing the legislation is demanding. Training and the development of best practice guidance (see: http://www.animaltransportguides.eu) is designed to improve compliance. There are requirements for vehicle design in relation to materials (e.g. non-slip flooring) and operation (e.g. ventilation systems and hygiene measures). In many cases (depending on journey distance) a route plan is required which should allow for contingencies such as delays or injury to any of the animals. EU transport regulations require that in 'basic' standard vehicles, the maximum journey time is 8 hours. In vehicles of higher specification, the maximum journey time for adult sheep is 14 hours' travel, at least 1 hour of rest (and the provision of water, and feed if deemed necessary) and then a further 14 hours' travel. In particular circumstances the journey can extend a further 2 hours if close to the destination at the end of the prescribed time. Otherwise, a 24-hour rest period must follow before further transport is possible. Rules also include an assessment of driver competence; one of the main impacts on the welfare of transported sheep is the care with which a vehicle is driven, e.g. avoiding rapid acceleration and sharp cornering in order that sheep may more easily retain their balance. This reduces energy demand (and possible fatigue) and the chance of injury. The road quality is also important, and drivers should avoid minor or unmade roads with many corners.

In addition to driving quality, the care taken on loading and unloading will have a major impact on sheep welfare. Sheep should be allowed to load at their own pace, and this is encouraged by the provision of suitable handling pens and loading bays. Fitness to travel for the whole journey also needs to be assured prior to departure. This is an issue for many cast-age ewes, some of which should be euthanized on-farm.

5.14.4 Markets

Livestock markets present sheep with a range of novel experiences, many of which may be stressful. There are often many humans in close proximity to pens and raceways, animals may be mixed with unfamiliar animals, the market can be very noisy, and feed, water and bedding may be unavailable. Handling and movement of animals also involves unfamiliar people, and usually pushing animals through unfamiliar systems. There must be adequate provision for the care of sick or injured sheep and all facilities must be well-designed and maintained to prevent injury and the build-up of disease organisms. A range of agencies have representatives at markets to ensure animal welfare but it is not always entirely clear who is explicitly responsible. Because of the high visibility of market activities, it is in everyone's interest to ensure that standards of animal welfare are maintained at a high level.

While markets may be required to set a price for classes of livestock and to batch up small numbers of animals, it is preferable if animals for slaughter go directly from farm to abattoir. For breeding stock, internet sales may reduce the opportunity for disease transmission. Internet marketing is more attractive where purchasers place greater weight on performance records rather than phenotypic appearance.

5.14.5 Shearing

Shearing presents a cluster of aversive elements, from gathering, penning, possible food and water deprivation, individual handling, noise of clippers and the shearing process. Individual animal care is difficult to deliver when large mobs of sheep are handled in a situation that is stressful for the handlers, and where speed is encouraged. While wool in some countries is a valuable commodity, such as Australia where Merino sheep produce up to 8 kg of fine apparel wool per clip, in others the value is sometimes too low to offset the shearing cost (e.g. 2 kg of carpet wool from hill sheep). In these situations, shearing is undertaken primarily to protect sheep welfare and as a result there is increasing interest in using breeds of sheep with a natural propensity to shed their fleece in the summer (such as Easy Care sheep). Failure to shear sheep on an annual basis due to economic pressures can lead to welfare problems (e.g. greater risk of ectoparasitic disease or the inability to regain their footing if they become cast with a heavy, wet fleece).

Wool removal itself appears to be the most stressful component overall. Shearing must be conducted skilfully to minimize injuries to sheep (primarily cuts from the shears). Systems where shearers are paid to shear as many animals as possible in the shortest time tend to encourage poorer quality of care, and greater risks of injuries. Some stockpersons house sheep the night before shearing to ensure that fleeces are dry. Shearing should not be undertaken on days when adverse weather is forecast, particularly if undertaken early in the season when shorn sheep can become severely chilled and may even die. Winter shearing of sheep prior to housing allows animals to be kept at a lower space allowance (especially at the feeding face) and facilitates supervision at lambing but must not be undertaken in the absence of housing. Winter-shorn sheep should not be turned out until at least 15–20 mm of fleece has regrown.

5.14.6 Castration

Male lambs are castrated to prevent indiscriminate breeding, particularly of ewe lambs, unwanted behaviours, such as aggression, to improve handling safety, and to improve carcass quality in older lambs. However, with faster growing breeds and good nutrition this practice is decreasing for lowland farmers in the UK, and increasing numbers of male lambs are left entire, reaching market weights before puberty. For hill farms, however, with slower growing breeds and limited options to manage male and female lambs separately, the need for castration is still an issue. Since castration is an action primarily for management benefit, it should only be conducted when absolutely necessary and then with the least possible welfare disbenefit to the lamb.

Castration can be performed by several methods, including surgical approaches, methods to restrict the flow of blood to the testes, methods designed to crush the spermatic cords, and by immunocastration. The most common method in the UK is the application of tight rubber rings, placed around the scrotum by use of a device called an elastrator. The ring constricts to restrict the blood supply to the scrotum and its contents, which die and eventually drop off distal to the ring. Rubber rings are typically applied without anaesthesia or analgesia, and lambs express pain-related behaviours, such as abnormal standing and lying postures, kicking, rolling and restlessness for up to 2 hours following application. Infection can form around the site of the ring. The testes are shed after about 4 weeks. Short scrotum castration can also be undertaken whereby the ring is applied distal to the testes to force them into the lamb's body, where increased temperature restricts sperm production and renders the lamb infertile. Lambs castrated by this method express a lower pain response compared to lambs with a full bilateral castration. Less commonly, the spermatic cords are crushed using a bloodless castration device (Burdizzo). This causes an instant pain response from the lamb, but this is much shorter in duration than the response to the rubber ring as the nerves are crushed at the same time as the spermatic cords. Local anaesthetic reduces the behavioural and physiological response of lambs to castration by any method, but it is not often applied and will not provide analgesia extending beyond the duration of the acute pain. More recently, newer devices, that can deliver local anaesthetic as the ring is applied have been developed and may offer a viable solution for farmers. The availability of anti-inflammatory drugs and analgesics for sheep is generally poor and their use is not widespread; they are rarely, if ever, used following castration.

Methods are prescribed in legislation and are often time-limited. For example, in the UK the use of rubber elastrator rings is not permitted after seven days of age, which presents problems for hill farmers who usually do not want to disturb the lambing flock until lambs are older. There is no evidence to support the implication that pain perception is less during the first week of life than at a later age, although in larger lambs the volume of tissue to be shed is greater and lesions are larger. In the UK, for lambs older than three months, an anaesthetic must be used and castration undertaken by a veterinary surgeon.

Recent developments in immunocastration, where the lamb is vaccinated with antibodies against components of the reproductive pathways, have been shown to be effective in reducing circulating testosterone and preventing the development of the testes. This approach could allow older lambs to be castrated as required, but a commercial product has not yet been licensed for use in sheep.

5.14.7 Tail Docking

This procedure, involving removal of the distal part of the tail, is performed to reduce the risk of flystrike (myiasis): a serious, debilitating, sometimes life-threatening condition. If practiced, all sheep in a flock are typically docked, yet the potential benefit is unpredictable as some sheep would never have suffered flystrike. Predisposing factors include soiled breech areas often because of heavy burdens of gut parasites. Thus, good parasite control (e.g. through selection of sheep with genetic resistance to nematode parasites) is an effective way of reducing the chance of strike. Equally, effective prophylaxis against blowfly attack is important. Some breeds of sheep have reduced fleece in the breech area or shorter tails and selective breeding could be better employed to increase the penetration of these desirable traits. Tail docking is rare in hill flocks, where the chance of myiasis is less and the tail provides additional protection against the cold.

Methods include the use of elastrator rings within the first week of life, cauterization using a hot docking iron, or the combination of Burdizzo and elastrator rings. Many lambs are docked surgically using a sharp knife. The pain and distress caused by tail docking appears to be less than following castration, and hot iron docking is considered less painful than the use of rubber rings. Enough tail must be left to cover the vulva in females and the anus in males.

For Merino and Merino-type sheep bred with deep skin folds to increase skin surface area and thus yield of wool, the technique of mulesing has been adopted in Australia whereby some of the folded skin around the breech and tail regions is surgically removed. The contraction of resultant wool-free scar tissue reduces the chance of subsequent faecal soiling. Topical application of anaesthetic to the wound is increasingly used to treat lambs following mulesing, following evidence that lambs find the procedure extremely aversive, and public opposition to the procedure is considerable. Selective breeding of sheep with reduced fleece or less skin folding in this area is a solution to be exploited, together with selection of strains of sheep more resistant to internal parasites, as noted above. However, these measures may be insufficient, particularly during long spells of warm, wet weather.

Dagging of sheep using clippers removes excess wool around the breech area, tail and down the inside of the hind limbs to discourage faecal soiling. It is often undertaken prior to shearing to ensure that a clean fleece can be produced for sale, but also on a more individual needs basis if excessive soiling is evident at any time to reduce the risk of flystrike.

5.14.8 Slaughter

Methods of commercial slaughter involve two phases: pre-slaughter stunning, using captive bolt, or electrical current, and killing by cutting arteries in the neck and exsanguination. The slaughter process itself should render the sheep insensible as rapidly as possible and ensure that death through exsanguination occurs before consciousness returns. With few exceptions, for religious purposes, all sheep are required to be stunned before killing in the UK and in many other countries. Slaughter processes, including related operations inside and outside the slaughterhouse, are prescribed in legislation and have a primary purpose to reduce distress, pain or suffering during pre-slaughter handling and killing.

5.14.8.1 Emergency Slaughter

There may be situations in which a sheep that has sustained an injury or a disease has progressed to the point when slaughter is the most humane option, and animals are not fit to be legally transported to a slaughterhouse. Flock health and welfare plans should consider, in advance, the inevitable need to destroy sheep on-farm. In most cases, the method of choice is to use a shotgun to shoot sheep at close range. For those with a slaughterman's licence, a captive bolt pistol could be used. The animal should then be promptly bled out to ensure rapid death.

5.15   Welfare Assessment in Sheep

Welfare assessment is typically used to assess compliance with legislation, or with standards and practices in assurance schemes, although welfare assessment can also be used for continuous improvements or to assess the impact of changes in management. Often assessment of compliance involves a 'snapshot'-type assessment where measures are made by an external assessor, whereas farmer assessments allow a more longitudinal approach. Welfare assessment can be through assessing inputs (resource-based) where the facilities, food, space and other inputs available to the sheep are assessed, or outcomes (animal-based), where measures are made on the animals themselves. It is generally considered that outcome measures are more reflective of the animal's actual experience, and have become the preferred method of assessing welfare, although resource-based measures are still largely used for assurance schemes.

5.15.1   Animal-based Welfare Indicators

Outcome-based assessment methods have now been developed for many farmed species, including sheep. To provide an overall assessment, several animals are assessed individually, or as a group, focusing on assessing the different aspects of welfare: feeding, environment, health and behaviour. The approach taken by the EU Welfare Quality® project, and then subsequently in the Animal Welfare Indicators (AWIN) project, which included sheep, has defined twelve criteria for welfare, within the four main principles, and then developed suitable indicators for each. Selection of appropriate animal-based indicators for inclusion involves assessing that they are valid (that they measure what they are supposed to), reliable (that they can be measured in the same way by different assessors, or by the same assessor on different days/farms) and can feasibly be measured on all farms. The ability of the welfare assessment protocol to consider positive welfare aspects, as well as negative, is also important. The AWIN protocol provides an example of a welfare assessment protocol developed for sheep.

An alternative to providing on farm assessment of the living animals is to use abattoir measures, which can be fed back to the farm (e.g. Llonch et al. 2015). These can be limited to a number of key disease measures, but can provide information that is not available from inspection of the live sheep. This allows welfare improvement to be made at the farm level, and for animals still in the flock, but clearly does not allow mitigation of welfare issues for the assessed animal.

There is increasing interest in the use of technology and sensors to collect continuous monitoring data on the behaviour, health or feed intake of individual animals, or to monitor the overall group welfare. These can involve on-animal technology, such as GPS or accelerometers, or off-animal approaches such as the use of cameras or automated weighing machines. Use of these technologies is still in its infancy in the sheep sector but has the potential to allow much more monitoring and early assessment of welfare issues for sheep.

5.15.2 Welfare Assurance Schemes

Minimum standards of welfare are covered by legislation. However, farm assurance schemes and retailers may seek a higher standard of welfare, to meet consumer demands for good welfare. This may also attract a higher price premium for sheep products. As the public already considers that sheep benefit from a high standard of welfare (not least because of the 'naturalness' aspects of sheep production), there is less scope for producers to further enhance their systems in the public's view. Many initiatives, such as organic standards, include animal welfare within a group of attributes that include environmental stewardship, and may focus on a few important welfare compromises for sheep (e.g. lameness, avoidance of castration and tail docking). Most assurance schemes still rely mainly on resource-based indicators of welfare, to assess compliance with designated standards or provisions, although some will include a small number of additional animal-based assessments of key metrics (e.g. RSPCA-Assured lamb).

References and Further Reading

Agriculture and Horticulture Development Board. (2015). Improving Ewe Nutrition of Better Returns. https://ahdb.org.uk/knowledge-library/improving-ewe-nutrition-for-better-returns.

Aitken, I.D. (ed.) (2007). *Diseases of Sheep*, 4e. Oxford: Blackwell Publishing.

Animal Transport Guides. http://www.animaltransportguides.eu.

Animal Welfare Indicators Sheep Welfare Assessment Protocol. https://www.researchgate.net/publication/275887069_AWIN_Welfare_Assessment_Protocol_for_Sheep.

Appleby, M.C., Cussen, V., Garces, L., Lambert, J.A., and Turner, J. (eds.) (2008). *Long Distance Transport and Welfare of Farm Animals*. Wallingford: CABI Publishing.

Beef+Lamb New Zealand: principles of feeding: from mating to lambing (sheep). https://beeflambnz.com/knowledge-hub/module/principles-feeding-mating-lambing-sheep.

DEFRA Codes of Recommendations for the Welfare of Livestock: Sheep. https://assets.publishing.service.gov.uk/government/uploads/system/uploads/attachment_data/file/69365/pb5162-sheep-041028.pdf.

Dwyer, C. (ed.) (2008). *The Welfare of Sheep*. New York: Springer.

Farm Animal Welfare Council. (2011). *Opinion on Sheep Lameness*. London: FAWC. https://www.gov.uk/government/publications/fawc-opinion-on-sheep-lameness.

Grandin, T. (ed.) (2019). *Livestock Handling and Transport*, 5e. Wallingford: CABI Publishing.

Hemsworth, P.H. and Coleman, G.J. (2011). *Human-Livestock Interactions: The Stockperson and the Productivity and Welfare of Intensively Farmed Animals*, 2e. Wallingford: CABI Publishing.

Henderson, D.C. (2002). *The Veterinary Book for Sheep Farmers*. Ipswich, UK: Old Pond Publishing.

Jensen, P. (ed.) (2017). *The Ethology of Domestic Animals*, 3e. Wallingford: CABI Publishing.

Llonch, P., King, E.M., Clarke, K.A., Downes, J.M., and Green, L.E. (2015). A systematic review of animal-based indicators of sheep welfare on farm, at market and during transport, and qualitative appraisal of their validity and feasibility for use in UK abattoirs. *The Veterinary Journal* 206: 289–297.

Mellor, D.J. (et al.). (2020). The 2020 Five Domains Model: including human-animal interactions in assessments of animal welfare. *Animals* 10: 1870.

National Animal Disease Information Service. https://www.nadis.org.uk.

National Sheep Association. www.nationalsheep.org.uk.

Quality Meat Scotland: Ewe nutrition and body condition scoring timeline. https://www.qmscotland.co.uk/sites/default/files/ewe_nutrition_timeline_poster_0.pdf (accessed 01 June 2021).

Sargison, N. (2008). *Sheep Flock Health: A Planned Approach*. Oxford: Blackwell Publishing.

Sargison, N., Crilly, J.P., and Hopker, A. (2018). *Practical Lambing and Lamb Care: A Veterinary Guide*, 4e. Oxford: Wiley Blackwell Publishing.

Sustainable Control of Parasites (SCOPS). https://www.scops.org.uk.

6

Pigs

Sandra Edwards

6.1   The Natural Biology of the Pig

Modern agricultural pigs have descended from the European wild boar (*Sus scrofa*). While their appearance and productive characteristics have been greatly changed by selective breeding, many of their basic behavioural instincts have been largely conserved despite many generations of domestication. An understanding of the basic biology of their wild ancestors is therefore very important in designing good management and husbandry systems.

Management and Welfare of Farm Animals: The UFAW Farm Handbook, Sixth Edition.
Edited by John Webster and Jean Margerison.
© Universities Federation for Animal Welfare 2022. Published 2022 by John Wiley & Sons Ltd.

Wild boars are omnivores living in forest margins in small family groups of four to six related sows and their offspring of the last one to two years. Males live as solitary individuals or in bachelor groups, joining the sows only at the time of breeding. The wild pig is a seasonal breeder, coming into heat and mating in the autumn, and farrowing four months later in early spring. Sometimes a second farrowing may occur later in the year in August and September. This seasonality appears to be primarily determined by photoperiod, but food supply has also been shown to influence the timing of onset of ovarian activity in the autumn. Sows about to give birth isolate themselves from the main group and build a nest, where they give birth and initially nurse their young. After one to two weeks, they abandon the nest and lead their young back to rejoin the main group. The piglets show a gradually reducing frequency of suckling and increase in foraging for solid food, until they are finally weaned at an age of three to four months. Wild boars are not territorial but have home ranges without a well-defined boundary. The family groups range over an area of 100 to 2,500 hectares, depending on season and food availability. These areas contain resting places and nests, watering places and wallows, rubbing and scratching places, regular rooting areas, and a network of regularly used interconnecting paths. The family disperses over a wide area while foraging but comes back together for communal resting during the day and at night in simple nests made in areas of dense cover. Foraging activity occupies more than 50% of their active time, with a diurnal pattern of activity peaks at dawn and dusk and comprises a mixture of grazing and rooting behaviour. The principal feeds are grasses, roots and tubers in the summer and mast crops, nuts and fruits in the autumn and winter, supplemented by invertebrates and carrion when these can be found.

Because of wild boars' forest habitat, their need to seek out food which is hidden or underground and to be aware of approaching predators, the senses of smell, touch and hearing are more important than vision. The snout is a highly developed organ for olfaction and rooting. Scent marks from glands on the face and neck, anogenital region, and feet are used to map their home range, and to identify members of the group. The pigs also have a complex repertoire of vocalizations, with grunts used in maintaining social contact, barks indicating alarm and squeals indicating distress. Within the group, overt aggression is rare because of the existence of a dominance hierarchy based on age and size which gives priority of access to resources without conflict. This is maintained by use of signals based on threatening and submissive postures. Physical aggression occurs only if there is competition for some highly prized resource, such as when males compete for breeding opportunities, or when unfamiliar animals encounter each other.

These patterns of behaviour seen in the wild boar can all be observed in modern feral pigs, or when modern domestic pigs are placed in semi-natural environments. They can also be seen in some traditional extensive farming systems, such as those for indigenous Iberian pigs grazing in the oak forest 'dehesa' regions of Mediterranean countries. In more intensive farming conditions, expression of many of these patterns of natural behaviour is limited, and this can give rise to some animal welfare problems, even where the physical needs of the animals are met by other means.

6.2 Domestication and Adaptability

Domestication of the pig was favoured by its social nature, adaptability and omnivorous habits. It occurred in Neolithic times, possibly by capture and habituation of wild pigs foraging on sown crops. Their ability to reproduce prolifically and deposit large stores of body fat favoured their value to humans. The development of distinct breeds of pig involved the promotion of these characteristics by the introduction of genes from smaller, early maturing breeds (*Sus vittatus*), originating in Southeast Asia. In medieval times, village pigs were driven in groups to forage in woodlands and fatten in the autumn on mast, berries and roots. This system, known as pannage, gradually reduced in the Middle Ages as access to woodlands became more restricted and the role of the pig changed to utilize their ability to exploit human food wastes. Pigs were more often housed on a household basis and fed on kitchen wastes, while pigs kept in towns were often allowed to scavenge for food during the day. These keeping styles can still be seen around the world in subsistence living conditions. The intensification of pig production initially developed in conjunction with availability of specialized sources of by-product feeds such as dairy or brewery wastes. As the nineteenth and twentieth centuries progressed, the growing demand for pig meat and availability of cheaper cereals gave rise to the current systems of specialized farms, with permanently housed animals fed predominantly on cereal-based diets.

Because of their adaptability, farmed pigs are found in almost all regions of the world, although their use for human food is restricted in some regions by religious taboos. Both Moslems and Jews believe their meat to be unsuitable for human consumption. Over the world as a whole, pigs constitute the most important source of meat, supplying about 40% of world meat supply. The global distribution of pig numbers and their trends are shown in Table 6.1.

Table 6.1 Pig population in the world (million head).

	1997	2007	2017
Africa	20	27	38
Asia	463	532	558
(incl. China)	(374)	(426)	(441)
Europe	203	198	186
Americas	143	157	181
(incl. North America)	(73)	(77)	(88)
Oceania	5	6	6
World total	**835**	**919**	**967**

(*Source*: FAO statistics (http://faostat.fao.org).

6.3 The Basic Pig Production Cycle

The basic production cycle of the pig under modern farmed conditions is shown in Figure 6.1. Piglets are now born all year round to ensure a reliable source of meat in all seasons. On many farms, production is organized so that a regular proportion of the farrowings take place on a weekly basis, although on some smaller farms a batched system may operate, with animals grouped to farrow in cohorts, typically every 3 or 6 weeks. This allows staff to specialize weekly in specific tasks and the larger batch size facilitates all-in all-out management to reduce risk of vertical disease spread. The breeding animals reach puberty at about 6 months of age. In the female, the oestrous cycle lasts 21 days and animals will continue to cycle at all times of the year until pregnant. Pregnancy lasts approximately 115 days (3 months, 3 weeks, 3 days), after which the female gives birth to a litter of typically 8 to 16 piglets, although litter sizes in modern hybrid lines can now often exceed 20. These piglets suckle for a period of 2 to 6 weeks, most typically 3 to 4 weeks, before being abruptly weaned and housed separately from their mother. The sow then comes back into oestrus in 5 to 7 days and is bred again. The weaned piglets grow on for meat production, reaching a typical slaughter weight of 90 to 120 kg by 5 to 6 months of age.

The farm may buy in replacement breeding animals or may breed its own in a specialized within-herd system. It will sell cull sows at the end of their reproductive life, and the progeny at a defined stage of growth. Many farms are 'farrow to finish', keeping the progeny until slaughter for meat production. While this is most typically at 100 to 120 kg live-weight, slaughter may take place at lighter weights in some specialist markets for fresh meat (the pork pig) or at heaver weights in markets for processed meat and ham (e.g. the Italian Parma ham pig may be 170 kg at slaughter). Some farms specialize only in piglet production and sell their progeny soon after weaning at 20 to 30 kg live eight. These pigs are purchased by specialist finishing farms, who complete the rearing period until slaughter for meat. Occasionally farms sell newly weaned piglets directly from the sow, but this is less common because of the greater vulnerability of the animals currently.

Typical levels of pig performance are shown in Table 6.2. These are based on national recording schemes in different European and American countries. They demonstrate that the

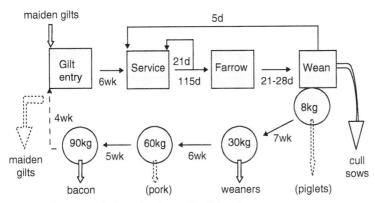

Figure 6.1 The typical production cycle of the pig.

Table 6.2 Pig performance standards for different countries in 2017 and trends over time.

	EU average 2007	EU average 2017	Denmark 2017	USA 2017
Pigs born alive per litter	11.9	13.9	16.9	12.7
Pre-weaning mortality (%)	12.9	13.0	13.6	14.7
Litters/sow/year	2.25	2.30	2.28	2.44
Pigs weaned/sow/year	23.2	27.8	33.3	26.4
Post weaning mortality (%)	5.8	5.8	6.2	8.8
Finishing daily live-weight gain (g/day)	759	819	971	857
Finishing feed conversion ratio (kg feed/kg gain)	2.92	2.83	2.66	2.71
Average live weight at slaughter (kg)	117	120	114	127
Carcass meat production/sow/year (kg)	1956	2427	2683	2287

(*Source*: AHDB, SEGES, PigChamp, 2018).

production processes and outcomes are very similar in intensive systems around the world, with sows producing on average 26 to 28 weaned piglets each year. However, in some countries such as Denmark, a combination of breeding for greater litter size and good management has now resulted in a national average of more than 33 weaned pigs per sow annually, a figure reached only by herds in the top 10% of achievement in other countries.

6.4 Housing Systems for Pigs

The housing systems for the pigs are typically, but not always, divided up by reproductive stage for breeding animals, and by age for growing and finishing animals. In intensive pig farming throughout the world, the systems used for production are relatively similar, although with some variations in housing design dependent on the regional climate. Less intensive systems also occur, ranging from traditional silvo-pastoral systems in Mediterranean countries, backyard pigs in developing countries or large-scale outdoor systems found in some parts of Europe and America.

In some countries, constraints on housing are set by legislation. This is generally the case in Europe, where the EU member states have agreed Directives to safeguard pig welfare. The first of these to specifically address pig housing systems was agreed in 1991 and, following further Directives in 2001 which increased legislative requirements, requirements were consolidated in Council Directive 2008/120/EC. Additional constraints on systems of pig housing and management have arisen from public concern about the environmental impact of large livestock enterprises. Such concerns relate to the emission of ammonia, which can cause acid rain, and the entry into watercourses of excess nitrogen and phosphorus from manure which can cause algal bloom. In the EU, progressively increasing legislation to protect air and water quality against such threats has culminated in Directive 2010/75/EU and the Commission implementing decision 2017/302 establishing best available techniques (BAT) for the intensive rearing of poultry or pigs. This lays out stringent measures for the design and management of pig buildings which should be adopted to reduce pollution risk. Some individual countries have even more demanding national legislation, either for environmental or animal welfare reasons, as will be highlighted in individual sections of this chapter. Production systems may also be determined by the requirements of special labelling schemes. Some of these, such as organic production, have agreed international standards. For example, within the EU, the rules for organic pig production were first defined in 1999 and then further elaborated in Regulation EC 834/2007. Other schemes are voluntary and may focus on different traits of interest to consumers. Examples of schemes which are designed to provide higher welfare for the animals, by specifying more extensive housing systems and limiting certain contentious managements practices, include the RSPCA Assured Scheme in the UK, and similar initiatives such as the 'Bedre Dyrevelfærd' (3 hearts) scheme in Denmark, 'Beter Leven' scheme in The Netherlands, 'Tierschutz' scheme in Germany and 'Certified Humane' scheme in North America. There are also larger-scale schemes run by industry bodies such as the Red Tractor Farm Assurance Pigs scheme in the UK, the QSG scheme in Denmark, IKB scheme in the Netherlands and QS scheme in Germany. Such schemes typically require evidence of good practice within the current legislative framework, rather than setting additional constraints to building type or management system. They operate according to European requirements for quality assurance of products under the framework of ISO 17065, combining a set of specific published standards with regular independent inspection of the farm to check compliance.

Housing systems adopted by pig-keepers can be divided into three major categories: outdoor systems, bedded indoor systems handling solid manure and slatted indoor systems handling liquid manure.

6.4.1 Outdoor Systems

Large-scale outdoor production typically occurs in more temperate regions and comes in two distinctive forms – those supplying the commodity pig-meat market and those supplying specialist niche markets. In some European countries, particularly the UK but also to a lesser extent in France, and in some regions of North and South America, there are a significant number of outdoor herds contributing to conventional pig-meat supplies. These developed because of low establishment and overhead cost. Most commonly only the breeding animals are maintained outside, with the progeny transferred to more intensive housing at the time of weaning. These systems stock the sows relatively densely, at 12 to 15 sows per hectare, as part of an annual rotation with arable cropping. They function well only in areas with light, free-draining soils of sand or chalk and low annual rainfall of < 750 mm. The pigs are kept in groups according to reproductive stage, in paddocks separated by electrified fencing and with simple wooden or metal shelters.

This conventional outdoor production contrasts with a smaller number of farms keeping pigs outdoors for production to supply local niche markets or according to organic standards. It is a requirement of the EU Directive on organic standards that breeding animals have access to pasture. Some national certification schemes also require that the progeny be kept at pasture, but this is not universal and, in many countries, the growing and finishing pigs are kept in housing with an outdoor run area which may be of concrete. It is not possible to have an organic pig enterprise in isolation, since they must be kept within an organic whole-farm system. In general, breeding sows and boars are kept in outdoor paddocks with simple shelters in the same way as conventional outdoor production. Weaned and growing pigs can be kept in similar paddock systems, in outdoor hut-and-run systems, or in more permanent housing with an outdoor exercise and dunging area.

A third major European outdoor system is the traditional Mediterranean silvo-pastoral system. This system, found most commonly in Spain, Portugal and Corsica, involves indigenous breeds that are extensively pastured in natural forests of oak or chestnut for the production of high-value dry-cured hams. Typically, all phases of production take place outdoors, with the finishing period taking place during the autumn when animals convert large quantities of acorns or chestnuts into fat deposits.

6.4.2 Indoor Systems

Indoor housing is most commonly classified according to the method of manure management. The most common system throughout the world is to have pigs kept on fully or partly slatted flooring, so that the faeces and urine fall through the floor into a collection pit below and are handled as a liquid slurry by pumping systems. In smaller, more traditional or high-welfare systems, the pigs are housed in pens with bedding and produce solid manure, or muck, which must be removed by hand in small herd systems or by machinery in larger enterprises. The most common bedding is straw, but in some countries other materials such as sawdust, wood shavings or rice hulls may be used. Bedded systems may take the form of deep litter pens, where the animals determine their own zones for resting and for dunging, and manure removal is done relatively infrequently, or minimally bedded pens in which the material is largely confined to a specific lying area while the dunging area is cleaned out on a more regular basis.

6.5   Breeds and Replacement Policy

While a wide variety of indigenous breeds exist in the different countries of the world, modern intensive production has focused almost completely on a few specialized breeds. The Landrace and Large White (or Yorkshire) breeds predominate in maternal lines, with breeds including the Duroc, Hampshire and Pietrain used extensively in sire lines for their carcass conformation and meat quality characteristics. The indigenous breeds survive in specialized production systems, such as the Iberian breeds in the extensive Mediterranean systems, and in smaller farms producing for niche markets. In particular, the use of traditional breeds is recommended in organic standards and a UK survey of organic farms found a wide range of such breeds still in use in the UK, including the British Saddleback, Tamworth, Gloucester Old Spot, Large Black, Welsh and Berkshire breeds. These traditional breeds are hardy and often have good maternal traits but have largely disappeared from conventional production because of their early maturing characteristics and consequent tendency to become over-fat at a very young age. This usually means that they need to have their feed carefully restricted and to be slaughtered younger and at lighter weights and are hence less profitable for conventional markets.

While pure-bred animals are still used in these niche systems, large-scale intensive systems typically use crossbred animals to exploit the benefits of hybrid vigour. Breeding females are most commonly first crosses between the Landrace and Large White breeds. However, in outdoor production systems the Duroc breed is often included, to supply 25 or 50% of genes in a three-way cross with these breeds, to give the greater robustness necessary to cope with the varying climate and greater social competition. Boars used in both intensive and extensive systems may be pure-bred Large White (Yorkshire), but are commonly synthetic lines blending a range of different breeds to give a 'terminal sire'. Although breeds are still described by their traditional names, in reality much of the selection and differentiation in recent decades has taken place within breed. Thus, a Large White line selected as a 'damline' for maternal characteristics of prolificacy and good lactation performance will vary markedly from a 'sireline' selected more heavily for traits of growth, feed efficiency and carcass conformation. The development of these specialist lines and synthetic breeds has been carried out very effectively by large international breeding companies, who can use sophisticated statistical methods to select animals for the most desirable combination of traits over large populations. By these means, rapid genetic progress can be made. For example, carcass backfat thickness in the UK slaughter pig was reduced in the late twentieth century by 0.4 mm per year, or 50% over 25 years, in response to consumer demand for leaner and healthier meat. More recently, litter size in Danish pigs was increased by 15% in only 5 years. Such approaches also make it possible to select for new traits which can enhance health and welfare in the population. These include resistance to disease, improved piglet survival and, most recently, reduction in aggressiveness and a beneficial social influence on other animals within the group. Genetic modification of pigs, such as the introduction of new genes to improve growth and feed utilization, has not found public acceptance. However, the new technology of 'gene editing', the targeted modification of gene expression, has already been able to produce pigs with resistance against one major endemic disease (PRRS) and is currently under discussion in many countries.

To exploit this rate of progress, many farms purchase their replacement breeding animals from a specialized breeding company. The maintenance and development of the pure-bred 'grandparent' lines takes place in nucleus units owned by these companies. Animals from these units are transferred to multiplication units, also usually owned or managed on contract for the breeding companies, where the appropriate crosses are carried out to produce the crossbred production animals sold as breeding stock to meat-producing farms (Figure 6.2).

To minimize the risk of introduction of disease, some farms breed their own replacement females. In order to do this, they must either maintain a nucleus of pure-bred animals in the herd, to generate the most productive first-cross gilts, or adopt a reciprocal crossing policy between two breeds, known as 'criss-cross breeding'. In this system, boars of two different breeds (e.g. Landrace and Large White) are used in alternate generations so that a sow is always mated to the breed which was not her father. In this way, each generation has some

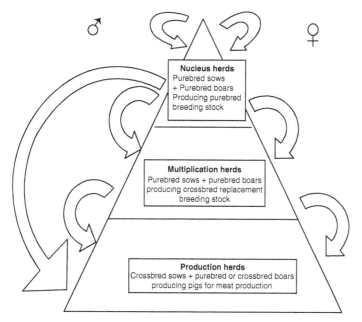

Figure 6.2 The typical breeding 'pyramid' in intensive pig production.

hybrid vigour, having one-third of the genes from one breed and two-thirds from the other. This is an attractive option for a smaller unit, since no specialist pure-bred animals need to be maintained, but does require good animal identification and record-keeping to ensure the correct cross is always made, and gives a slight reduction in hybrid vigour which is equivalent to 0.5–1.0 fewer pigs produced per sow per year.

6.6   The Breeding Phase

Domestication has largely abolished the seasonal breeding characteristics of the wild boar, and females will now come into oestrus year-round. However, some vestiges of their ancestral propensity to seasonality still exist, as shown by the occurrence of summer infertility which is especially pronounced in outdoor animals subject to natural photoperiod and in animals in hot climates. On any pig unit, the most important phase of production is the mating, since poor management here will result in poor conception or litter size and under-utilization of all the other buildings on the farm. A well-managed farm will have a calculated pig flow pattern, working out the building capacity at each production stage, and planning the number of weekly matings accordingly. To maintain this correct number of matings, new gilts must be introduced to the herd to replace older sows which are culled for poor production or age. While sows can continue to breed for many years, the modern sow is usually replaced after six litters, when her productivity starts to decline. The maintenance of a stable herd size typically requires the introduction of 40% of the herd size as new gilts each year.

Breeding gilts (nulliparous females) are typically delivered to the farm at about six months of age and 100 kg live-weight, and at the point of puberty. Since, when imminent, puberty can be triggered by mild stressors, the stimuli from the journey, handling and new housing often result in oestrus within a week of arrival. However, animals are seldom bred at this first oestrus, for several reasons. The first is that newly introduced animals are typically held in quarantine for a period of six weeks. This allows the new owner to be sure that they are not incubating any disease before they are introduced to the main herd, and also gives the animals the possibility to settle in their new location and be gradually adapted to the microbial challenges on that farm. For this purpose, cull sows or finishing pigs are sometimes introduced into the quarantine accommodation. Breeding gilts can also be purchased and introduced to the farm at a younger age, typically at 3 months of age and 30 kg. This gives them a longer period to adapt to the herd and has been associated with an increase in reproductive performance when bred. However, the extra housing demands make this option unattractive for many farms. The second reason for delaying breeding is that litter size increases with each successive oestrous cycle in these young animals, so that delaying until the second or third oestrus is usually cost-effective and also gives an animal which is older at farrowing and better able to meet the heavy demands of lactation.

Sows which are already in production enter the service house after weaning, and the cessation of the suckling stimulus normally induces a return to oestrus in five to seven days. However, a number of management procedures will ensure that this process is not delayed and will optimize the expression of oestrous behaviour and the ovulation rate. Group housing of sows, as opposed to individual housing in stalls, and daily physical contact with a boar both reduce the weaning to oestrus interval in an additive way, while isolation of weaned sows from boars can delay the onset of oestrus. Gilts tested for oestrus by a stockperson show a stronger behavioural response when adjacent to a boar than when tested in the home pen. However, young females housed permanently adjacent to boars appear to habituate to boar stimulation, showing shorter duration of oestrous behaviour and reduced response to a back-pressure test during oestrus.

The oestrous and mating behaviours of the domestic pig show few changes from those exhibited by their wild counterparts. The oestrous cycle can be divided into four phases, each characterized by certain physical and behavioural symptoms. Dioestrus or anoestrus is the period when the ovary is least active and there are no external symptoms. Pro-oestrus is a period of increasing ovarian activity in which symptoms of approaching heat can be observed, such as reddening and swelling of the vulva. At this stage, behavioural changes are also seen as sows increase their level of activity, begin to nose and lever the flanks of other females and try to mount other sows. Where the possibility exists, oestrous sows will seek out and associate with a boar. Follicular ripening reaches its peak at oestrus and then ovulation takes place. At this time the behaviour of the female is characterized by willingness to adopt the standing reflex, necessary to allow mating by the boar.

The reflex is characterized by a flattening of the back and elevation of the perianal region, a posture also called lordosis, with a characteristic pricking of the ears in some breed types.

This behaviour is shown most strongly in response to stimuli provided by the boar, but at the time of peak oestrus can also be induced by other sows or by a human who provides the appropriate tactile stimulus of pressure on the back. This period, often called 'standing oestrus, when the female accepts copulation, lasts on average 48 hours.

The most fertile period for the sow is towards the end of standing oestrus, when ovulation occurs. Detailed studies of ovulation by ultrasonography in the sow have shown that, irrespective of the total duration of standing oestrus, ovulation occurs after approximately two-thirds of the duration of oestrus. Where boars and sows are housed separately, it is normal to allow natural service or artificial insemination of sows once or twice daily throughout the period of standing oestrus, so as to maximize the chances of hitting this fertile period (Figure 6.3).

Although sows may be bred by natural service or artificial insemination, some boars are always needed on the farm to ensure good oestrus stimulation. Where natural service is used, it is normal to keep one boar for every 20 sows in the herd. However, where group mating systems are used, such as in outdoor production, a higher ratio of one boar to 15 sows is

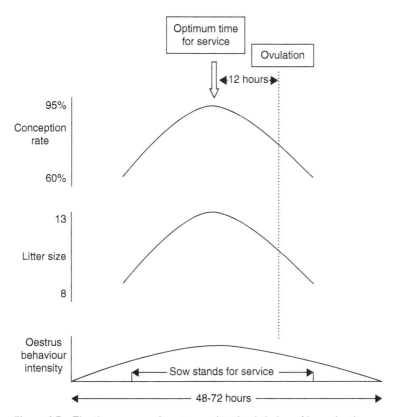

Figure 6.3 The time course of oestrus and optimal timing of insemination.

required. The number of sperm and volume of an ejaculation increases from puberty until 18 months of age. This production level is maintained for about 5 years and then declines. Boars are normally culled after 2 to 3 years because of large size and the need for continuous genetic improvement. Indoor boars are normally housed singly and fed 2–3 kg of pregnant-sow diet. Present EU legislation specifies a minimum pen area allowance of 6 m^2 per animal and 10 m^2 if this pen is also used for service. It is possible to house familiar boars together in pairs or groups, but their management and handling is then more difficult. Mature boars will fight if unfamiliar animals are mixed and severe injury can result.

Domestic pigs show the same patterns of courtship behaviour as wild boar, with chanting (rhythmic grunting), sniffing and licking of the vulva, and pushing and nudging of the flanks preceding mounting, intromission and ejaculation. In commercial circumstances, where an oestrous sow is introduced to a boar in a limited area, boar courtship behaviour sometimes lasts less than 1 minute, but is very important as a higher level of courtship has been shown to increase conception and litter size. When the female shows the standing response, the male mounts and makes thrusting actions with the penis. Ejaculation occurs after 3 to 20 minutes (average 4.5 min). The use of a specially designed mating area of 10 m^2 with no obstructions, a non-slip floor and stimulation from other adjacent boars has been shown to give better breeding results than allowing mating to take place in the boar's home pen.

The use of group mating systems, in which a team of boars are placed with the weaned sows and mating takes place without significant supervision, is also adopted in some situations. While mating systems involving groups of boars housed together are still relatively uncommon in indoor production, this is historically the most common method used in outdoor production. However, a detailed study of this system highlighted its weaknesses, since the number of successful matings per sow varied from 0 to 7, while the number of matings performed by individual boars over the peak four-day oestrous period varied from 0 to 13. Of the 45% of all mating attempts which failed to achieve copulation, half were due to intervention of a second boar. In a UK survey of breeding records from outdoor herds, it was found that 80 herds using outdoor group mating with three or more boars per group had an average farrowing percentage of 73%, 18 herds using outdoor mating with 1 or 2 boars achieved 75%, while herds adopting indoor mating achieved 79% success. For this reason, an increasing number of outdoor herds now house the sows temporarily during the breeding phase in nearby buildings or tents in the field, where individual boars are kept, and controlled mating or artificial insemination can be carried out.

To allow exploitation of the best genetics, most mating in large conventional units is carried out by artificial insemination (AI). Since one ejaculate of semen can be used to inseminate 20 sows, AI offers the advantages of purchasing and keeping fewer boars, and the ability to invest in fewer but genetically superior boars. It also allows the semen to be checked for quality before use. While some larger farms will collect and process semen from their own boars, the majority will purchase the semen from a specialized stud. Semen from boars with the highest breeding values for desirable traits is made available by breeding companies, or in some countries by government-owned studs. In pigs, a large volume of semen is required for insemination relative to other species and, because the sperm do not survive well after freezing as a result of their higher lipid content than other species, most semen is delivered and used fresh. The development of special diluents with which the semen is mixed can prolong its effective lifetime for a period of five to seven days, but this means that correct prediction of the time of oestrus in the sow and correct handling and storage of the temperature-sensitive semen is vital for good conception and litter size. Successful use of AI requires good operator skill for oestrus detection and insemination. The close proximity of a boar helps to elicit clear signs of oestrus, provide olfactory and auditory stimulation at the time of insemination and promote good conception.

6.7 The Gestation Phase

The two major objectives of management of the pregnant sow are to establish large numbers of embryos in the uterus and to feed the sow in such a way that she is best prepared for the high demands of the subsequent lactation. It is important to avoid stress during the implantation period (10 to 18 days after service is a particularly sensitive time) as this can increase embryo mortality and reduce litter size. This can be helped by avoiding mixing or a change of environment during this period. If the sow does not return to oestrus at 21 days after service, she is likely to be pregnant, but this is generally checked by ultrasound pregnancy diagnosis at 4 weeks after service. The equipment most used detects the increased blood flow in the uterine vessels using the Doppler effect. It is now possible to carry out pregnancy detection at 19 days after service using ultrasound scanning to observe changes in the appearance of the uterus, but this equipment is expensive, and the method requires more skill.

6.7.1 Pregnancy Stalls

Gestation in the pig lasts for 115 days, with little variation about this average. This period of the sow's life has been the subject of much debate about welfare issues. Traditional systems, in which groups of pregnant sows were housed in outdoor paddocks or in covered straw yards, fell out of favour as herd sizes increased and they became more difficult to manage. The 1960s saw the large-scale development and adoption of individual housing systems for sows, and these rapidly became the norm in many pig-producing countries. Such systems offered the attraction of low space requirement and ease of management. Sows could no longer fight, and individual feeding could ensure that the nutritional needs of all animals were precisely met. With the small space allowances and enclosed buildings associated with individual housing, automated air temperature control was possible, but provision of bedding and daily cleaning out presented a difficult and laborious manual task. In consequence, this was automated in many buildings by using fully or partly slatted floors, through which all excreta passed for storage away from the animals as a slurry. The slurry could then be mechanically removed from the building at any convenient time. To ensure that all urine and faeces were deposited over the slurry collection area, which was essential to avoid manual pen cleaning and keep the animals clean and dry, it was necessary to prevent sows from turning around in their pen. This was achieved either by enclosing them in a stall too narrow to permit this or by tethering them within their pen by means of a neck collar or girth strap. The resulting form of housing offered a relatively low-cost, simply managed system for large-scale pig production enterprises under all farming conditions. However, the very restrictive nature of such systems has given rise to serious public concern about sow welfare, and individually confined sows are often seen to develop stereotyped behaviours such as bar biting or vacuum chewing. As a result of these concerns, legislation to ban such housing systems has now been passed in many countries. A total ban has existed for many years in Sweden, Switzerland, Norway, Finland and the UK. In the rest of the EU, tether systems were banned from 2005 and gestation stall systems only permitted for the period between weaning and the first four weeks after service since 2012. Elsewhere in the world, stalls are still the predominant housing system for gestation although their use is being reviewed in many countries. Partial stall bans have been voluntarily adopted by the New Zealand, Australian and Canadian industries and have been the subject of public votes in several states in the USA. As pressures from consumers and retailers increase worldwide, group housing systems are increasingly being adopted.

6.7.2 Group Housing for Pregnant Sows

There is a wide variety of alternative group housing systems in use during the gestation stage, made up from all combinations of their key components of group size, floor type, lying area design and feeding system. Group sizes vary depending on herd size, frequency of batch farrowing and whether small stable groups or large dynamic groups are adopted. Stable groups are formed at the time of weaning and remain together throughout pregnancy. This avoids any mixing and fighting to re-establish the dominance hierarchy. Dynamic groups have sows at all stages of pregnancy, with animals added, after service or pregnancy diagnosis, and removed, shortly prior to farrowing, on a regular (often weekly) basis. These large groups allow cheaper housing cost and provide more total space for exercise, escape from aggression and choice of location for the animals. However, because of the regular introduction of unfamiliar animals, they tend to have more aggression as the dominance relationships are repeatedly being re-established, and therefore need a higher standard of management.

As with all production stages, pens can be deep-bedded, shallow-bedded or without bedding, in the latter case usually having fully or partly slatted flooring. Slatted floors reduce labour and cost of bedding but must be of good quality if lameness is to be avoided. In the EU, legislation now requires a minimum slat width of 80 mm and a maximum gap of 20 mm for concrete floors to reduce the risk of foot injury. Straw-based systems are often preferred because the straw provides not only additional thermal and physical comfort, but also a source of gut fill and occupation which is particularly important to reduce aggression in the pregnant sow.

Because of their restricted feeding level, the thermal comfort zone for a pregnant sow is relatively high (18–20°C when individually housed without bedding). While this does not pose a problem in tropical countries, in more temperate regions ambient temperature often falls below this. To avoid the wasteful use of feed to maintain body temperature, sows in stalls or slatted systems are usually kept in insulated, controlled environment buildings, where the air temperature is regulated by changing ventilation rates of fans. However, systems in which animals are housed in larger groups on straw require access for machinery to enter the building to deliver straw and remove muck. These systems are therefore often found in large, uninsulated buildings where temperature is difficult to regulate. Covering the lying area with a false roof to form a kennel allows the sows to make a microclimate and conserve heat. These benefit sow welfare and feed efficiency but make inspection and access to animals for routine tasks such as vaccination or pregnancy diagnosis more difficult.

6.7.3 Feeding Systems for Sows

Feeding of the non-lactating sow is an area of great importance. There are specific times when the level of feeding can directly impact on productivity, while at other times the objective is to minimize feed cost. Between weaning and breeding, a high plane of nutrition is important to stimulate a high ovulation rate. It is usual to continue feeding with the higher-quality lactation diet during this period and to feed *ad libitum* or at a generous allowance of 3–4 kg/day. For gilts coming up to their first service, this 'flushing' should be applied for 12 to 14 days before ovulation, since this can increase litter size by one or two piglets. However, once mating has occurred, continuation of this high feed level can adversely affect the hormonal balance and impair embryo implantation, especially in young animals. It is therefore advised to reduce feed level to 2–2.5 kg from the day after mating until pregnancy diagnosis is positive. After this time, the objective is to feed the minimum amount necessary to achieve optimal body condition at farrowing of 3–3.5 on a 0–5 scale (see Figure 6.4). A sow which is thinner at farrowing will have lower birthweight piglets and fewer body reserves to support high milk output during lactation. Conversely, a sow which is too fat will have greater risk of prolonged parturition and increased stillbirths, and a lower appetite during lactation which will make her utilize body reserves to produce milk and adversely affect her subsequent breeding. To achieve the ideal body condition, sows are typically fed 2–3 kg of a gestation diet with 13 MJ/kg of digestible energy (9.2 MJ/kg of net energy) and 13 to 14% crude protein (4–5 g/kg of ileal digestible lysine). The exact amount of feed will depend on their size, body condition and housing, where the needs for exercise and keeping warm may differ. In the final stages of pregnancy, the foetal piglets show exponential growth rate. The birthweight of the piglets can be influenced by the feed level of the sow but the response is quite small (it takes ~ 100 kg of sow feed to increase individual piglet birthweight by 100 g). However, it is common practice to increase the feed level for the pregnant sow in the last three weeks before farrowing to 3–3.5 kg to reduce her mobilization of body reserves at this time of high demand. The food is typically reduced again to 2–2.5 kg in the last three days before farrowing, since this can reduce the risk of health problems in the immediate post-partum period.

Outdoor sows have higher feed requirements because of greater activity and the lower temperatures experienced during winter. Their annual feed use in temperate regions is typically 15% higher than that of animals living indoors. Because the feed is usually scattered widely on the ground, so that all sows in the group can obtain access, a special large pellet or 'cob' is

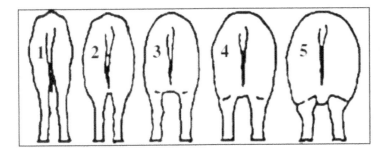

Score	Body condition	Prominence of backbone, ribs and pelvic bones
1	Emaciated	Bones visible
2	Thin	Bones felt by flat of hand without pressure
3	Optimal	Bones felt by flat of hand only with pressure
4	Fat	Bones felt only by pushing with finger tips
5	Obese	Bones cannot be felt

Figure 6.4 Body condition scoring in sows.

manufactured to prevent wastage from blowing away in the wind, becoming lost in mud or carried off by small birds. The outdoor conditions give sows the advantage of a more natural environment, allowing them to forage for vegetation and invertebrates. However, for much of the year they obtain little additional nutrition from these activities and their vigorous rooting can rapidly destroy any vegetation cover on their paddock, leaving a bare surface which can become very muddy in wet weather. To prevent this, some farms insert nose rings in the sows to prevent them from rooting. Traditionally, two or three small rings were clipped through the upper rim of the nasal disc. While initially very effective in preventing rooting without impairing grazing, these rings are easily dislodged and may need to be replaced a number of times during the life of the sow. Consequently, an alternative design has been favoured in which a larger 'bull ring' is fastened through the nasal septum and protrudes in front of the snout. The welfare implications of nose ringing are the subject of debate. The insertion of the rings is a painful procedure and the inability to express motivated rooting behaviour when hungry can be a source of frustration. These adverse effects for the animal must be offset against the better living conditions if a dry and grassy paddock can be preserved. The maintenance of vegetative cover also has important environmental benefits, since it allows plant capture of excreted nutrients throughout the growing season and helps to maintain soil structure. This reduces the risk of leaching and run-off of nitrogen and phosphorus which can pollute waterways, and the undesirable emissions of gases such as ammonia and nitrous oxide into the atmosphere. At present there is no legislation against the use of nose rings and they are widely used in both intensive and more traditional outdoor systems according to environmental needs and the preferences of individual farms. Their use is even permitted in some organic schemes, where utilizing natural vegetation as a contribution to nutritional requirements is favoured.

The concentrate feed allowance for the pregnant sow is designed to meet all her nutrient requirements (typically about 1.3 times maintenance need) and is adequate for good health and performance but does not satisfy her appetite and leaves her in a state of chronic hunger. This situation is now known to give rise to the stereotyped behaviours in sows in restrictive environments, where the food-seeking behaviours generated by this hunger have no appropriate outlet for expression. In group housing, it also causes aggression during competition for feed, and the abnormal injurious behaviour of vulva biting. To minimize these problems, it is recommended to feed the sow once daily, since one large meal is more satisfying both physically and physiologically than a number of smaller meals, and to provide additional roughage which can give greater gut fill and feelings of satiety. This can be in the form of supplementary hay or silage, or fresh straw bedding or by formulating the compound diet to have a higher fibre content.

Because the feed amount is so limited, it is important to ensure that each individual is able to eat her own appropriate share. This need has given rise to a variety of housing systems with different methods of feed provision designed to meet this challenge. More traditional systems often adopt simple group feeding options, placing the allowance for a number of sows in a long trough or spreading it widely over the ground. This approach can be mechanized using automated canisters, suspended over each pen and filled from a pipeline, to measure the group feed allowance and then dump it onto the floor at feeding time (dump feed systems) or with spinning discs which spread the food over a much wider area (spin feed systems). While this is a cheap housing option, it can cause significant welfare problems for the animals. Older and larger sows eat at least twice as fast as small ones and can dominate areas of food resource. This can result in uneven sow condition, aggression as the hungry sows compete for the limited feed and the failure of young and timid sows to thrive. Housing systems with provision for individual rationing, while more costly in terms of space and equipment, prevent aggression over food and allow all sows to reach the time of farrowing in ideal body condition. Because of these advantages, many different systems of ensuring individual feed intake have been developed.

The most traditional method is to house sows in pens with individual feeding stalls in which the animals are enclosed only during the feeding period. Each animal can then be offered the appropriate amount of food and remains protected while she consumes it. The communal area may be deep bedded, comprise a kennelled lying area and scraped dunging passage, or be unbedded with a slatted dunging area. While this is perhaps the ideal system from the perspective of sow welfare, it has a high labour requirement for confining and releasing sows each day and hand feeding the correct ration for each animal. It also has a high space requirement for provision of individual feeding stalls which are used for only a short period each day, and hence a high capital cost. Space allowance and cost can be greatly reduced by combining the feeding stall and lying area, as is done in systems with cubicles or free access stalls. Animals are free to leave the stalls during the day to spend time in a communal exercise and dunging area, but the space provided for this is very limited. If aggression occurs, it is difficult for the lower-ranking sow to escape and there is a danger that she becomes trapped in a stall by a following aggressor. This risk is lessened in systems where the length of the feeding stall is reduced, such that only partial barriers separating the head and shoulder are used. However, this increases the risk that faster-eating sows will finish their own ration and then bully their slower-eating groupmates away from their feeding place to steal additional food. To minimize this possibility, a more complex feed delivery system known as the trickle-feed system has been developed. This uses a method of 'biological fixation', in which feed is dribbled out by an auger at the same controlled rate to each individual place. Since the sows cannot then eat at a differential speed, movement between feeding places gives no benefit and only short partitions along the trough are necessary to protect the feeding sows. Correct selection of the dispensing rate is essential to the success of the system, since too slow a rate will lead to restlessness in fast-eating sows, while too fast a rate will overwhelm the slow-eating animals. Experiments have shown that the number of aggressive interactions and changes of place during feeding increase as the dispensing feed drops below 100 g of pellets per minute. However, with rates of above 120 g per minute more sows have food accumulating in the trough and the number of aggressive interactions when feed dispensing stops is increased. This system has the disadvantage that it is a flat-rate delivery and it is not possible to feed different amounts to individuals within the same group. It is therefore best used with small groups of sows where size and condition of animals within the group can be closely matched.

Because the nutritional requirements of individual sows can vary significantly, depending on such factors as live-weight, body condition and stage of pregnancy, the development of a system in which individual rationing could be automated was highly desirable. This was made possible by the development of electronic sow feeding, or transponder feeding, systems (Figure 6.5). In this system animals are identified electronically by a device, usually placed in an ear tag, and feed sequentially at one or more feeding stations controlled by a central computer. The sow entering the feeder is automatically locked into a protective stall, recognized by her electronic tag and dispensed the appropriate amount of food according to her preset ration. On completion of her feeding period, the gates are unlocked, and she is replaced by the next sow. Sows in stable groups using this system soon develop a relatively stable feeding order, with dominant sows feeding at the start of the cycle and low-ranking sows waiting until a quieter time of day. However, to maximize use of this expensive feeding technology, many sows (typically 40 to 60) must share each station. This means that, except in very large herds, the system must operate with dynamic groups. Sows newly introduced to the group generally begin low in the feeding order, establishing themselves over time as longer-term group members are removed to farrow and other new sows are introduced. However, the constant introduction of new sows can disrupt the settled feeding order and cause more aggression and competition for feeder entry. There can also be problems when sows which have already consumed their daily ration return to the station in the hope of obtaining further food. These may try to circumvent protective devices to eject a feeding animal or may occupy the feeder for long periods of time and prevent unfed sows from entering.

In general, as summarized in Table 6.3, the different systems offer a trade-off between simplicity and the ability to provide for individual sow needs, and between mechanization, and

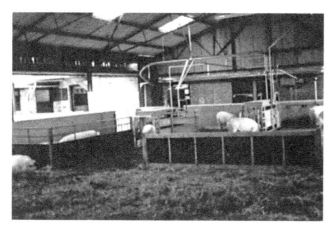

Figure 6.5   An electronic feeding system for gestating sows.

Table 6.3   A comparison of dry sow housing systems.

System	Advantages	Disadvantages
Outdoor production	Low capital cost Large space and enriched environment	Group feeding on ground Exposure to climatic variation Higher feed wastage
Floor feeding (by hand, dump or spin feeding)	Simple and flexible Lowest capital cost	Group feeding only High aggression during feeding Higher feed wastage
Small groups with individual feeding stalls	Stable groups Individual rationing	High space requirement High capital cost
Cubicles	Individual rationing	Limited social space
Free access stalls	Lower space requirement	Visibility poor in covered cubicles
Trickle feed Biofix	Reduced space requirement with only partial feeding stalls Individual feeding	All sows in group receive same feed level Correct feed delivery rate critical
Electronic sow feeding	Individual rationing controlled by computer Low cost because feed station shared between many sows	Large groups often involve dynamic grouping Individual sows harder to check Equipment failure causes aggression
Wet feeding	Greater bulk gives quieter sows Cheap liquid by-products can reduce feed cost	Group feeding only High initial capital investment

hence capital cost, and labour input. However, it must be recognized that mechanization always carries a greater risk of malfunction and cannot fully replace the inputs of a skilled stockperson.

6.8 Farrowing and Lactation

The main objective for the farrowing and lactation period is to rear as large numbers of piglets as possible, to achieve an even and adequate weaning weight and to leave the sow in good condition to commence the next breeding cycle. Because sows have been genetically selected to become much more prolific in recent years, these objectives now pose a greater challenge.

Sows are usually moved to special accommodation five to seven days before their expected farrowing date to allow them time to settle before farrowing commences. In the wild, sows leave their group and walk long distances (10 to 30 km) in the days immediately prior to farrowing, before selecting a nest site and building a farrowing nest. In commercial conditions, the exact time of farrowing can be difficult to predict but the signs of imminent farrowing are restlessness, which typically occurs from about 24 hours before farrowing, and nest building which typically peaks at 6 to 12 hours before farrowing but can be very variable in time of onset. Shortly before farrowing, typically 6 to 8 hours but sometimes as early as 24 to 48 hours, it is possible to express milk from the teats of the sow and this is one of the more reliable signs that farrowing is imminent. Contractions can usually be seen from 3 hours prior to farrowing, but sometimes as early as 10 hours. Farrowing typically lasts 2 to 4 hours, being shorter in gilts than in older sows, with piglets delivered at varying intervals, averaging about 20 minutes. However, in very prolific lines of sow farrowing duration can now be as long as 8 to 10 hours.

The newborn piglet is born in a very vulnerable state. It is small, weighing typically 1 to 1.5 kg, and wet with birth fluid, and thus loses heat very rapidly. At the time of birth, it has very low body fat reserves and therefore limited ability to maintain its core body temperature. Unless it suckles quickly it will become hypothermic, lethargic and likely to die. However, suckling is not a simple activity. The newborn piglet must compete against its littermates for access to a limited number of teats, which can be difficult for small piglets born later in the birth order when older siblings are already well established. It also runs the risk of being crushed if its mother, weighing at least 200 times as much as the piglet, should move and trap it between her body and the floor. Occasionally, usually in gilts giving birth for the first time, the mother will be fearful and aggressive towards her piglets and may savage them. Given this scenario, it is not surprising that many piglets fail to survive the first few days of life. In the wild, the pig has evolved a strategy of producing a large number of young with low pregnancy investment. This allows the mother to rear a large litter in a good year, when food is plentiful, or to limit her efforts to fewer offspring if resources are scarce. For this strategy to work efficiently, surplus piglets should die quickly with least investment of resources, without compromising the survival of their littermates, and be those of poorest quality. The objectives of modern farming in keeping every piglet alive are therefore working against a long-term evolutionary strategy.

In modern farming, 18 to 20% of the piglets born do not survive until weaning and this mortality level has seen little improvement over recent years. Indeed, the introduction of hyper-prolific sow lines has made piglet survival even more challenging. More than half of these deaths happen during the farrowing period or within the first 48 hours. Stillbirths (piglets which die without ever breathing) account for 30–40% of all losses. Some of these piglets die during gestation as a result of infections and are born in mummified form if this death happens a long time before farrowing. Others may die as a result of lack of adequate nutrients because of crowding in the uterus and lack of good placental support. However, many die during the actual farrowing process as a result of asphyxia. This is a particular risk for those born later in the birth order, because the contractions of the uterus can disrupt their placental blood supply before they emerge and are able to breathe for themselves. Prolonged parturition as a result of sows being too old, too fat, too hot or experiencing too much disturbance during farrowing can exacerbate the problem. The level of stillbirth losses can be minimized by monitoring the progress of parturition and giving assistance if the inter-birth interval is too long (typically > 40–60 minutes). To facilitate supervision of farrowing, sows can be induced to farrow in more predictable, synchronous batches by injection of a prostaglandin analogue, which will induce farrowing in 12 to 24 hours. However, sows should never be induced earlier than 2 days before their expected farrowing date, or piglet viability will be seriously impaired.

For the piglets which are born alive, most deaths are attributed to crushing by the sow. However, as described earlier, this is part of an interacting complex of risk factors (Figure 6.6) and is often only the final endpoint of a path to mortality predisposed by other events. To prevent crushing, most farms house the farrowing sow in a crate, only slightly larger than her body size, designed to control her movements when lying down and prevent her from 'flopping' onto her piglets. The farrowing crate also offers other advantages when trying to improve piglet survival. Because the sow is fixed in one location, it is possible to predict exactly where the piglets will be born and to provide temporary extra heat at this place, thus reducing risk of hypothermia before suckling. A more permanent specialized resting area for the piglets, usually referred to as the 'creep area', can be provided close to the sow with supplementary heating by lamps or heat pads. This proximity of a warm area helps to encourage the piglets to lie away from the sow between sucklings, at a location where they are at less risk of crushing. Confinement of the sow in a crate also means that small or weak piglets can be assisted by stock people in safety, without fear of maternal aggression.

6.8.1 Housing Systems for Lactating Sows

When first introduced, the farrowing crate led to significant improvements in piglet survival and ease of management. However, it has also raised concerns about the welfare implications for the sow. The crate imposes severe restriction on movement during the period before farrowing when the sow is very active and motivated to build a nest. The nest-building behaviours are further thwarted if, as is commonly the case to facilitate management and hygiene, fully or partly slatted floors are used with little or no bedding provided to act as a

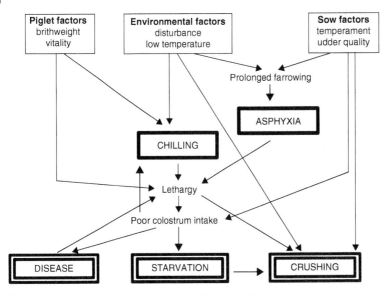

Figure 6.6 The interacting causes of piglet mortality.

substrate for the behaviour. It has been demonstrated that inability to express nest-building behaviour at this time causes expression of abnormal behaviours and a physiological stress response in the sow. Furthermore, as lactation progresses, the inability of the sow to escape from the attentions of her large litter can again induce stress. For these reasons, use of the farrowing crate has been banned in some countries, such as Switzerland, and its continued use is under debate in many others. However, finding an acceptable commercial alternative has not been simple.

Although it is the case that, in the UK, outdoor systems can achieve comparable levels of piglet survival in very simple huts without any supplementary piglet protection or heating (Figure 6.7), this is probably due to a unique combination of circumstances. The genotypes used in outdoor production tend to produce a larger and more viable piglet, but the system itself also favours survival. The large space in the paddock means that the sow can farrow with minimal disturbance. The importance of this factor is shown by the increase in mortality which occurs in group, rather than individual, farrowing paddocks or when predators such as foxes are in the vicinity. Most importantly, the provision of a deep bed of clean dry straw allows the sow to fully express nest-building behaviour, which has been shown to lead to less restlessness during farrowing and better maternal behaviour. The sloping walls of a well-designed farrowing hut help to control the lying movements of the sow and provide escape routes for the piglets, while, if crushing does occur, the cushioning properties of the deep bedding can reduce the risk of injury.

Attempts to reproduce this non-crate approach in indoor conditions have so far met with only limited success. Where sows have been housed in groups, with free access to individual

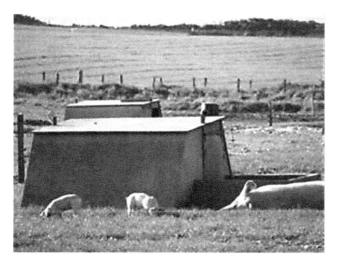

Figure 6.7 A typical farrowing system for outdoor production.

nests, there have been problems with animals which have given birth outside the nest in an inappropriate place, with disturbance of farrowing sows by others in the group, and with early desertion of the litter by some mothers. Where sows have been housed in individual pens without a crate, crushing of piglets has frequently been higher and the workload and safety of stock-people has been compromised. Many different designs of non-crate system have been tried (Table 6.4). Sometimes these have given promising results during the development stage but failed to be sufficiently robust under the more demanding conditions on large commercial farms. However, it is the case that countries which have banned, or restricted use of the farrowing crate can achieve an acceptable level of survival, albeit usually on smaller family-run farms. New research and trialling of prototypes at the current time (such as the PigSAFE system, Figure 6.8, where survival levels similar to those in creates have been achieved) suggests that acceptable commercial alternatives might soon develop but these are likely to require higher capital cost and greater stockperson expertise in order to be successful. For a free farrowing pen to achieve good piglet survival, careful attention to the design features is essential. Critical factors include the size of nest area, a well-drained floor, piglet protection features such as sloped walls, and easy accessibility of the heated creep area (see www.freefarrowing.org for more detailed discussion). It is also important to consider the selection of sows which show good maternal traits suited to free farrowing systems and staff with the confidence and ability to work in these conditions.

Another approach used on some farms is to retain the farrowing crate for the period around parturition, but then to either give the sow more freedom of movement by opening up one of the crate sides so that the whole pen is available, a so-called temporary crating system, or to move the sow and her litter to different accommodation where she is grouped with other animals at the same stage. This 'multi-suckling' system allows both sows and piglets to

Table 6.4 A comparison of farrowing and lactation systems.

System	Advantages	Disadvantages
Farrowing crate	Control of sow lying Facilitates localized heating Protection for stock-people Low space requirement Low labour requirement	Sow movement highly restricted Prevents sow nest building behaviour Sow cannot escape older litter
Modified crates (e.g. turn-around crate, Ottawa crate, ellipsoid crate)	Greater possibility for sow movement Control of sow lying Protection for stock-people Low space requirement	Prevents sow nest building behaviour Sow cannot escape older litter
Temporary crating (crate opened after the farrowing period)	Benefits of crate during first days after farrowing Greater sow freedom in later lactation Feed intake and milk yield often improved	Prevents sow nest building behaviour Hygiene problematic unless slatted flooring
Open pens	Behavioural freedom for sow Simple, low cost housing	Little warmth or protection for newborn piglets High crushing levels common No protection for stock-people Hygiene problematic unless slatted flooring
Designed pens (e.g. Schmid box, FAT pen, Werribee pen)	Behavioural freedom for sow Greater protection against piglet crushing Heated creep areas for piglets Zoned areas facilitate hygiene	Greater space requirement High capital cost
Indoor group farrowing (get-away pens, Freedom farrowing, Thorstensson system)	Large space for sow Individual nests for farrowing Social integration possible	Sows may farrow outside nest Farrowing may be disturbed Sows may desert litter Piglet mortality often high
Multi-suckling systems	Benefits of crate during first days after farrowing Behavioural freedom and social integration in later lactation Low cost lactation housing	Animals must be moved during lactation Suckling is disrupted when litters are grouped Lactational oestrus may occur
Outdoor farrowing (group or individual paddocks)	Plentiful space and enriched environment Isolation reduces disturbance Low capital cost	Exposure to climatic extremes Predators may take piglets Working conditions often challenging

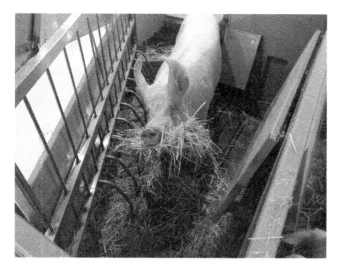

Figure 6.8   The PigSAFE free farrowing pen (Courtesy of M. Farish, SRUC).

co-mingle, typically from about two weeks after farrowing, so that no mixing and aggression occur at the time of weaning. However, there can be a major disruption of suckling at the time when grouping occurs which can increase risk of mortality for the piglets and induce a premature return to oestrus during lactation by the sows.

6.8.2   Management of the Newborn Piglet

The inputs of the skilled stockperson in the first days after farrowing are the key to good piglet survival. The importance of rapid suckling after birth has been emphasized for nutrition and thermoregulation of the piglet, but it is also important for longer-term survival and health. Because of the nature of the porcine placenta, large molecules such as immunoglobulins cannot cross from the maternal blood supply. This means that the piglet is born without any protective immunity against infection. Until it starts to synthesize its own immunoglobulins in sufficient amounts at four to six weeks of age, it is dependent on the passive transfer of immunity via maternal colostrum. The colostrum produced by the mammary glands at the time of farrowing is a very concentrated source of immunoglobulin, providing both general protection and specific protection against the infectious diseases that the sow has experienced on that farm, or has been vaccinated against. For the first 24 hours after birth, the gut of the newborn piglet is permeable to these large molecules, allowing them to be taken up from the colostrum into the bloodstream of the piglet. This permeability gradually reduces with time, a process hastened by the ingestion of food, until closure is complete, and no further transfer is possible. If the piglet fails to suckle, or suckles only poorly in the immediate post-partum period, it will be at much greater risk of succumbing to infectious disease during the lactation period and may even be compromised throughout its lifetime. The skilled stockperson will therefore intervene if necessary, to ensure that weak piglets, or small piglets in large litters, are able to obtain their adequate share of colostrum during the critical period. With very weak piglets, it is possible to feed them by hand after milking the sow, or to use colostrum which has previously been obtained and frozen for emergencies. However, a better solution for large litters of healthy pigs can be to adopt 'split suckling' where the bigger pigs in the litter which have already had a good feed are closed into a heated creep area for an hour to allow the less strong piglets the opportunity to suckle without competition.

This can be important because, from the minute of birth, each piglet tries to locate and defend the best teat on its mother. The sow typically has 14 functional teats, but not all are equally productive. Those at the rear of the udder are more likely to be low-yielding or damaged in older sows. Very early in life each litter forms a 'teat order' whereby each individual piglet always goes to the same teat to suckle and defends this teat vigorously against its siblings. The stronger piglets are able to appropriate the most productive teats, while the smaller and weaker piglets are relegated to the poorer-quality teats. In nature, this strategy is logical, giving the best chance to the fittest individuals, but in modern farming it is yet another challenge to the production of a large and even litter. To promote this teat fidelity, the pig has developed a complex suckling behaviour with a fixed sequence of interacting events. Milk is not available on demand, as is the case in many other species, except in the first few hours after birth. After this time, the availability of milk is restricted to a 20-second letdown period occurring during short suckling bouts taking place every 40 to 60 minutes. These bouts are initiated either by characteristic nursing grunts from the sow, or by the demands of many hungry piglets massaging the udder. As the whole litter assembles at the udder and starts vigorous massage, the nursing grunts increase in frequency until milk letdown occurs. After a period of quiet and intense suckling, the piglets again show active massaging of their teats once milk supply has ceased. The vigour of this massage has been shown to influence subsequent teat productivity and provides a mechanism whereby the larger and stronger piglets can stimulate better yield from their own teats. To defend its teat, the piglet uses its well-developed, and needle-sharp, canine teeth which can inflict serious facial wounds on its littermates. This can be problematic in large litters, where competition is higher, and is often prevented by the clipping off or grinding down of these teeth on the first day of life by the stockperson. Once again, the welfare implications of this procedure have been questioned; according to EU legislation it can be carried out only where the welfare risk of pain or gum damage during the procedure is outweighed by the reduction in injury to the faces of littermates and the udder of the sow if it is performed.

Where the number of piglets in the litter exceeds the number of functional teats, the surplus piglets have a high probability of mortality since supplementary feeding at this very young age is seldom adequate to sustain them. The best chance to reduce mortality in this situation is to cross-foster some piglets onto another sow, which has spare capacity. Skilful cross-fostering allows litter numbers to be evened up and matched to the rearing capacity of each sow and allows the size of piglets within each litter to be matched. This gives small piglets a better chance of survival because they are competing with piglets of similar size.

Fostering should ideally be done soon after the end of the colostrum period, and before the teat order becomes well established. It is better to move the large, strong piglets when fostering, rather than disturbing the establishment of the smaller or weaker piglets, and to close the new litter together in the creep area for a period to give them a more uniform smell and make the process less apparent to the foster sow. As lactation progresses, some piglets may start to fall behind in size because of a poor-quality teat. While it is possible to foster piglets between older litters, this is best done only when essential. Because the teat order is strongly formed by this time, and any unused teats will have dried off within about two days, introducing a new piglet causes a major disruption of suckling and litter disturbance, which can increase crushing and starvation risk for both the newcomer and the resident piglets.

With the modern trend for use of highly prolific sows, it can often be the case that the number of piglets born in a farrowing batch exceeds the number of available teats. Where this occurs, there are two possibilities to accommodate these supernumerary piglets. The first involves the use of nurse sows, in either a one or two stage fostering process. In a one stage process, a suitable quiet sow with a strong litter is weaned early and given a new litter made up of the stronger newborn piglets. However, because this gives a big mismatch between the lactation stage of the sow and the age of the piglets, it is becoming more common to use an intermediate step, whereby the weaned sow is given the whole litter from a sow which is one week post-farrowing and this sow then receives the surplus newborn. In some countries, rather than using a nurse sow strategy, an artificial rearing system is used for surplus newborn piglets once they have received colostrum. Such a strategy can only work with the highest level of hygiene and management, and even then, these piglets often show long term behavioural abnormalities.

In addition to teeth clipping, other procedures may be carried out on young piglets according to the needs of the individual farm. Tail docking involves removal of the distal part of the piglet's tail using a scalpel, clippers or cauterizing iron. This is done to reduce the risk of tail biting later in life, which can be a major welfare issue on some units. It is believed that the shorter tail is either less attractive as a stimulus for this behaviour, or more sensitive to the initial nibbling which is not then allowed to progress to a damaging phase. Once again, EU legislation requires assessment of the welfare balance between the pain of carrying out the procedure and the known degree of risk of later tail-biting injury. Recent evidence suggests that tail docking is not only painful at the time but can also cause longer term pain from the damaged nerves in the remaining stump, and there is now strong political pressure to reduce the tail biting risk factors present in later life rather than resorting to this procedure. Another surgical procedure carried out on the suckling animal in most countries is the castration of male piglets, which involves incision of the scrotum and removal of the testicles. This is done primarily to reduce the risk of 'boar taint' in the meat resulting from the presence of androstenone and skatole, induced by the hormonal state of the male after puberty. Only a few countries, including the UK and Ireland, currently produce a significant amount of pig meat from entire male animals, although this is now increasing in several other European countries. In most countries, castration is performed in the first week of life without any anaesthesia or analgesia. However, this is the subject of great debate within the EU, and a growing number of counties have already put in place legislation or industry codes requiring that some form of general or local anaesthesia be used. A new alternative of immunological castration has also recently become available, though is not yet accepted in all markets. This involves two injections in later life of an antibody which inactivates the production of male reproductive hormones, effectively castrating the animal only for a few weeks between the second injection and slaughter, without any surgical intervention.

The final procedure usually carried out on young piglets is the administration of iron. Iron is needed as one of the essential constituents of haemoglobin (the oxygen-carrying molecule in the blood) in the rapidly growing young pig. Sow's milk contains a very low level of iron, supplying only 1 mg/day against a requirement of 7 mg/day. Because of limited body reserves at birth, the piglet therefore begins to become anaemic after about seven days. In the wild, piglets get iron from rooting in the soil, as do piglets in outdoor herds unless on very sandy ground. In indoor herds, it is normal practice to supply iron to the suckling piglet at three to six days of age by intramuscular injection, although oral dosing is also possible. This is necessary because piglets will eat very little solid food before about three weeks of age, although they will drink substantial amounts of water, electrolyte solution or milk substitute if this is offered, especially if the sow is lactating poorly. By three weeks after farrowing, the milk yield of the sow reaches a plateau and then begins to decrease, and no longer supplies the needs of the growing piglets. It is therefore normal to supply a palatable, high-quality creep feed, starting from 10 to 14 days of age, to supplement the milk supply and make piglets familiar with solid food before weaning. If this is supplied in a location where the sow and piglets can feed in close proximity, learning from the mother helps to stimulate early intake.

The best determinant of good piglet weaning weights is a good milk yield from the sow. This is achieved by ensuring that the sow farrows in the correct body condition, neither too thin nor too fat, and achieves a high intake of a good-quality diet during lactation. If the sow is nursing a large litter, it is common for her to mobilize some body reserves in early lactation to support milk production. However, if this mobilization is excessive or prolonged, she will be weaned in poor body condition and her next reproductive cycle will be compromised. Either she will fail to come back into oestrus after the expected period of five or six days, or she will fail to conceive to the first mating, or she will produce a small litter at her next farrowing. To avoid these risks, everything possible should be done to encourage a high feed intake. The sow should be given fresh feed twice daily, building up the amount offered as her appetite increases over the week after farrowing until *ad libitum* intake is achieved. By the middle of the second week she should be eating 6 to 8 kg/day of a high-quality diet containing 14 MJ/kg of digestible energy (9.9 MJ/kg of net energy) and 16–18% crude protein (providing at least 8 g/kg of ileal digestible lysine). Intake can be promoted by ensuring good feed hygiene, removing any uneaten stale food, and by ready access to fresh water, adding water to the daily feed and ensuring that the drinker has an adequate flow rate of at least 1 litre/minute. It is also important to avoid excessive room temperature. While a room temperature of 20°C is often maintained during the farrowing period to reduce chilling risk for the piglets, reducing this to 18°C as soon as the piglets have learnt to use a heated creep area will benefit the sow because of her high metabolic heat production. In hot climates, feeding in the early morning and late evening when air temperatures are cooler can also be beneficial.

6.9   The Weaning Phase

The age at which piglets are weaned is a compromise between the need to have a robust piglet, able to weather the nutritional and social changes inherent in the process, and the desire to minimize the time between successive farrowings of the sow to obtain maximum piglet production and profitability. In most commercial systems, this compromise is at three to five weeks after farrowing, depending on housing and nutritional circumstances. Under natural conditions, weaning is a gradual process in which the frequency of sucklings gradually reduces and the intake of solid food gradually increases until final completion at 12 to 16 weeks of age. During later lactation the sow comes back into oestrus and becomes pregnant again while still nursing. Oestrus is suppressed by suckling and, although it is possible to induce oestrus during lactation under commercial conditions by a high plane of nutrition, disruption of regular suckling and the stimulus of a boar, the timing of this event is not always predictable and it is seldom attempted.

In commercial production, operating a well-controlled batch system is very important for health management and efficient utilization of buildings. This means that all sows in the batch should be served at a similar time so that stable groups can be maintained and entry and exit from farrowing rooms can be synchronous, allowing thorough cleaning and disinfection between batches to avoid carry-over of any infectious agents. A similar 'all in, all out' policy is very important for the newly weaned piglet, which is particularly vulnerable to health challenges because of its immature digestive and immune systems. The key to maintaining this planned batch schedule is the weaning time, since correctly managed sows weaned in the first month of lactation are unlikely to show lactational oestrus, and a synchronized oestrus will be stimulated to occur five to six days after weaning.

Theoretically, each extra week of lactation reduces the average sow output by about one piglet per year. However, research has demonstrated that weaning earlier than three weeks can be counterproductive because the recovery period after farrowing is too short, resulting in increased rebreeding interval and poorer conception rate. The optimal weaning time to maximize sow output is therefore between three and four weeks. However, the piglet is still quite immature at this stage, since it only starts to eat significant quantities of solid food at about three weeks of age and its digestive enzyme capacity to deal with non-milk diets is very limited. When weaned at less than three weeks, the piglet experiences a significant growth check while the transition to solid food takes place. During this period, the limited digestive capacity makes it very prone to enteric disease, while its poorly developed immune system means it is also at higher risk of other infectious challenges. By four or five weeks, the piglet is much more robust, and the weaning process involves less growth check and health risk. For these reasons, current EU legislation specifies that piglets should not be weaned at less than four weeks of age, although a special clause allows litters to be weaned up to seven days earlier to facilitate all-in all-out batch management. In organic systems, weaning is not allowed at less than six weeks of age and some national certification schemes recommend eight weeks of age.

There are situations in which weaning before this time may be permitted and may give some benefits. Because the passive immunity of the piglet declines with time after colostrum ingestion, and because a number of endemic disease agent are passed from the sow to her piglets during the suckling period, it can sometimes be advantageous in breaking a disease cycle to wean the piglets at 10 to 14 days of age, while their immune protection is still high, and remove them from the vicinity of the sow to prevent cross-infection. This system, known as segregated early weaning (SEW) or 'isowean', has been widely adopted in large enterprises in some countries such as the USA, but poses particular challenges in both the rebreeding of the early weaned sow and the establishment of the immature piglet.

Abrupt weaning at any age younger than the natural weaning age imposes some degree of challenge for the piglet. As the change from milk to solid feed generally involves a break in the regular pattern of feeding and a reduction in total nutrient intake, the piglet generates less body heat and requires a higher environmental temperature to be comfortable and less susceptible to disease. It can take up to two weeks for nutrient intake to regain the level previously achieved during suckling, during which period the piglet needs a temperature of 27 to 30°C to achieve thermal neutrality. Its susceptibility to enteric disease at this time also means that a high standard of hygiene is essential. For these reasons, newly weaned piglets are often housed in heated, controlled-environment buildings on fully slatted floors called flat-decks. A cheaper alternative to heating up the whole airspace of a room is to create a lying area with a microclimate by providing a kennelled system. Such systems include 'bungalows' with an enclosed insulated lying area and an outdoor slatted dunging area, or the provision of a kennel within a strawed system inside a simple building shell. On larger units, it is possible to house large groups of weaners together in deep litter systems, with a temporary kennel made of straw bales which can be broken down for bedding as the pigs grow. The use of large group systems (100 or more pigs in a group) for newly weaned pigs has been quite widely adopted in larger herds because they offer the scope to cheapen housing and simplify management, as well as avoiding the need for regrouping of unfamiliar pigs in later growing stages when fighting is likely to result in lost performance. Although initially used in straw-based housing in large kennelled yards, such systems have also been developed for controlled-environment, fully slatted nurseries. Trial results have sometimes indicated reduced growth rate in controlled-environment large group nurseries compared with smaller groups, but this reduced growth can be compensated by better subsequent growth, resulting in no reduction in overall lifetime performance. The poorer initial growth in large groups seems to be related to the ease of accessing resources. The newly weaned piglets are less willing to move long distances to find food on a frequent basis, instead reducing their total daily intake.

The housing of large groups of piglets in deep litter systems was most popular for the weaners from outdoor breeding herds, which already form large groups for exploratory activities in the field while still suckling. Mobile outdoor kennel-and-run systems are also used by such enterprises, and generally give performance as good as that seen in more intensive systems. Piglets weaned from outdoor systems are better able to manage the weaning transition, being faster to explore and ingest food and experiencing less growth check, despite the fact that practicalities dictate that they do not receive any special creep feed before this time. It may be that the greater experience of separation from the sow and exploration of a diverse environment are of benefit.

The most critical part of an early weaning system is correct nutrition. The sucking piglet has an enzyme system specialized for digesting the components of a milk diet, and the ability to digest starch and plant proteins is poorly developed. Only after it starts to eat significant quantities of solid food is the induction of these enzymes triggered. If given a poor-quality diet at the time of weaning this can only be partially digested, limiting the nutritional value and inducing diarrhoea. It is therefore necessary to formulate special diets for the weaned piglet containing milk or whey powder and readily digestible protein such as fish meal. The starch component can be made more digestible by cooking the cereals to break up their starch molecules, while a highly digestible fat source provides concentrated energy. Such ingredients are expensive but are important for successful weaning at an early age. This is particularly true now that political or market pressures in many countries have led to cessation of the routine inclusion of prophylactic antibiotics in the diet. As the pig becomes older, the inclusion level of cheaper ingredients such as uncooked cereals and plant proteins can be gradually increased, and nutrient density reduced, until the pig can thrive on these components alone. When pigs are produced according to organic standards, the choice of dietary ingredients is more limited and many of the high-quality ingredients needed for successful early weaning, such as synthetic amino acids, are not permitted. Organic weaner diets consequently tend to be of simpler formulation and lower digestibility, but the greater weaning age of the piglets can offset these disadvantages.

6.10 The Growing and Finishing Phase

Once the weaned piglet is established, the main objective is to grow the pig to slaughter as rapidly and efficiently as possible. This requires attention to disease prevention, environmental quality and nutritional specification.

DE, digestible energy; NE, net energy; CP, crude protein; idL, ileal digestible lysine.

As with the other stages of pig production, housing for growing and finishing pigs varies widely. The most common form of housing across Europe is in controlled-environment buildings with fully or partly slatted flooring. This has the advantage that pigs can be maintained at the optimal temperature to maximize efficient use of feed (see Table 6.5), while labour for cleaning is minimized and the separation of the pig from its manure helps to maintain good health and reduce risk of zoonotic diseases such as salmonellosis. Temperature and air quality are regulated by use of thermostatically controlled fan systems, or by automatically controlled natural ventilation (ACNV) in which ventilation flaps open or close according to internal temperature levels. In more tropical regions, building construction tends to be simpler, with open-sided buildings to maximize air flow or the use of curtains in colder seasons. Finishing pigs fed *ad libitum* can be particularly prone to heat stress, since they possess no sweat glands in the skin, and the provision of showers or wallows when ambient temperature is high can be beneficial to both welfare and performance. If they have no other possibility for cooling, they will seek to wallow in their own excreta, increasing risk of disease transmission.

Table 6.5 Guideline temperatures and feed specifications for growing pigs.

Category of pig	Temperature range (°C)[†]	Diet specification[‡]	
		Energy (MJ/kg)	Protein (g/kg)
Newly weaned piglets (weaned at 3 to 4 weeks of age)	25 to 30	16.0 DE *11.0 NE*	220 CP *13 idL*
Weaners (15 to 25 kg)	21 to 24	15.0 DE *10.5 NE*	210 CP *12 idL*
Growing pigs (25 to 50 kg)	18 to 21	14.0 DE *9.8 NE*	200 CP *10 idL*
Finishing pigs (50 to 100 kg)	15 to 18	13.0 DE *9.0 NE*	180 CP *8 idL*

[†]Lower temperatures are required if pigs are housed on deep bedding.

[‡]Assuming entire males and females of improved genotype fed *ad libitum*. Traditional breeds have lower requirement.

Table 6.6 Space requirements and flooring specifications for pigs (to comply with EU Directive 2008/120/EC).

Category of pig	Space requirement (m²)	Specifications for slatted floors (mm)	
		Maximum void width	Minimum slat width
Breeding boar	6.0 (10.0 if service pen)		
Sow (group housed)	2.25	20	80
Growing pig:			
<10 kg	0.15	11	50
10 to 20 kg	0.20	14	50
20 to 30 kg	0.30	18	80
30 to 50 kg	0.40	18	80
50 to 86 kg	0.55	18	80
85 to 110 kg	0.65	18	80
>110 kg	1.00	18	80

Within the EU, legislation exists about the minimum space requirement at each production stage and design of slatted flooring to avoid injuries to pigs' feet (Table 6.6). Controlled-environment buildings can also be designed to incorporate solid flooring and use of some bedding material, when cleaned out regularly by tractor scraping of dunging passages or under-slat scrapers, or by use of sloping floors in 'straw flow' systems where the straw gradually moves down the sloped lying area into a scraped dunging channel at its base. More extensive forms of housing are provided by kennelled housing with tractor-scraped passages or deep litter systems in cheaper, naturally ventilated buildings. These incur additional costs in purchase of bedding material and labour to provide straw and remove manure but offer some benefits for pig welfare if managed in a hygienic way. Comparison of fully slatted and straw-bedding housing for growing and finishing pigs has shown that risk of enteric and respiratory disease is greater in the bedded housing, where the pig is in contact with its manure and dust levels can be higher, but the risk of lameness, gastric ulcers and tail biting is greater in slatted housing.

6.10.1 Tail Biting

Tail biting is an injurious abnormal behaviour which occurs sporadically and unpredictably on many farms, usually first seen in the later stages of nursery accommodation or the finishing accommodation. It involves progressive chewing of the tail from a mildly scratched condition to one in which the whole tail is removed and the flesh of the victim may be eaten away up into the spine. Similar but less common abnormal behaviours causing lesions on other parts of the body include ear biting or flank biting. These behaviours are a major economic as well as a welfare issue, since they involve veterinary treatment of injury, mortality and condemnation of carcasses through infection. The widely used preventive measure of tail docking piglets soon after birth can reduce the risk of tail biting but does not abolish it and a prevalence of about 5% is still recorded in most countries. The causes of tail biting, and its related injurious behaviours, appear to be multifactorial, with a genetic predisposition triggered by environmental or nutritional factors. It has been suggested that more than one type of causation may contribute to the expression of the behaviour. One form seems to be a result of redirected foraging behaviour in a barren environment. In this form, initial nibbling and chewing which might otherwise be directed to environmental substrates is directed towards the tails of pen-mates and gradually becomes more severe until blood is drawn. At this point, the attraction of other pigs to the blood results in a rapid escalation of the problem. Dietary deficiencies in protein and minerals, particularly salt, have been shown to increase tail-biting risk, possibly through enhanced attraction to blood. Another form of tail biting appears to erupt without a gradual build-up in chewing and may be linked to frustration of animals unable to access resources such as food, water or preferred lying places. This sudden initial event is seldom directly observed but, again, once blood is drawn the behaviour spreads and escalates. It is often apparent that certain individual pigs, usually the smaller and unthrifty individuals, develop chronic tail-biting behaviour and move from tail to tail in an apparently obsessive way. Exactly what causes such pigs to develop is currently unknown, but their rapid identification and removal from the group is vital in controlling any outbreak. Other remedial measures involve removing all bitten pigs to eliminate traces of blood, painting the tails with unpalatable Stockholm tar, increasing the salt content of the diet to 0.4%, putting salt blocks into the pen and giving straw and playthings to distract the animals. Controlling an outbreak once under way is very difficult, and the objective should always be to prevent the onset of the problem by careful attention to housing and management. Decision support systems which can be used to assess the risk areas on an individual farm are now available (see for example https://webhat.ahdb.org.uk). Outbreaks can sometimes be averted if detected at a very early stage, by removing a causal factor, moving the pigs to a new pen or providing additional enrichment. New automated methods to detect the early signs of tail biting, such as an increase in restlessness or vocalization and the presence of lowered tails tucked close to the rump, are therefore currently under development.

The demonstrated role of barren environments in increasing tail-biting risk highlights the importance of environmental enrichment for the pig. Pigs are highly intelligent and exploratory animals and, although spending 70–80% of the day lying and resting when well fed, have a requirement for functional occupation during the remaining period if abnormal behaviours are to be avoided. When housed with straw bedding, the chewing and rooting of this material provides a good outlet for exploratory motivation. Even a relatively limited amount of chopped straw given fresh each day appears to fulfil this function adequately. However, in slatted systems the provision of bedding may not be possible because it interferes with the management of the liquid manure if it falls through the slats and blocks up pipelines and pumps. Finding alternative forms of enrichment in these systems has proved to be a major challenge. Many items such as footballs and rubber tyres are initially stimulating but soon become ignored as lacking in novelty. In the same way, hanging chains, which were widely used in the past, appear to generate only limited interest. The properties of enrichment that attract and hold the attention of the animals have been shown to include novelty, deformability and destructibility, nutritional content, and lack of soiling. EU legislation suggests straw, hay, wood, sawdust, mushroom compost, peat or a mixture of these materials to be appropriate substrates for proper expression of investigation and manipulation activities. However, ropes, paper sacks and root vegetables have also been shown to be very effective.

Other forms of aggression within the group are usually uncommon, provided that a stable group is maintained without introduction of unfamiliar animals and access to resources is adequate. Where this is not the case, serious fighting can occur to establish and maintain social ranking and may even result in death in these larger and stronger animals. It has recently been shown that aggressive predisposition also has some genetic basis, and new breeding strategies may reduce the severity of aggression if mixing is unavoidable. However, with good planning and batch management this should not be necessary.

6.10.2 Feeding the Finishing Pig

The major nutritional objective of the finishing phase is to produce pigs at market weight which meet the specification for best carcass price. In most markets, this involves meeting a contract grading specification for both carcass weight and leanness, usually measured as subcutaneous fat thickness at one or more specified points on the back. Because they have been bred for leanness, it is possible for genetically superior pigs to be fed *ad libitum* through to slaughter and still give acceptable grading. This greatly simplifies the management of feeding since automated filling of feed reservoirs in each pen, which the pigs can access on a 24-hour basis, means that many pigs can share a limited feeding area provided from linear hoppers, circular pans or single space feeders. Such feeders vary widely in design and may supply dry meal or pelleted feed, liquid feed as a soup or incorporate integral watering devices in combination with dry food. Current recommendations in such systems are that up to 12 pigs can share a feeding place with dry food, and up to 20 with feeders which wet the food at point of delivery or provide liquid food. However, it has been suggested that some modern genotypes may eat more slowly, making more generous feed space allowance beneficial in improving growth and avoiding behavioural problems. *Ad libitum* feeding without development of excessive carcass fatness may not be possible with less improved genotypes, and particularly the castrated males, or when pigs are kept up until much heavier weights before slaughter for some specialized markets such as Italian Parma ham. In these circumstances, feed restriction in the final stages of fattening may be necessary. When this is the case, adequate feed distribution is essential to ensure evenness of weight is maintained within the group and to minimize aggression at feeding time. The feed can be provided in long troughs or scattered widely on the floor. When troughs are used, the feeding space allowance per pig must be at least the width of an animal across the shoulders so that all can feed simultaneously. However, even when this space is provided, some individuals may dominate greater areas of the trough unless head, or head and shoulder, barriers are incorporated.

Feeds for the growing-finishing pig are usually based on cereals and plant proteins, most commonly soya bean meal. However, feed costs can be reduced by the inclusion of industrial by-products from the human food and drink sector such as wheat feed, vegetable wastes and brewery and distillery products. Many of these products come in liquid form and can only be utilized with specialized feeding systems designed for this purpose. It used to be common practice to feed pigs on kitchen waste, particularly in smallholder systems. However, the disease risks associated with this procedure, where infected meat might be fed back into the food chain, have resulted in an EU ban on this practice. As the pig becomes older, its appetite increases and its need for protein relative to energy in the diet decreases. To maximize use of nutrients, it is therefore normal to feed a series of diets over the growing period which change in specification as the pig ages (Table 6.5).

6.10.3 Outdoor Systems

While outdoor production systems for breeding sows are common in some countries, and outdoor systems for weaned pigs have increased, the outdoor finishing of pigs is still very uncommon. Constraints include land availability and soil damage, pollution potential, loss of performance and logistics of supplying the large daily requirement for feed and water in all weather conditions. A small number of herds have operated such systems for organic pig production, but information and experience outside this context is very limited. Outdoor finishing can be divided into two types. In the first, free-range pigs are provided with a large paddock and simple shelter, while in the second they are confined within an outdoor hut-and-run system. Paddock systems are the least common, requiring more land and being more difficult to manage.

In true paddock systems, pigs have the free run of a fenced paddock area. They are normally contained by a two-strand electric fence. The stocking rate suggested has been approximately 4,000 kg/ha, giving 40 to 50 finishing pigs per hectare, although this will depend on soil type and climatic conditions. In practice, even higher stocking densities have been used for limited periods in arable rotations (up to 500 pigs/ha) but have generally resulted in a high level of paddock damage. Housing for free-range pigs will depend on climate and group size. It must provide a warm, dry lying area in winter and, unless other provision is made, must also provide shade in summer. A minimum lying area of 0.5 m^2 for a 100 kg pig (0.3 m^2 for a 50 kg pig) should be provided. Bedding should be provided in winter to provide floor insulation, and replenished frequently enough to maintain a clean, dry surface. Under UK conditions, a straw usage of 20–60 kg per growing-finishing pig per cycle has been reported. Housing is generally moveable, so that each new batch of pigs can begin in a clean paddock with a newly re-sited house. In UK conditions, housing comprising corrugated iron arcs or wooden sheds has generally been used, although tents have more recently been adopted on a few farms. These can have walls made of large straw bales, protected by wire mesh, and a canvas roof. Feed is generally provided *ad libitum* via bulk hoppers, which can be filled mechanically (a group of 50 pigs requiring up to 1 tonne of feed per week). Water is generally provided from open troughs, allowing at least 12 mm of trough space per pig. These troughs need to have an adequate capacity and/or filling rate to provide at least 5 litres of water per pig per day, although this will vary with size of pig and environmental temperature.

The most common system of outdoor finishing in the UK involves a hut-and-run system, where pigs are provided with a hut and small outdoor run area bounded by solid fencing and bedded with straw to maintain hygiene. One common type features a wooden hut of 2.4 m by 6.1 m with an insulated steel roof, and an outdoor run of approximately 33 m^2 to house 25 pigs from 30 to 90 kg The hut has an adjustable ventilator and contains and integral feed hopper with large capacity and water tank holding a one-day reserve supply. Between each batch of pigs, and even within-batch if the run becomes very soiled, the hut can be lifted and towed to a clean area of ground to reduce risk of infection. A further option for easier management and mechanization of feed and water supply is to place such units on a permanent concrete base. In this situation, the units are dismantled between batches, and reassembled after the base has been cleaned. Such systems start to resemble in approach the traditional brick pig houses with outdoor concrete runs which were used on small farms early in the twentieth century, or the systems used in many countries for organic pig production at the present time.

Information on performance levels of outdoor pigs is scarce, and controlled performance comparisons between indoor and outdoor finishing pig production are even less common. It would be expected that outdoor finishing systems would have poorer pig performance because of the additional energy losses associated with lower temperatures and greater amount of exercise, and limited trial data suggest a 5–10% poorer feed efficiency. Additionally, the genotypes of pigs commonly used in outdoor systems have been selected to better withstand adverse climatic conditions and, in consequence, have poorer lean tissue deposition potential and greater propensity to fatness than those used in intensive indoor systems. This results in poorer feed conversion ratios because of the higher energetic cost of fat deposition compared to lean deposition. However, respiratory health of the animals is generally better because of the plentiful supply of fresh air and lack of noxious gases which irritate lung tissue.

6.10.4 Handling and Transport

The greatest challenges to the welfare of finishing pigs come during human interventions for procedures such as moving, weighing, transporting, catching and injecting. To facilitate ease of handling and minimize the number of negative behaviours which the stockperson must carry out during the process, good housing design is critical. A thorough knowledge of pig behaviour can aid both the design of pig housing and the way in which animals are handled with least difficulty. The application of behaviourally based design criteria to pig movement facilities has been studied in some detail. Since pigs have poor depth perception, they are unwilling to cross shadows or high-contrast objects. Entering a strange dark space can take three times as long as entering a strange, brightly lit space. Therefore, provision of even lighting and uniform flooring will facilitate movement. Since pigs have a wide-angled visual field, they can be easily distracted and hence solid-sided, gently curved races prevent movement being disturbed by outside events. Pigs raised in very confined and uniform environments have often proved more easily baulked and difficult to drive than those reared in more enriched environments. While pigs have less pronounced following behaviour than ruminants, they will follow a leader when it is an established member of their social group. Isolation from the group is very stressful and they will often panic if they become separated. Prevention of jamming at the entrance to a single-file race can be prevented by using an offset step at the race entrance but use of a double race where two pigs can progress side by side is better. One of the greatest physical stressors is walking up a ramp, such as a loading bridge for transport. According to the behaviour of inexperienced pigs, a ramp with an angle of 30 degrees appears inaccessible.

The degree of stress during loading, transport, lairage and slaughter is important not only for the welfare of the animals but also for the quality of the meat. To assess the relative stressfulness of procedures carried out during transport, an artificial simulator has been used. Starting the motor which generated vibration and noise caused the greatest increase in heart rate, but this gradually declined as the test progressed, indicating some degree of adaptation. Similar results were obtained during real road journeys. By placing a switch panel inside the transport simulator, it was possible to study the motivation of pigs to avoid vibration and noise. Pigs quickly learnt to press the panel and temporarily switch off the simulator, indicating that they found it aversive. They pressed the panel more often if the level of noise and vibration was more intense, and continued to do so throughout the test period, indicating no degree of habituation. Pigs did not learn to press the panel to switch off noise alone, suggesting that it was the vibration which was important. When tested just after a large meal, they switched off the simulator more often, suggesting that transport was even more aversive at this time. Pigs appear to be particularly sensitive to travel sickness and fasting them overnight before a journey is recommended.

6.11 Pig Diseases, Disease Detection and Health Management

Pigs, especially when kept intensively, are susceptible to a number of infectious diseases which can spread rapidly within and between herds. Highly infectious exotic diseases, such as foot and mouth disease, classical swine fever and African swine fever, are controlled in many countries by national eradication programmes, in which all pigs in any herd where the disease is detected are slaughtered and their carcasses buried or burnt to prevent disease spread. Other, less serious diseases can exist endemically within herds where their effects on health and welfare can be minimized by good management. Many of these can be controlled by a vaccination programme within the herd. Use of vaccines against enzootic pneumonia (EP), porcine respiratory and reproductive syndrome (PRRS), erysipelas, *Escherichia coli* and postweaning multisystemic wasting disease (PMWS) is now widespread. However, for many respiratory and enteric diseases, maintaining a good level of hygiene and minimizing stressors for the animals, combined with rapid diagnosis and antibiotic treatment of clinical cases, prevents occurrence of serious herd losses. By maintaining a strictly controlled pig flow, with all-in all-out management of accommodation, thorough cleaning and disinfection between batches, and no mixing of cohorts of different ages, and paying strict attention to pen hygiene and air quality, the infection pressure can be kept at a low level. The widespread adoption of these approaches has made it possible to reduce reliance on prophylactic use of antibiotics in feed or water, which has become unacceptable in many countries because of a possible association with the development of antibiotic-resistant strains of pathogen which might pose a threat to human health.

The early detection and treatment of sick animals is very important in this situation and the rapid developments in Precision Livestock Farming are now being harnessed for this purpose. The use of electronic RFID tags to identify individual pigs allows the monitoring of their liveweight and feed intake at computer-linked feeding stations. Sudden changes, or progressive deviations from the normal pattern of growth, provide early warning of a health problem. More recently, systems employing visual image analysis from strategically placed cameras are being developed to track growth profiles and behaviour patterns in groups of pigs. Machine learning techniques are being applied to detect deviations in feeding, drinking and resting patterns occurring at disease onset, or changes in gait indicative of lameness.

Because even well-managed endemic diseases result in slower growth and poorer feed efficiency, and hence significant economic losses, many herds seek to maintain a high health status. Provided that they are located far enough away from other infected herds, since some disease agents can easily be carried for distances of 3 to 4 km on the wind, good biosecurity precautions can prevent ingress of disease. The most important precautions relate to importation of diseased animals, or animal products. Therefore, high health herds will either run a closed breeding replacement system, or only take in animals and semen from specific pathogen free (SPF) herds of known and tested high health status. Any incoming animals must undergo a quarantine period, so that any incubating disease has time to be expressed. A perimeter fence around the unit, a good rodent control programme and bird-proofing of buildings prevent wildlife from bringing in disease. This fencing also allows control of visitors, with only those who have had no contact with other pigs in at least the last 48 hours being considered low risk. A requirement to shower at the entry point, and the provision of clean protective clothing and boots, further reduce the likelihood of importing disease agents. Similarly, all but essential vehicles are excluded, with feed deliveries and pig removal vehicles all operating from outside the perimeter. The use of disinfectant wheel dips and sprays at the unit entrance ensures that manure picked up on other farms is not brought in on vehicles, and foot dips outside each building prevent tracking around the unit. Where such precautions are rigorously enforced, high health status can be maintained with major benefits for both profitability and animal welfare.

6.12 Animal Welfare in Different Systems

The many welfare problems described with intensive indoor housing systems for pigs do not mean that welfare can only be good in an extensive situation; indeed, the opposite can sometimes be the case. The favourable consumer perception of outdoor systems results from the large area of free space, the environmental complexity and the choice of physical and social environment which is possible in these circumstances. There is evidence that outdoor systems may be better for health in some respects, since veterinary and medicine costs per pig are 10–20% lower in outdoor than in indoor herds. However, parasitism may be greater in the outdoor situation, where worm eggs can remain viable in the soil for extended periods and constitute a source of reinfection. This is a particular issue in organic herds, where routine use of anthelminthics is prohibited. Outdoor pigs face other welfare problems, particularly in relation to thermal stress and social competition. Low-ranking animals may be particularly disadvantaged in outdoor systems in comparison with the more controlled indoor situation, since they can receive only limited human assistance in attaining adequate access to resources such as shelter and food. Thus, when considered in the welfare framework of the 'five freedoms', the following conclusions about outdoor production systems can be drawn:

- freedom from hunger and thirst – no effect, or possible negative effect if reliant on natural foraging;
- freedom from thermal and physical discomfort – possible negative effect from climatic extremes;
- freedom from injury and disease – positive effect from reduced infection intensity, but possible negative effect from reduced biosecurity and increased parasitic burden;
- freedom from fear and stress – positive effect from greater space allowance and enriched behavioural development, but less human assistance for subordinate animals and possible negative effects at time of slaughter from unfamiliarity with confinement and handling;
- freedom to express normal behaviour – clear positive effects, although nose-ringing of breeding stock is an issue.

Organic production systems specify specific conditions that are thought to improve the welfare of pigs. Permanent indoor housing of organic livestock is not permitted. Animals can be housed indoors for a maximum of 20% of their lifetime, but at other times must be kept either in fields or in housing where they have permanent access to an outdoor run. All housing must have a bedded lying area and slats, while permitted, must not exceed 50% of the total floor area (25% in some schemes). The space requirements for organic pigs are greater than those conventionally used. All pigs must be given access to roughage or fodder, and at present farmers use grazed grass/clover swards, conserved silage from such swards, from whole-crop cereals or from maize, and root crops such as fodder beet. However, a major current challenge for organic pig producers is to find enough organically produced feed of appropriate quality, especially for the newly weaned piglets. The objective of organic production is to maintain good health through the adoption of effective management practices. Organic production forbids the routine use of antibiotics, although it does not preclude their use for individual animals where there is a veterinary need. In such circumstances, longer withdrawal periods are specified (twice that required by law) before the animal can be slaughtered for meat. Animals which have received repeated antibiotic treatment cannot be sold for organic meat, presenting the risk that producers may withhold treatments to maintain their organic premium. Routine use of anthelminthics is not allowed, and the emphasis is on good pasture management and regular rotation to control parasite build-up. However, survey data suggest that parasitism can be a major problem in organic pig herds.

Build-up of parasites and other infectious agents can also pose greater challenges in bedded systems than in those where pigs are kept on slatted floors, and hence separated from their manure. However, such health benefits must be considered in opposition to many beneficial roles of bedding in provision of physical comfort, thermal comfort and environmental enrichment. As discussed throughout this chapter, each system has its own strengths and weaknesses which need to be addressed in the most appropriate way to ensure good pig welfare.

No matter which system is adopted, one of the most important determinants of pig welfare is the quality of the management and stockperson ship that they receive. The importance of the relationship between the stockperson and their animals for productivity was first highlighted in a study carried out in the Netherlands. Twelve commercial units, each run by a single stockperson, were controlled by a large integrated company which dictated that all outside inputs (source of pigs, feed, management and veterinary advice) were similar. Despite this, the farms showed large differences in reproductive performance, with averages ranging from 17.9 to 22.5 pigs born per sow per year. To seek some explanation for this, the sows on each unit were subject to behavioural tests assessing their response to humans. It was found that sows on farms with poor reproductive performance showed more signs of fear of humans. When tested in their stalls, they had a greater withdrawal response to the approach of an experimenter's hand, and when confronted with a strange person in an open arena they showed less approach behaviour. This phenomenon was subsequently investigated in a series of controlled experiments, which demonstrated that pigs subjected to repeated negative or inconsistent handling developed a chronic stress response. This was reflected in poorer growth rate and reproductive performance. Subsequent studies have shown a relationship between the attitudinal and behavioural profiles of stockpersons and the level of fear of humans seen in their pigs. In Australia, implementing a training procedure which involved providing stock-people with information on the sensitivity of pigs to negative handling and the practical benefits in ease of management and productivity when positive handling procedures are adopted, markedly reduced fear levels in the pigs and increased performance by five pigs per sow per year. Growing awareness of such benefits has led to the introduction of certified training programmes in many countries, and the highlighting of the importance of the human–animal interaction in both legislation and codes of good practice.

References and Further Reading

AHDB. (2018). *2017 Pig Cost of Production in Selected Countries*. Kenilworth, UK: Agriculture and Horticulture Development Board. https://pork.ahdb.org.uk.

English, P., Smith, W., and MacLean, A. (1982). *The Sow: Improving Her Efficiency*. Ipswich, UK: Farming Press.

English, P.R., Fowler, V.R., Baxter, S., and Smith, B. (1988). *The Growing and Finishing Pig: Improving Efficiency*. Ipswich, UK: Farming Press.

Marchant-Forde, J.N. (ed.) (2009). *The Welfare of Pigs*. Springer Netherlands.

Red Tractor Assurance. (2019). *Pig Standards*. London, UK: Red Tractor Assurance.

RSPCA. (2016). *RSPCA Welfare Standards for Pigs*. Horsham, UK: RSPCA.

Thornton, K. (1988). *Outdoor Pig Production*. Ipswich, UK: Farming Press.

Vaarst, M., Roderick, S., Lund, V., and Lockeretz, W. (2003). *Animal Health and Welfare in Organic Agriculture*. Wallingford: CABI Publishing.

Varley, M.A. and Wiseman, J. (eds.) (2001). *The Weaner Pig: Nutrition and Management*. Wallingford, UK: CABI Publishing.

Wiseman, J. (2000). *The Pig: A British History*. London: Duckworth.

Wiseman, J. (ed.) (2018). *Achieving Sustainable Production of Pig Meat. Volume 3: Animal Health and Welfare*. Cambridge, UK: Burleigh Dodds.

Zimmerman, J.J., Karriker, L.A., Ramirez, A., Schwartz, K.J., Stevenson, G.W., and Zhang, J. (eds.) (2019). *Diseases of Swine*, 11e. Hoboken, NI, USA: John Wiley & Sons.

7

Laying Hens

Graham Scott

Management and Welfare of Farm Animals: The UFAW Farm Handbook, Sixth Edition.
Edited by John Webster and Jean Margerison.
© Universities Federation for Animal Welfare 2022. Published 2022 by John Wiley & Sons Ltd.

7.1 Introduction

When considering the welfare of laying hens it is essential to remember that birds are not egg-producing machines. They are living, sentient creatures and human conscience should dictate that they be treated with respect. Chickens are capable of adapting to a wide variety of environmental conditions, mainly through adaption; they can become accustomed and cope with many types of change to their environment. Animal welfare is increasingly described in terms of animals being able to cope with such changes; if the animals cannot adapt and cope, then welfare is negatively affected. If humans can establish the limits of adaptability of laying hens we can provide a suitable environment that birds can adapt to easily and does not negatively affect the birds' welfare. Similarly, humans can modify the production expectations (egg production per bird) so that welfare is not threatened. To do this we need an in-depth knowledge of the needs of the birds that we use.

In order to care properly for laying hens, it is important to understand the basic biology of the bird (in terms of anatomy and physiology). Chickens are complex organisms. Knowledge of the fundamental systems can assist in providing for the welfare requirements of the species. Since laying hens are producing eggs on a regular basis, the reproductive system of the female (hen) will be described in some detail, along with the skeletal and digestive systems. Behavioural needs of the hens may also relate to how birds perceive their environment and so sensory perception will be considered.

The keeping of hens for egg production will be put into context in terms of both the historical relationship between humans and hens for egg production, and the UK and global egg production industries. The permitted systems for the egg industry will be described and explained. This will include the rearing of pullets from day-old chicks to point of lay and then on to the production systems. The management requirements, biosecurity, disease control and common problems, including behavioural problems, and issues will be addressed. Bird welfare and larger welfare issues will be assessed. Egg quality systems, including provision for bird welfare, will be included before speculation on how egg production may evolve in the future brings the chapter to a close. While this chapter is addressed at an international audience, many of the descriptions of regulations and welfare organizations use the UK situation as an example.

7.2 Chicken Physiology

7.2.1 The Reproductive System

Before discussing the way that chickens are kept, it is important to grasp the basic biology of the chicken to enable a better understanding of the birds. In birds (unlike mammals) it is the male that is homogametic, carrying two of the same sex chromosomes. So, at the point of fertilization there are males (ZZ) and females (Z-). The female chick carries all of her undeveloped ova at hatch. However, only one of the female's ovaries (the left) is functional. At sexual maturity, under the control of hormones from the anterior pituitary gland, these Graafian follicles develop into mature ova, attached to part of the egg yolk. The yolk contains phospholipids (from the liver) which provide most of the nutrients required for a developing chick in the fertile egg. In the functioning ovary the follicles are different in size as they develop their attachment to the phospholipids. The larger yolks are the first to be shed from the ovary (Figure 7.1). The oviduct also changes at sexual maturity for it is here that the albumen (egg white), shell membranes, water and eggshells are attached. The pelvis of the bird widens to allow the passage of the egg and the cloaca (vent) changes to allow easy oviposition (egg-laying).

When the hen is in lay, this left oviduct will occupy most of the left side of the abdomen. Ovulation occurs daily and egg production (ovulation) is independent of mating. Hence there are no cockerels on most commercial egg production systems. It takes about 25 hours between ovulation and egg-laying (oviposition) so each egg is laid later each day. Most eggs are laid within 4 hours of dawn (or when the artificial lighting is turned on after the longest dark period for housed birds). Birds tend not to lay eggs in the dark period, retaining them to be laid early the following day. Thus, we talk of birds laying 'clutches' of about nine eggs. Egg-laying behaviour is not related to the presence of an egg in the shell gland but is connected to ovulation at least 24 hours earlier. Ovulation is controlled by luteinizing hormone from the pituitary gland. Once the egg is released from the ovary, it travels to the infundibulum where a thin layer of albumin surrounds the yolk. At the magnum, thick albumen, calcium, sodium and magnesium are introduced to the developing egg. Egg weight doubles until the two shell membranes are attached. In the uterus the egg spins and the calcium carbonate shell is added. This is usually done during the night as the bird is roosting. Finally, the waxy cuticle is added in the vagina before the egg is ready to be laid. The non-functioning ovary remains dormant. However, in a small number of cases, it can become active. The outcome is that the hen will cease to lay eggs. The comb will grow and the hen will commence crowing like a cockerel.

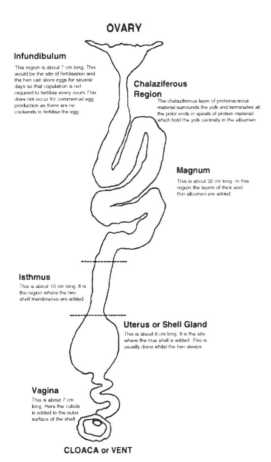

OVARY

Infundibulum
This region is about 7 cm long. This would be the site of fertilisation and the hen can store eggs for several days so that copulation is not required to fertilise every ovum. This does not occur for commercial egg production as there are no cockerels to fertilise the egg

Chalaziferous Region
The chalaziferous layer of proteinaceous material surrounds the yolk and terminates at the polar ends in spirals of protein material which hold the yolk centrally in the albumen

Magnum
This is about 32 cm long. In this region the layers of thick and thin albumen are added

Isthmus
This is about 10 cm long. It is this region where the two shell membranes are added

Uterus or Shell Gland
This is about 6 cm long. It is the site where the true shell is added. This is usually done whilst the hen sleeps

Vagina
This is about 7 cm long. Here the cuticle is added to the outer surface of the shell

CLOACA or VENT

Figure 7.1 The oviduct of a laying hen.

Daily egg production puts a great burden on the hen. Her daily food intake will increase by about 35% from pre-lay to peak lay and the bird will need a great deal of calcium to provide for the eggshell formation. This is particularly important in later life as hens can mobilize the stored calcium from the skeleton, particularly from the long bones such as the tibia (Figure 7.2).

7.2.2 The Skeleton

The skeleton of the chicken (like other flying birds) combines strength with lightness. The large sternum has a deep keel to accommodate the flight muscles. This keel can be vulnerable to damage when being handled, particularly during any rough handling when being extracted from the cage. It is important that birds are held properly and that the keel is supported (Figure 7.3).

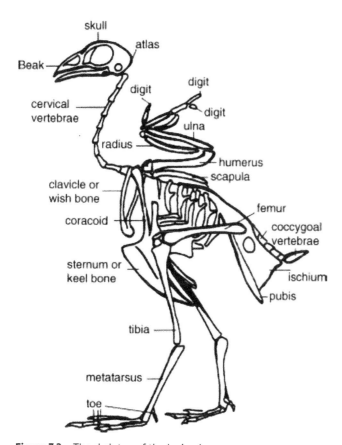

Figure 7.2 The skeleton of the laying hen.

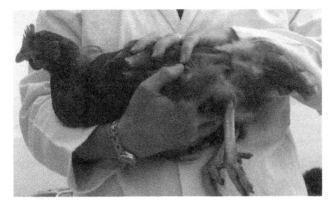

Figure 7.3 The correct way to hold a chicken, supporting the sternum and holding the legs with one hand with the other hand covering the wings.

On the ground, the whole weight of the bird is supported by the pelvic girdle and hips. The body weight is maintained close to the centre of gravity. Many of the bones are hollow (reducing weight). The long bones, such as the tibia, contain calcium which can be utilized by the hen for shell formation if there is insufficient other calcium available in the diet or other body reserves. Over a prolonged period, this can lead to osteoporosis, or brittle bones, which has been termed 'caged layer fatigue'.

In general, during egg production in controlled-environment houses, feather growth is almost halted. In more traditional systems, during the 'winter months' when egg production stopped the birds would moult. Moulting involves new feathers pushing out old ones, calcium depletion in the long bones stops and calcium levels in these bones recover during the non-lay period. After about 3 months the birds come back in to lay, laying large numbers of eggs, larger than the corresponding eggs during the first period of egg production as point-of-lay pullets. Although laying hens can live up to 13 years, commercial laying hens are usually replaced after their first year of egg production (about 74 weeks of age).

7.2.3 The Digestive System

Diet is particularly important to maintain output of good-quality eggs. Hens, like humans, are monogastric. They obtain nutrients directly by absorbing material from the food they eat, rather than relying on cellulose-digesting bacteria, like ruminants. The digestive system of the chicken is illustrated in Figure 7.4. The beak and tongue are used to investigate the environment and the taste of food. The beak tip is very sensitive with many nerves. Taste buds have been found on the base of the tongue and floor of the pharynx. The chicken's taste buds are morphologically like, but not identical to, those of mammals. Chickens apparently avoid saccharine and sweet flavours, such as honey and strawberry, though they show a preference for sucrose and the butter-type flavours. Some producers use the appeal of ascorbic acid in water to get the birds to drink on arrival at the production system and to offset the effects of heat stress.

The crop is positioned in the neck region. It is an extension of the oesophagus with a thin, elastic membranous wall. Thus, it is able to expand and act as a storage facility for food prior to digestion. This can be useful for flock-keepers since the neck can be palpated to determine if the birds are eating (a full crop). Occasionally birds can suffer a compacted crop, possibly from eating long grass. This can be treated by massaging after giving the bird a syringe of warm water, vegetable oil (or olive oil), melted butter or a yoghurt-type product. If this fails, veterinary assistance can be sought in order to make a small incision at the crop to remove the impacted material. Compacted crops can be fatal.

The proventriculus is at the anterior end of the stomach. This glandular section secretes hydrochloric acid and digestive enzymes into the food mix before the food moves down to the thick-walled muscular gizzard. Since birds do not have teeth and are unable to chew or mix their food prior to digestion, the gizzard performs a similar function. Birds deliberately swallow grit or stones and anything over 4 mm in diameter remains in the gizzard. The churning action of the muscular gizzard helps to break down the food particles by the mechanical, grinding action of these stones along with the digestive action of the material secreted from the proventriculus. The controlled release of the resulting fluid into the duodenum enables the beginning of absorption. The bile and pancreatic ducts add further digestive enzymes or modify the pH in the gut to promote enzyme activity. The ileum (small intestine) is the major site of food absorption. Two blind-ended caeca occur at the junction between the small and large intestine. These caeca are involved in bacterial breakdown of cellulose, though the contribution to total food absorption by the bird is unlikely to be significant except in undeveloped village systems where the birds are expected to scavenge for most or all their food. About every fortieth evacuation of faeces from the cloaca includes the watery contents of the caeca. It is wrong to believe that chickens urinate, though the kidneys do function as part of the waste removal system. They do not possess the essential metabolic pathways to produce urea. Nitrogenous waste from birds is in the form of solid uric acid (the white part of bird faeces). Some water reabsorption takes place in the large intestine along with storage of faecal material until evacuation takes place through the cloaca.

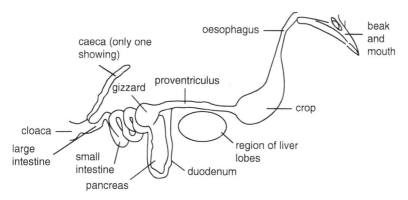

Figure 7.4 Pictorial representation of the digestive system of the laying hen. Note: the duodenal loop has been distended for clarity.

7.2.4 Sensory Perception

The skin of a chicken possesses thermal and mechano-receptors (for pressure or 'touch') and receptors for vibration, particularly in the legs. This may allow rapid changes in body position when perched on a swaying branch but could also be a warning mechanism if an unseen predator is approaching. Birds have a relatively large brain. They rely heavily on muscular coordination (for flight) and vision systems (eyes and visual acuity) for information about their environment. Hens have similar colour vision to humans, but their visual acuity covers a wide field, enabling large amounts of visual information, particularly movement, to be collected and assessed. Chickens perform rapid head movement to determine the location and distance of specific objects in their field of vision. The eye also appears to be capable of sharp focus, which is important during flight or moving between perches to avoid collision and injury.

Chickens possess olfactory receptors in the base of the upper jaw though smell does not seem to be an important stimulus compared to other types of stimuli for poultry. For example, birds can hear over a relatively narrow range of wavelengths but have very sensitive hearing (to pitch and volume) over that range. The ear system is similar to humans in that it is involved in hearing and balance. The outer ear has very little specialized structure. However, often producers use the colour of the feathers on the ear lobes as an indication of the colour of the eggshell. Chickens are capable of communication through body position and some vocalization. Vocal calls are produced at the syrinx, where the trachea forks into the bronchi.

7.3 The Poultry Industry

7.3.1 History of Poultry in Human Society

The keeping of poultry dates back to classical societies such as Egyptian, Roman and ancient Chinese. Romans brought poultry to Britain when the Roman Empire expanded. It is possible that poultry remained in Britain through the centuries, but right up to the early 1900s poultry-keeping does not appear to have had the same cultural importance as, say, the keeping of swine, sheep or cattle. Even today, some influential agriculturalists appear to have a blind spot when considering poultry, compared to, say, dairy or other, more traditional, larger livestock. Yet, the poultry industry, of all livestock, is an expanding global industry with all of the sophistication of worldwide trading and supply chains, not seen in some of the more traditional livestock industries. The view that poultry is not important may result from outdated ideas of wealth and 'snobbery'. Presumably, being of lower individual value, there would not be the same prestige in owning a chicken compared to, perhaps, the ownership of a cow! Right up to the time of World War I, farmers' wives took care of chickens in the farmyard. Presumably, it was demeaning for the farmer (the man) to lower himself to do 'woman's work', looking after the farm chickens. Nevertheless, chickens seem to have a place deep in human culture.

From the days of Aesop, infants have been warned not to 'count the chickens before they hatch' or not to 'put all of our eggs in one basket'. We learned the importance of sharing from 'the Little Red Hen' and the foolishness of 'Chicken Licken' who thought the sky was falling. Male prowess has been likened to 'strutting roosters' and fussing mothers have been likened to mother hens. Eggs and chicks have become associated with Spring religious festivals and have come to symbolize new birth and fertility.

7.3.2 Poultry-Keeping in the UK

A cultural shift, to raise the profile of poultry production in Britain, occurred after World War I. The government realized the threat posed by submarine warfare, with the potential to disrupt food supply to the British Isles, and so looked favourably on any project that might improve self-sufficiency in food supply. At the same time, soldiers, sickened by their experiences in the trenches and the prospect of returning to a class-ridden society, expressed a desire to become (chicken) farmers. With government assistance several free-range units of about 500 dual-purpose birds were established. There was minimal environmental control for these flocks and pure strains such as Rhode Island Red and Light Sussex were common. The management of these relatively small flocks relied heavily on experience and intuition. The Egg Marketing Board ensured that all eggs were sold, and prices were more-or-less guaranteed. This situation continued through World War II. There was no real black market in eggs during the war since the Egg Marketing Board continued to purchase and distribute eggs.

Since the early 1900s some entrepreneurs in the UK had realized the potential gains to be had from properly organized poultry farming, following examples in the USA. Around this time poultry research was beginning to blossom, particularly in standardizing management techniques. Research was undertaken to increase production through breed selection, formulation of balanced diets and the development of improved, more intensive management techniques. Such research assisted in increasing production, but a number of significant events occurred in the 1950s which laid the foundation for the modern egg production industry.

Perhaps the most important event of the decade was the derationing of wheat after World War II. The amount of feed wheat available effectively restricted the number of birds in a flock. Once this restriction was withdrawn, individuals could manage much larger flocks since it was this, and not labour, that was limiting at the time. A second, important event was the introduction of electricity on farms. This was probably of most significance in the later development of the egg production systems that relied on motorized automated delivery and egg collection apparatus. The third watershed occurred after a study group visited the USA and returned with a fast-growing strain of chicken 'designed' exclusively for the poultry meat trade. (One of the groups smuggled hatching eggs in his luggage and these became the first broilers in Britain!) This effectively led to the parting of the ways for the poultry egg and the poultry meat industries. Instead of the dual-purpose birds, this enabled concentrated efforts in the development of birds selected either for egg output or for rapid muscle growth. These developments acting in unison with the research led to significant steps forward in terms of output.

The most significant consequences of research to improve egg numbers and quality have been the development of balanced, least-cost diets, notably incorporating the essential amino acids, lysine and methionine, and the establishment of management regimes in controlled-environment buildings. Perhaps the most significant was the determination of the importance of lighting on sexual maturity and egg production. Chickens possess a pineal gland which is associated with melatonin production. Since this hormone is produced during darkness, melatonin levels in the body are associated with daylength. Melatonin is involved in controlling other hormones and body systems. The detail will not be discussed here but can be found in any good chicken physiology text (e.g. Reece 2009). There are critical levels of melatonin for the control of sexual maturity and sexual cycling (egg production). This is why such a discovery was critical for commercial egg production. Up to the 1950s or so, it was accepted that chickens generally stopped egg production during the autumn and winter months in Britain. Unfortunately, this clashed with one of the two main peaks in demand for eggs (i.e. Christmas, for cakes and puddings, and Easter, with egg-related festivities).

Putting the birds in sheds with electric lighting allowed for extended daylength with year-round egg production (with a significant economic advantage). The first indoor systems were simple 'deep litter' systems where the chickens were taken into a shed with an open-plan arrangement with a litter material on the floor (e.g. straw, sawdust or wood shavings), manually filled water and food dispensers, and nest boxes. This enabled housing of the birds for relatively little capital expense. However, the coprophagic birds suffered from disease and, in cases of panic, smothered each other in their attempts to escape. Also, in large flocks, birds were aggressive and even cannibalistic. Such cannibalism was not found in cages and so caged birds were introduced into the controlled environment indoors. The more 'modern' egg-laying bird was relatively smaller than the previous dual-purpose birds and so producers put more than one bird in each cage. Since chickens are reasonably gregarious the birds were less frightened than birds kept individually, and output increased. Although simplified management and increased output with reduced marginal costs may have been the driving force, it could be argued that the caged system also improved the welfare of the birds by reduced aggression, reduced disease, lowered risks from predation and the provision of healthy food and a cleaner environment. The logical flow, however, was to increase the number of birds in cages and to put cages on top of each other to maximize the usage of the building. The increased use of electrical systems for environmental management and automated delivery of foodstuff and egg removal enabled increasing numbers of birds to be managed by a relatively small labour force. Eggs became more freely available at a lower cost and consumption grew.

As with any growing and developing industry, take-overs and mergers occurred. Relatively easy money was to be made and some of the businesses were bought by financial speculators. Strategic expansion within the industry led to vertically integrated companies, with more control over resources and quality control (Figure 7.5).

A number of 'breeders' emerged on the international market, providing birds best suited to the requirements of egg production. These egg production companies expanded horizontally,

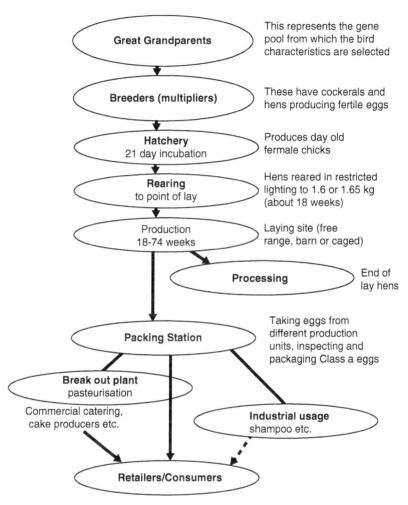

Figure 7.5 Diagrammatic representation of the vertically integrated laying hen egg industry. Note: breeders typically own all stages to the hatchery and producers from the rearing stage to the packing station.

purchasing other egg production units, and also purchased feed mills, rearing facilities, egg grading and supply chains to the newly developing supermarkets.

7.3.2.1 The Structure of the Egg Production Industry in the UK

The UK industry uses, almost exclusively, medium hybrid brown birds, supplied by well-established breeding companies. During the 1960s, a marketing decision assumed that consumers preferred a brown-shelled egg from brown-feathered birds (on the basis that they appear more 'natural' than the white-shelled variety). In the USA, the reverse is the case;

white-shelled eggs are the standard (presumably on the basis that they appear more 'hygienic' than brown eggs). From the 1960s the birds were selected for several phenotypic characteristics such as egg output (in terms of numbers and quality), good food conversion (to eggs rather than muscle development and increased growth), hardiness (disease resistance) and docility (rather than aggressiveness). Once the breeding companies establish the bird type it is then the role of the multiplier farms to breed sufficient birds to meet the demands of the egg producers (Figure 7.5). These multiplier farms produce fertile eggs, having cockerels running with the hens (one cockerel for every 10 to 12 females). Sperm transfer is by natural copulation. Since the cockerels' testes are situated within the body cavity, there is little thermal shock at transfer into the females' bodies. Hence the sperm can survive in the females' bodies and go on to fertilize the successive eggs for several days without further copulation being required. These birds are maintained in these conditions from about 24 weeks to about 68 to 70 weeks. In this time the hens will lay over 200 fertile eggs. The eggs are taken to the hatchery and incubated for about 21 days. About 80% of the eggs placed in the incubators survive to hatch properly.

In modern commercial strains it is possible to identify the sex of day-old chicks from the down colour. Male chicks are removed and, since they do not lay eggs, are humanely killed by gassing at the hatchery. They are often sold as frozen chicks for food for captive birds of prey. The female day-old chicks are transported to rearing units.

7.3.3 World Poultry Keeping and Egg Production

Between 1970 and 2005 global egg production tripled and from that date has increased by 18% to 2016. Most of the world's eggs are produced in China (Table 7.1) and the UK is no

Table 7.1 Approximate Global Egg Production (Billion Eggs) in 2016 (based on FAOSTAT data 2018).

Country	Approximate egg output (billion eggs)(±10%)
China	550
USA	105
India	100
Mexico	80
Brazil	50
Russia	50
Japan	50
Indonesia	40
Iran	10
Turkey	10

longer included in the top ten producers. The majority of the countries in the top ten producers (Table 7.1) do not necessarily prioritize animal welfare, since food provision and security are possibly more important. The practices and problems of poultry-keeping are not the same between countries. Some of the main problems are often temperature dependent. For example, in tropical countries keeping the birds sufficiently cool can be a problem. Although the ancestor to the modern chicken was the Burmese jungle-fowl, it can be difficult for a large number of birds to regulate their thermal environment. In poorly ventilated sheds or in regions where air temperature and relative humidity are high (e.g. tropical countries) this is especially difficult. Some of the problems can be overcome to a degree by the breeding of birds adapted to these environments. Some keepers deliberately use, for example, naked-necked birds or birds with 'frizzle feathers'; genetic strains producing relatively poorly feathered birds which may be less prone to heat stress. Some modifications to housing can also assist in maintaining the birds' environment. In some countries, curtain-sided buildings are used where netting material replaces solid walls so that air can circulate relatively freely. In other circumstances water or mist sprays are used as part of the control of the thermal environment. In some countries, birds are kept on soil floors. Since it is difficult to disinfect these systems properly, they can often suffer relatively high levels of infection, parasitism and other health problems.

In many countries such as in Africa and Asia, where refrigeration units are not commonplace, chickens are kept in relatively small numbers in close proximity to the household. These birds are used to provide fresh eggs and meat and are not slaughtered until they are required for the table. These birds are often fed scraps or are allowed to forage for food items and insects. Birds are sold live at markets coming into contact with many other birds. Biosecurity is difficult, if not non-existent.

Public concern as to the welfare of the laying hen seems to be most prevalent in northern European countries. This concern is directed mainly at the keeping of hens in the unenriched 'battery cage'. Some argue that this concern is the prerogative of more affluent, relatively well-fed societies whereas, in poorer countries, the need for food is more pressing. In other developed societies, such as the USA, the majority view, supported by legislation, continues to support the most intensive systems (although this view is strongly opposed by welfare groups within the same country). Where this approach prevails, extremely large numbers of laying hens are maintained to achieve the economies of scale that can arise from large intensive systems, producing large numbers of eggs.

7.4 Production Systems for Laying Hens

7.4.1 Pullet Rearing

Flock rearers take the day-old female chicks and rear them to point of lay, usually around 18 weeks, though there are some variations, such as rearing to 16 weeks, before transferring to the production site. Generally, it is not the age of the bird that is important as much as the body mass. The target for hens for caged egg production is about 1.6 kg and, for free-range, 1.65 kg If a bird is small when she lays her first egg, it is likely that she will lay smaller eggs (compared to her flock mates) for the rest of her life. Because there is such a strong link between daylength and sexual maturity in birds, these young birds are raised in lightproof sheds with restricted daylength (Table 7.2).

As the birds approach sexual maturity daylight hours are restricted to postpone the onset of sexual maturity. Because this involves artificial light restriction, some individuals have argued that it poses a welfare insult. However, eight hours of light is similar to a winter day in the UK, thus not inherently unnatural. The argument that the birds never receive natural daylight depends on how important 'natural' light is to a species. Animals can adapt and so 'natural' light may be satisfactorily replaced with artificial light in terms of welfare 'needs'. However, hens are diurnal and are capable of utilizing sunlight for vitamin synthesis, suggesting that sunlight may be important to the birds. More research is required before 'natural' light is considered a welfare 'need' (rather than relying on an anthropomorphic 'natural is best' approach). Nevertheless, restricting birds to reduced light intensity may be another matter. Birds are often subjected to light intensities where they can see to eat and drink but to reduce 'vices' such as aggression and feather pecking or feather pulling. Keeping the birds under low light conditions has been a traditional management approach to minimize such problems. This may be more difficult to justify when reduced stocking, or some environmental enrichment, may be a more welfare-friendly strategy. Similarly, in production systems, interrupted lighting patterns have been used to reduce fuel and feed costs. In such situations light and dark periods throughout the day do not follow a 'natural' rhythm of one light and one dark period in 24 hours but have shorter light periods with intermittent darkness. These can prevent birds from having extended dark, rest periods. This is of concern to welfare groups who campaign for at least 8 hours of uninterrupted darkness for the birds.

Table 7.2 Lighting patterns for laying hens.

Age (days)	Light period (hours)	Light intensity (lux)
1–2	22	20–40
3–4	20	15–30
5–6	18	15–30
7–14	16	10–20
15–21	15	10
22–28	14	10
29–35	13	10
36–42	12	10
43–49	11	10
50–105	10	10
From 133 days	Increase 0.5 h per week to 16 h	15–30

Source: ISA (2009–10).

Some chick rearers use chick cages to rear the birds to point of lay (particularly for birds destined for the caged sector). These are relatively large cages for communities of chicks. As they grow, a proportion of the chicks are removed to adjacent cages to prevent overcrowding. Other chick rearers raise chicks on litter (such as white wood shavings) using systems which are similar to broiler rearing sheds. During rearing the birds may be subject to beak trimming.

Once the birds are light stimulated (Brambell Report' 7.2), it takes about 10–14 days before they commence ovulation. This usually allows the birds to be transferred to the production site and settle in (finding the feeder and drinker systems, and so on) before the stress associated with laying an egg for the first time. The birds are often introduced at 18 weeks of age and come into lay in the following 2 weeks. Most birds are kept in controlled environments. The operating temperature in laying shed is around 23°C. Of all the environmental controls it is, perhaps, lighting that has the most direct effect on egg production.

7.4.1.1 Vaccination

During the rearing period, mainstream commercial birds (but not organic birds) receive prophylactic vaccination. Some vaccines are administered at the hatchery either as a mist, allowing the birds to receive the vaccines by inhalation, through the conjunctiva or by ingestion from pecking at droplets on the down of their hatchery mates. Some may be given by injection (e.g. Marek's vaccine by injection at the back of the neck). Common vaccines in a typical vaccination program for laying hens are listed in Table 7.3.

Such prophylactic vaccination programs ensure that the hens are protected against disease outbreaks. It is not usual to routinely vaccinate hens once they are in lay (though some

Table 7.3 A typical vaccination schedule for laying hens.

Week of vaccination	Type of vaccination
Day old	Marek's
15 days (1/2 dose)	Infectious bursal (IB)
20 days (1/2 dose)	Infectious bursal (IB)
25 days	Bronchitis, Newcastle disease, infectious bursal (typical brand name Combo Vec. 30)
30 days	Bronchitis, Newcastle disease, infectious bursal (typical brand name Combo Vec. 30)
49 days	Bronchitis, Newcastle disease, infectious bursal (typical brand name Combo Vec. 30)
10 weeks	Fowl pox and laryngotracheitis (commonly referred to as LT)
12 weeks	Combo Vac 30
13 weeks	Avian encephalomyelitis (commonly referred to as AE)
16 weeks	Newcastle disease

Source: Meunier and Latour (undated).

free-range flocks are vaccinated because of the greater risk of disease with the outdoor life-style). A major problem for free-range hens (or birds indoors on litter) is coccidiosis. This is only a risk where birds are liable to encounter poultry faeces or equipment (feeders and drinkers) contaminated with birds' faeces. The causative gut parasite produces fertile eggs as a contaminant of faeces from infected birds. Other 'clean' birds then ingest the eggs and become contaminated themselves (producing contaminated faeces). This disease, along with other gut parasites, can build up to the point where 'fowl sick land' is a problem (with a very high risk of contamination between birds and between successive flocks.

As part of the Lion Code, commercial laying hens are vaccinated against Salmonella to ensure the safety of table eggs against infection

7.4.1.2 Use of Antibiotics

Several opponents to intensive egg production claim that there is unrestricted use of antibiotics for the birds. Specific bacterial diseases such as *E. coli*, *Brachyspira* spp., *Erysipelothrix*, *Enterococcus* sp and *Pasteurella* sp do require antibiotic use, as prescribed by veterinarians. This is essential to ensure the health and welfare of the birds. However routine usage does not occur. This is not permitted under the Lion Scheme of quality assurance, which includes over 90% of UK egg production. Specifically, the scheme includes: an obligatory system of detailed reporting of all antibiotic use, from January 2015; third- and fourth-generation Cephalosporins may not be used; Fluoroquinolones may not be used at one day of age and, from 6 June 2016, Colistin may not be used. Such measures are to ensure that bird health and welfare can be maintained and human health is not negatively affected or antibiotic use for human medication is not compromised. In the main poultry health and welfare is maintained by high standards of biosecurity.

7.4.2 Production Systems

The permitted egg production systems are:

- eggs from caged hens;
- barn eggs;
- free range;
- organic.

The requirements for these systems will be explained later. The initial eggs are quite small, though egg size can be manipulated, e.g. by increasing the oil components in the food. The birds will maintain egg output above 90% per day for up to 40 weeks. As the birds age, the egg numbers decrease but egg size increases. The birds remain in the shed until the egg numbers reduce to a level that the system becomes uneconomic (bearing in mind that the birds continue food consumption at around 110–120 g per bird per day) at about 72 to 74 weeks of age. Currently there are about 40 million laying hens in the UK, each bird producing between about 280 and 310 eggs. The systems will now be considered in detail.

7.4.2.1 Cage Systems

According to classical scripts the Romans kept chickens in what we might recognize as a form of battery cage system. In the UK the first cages were introduced early in the twentieth century. Some of the first research cage systems were placed at the National Institute for Poultry Husbandry (NIPH). Chickens were put into cages to protect them from predators and to prevent coprophagy (muck eating) by the birds, which improved the welfare of the birds by reducing disease and mortality. The quality of the eggs was also improved since the contact of the eggs with the birds' faeces was reduced. The first cages were outdoors but these proved unsuccessful since it was difficult to maintain feeding for the birds, and the British climate meant that the birds ate more in the winter cold and less in the summer heat in order to maintain body temperature by adjusting metabolic heat production to meet the varying thermal changes of the environment.

In the early systems individuals were caged singly, enabling output to be monitored easily. If a bird ceased laying it was obvious and she could be replaced. However, when a second bird was added to the cage, productivity increased because the birds preferred the presence of conspecifics. To overcome the problems of the British weather, and to extend the laying period in an artificial lighting regime, birds were relatively quickly brought indoors (in cages) once electricity supplies became available on farms. The benefits of caged systems over deep litter systems quickly became apparent, in terms of bird health, egg quality and labour saving. Through the late 1950s and early 1960s the number of birds in individual cages and the number of cages in a shed grew quickly.

This escalation of large numbers of individual birds in large groups in a caged environment has obvious visual impact, and such intensive systems caused individuals and groups concerned with animal welfare to become increasingly alarmed. The need for legislative control to preserve the welfare of the laying hens was obvious and, as a result, the UK government set up a committee, which produced the 'Brambell Report, 1965 which considered the welfare of farmed animals. The Farm Animal Welfare Council was established, based on the recommendations of the report and successive governments have introduced legislation to improve the welfare of caged laying hens. In the mid-1990s floor space was increased to 450 cm^2 per bird. The 1999 EU Directive was incorporated into UK law in 2002 to create a major welfare improvement in 'enriched cages' in 2012. In the UK from 2012 unenriched (conventional) battery cages were banned and so will not be considered in detail here. Differences between the banned cages and the post-2012 cages are presented in Table 7.4

7.4.2.2 Enriched Cages (Colonies)

Enriched cages attempt to meet all of the behavioural and welfare needs of the hens. They were developed based on research from several countries. In the early 1990s, UK researchers such as Appleby in Edinburgh and Nicol in Bristol considered the inclusion of nesting devices in cages (Appleby et al. 2004). As part of the normal behavioural repertoire during egg-laying, hens need to find and investigate suitable nesting sites before the normal behaviour patterns continue. Where nesting sites are available the whole routine takes about two hours from the first signs of egg-laying behaviour and oviposition. In non-enriched cages the behaviours

Table 7.4 The differences in cages for laying hens *before* and *after* 2012.

Cage feature	Before 2012	New cages from 2003 and all cages from 2012
Stocking density (cm² per bird)	550	750 (600 usable area; at least 45 cm high)
Minimum total area (cm²)	550 × no of birds	2000
Perch	x	✓(15 cm per bird)
Dust-bathing/scratch area	x	✓
Nesting area	x	✓
Claw shortening device	From 2003	✓
Feeder space/bird (cm)	10	12
Drinker space/bird (cm)	10 (or access to 2 nipples)	Suitable for group size (or access to 2 nipples)
Minimum height (cm)	35 (at least 40 over 65% area)	20
Slope (rectangular mesh) (degrees)	8	Not specified
Slope (other floors) (degrees)	12	Not specified
Illegal after 2011	✓	x

appear thwarted and the routine can continue for four hours until oviposition has to occur. Similarly, in barren cages dustbathing behaviour (usually associated with maintenance of feather condition) occurs in the absence of substrate as a vacuum behaviour, indicating that this is a behavioural need.

The Farm Animal Welfare Council produced their opinion on enriched cages in 2007. The Council was concerned that some designs of enriched cages continue to keep the hens continuously confined and do not allow expression of the full behavioural repertoire of the hens but, with adequate designs which pay attention to the needs of the hens, a more welfare-friendly system should result. The EU funded 'LayWel Project (2006) compared conventional cages; 'small', 'medium' and 'large' enriched cages and non-caged systems (Table 7.5). The main conclusions were that (apart from conventional cages which restrict behaviour to an unacceptable level) all systems had the potential to provide satisfactory welfare for laying hens (though the potential may not always be realized). Also, all cage systems tend to provide a more hygienic environment with low risks of parasitic disease.

7.4.2.3 Barn Systems

Until 2004 barn systems were also called perchery systems, but this is no longer included as a special marketing term (SMT) in the UK. Barn systems can trace their development from the deep litter systems that became common in the 1950s when electricity was introduced on farms. In order to improve management of the flocks, remove the effects of season and day-length on egg production, birds were brought indoors in an enclosed system. It was very simple and was similar to how modern broiler systems operate, apart from the provision of nest

Table 7.5 Welfare risks in different laying systems. Adapted from Laywel (2006).

	Caged				Non-cage		Outdoor
	Conventional		Enriched		Single-level	Multi-level	
		Small	Medium	Large			
Mortality (%)							
Mortality from feather pecking & cannibalism							
Red mite							
Bumble foot							
Feather loss							
Use of nest boxes							
Use of perches							
Foraging behaviour							
Dustbathing behaviour							
Air quality							
Water intake							
Welfare risk: code			Low			Medium	High

boxes and perches. The deep litter system required relatively low capital investment for a significant increase in production in a controlled environment. Birds were kept on a litter material (sawdust, wood shavings, etc.). The birds were stocked at seven birds per m². The system was very labour intensive, with manual egg collection and bird feeding systems. Nevertheless, the increased production and the levels of control made it a more attractive option. However, the high levels of labour requirements in the first systems (with manual feeding and egg collection), the relative high levels of floor-laid or dirty eggs and the disease risks to the birds in contact with their faeces meant that cage systems were preferred. More latterly, the legal requirement for no perches over litter made the pure deep litter system illegal.

Other non-cage systems developed with slatted areas (improving manure management). Some systems included perches and some had mesh-floored tiered systems or platforms to utilize the height of the building and increase stocking in the sheds. The permitted stocking density of such systems was set at about 25 birds per m². However, such high stocking often led to problems such as aggression, and in the early 1990s the author visited one site where over 30% of the birds were lost due to cannibalism. Many producers stocked at around 11–13 birds per m². This proved a bonus when in the 2002 legislation in the UK such producers were allowed to continue to stock at 12 birds per m² up to 2012, while anyone else had to stock at 9 birds per m². The feeder and drinking space per bird is strictly controlled. Nest boxes can be individual nests (1 per 7 hens) or communal (1 m^2 for up to 120 hens). The perch allocation (15 cm per hen) and location (at least 30 cm apart and at least 20 cm from a wall) ensures that slatted floors cannot be included in perch calculations and allows easier use by the birds. Since birds need to dust-bathe and scratch, 250 cm^2 per hen (at least one-third of the floor area) must provide a litter material. Any tiered system can have a maximum of four tiers (with 45 cm headroom between tiers) and faeces cannot fall on to birds on lower tiers.

In terms of market share, barn eggs do not appear to have caught the imagination of the UK purchaser, with a polarization between eggs from caged hens or eggs from free-range systems. The share for barn eggs remains between about 5% and 7% of egg sales. However, all free-range systems have to provide internal accommodation that meets the legal standard for barn eggs (the difference being that birds must have access to range).

7.4.2.4 Free Range

For many consumers, free-range egg production conjures up ideas of traditional, non-intensive, low capital systems with relatively small flocks. The modern commercial systems may be very different but are still strictly controlled in legislation. Birds must have daytime access to land mostly covered with vegetation. The pop-holes to the range must be at least 35 cm high by 40 cm wide and along the entire length of the building, with 2 m opening per 1000 birds. This was important because, in the past when the pop-holes were smaller, there was a tendency for the dominant birds to patrol the pop-holes and aggressively prevent subordinate birds accessing the range area. The maximum permitted stocking on the land was raised for 2004 from 1000 birds to 2500 birds per hectare (since at that time the term 'free range' was a merging of the existing 'free range' and 'semi-intensive' marketing terms). This caused some controversy at the time since welfare groups considered this a retrograde step in welfare terms. The RSPCA maintained the 10 m^2 per bird stocking, though they are now considering a higher stocking rate for their Freedom Food farms.

Currently several UK retailers are stating that they will source all of their eggs from the non-cage sector. As a result of this, and the changes in legislation, the market share is increasing and currently accounts for about 50% of the UK market.

7.4.2.5 Organic Production

Over the past few decades consumers have become increasingly concerned by management practices in agricultural production. The supposed widespread use of growth promoters, medication and chemicals fuelled a backlash with some small-scale producers seeking an alternative. The United Kingdom Register of Organic Food Standards (UKROFS) (later superseded by Advisory Committee on Organic Standards (ACOS) in 2003, under the Department for Food, Environment and Rural Affairs; DEFRA) established standards for UK organic production. Current organic standards for laying hens state that no birds are kept in cages and there must be no more than 3000 in the shed. There should be six birds per m^2, with 18 cm perch per bird. One individual nest is required per eight birds or 120 cm^2 of communal nest per bird. There must be 4 m length of pop-hole per 100 m^2 of the floor in the house. There should be 4 m^2 per bird of range (with rotational land use). Permitted medicines rely heavily on homeopathic remedies. The use of disinfectants is strictly controlled, as are the permitted feedstuffs. Although the eggs are classed as organic, the birds, from non-organically produced parents, are not. Poultry must have access to an open-air area for at least one-third of their life. These areas for poultry must be mainly covered with vegetation and be provided with protective facilities and permit easy access to adequate numbers of drinking and feeding troughs. In the UK the Soil Association is an association of organic producers. The standards set are often in excess of those required in law. Members can use the Soil Association logo to demonstrate that the standards are met.

7.4.2.6 Backyard Systems

In recent years poultry has become a popular gift in the UK (e.g. as a wedding gift, particularly in middle-class society) to be kept almost as pets. The birds are often pure breeds; the selling on of birds that have been 'rescued' at end of lay from caged systems is also a thriving (though small) business. DEFRA require that owners of 50 or more birds are registered. As of 16 June 2009, the GB Poultry Register holds details of 24,677 premises. A total of 262,937,612 birds have been registered. Small, backyard systems occur everywhere in the UK, mainly for showing purposes, pets or for production of fresh eggs for the kitchen. Bird pairs or trios are often kept in wooden arks or similar which are about 2 m long by 0.75 m wide with accommodation for the birds and a wire-framed cover over the garden area. Larger groups may be contained within an area (again using chicken wire mesh) with a small shed for accommodation. Alternatively, the birds are allowed to range freely, returning at night to a secure shed for roosting. Paddocks may be fenced off to prevent entry by foxes and other predators. In such cases the mesh fence is often dug into the ground with the fence curved outwards so that any digging fox cannot dig under the fence and gain access to the birds. There is very little legislative control over these small flocks (particularly flocks of less than 350 birds). However, most of these flocks are not kept purely for commercial egg production and the care focused on individual birds is usually higher than that which may occur in larger flocks. In many cases cockerels are kept with these groups (unlike in commercial flocks). Many systems rely on manual labour for food and water delivery, though some do have water and power supplies to the sheds. The food and equipment can be purchased in manageable amounts from agricultural or countryside-based stores and, in the UK, there is a thriving trade in supporting such small-scale groups or flocks. Thus, such birds are generally fed balanced layer diets, supplemented with invertebrates and other scraps that the birds can forage.

In some countries, a few backyard chickens are kept as a source of both fresh eggs and meat for the family (rather than as a money-making enterprise). The birds live closely with their human keepers, often in their homes, and are generally free to roam and forage, feeding on scraps, etc. The level of direct care for the birds is relatively minimal as the birds tend to fend for themselves, but roost in close association with their keepers.

7.5 Management of the Laying Hen

7.5.1 Feeding and Watering

It is important that the laying hens have *ad libitum* access to clean and safe food and water. Balanced diets have been researched and are readily available for laying hens. During the rearing period it is essential that the birds are fed sufficient calcium to ensure that, when they reach point of lay, the bone density is as high as possible to offset the problems associated with the calcium demand of sustained egg-laying. Traditional, manual feeding systems include simple hoppers, suspended through the barn, but these are not suitable for caged systems, which use a trough system in front of the cages. These are not used in large commercial systems as they are very labour intensive, but they offer an inexpensive system for smallholders and backyard flocks.

Mechanized feeders are available. These include chain feeders where a flat chain in the feeding trough operates to distribute food from a hopper. In barn and free-range systems this can be problematic in that birds can perch on the feeder and defecate in the food, or if they are in the trough when it begins to operate can be dragged through the trough (causing injury). Auger-filled pan feeders are often preferred since there is less risk of spoilage of the food. These systems are less labour intensive since they can deliver food stored in bulk.

Similarly, water delivery can be inexpensive with manually filled free-standing drinkers for barn, free-range and smaller-scale systems. These are very labour intensive and are not used on larger systems. Bell drinkers offer a relatively cheap automated delivery system. These are connected to a water supply and a simple spring valve opens when the weight of the water is reduced in the suspended trough. This occurs when the birds drink. When the weight of water increases the valve is shut off, which prevents overfilling. The problems of water spillage and potential (faecal) contamination of the water have encouraged a greater use of nipple drinkers. These are simple ball-stoppers in a tube connected to the water supply. As the birds peck at the ball, water is delivered directly to their beaks. To ensure adequate provision and to reduce the incidence of competitive aggression, DEFRA has recommended minimal feeder and drinker space allocation per bird (Table 7.6).

Standing water can become contaminated and so many commercial egg producers are turning to regulated mains water delivery. In situations where water is delivered from boreholes, regular water testing is important to ensure that the minerals and constituents are not hazardous and there are no bacterial or other biological contaminants. Monitoring of food and water consumption can be used as a systems or flock health check where deviations from the expected can be first indicators of potential problems.

7.5.2 Lighting

Once the birds are in the laying accommodation, after a few days of continuous lighting the light duration is quickly reduced to match the lighting in the rearing accommodation. Once

Table 7.6 DEFRA Recommended water and food space per bird.

Feeders		Drinkers		
Linear	Circular	Continuous	Circular	Nipple/cups
10 cm	4 cm	2.5 cm	1 cm	1 per 10 hens OR (if plumbed in) at least 2

this is achieved the light duration is increased by between 20 and 30 minutes per week until about 15 hours of light per day is achieved. This is called a continuous lighting pattern. Birds produce eggs every 24.5 hours or so, so each bird lays her egg later in each consecutive day. Hens will generally lay eggs within the first 4 hours of 'dawn' so occasionally the bird does not lay but retains the egg to lay all the sooner the following day. Thus, we talk about birds laying clutches of between six and nine eggs. There has been a lot of research on the effects of alternative lighting patterns, summarized in Table 7.7, where the egg size and number will be used as the standard, allowing other patterns to be compared. In general, in interrupted patterns, 'dawn' is the first light period after the longest dark period. Some welfare groups are concerned with the manipulation of lighting. Ahemeral (non 24-h) lighting strategies are not permitted in the UK, since they interfere with the diurnal rhythm of the birds. Some welfarists consider that birds should have at least 8 hours of darkness to enable them to rest. In terms of management, the dark period allows proper shell formation.

7.5.3 Egg Collection

Manual egg collection is easy in small (e.g. backyard) flocks. In non-caged systems, eggs from places other than the nest boxes should be collected regularly to dissuade other birds from laying their eggs in the same location. If floor-laid eggs (in the litter) become a problem, agricultural electric fence wire can be used to stop the birds from laying eggs (particularly in corners or beside walls). Commercially only clean eggs laid in nest boxes can be sold as table

Table 7.7 Alternative lighting patterns and the influence on egg production.

Lighting pattern (light: dark (L:D)	Synchro- nized laying	Influence on egg size (egg mass)	Influence on egg number	Influence on shell	Main reason for use
15 : 9	Yes	Standard	Standard	Standard	Good number of medium-sized eggs
2 : 2 or 4 : 4, etc.	No	Standard	Standard	Standard	Better food efficiency. Reduced energy costs
4 × (2 L: 2D) 1 × (2 L: 6D)	Yes	Possible increase (if birds eat more)	Standard	Can be reduced if the birds retain shells in the shell gland for less time	Better food efficiency. Reduced energy costs
14 L: 14D (ahemeral)	Yes	Possible increase (if birds eat more)	Decrease	Can be increased if the birds retain shells in the shell gland for more time	Improve egg mass or shell quality/ thickness

eggs for 'in shell' consumption. In the UK it is illegal to wash or clean eggs from any contaminant if the eggs are to be in-shell table eggs. This is not the case in some EU countries and in the US, where a method has been developed to pasteurize eggs 'in shell'. Eggs should be stored 'pointed end' down, so that the air sac in the egg is at the upper end of the egg. In many larger commercial systems egg collection is carried out automatically. The birds stand on a sloping mesh floor so that the eggs roll to the front of the cage on to a conveyor belt. The conveyor operates at least once each day. It will operate more often during the period of peak lay (when the hens are between about 20 and 44 weeks old) to prevent a build-up of eggs on the belt and the risk of increased star cracks from collisions between eggs. In the UK, eggs are given their 'best before' date, which is ink-jet printed on to the shell (using food dye) at the time of sorting and grading, along with the code for the method of production (0 to 4, organic to eggs from caged hens) and a unique number associated with the farm or packing station from whence the eggs came. Legally the 'best before' date is 28 days from the day on which the eggs were laid and the sell-by date is 21 days from lay. Eggs sold commercially can only be packaged once and it is illegal to repackage them.

7.5.4 Disease Control

There are many types of poultry diseases, from many causes. A number of important poultry diseases, and the major causes, are listed in Table 7.8. Although controls are listed, some diseases are difficult to control and in some cases, mortality can be high (up to 100%). Note that in many cases the importance of good biosecurity is reinforced.

For those keeping small flocks it is important to take the greatest care not to introduce diseases to an established flock. If new birds are purchased or brought on to the site, a period of quarantine of up to 1 month is advised. If new birds are being introduced, it should be done carefully and strictly controlled, allowing birds to see each other, fenced off from each other.

Table 7.8 Important poultry diseases.

Disease	Cause	Control
Fatty liver syndrome	Imbalanced diet (sometimes seen with caged layer fatigue)	Correct diet at the correct point in bird's lifetime
Caged layer fatigue/rickets	Calcium related deficiency or imbalance in diet	Calcium phosphate, vitamin D3 (some medication and mould toxins)
Infectious bronchitis	Virus	Vaccination
Avian encephalomyelitis	Virus (mainly vertical transmission)	No treatment. Prevent exposure. Vaccination against
Avian Influenza	Virus (mainly waterfowl carriers)	Vaccination against some. Prevent exposure. Can be 100% fatal

(Continued)

Table 7.8 (Continued.)

Disease	Cause	Control
Chicken anaemia virus	Virus vertical transmission and horizontal (copraphagy of infected faeces)	Immunized parents. Prevention (biosecurity)
Infectious bursal disease (gumboro)	Virus	Vaccination against. Prevention (biosecurity)
Marek's disease	Virus	Vaccination against
Egg drop syndrome	Virus	Vaccination against. Prevention (biosecurity). EDS-free parents
Infectious laryngotracheitis	Virus	Vaccination
fowl pox	Virus	Vaccination. Prevention (biosecurity)
Lymphoid leukosis	Virus	Virus-free parents. Biosecurity
Newcastle disease	Virus	Slaughter. Vaccination. Biosecurity
Infectious coryza	Bacterial infection	Antibiotics. Vaccine. Biosecurity
Avian tuberculosis	Bacterial infection	Depopulation and biosecurity
Fowl cholera (pasteurellosis)	Bacterial infection	Sulphonamides and antibiotics. Vaccines. Biosecurity
Mycoplasmosis	Mycoplasmas	Mycoplasma-free parents. Antibiotics. Some vaccines. Biosecurity
Coccidiosis	Gut parasite	Anti-coccidial. Vaccines. Biosecurity. Natural immunity
Cryptosporidiosis	Gut parasite	Biosecurity
Histomoniasis (blackhead)	Gut parasite	Anthelminthics. Biosecurity
Toxoplasmosis (mainly backyard birds)	Protozoa in nervous, reproductive and musculoskeletal systems	Suppressing drugs. Biosecurity
Trichomoniasis	Protozoa in gut	Biosecurity
Round and flat worms	Gut	Medication. Biosecurity
Red mite	External	Topical treatments. Spray. Biosecurity
Lice	External	Topical treatments. Spray. Biosecurity

In an established flock there will be a hierarchy and new birds may cause an increase in aggression. This is not so pronounced if all the birds are at point of lay, as such social orders are generally created and quickly established around this time. In general it is the hobbyist's few birds and small pure-bred flocks that can pose a greater threat to the health of the nation's flocks: these tend to be the unvaccinated flocks and groups which are often transported around the country to shows and fairs.

Commercial flocks are managed to minimize disease risks. Breeding stock are valued highly and therefore are isolated; often such pedigree farms are situated in remote places or places where the sea borders the site to reduce the risk from airborne pathogens. In addition, access is strictly controlled, and potential visitors may be subjected to a microbial test (e.g. from rectal swabs) in advance of a proposed visit. Parent stock are also regularly assessed for *Salmonella* spp., after the outbreak of *Salmonella enteriditis* phage type IV in the 1980s when a junior health minister (Edwina Curry) claimed that all eggs carried *Salmonella*. This strain was of particular importance in that it infected the ovaries of the hen so that when eggs were laid there was a potential threat of *Salmonella* being incorporated in the yolk as the egg was formed. By registering and screening the parents the risk of laying hens being infected is minimized. The laying flocks are also regularly checked for infection and receive vaccines for *Salmonella* at least twice during the rearing programme. Key vaccines are administered during the rearing period (see Section 7.4.1.1). Birds generally do not receive vaccines or treatments during egg production, in keeping with the statement on egg boxes saying that the eggs are from birds free of medication. Subclinical levels of disease in laying flocks will be tolerated. However, if there is an apparent problem, the first response would be to collect blood samples from several birds for laboratory analysis. Appropriate treatment is then administered, based on the results.

Hens are susceptible to many disease risks (Figure 7.6) and can carry several gut parasites such as tapeworms and nematodes as well as pathogenic bacteria. Recently attention has focused on *Brachyspira* spp., which is a type of bacteria found in birds' caeca. Some species can affect egg-laying performance. They can live for long periods in puddles and are thus capable of infecting the birds. Many gut parasites eject eggs; some need to pass through other species as part of the life cycle, but the main problem is that eggs deposited in the range area can infect other birds. Enough build-up can lead to a high risk of bird infection. This 'fowl sick land' can cause many new birds or cleansed birds to quickly succumb to the parasites in the soil or on the grass. Because the risk of infection can be high for free-range birds it is usually free-range flocks that tend to receive vaccinations during their productive lifetime.

In the last decade attention has been focused on avian influenza H5N1, particularly following a number of deaths in Asia and Eastern Europe. The UK government has drawn up a strategy to deal with an outbreak of any zoonotic disease associated with poultry. Should there be an outbreak, flocks will be slaughtered, movement restrictions will be ordered, and free-range flocks will not be allowed to range (preventing exposure to wild birds). Since commercial hens are kept together in large flocks, avoidance of disease risk is the major strategy for the industry. Therefore, biosecurity is particularly important.

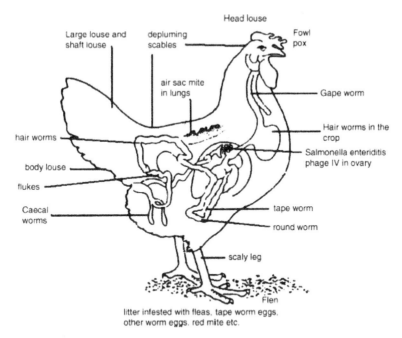

Figure 7.6 Pictorial representation of the potential threats to hens' health and welfare which can be spotted during bird (and environment) inspection. (*Source*: After ADAS undated).

7.5.5 Biosecurity and Hygiene

The benefits to be gained from economies of scale were quickly realized. Units of several hundred thousands of birds became the norm and units of up to 1.5 million or so exist nowadays. However, such large flocks can also be problematic. One of the major risks is disease, which might influence the entire flock, or infect the eggs that they produce, with significant economic consequences. The poultry industry pays particular attention to biosecurity where potential risks of infection are identified, and actions are taken to minimize the risk. Biosecurity activities are summarized in Table 7.9. The list is not exhaustive and some general hygiene has not been included.

7.5.6 Signs of Health and Disease

Good productivity and low mortality are obvious signs of good health. However, they cannot be taken as the only signs of a healthy flock. Simple health checks, such as checking water and food consumption, can be first indicators of possible problems, if there is any deviation from the norm. However, there are many potential causes (management of the thermal and physical environment and imbalanced diet, and so on) which can give the same results. A lot of information can be gleaned on entry to the flock. Listening to the birds can detect snicking (sneezing) or other unexpected sounds. A very quiet flock can also be suffering. By looking at

Table 7.9 Potential risks to birds or eggs and counter measures (biosecurity).

Carrier	Threat	Biosecurity measure
Human	Flock	Prevent unwanted visitors
		Make feed lorries/bird deliverers disinfect before delivery and on entry (disinfectant wheel dips)
		Single entry with gate guard
		Visitors' book (signed by every visitor)
		Prevent access if visitor has been with other poultry in the last few days
		Prevent entry of individuals with illness
		Prevent staff keeping birds at home
Human	Flock/eggs	Minimize visitors to packing facility (apply biosecurity systems listed above)
		Provide overalls, boots and hair cover
		Make visitors remove 'outdoor' clothes and shower before access
		Remove jewellery
		Hand washing/sanitizers on entry
		Boot disinfectant at every entrance
Vermin (rats/mice)	Flock/eggs	Keep weed-free
		Have an open space (concrete) around and between sheds
		Do not allow scrap/unused equipment to languish on site (to become infested)
		Ensure doors close and fit properly
		Do not leave spilled food (clean up immediately)
		Do not store (new) litter on site
		Remove soiled litter at least 1 mile from shed
		Have a vermin extermination program
		Maintain sheds properly (e.g. walls)
		Clean between flocks (birds of the same age in each shed allows thorough cleaning of the shed)
Micro-organisms and pathogens	Flock/eggs	Disinfect thoroughly
		Prevent contamination
		Regular cleaning with deep cleansing as appropriate
Insect/flies	Flock/eggs	Electric 'Insecticutors'
		Fly-killing poisons where possible
		Prevent ingress

(Continued)

Table 7.9 (Continued)

Carrier	Threat	Biosecurity measure
		Clean the environment to remove places where flies/fly eggs can survive
Wild birds	Flock/eggs	Ensure doors close and fit properly
		Do not leave spilled food (clean up immediately)
		Minimize exposure (bring free-range flocks indoors in times of risk (e.g. avian influenza outbreak)
Chickens	Flock/eggs	Remove dead/sick birds
		Dispose of dead birds quickly and efficiently (incineration)
		Test parents for *Salmonella* (if parents are free, offspring should be too)
		Regular cloacal swabs of laying flock to ensure free of *Salmonella* and other contamination

the birds, information can also be obtained about the health of the flock. A stationary bird, stooped and with eyes closed, may be in pain. Birds with swollen heads or with liquid around the eyes can be suffering from diseases such as influenza or bronchitis. Bad smells in the shed can be caused by birds showing signs of diarrhoea, resulting from gut parasitic problems (e.g. coccidiosis) or one of many diseases. In brown-egg laying flocks, the appearance of white shells may be an indicator of mite infestation or subclinical disease. Soft-shelled or shell-less eggs or a drop in egg numbers could be signs of calcium problems or egg drop syndrome. Increased levels of aggression, feather pulling and cannibalism can arise from frustration, overcrowding, poor drinker and feeder management or poor environmental control.

7.5.7 Production Disorders

7.5.7.1 Osteoporosis
Since the 1950s the physiological demands on the birds has increased remarkably. Expectations, in terms of egg numbers per bird, have almost doubled to the 300 eggs per bird expected from caged hens (or 280 or so from free range). The daily calcium requirements for eggshells are more than the diet can supply, or the bird can absorb, even though food is supplemented with granular calcium (traditionally as oyster shells). In times of calcium deficit, hens can mobilize skeletal calcium, particularly from the long bones (medullary bone) which become active as a calcium store around sexual maturity. Muscular paralysis and weak bones (osteoporosis) during peak egg production, caused by calcium deficiency, is known as caged layer fatigue. This can be offset by providing birds that have been light stimulated (i.e. about two weeks before the first egg, when medullary bone formation begins) with layer ration, rich in calcium. This allows birds to store calcium before the demands of egg-laying. A similar

problem can occur towards the end of lay where sustained calcium demand reduces the overall skeletal calcium. Eggshell thickness and quality are also compromised at this time if the shell glands are less efficient.

7.5.8 Behavioural Problems

7.5.8.1 Feather Pecking and Cannibalism

Feather pecking is not a problem in itself. Feather pecking is misdirected investigative pecking as the birds investigate their surrounds. However, when feather *pecking* becomes feather *pulling*, this can lead to problems, particularly if the victim bleeds and the pecking bird starts to peck at the wound. This can quickly lead to damaging aggressive pecking and cannibalism. Cannibalism can occur from many causes such as sudden changes or a poor environment (high temperature, high light intensity, poor ventilation, overstocking, competition for insufficient numbers of feeders or drinkers, access to prolapsed or sick and dying birds,) poor diet (e.g. salt imbalance, lack of trace element or lack of sodium) or aggressive strains of birds.

In large groups of birds, such as free-range or barn flocks of several thousand birds, a stable social order cannot be established and general aggression can be extended in duration. This is recognized by Farm Animal Welfare Council, who have declared that system design should make escape routes available for bullied birds. Cannibalism is generally more frequent in barns and free-range units compared to battery cages. However, it can occur in battery cages. In such cases it has to be combated quickly since birds in neighbouring cages seem to develop cannibalistic tendencies and it can sweep through the system unless checked. Currently the main method of control is beak trimming, though this will no longer be possible after 2010.

7.5.9 Beak Trimming

Chickens use their beaks for many different tasks. Apart from the obvious task of collecting food, it is used for aggression, investigation of the environment and as a gripping, breaking and ripping tool. The sharp beak has many nerve endings, suggesting that it also very sensitive. Because the beak is so sharp, poultry-keepers learned that the beak could be trimmed to remove the sharpness. This was found not only to reduce aggression (or at least reduce the potential damage birds did to each other), but it made the birds more careful when pecking for food. There was much less food wastage as the birds did not throw the food around as much. This is important to flock-keepers as food costs represent between 70% and 90% of production costs.

Trained beak trimmers can trim the beaks of young birds up to the age of 11 days. A maximum of one-third of the distance between the beak tip and the nostrils is permitted to be removed. This could be done for both the upper and lower beaks at a cost of about 3p per bird. This was often done with a hot wire or blade that not only cut the beak, but cauterized the wound at the same time. It was important that during the procedure the bird's tongue was protected to avoid any further damage. Beak trimming also prevented cannibalism from spreading in flocks and so flock-keepers were allowed to beak-trim mature birds if cannibalism occurred. It would be wrong to understate the problem of cannibalism in some flocks of poultry. The causes are complex, ranging from dietary imbalance, stocking density, bird 'poise' and the level of arousal of the flock, to sudden environmental changes. Birds in large colonies are unable to establish cohesive social hierarchies and aggression, to establish status, is more prevalent in large flocks. Birds can recognize 15 to 20 individuals and have a 'general recognition' for about 100 birds in order to create and sustain a hierarchy, usually around sexual maturity. So birds can relatively quickly establish a hierarchy and then the levels of aggression associated with creating a hierarchy are reduced. This is not to say that levels of aggression are reduced in smaller flocks. There is a significant body of evidence demonstrating that aggression in flocks of about 100 birds can often be greater than in larger flocks. Nevertheless, in larger commercial barn and free-range flocks, there can be prolonged aggression if a stable social order cannot be established. In such cases, there tends to be a more polarized social arrangement, with an apparent extreme between the 'despot' birds and the 'omega' or 'pariah' birds. Where cannibalism occurs, it is often the individuals at the bottom of the order that become the early victims (unless another bird is injured). Once cannibalism becomes established in a flock it becomes difficult to eradicate and so prevention is the best approach.

Beak trimming is one method that has been chosen in the past to prevent aggressive pecking, feather pulling and cannibalism. Since it is impossible to identify individual aggressors in a free-range flock of several thousand, birds destined for barn or free-range systems are more routinely beak-trimmed as a preventive measure than in cage systems. Research has shown that some (but not all) forms of beak trimming can cause chronic pain associated with neuroma formation (Gentle et al. 1990). Despite this there is a welfare argument to support beak trimming if it reduces the incidence of cannibalism. There is, however, no welfare argument to support beak trimming simply to prevent food wastage from birds flicking the food out of the feeders. Other techniques, including lasers and infra-red radiation, have been tested with varying degrees of success. Since June 2006, RSPCA Freedom Food has allowed commercial layer hatcheries to use an infrared beak-trimming device for chicks placed at Freedom Food laying farms and from December 2010 this is the only method permitted in the UK.

In 2007 the Farm Animal Welfare Council prepared a document advising the British government of the welfare implications of a ban on beak trimming, which was due to come into effect on 31 December 2010 but then postponed until 2016 and then continued to be permitted. The Beak trimming Action Group has been established to work with the Government to investigate alternatives to beak trimming.

The FAWC suggested that 'If injurious pecking could be eliminated by other means, for example through genetic selection, the use of controlled light for housed birds or other management practices, then the need for beak trimming would disappear and this mutilation would no longer be needed.' The current welfare codes for laying hens recommend that beak treatment should 'be restricted to beak tipping; that is the blunting of the beak to remove the sharp point which can be the cause of the most severe damage to other birds'. The FAWC view appears to be that beak trimming is a mutilation which goes against the 'five freedoms' of good animal welfare in that it causes pain and injury and possibly a deleterious change in behaviour. However, if this is not the case (particularly when it is done on young birds) then, if all other avenues of work (such as establishing a less aggressive strain of bird) are unsuccessful, beak tipping (of just the very end of the beak, and using the most humane techniques) should not be dismissed out of hand, if it prevents a worse welfare insult such as cannibalism.

7.5.10 Depopulation, Transport and Slaughter

Bird welfare during handling and transport is important. Birds should never be deprived of water before transport; however, feed may be withheld for up to 12 hours prior to slaughter (including catching, loading, transport, lairage and unloading times). This ensures that the birds do not have a full crop at slaughter. A full crop can burst and contaminate the carcass. The procedure should be coordinated to minimize the time that the birds are held in the handling crates or modules. Where possible any equipment (particularly equipment with sharp edges) should be removed if it may hinder the easy collection and transfer of the birds. The catching and handling of the birds must be done quietly, methodically and efficiently to prevent the birds from panicking, struggling or being injured. Reduced light intensity or blue lighting is often used to quieten the birds. The skilled catchers should be trained and demonstrate competence to ensure bird welfare throughout the procedure. If birds are in cages, they should be taken out individually from the cage, being held by both legs in one hand and the breast supported in the other hand. Similarly, birds in non-cage systems should be held by both legs. Any bird should be carried through the system by both legs and catchers must take care that the birds do not collide with anything in the system (particularly if the wings are flapping). Birds should never be carried by their wings, heads or necks and never more than three birds per hand. The distance birds are carried to the transport crates or modules must be minimized.

Although laying hens can survive longer than a decade, commercially most birds are removed from the laying site by about 75 weeks of age. Small, backyard flocks can be allowed to go through a moult, where egg production ceases and the birds refresh the plumage; the calcium in the bones is also replenished at this time. The birds return to almost peak egg production within a few weeks. This can occur several times and the birds can live a productive life for several years. Commercially, it is important that all of the birds in the same shed are removed at the same time to allow a thorough cleaning of the shed, for good biosecurity.

In the past, depopulation of laying hens from cages had significant welfare issues. End-of-lay hens have little economic value and the skill level of workers was low. Poor cage design meant that birds taken by the legs to be pulled from the cages risked significant damage to legs, wings and (in particular) keel bones. Studies showed that birds, already possibly suffering brittle bones (osteoporosis), risked bone breakage from poor handling when being taken from cages. Developments such as sliders over the food trough, better designed cage fronts and more careful handling have reduced the risks, but bird depopulation can still be a point where birds risk welfare insults. The depopulation of enriched cages may prove difficult in that the last few birds in the group have a relatively large space to avoid capture and in the ensuing struggle may be prone to injury. Also, once caught, the birds must be carried to the doors and then stacked in modules. Collision injuries are possible, and care has to be taken, even though catchers are compelled to complete the task as soon as possible.

The risk of injury is increased in barn and free-range systems where, as the population is reduced in the shed, the remaining birds can more easily avoid capture. Birds may be driven towards the catchers but seizing and restraining birds can be difficult and birds may be injured. Strategies, such as catching roosting birds in low light conditions, can be used so that the birds are less active.

Transport times are strictly controlled to avoid problems of hypo- or hyperthermia on board the lorries. As the number of slaughterhouses prepared to take end-of-lay hens has reduced in the UK over the last few years, distances and journey times have increased and the welfare of the hens during transport remains an important issue Commercially laying hens are slaughtered on lines usually used for broiler birds, though no broilers can be slaughtered on the line when it is used for laying hens. Smaller flocks can be slaughtered using hand-held stunners which render birds unconscious or dead by electrocution. Individuals may be killed by neck dislocation.

7.6   Welfare of the Laying Hen

There continue to be serious concerns for the welfare of animals used by humans for agricultural purposes. There are concerns for the welfare of the birds themselves, with continuing demands for increased productivity and efficiency (i.e. more eggs for less feed). A major historical problem with bird welfare and the poultry industry is one of profit. In the early development of the UK poultry egg industry, maximizing efficiency, producing more for least cost, was the driving force. Indeed, this was the aim of the UK government which provided minimal financial support for the developing industry but penalized the less efficient producers. When welfare issues were considered, from the 1960s onwards, any changes in production to improve bird welfare were seen as 'costs' to the industry, since it often meant that welfare requirements increased the costs of production, reduced stocking or negatively affected egg production per bird. Many producers argued that if the birds were alive and healthy then production itself demonstrated good welfare. The welfarists claimed that, while poor production was an indicator of poor welfare, high production levels were not indicators of good welfare per se. Another confounding problem for the industry has been that consumers may express a desire for higher welfare standards for laying hens (which would increase costs of production and therefore the price of eggs to the consumer) but actually elect to purchase cheaper eggs from caged hens. However, as stated earlier, the large increase in the sale of free-range eggs suggests that consumer demand is catching up with desire. Often proposed improvements for bird welfare have not been welcomed by an industry that perceives such moves as interference. Welfare improvements are often resented and the industry responds to minimize the effect of the proposals. For example, the response to the provision of 'litter' for dust-bathing in cages has been the use of Astroturf material, which is hardly a litter at all.

Similarly, a proposed increase in floor space per bird in cages was overcome not by reducing the number of birds per cage, but by the creation of an extension to the cage front.

Commercial free-range systems do not necessarily meet all of the welfare requirements of the laying hen. For example, large populations on inappropriate ground can cause birds to suffer disease risks, or smaller populations may exhibit high levels of aggression through frustration. The requirements of hens on range are not fully understood and there is a need to research birds' needs. The introduction of an enriched cage should be seen by the industry as an opportunity to create a system that not only meets the economic demands facing the industry but also best meets the welfare requirements of the birds. The compromise that often occurs between the scientific advice and the engineered systems means that the findings of academic research are not properly met and the expected welfare improvements are not guaranteed. This is apparently the case in some designs of enriched cages (e.g. where perches meet inappropriately and birds may be cramped) and some materials used may not provide the level of enrichment that might otherwise be provided (e.g. plastic matting instead of friable litter for dust-bathing). Despite such criticisms, it is important that producers are not seen as the villains. Ultimately, they will produce eggs however society demands, *provided that society is willing to meet the extra costs of production*, which is not always the case.

An oft-used argument by UK producers is that the cost of implementing welfare legislation creates an 'unlevel playing field' in terms of costs of home-produced eggs versus cheaper imports. The EU has some newer member states with weak economies where preparations for the changes in 2012 may be difficult to afford. The EU has also stated an intention not to trade with nations outside the EU that do not have the same levels of welfare for the birds. The resolution of these issues will not be easy. Whatever happens, it is essential that the progression to higher welfare standards for laying hens continues, in terms of both the demands on the birds and the methods of production.

7.6.1 Welfare Concerns for the Hen

Agricultural production in the UK responded to the needs of the population and the drive from government after World War I, i.e. to become self-sufficient in cheap food production. This need was reinforced following World War II. The push for efficiency meant that other issues such as welfare were secondary. Much of the research on poultry has been on production, and funding to research diet, food efficiency and alternative food sources has been more abundant than for welfare. Breeding companies are still primarily driven to maximize output and make the birds more efficient. This assumes that the selection of laying hens has not yet reached their genetic limits. Thus, with some manipulation, breeders assume that they can unlock some new, previously unrealized level of production from the birds. However, reason would predict that this is not sustainable. Pushing the birds beyond an unknown limit represents a serious welfare problem. Already, commercial laying hens suffer osteoporosis, often associated with calcium depletion in the skeleton in response to the physiological loading of eggshell formation for the 300 or so eggs expected from the bird in 13 months of production. However, osteoporosis can result from dietary imbalance (e.g. calcium and phosphorus levels and ratio in the food). Also, birds can recover bone strength and bone density during a moulting process. This is standard practice in the USA but it is not permitted in Lion Code flocks.

Birds in traditional cages generally display more fear responses to novel stimuli presented at the cage front, than birds in non-cage systems. Whether this is the case in enriched cages is not yet known. It seems that birds regularly exposed to changing novel (non-threatening) stimuli are more receptive and less fearful when exposed to some novel stimulus, though not to the possibly more extreme novelty of handling and transport.

Some of the hybrids used in the past for commercial egg production were known to be aggressive. The popularity of such strains has dwindled in the past 20 years or so. DEFRA are looking to the breeders to produce a more docile strain of bird which is less prone to aggressive behaviour. Commercial flock size may also cause increased levels of aggression, but there can be many other causes. A few producers, with non-caged systems, are including cockerels in the flock in an attempt to reduce levels of aggression among the hens.

7.6.2   Welfare Concerns in Society

In the UK it is probably the welfare of laying hens in battery cages that was foremost in the minds of animal welfarists when concerns for farmed animal welfare were first voiced. In the early 1960s Ruth Harrison wrote a book about 'animal machines', stating concerns about (intensive) factory farming techniques. Pressure from lobby groups caused the UK government to set up the Brambell Committee in the 1960s to assess animal welfare. Some of the committee's recommendations to improve animal welfare were based on anthropomorphic evaluations (e.g. the recommended floor for laying hens was solid metal with circular perforations, which the birds disliked, preferring a mesh floor). On the positive side, the committee came up with the notion of 'five freedoms' for animal welfare.

In the early 1970s the FAWC was established, which continued this theme of 'five freedoms' which, although not the same as those of the Brambell Committee, can trace their ancestry back to it. The FAWC was established to undertake investigations of welfare issues concerning farmed animals and their management (taking advice from the farming industry and scientific evidence) and then reported to government as an informed body, allowing government to create advised welfare codes and recommendations for good practice and also to incorporate welfare in legislation through DEFRA. Although the *Codes and Recommendations for the Welfare of Livestock: Laying Hens* is not legislation itself, failure to comply with the codes can be used in court as evidence of cruelty, should a prosecution occur. Since its foundation, the FAWC has reported on a number of issues relating to the egg industry, such as:

- advice to the Agriculture Ministers of Great Britain on the need to control certain mutilations of farm animals (1981);
- report on the welfare of poultry at the time of slaughter (1982);
- an assessment of egg production systems (1986);
- report on the welfare of laying hens in colony systems (1991);
- report on the welfare of laying hens (1997).

In general, the FAWC report to the Government and then the Government, through DEFRA, responds, stating whether the current provisions are sufficient or how the recommendations are to be acted up on. There have been several pieces of legislation since the mid-1960s to improve the welfare of laying hens. These include:

- The Agriculture (Miscellaneous Provisions) Act 1968;
- The Welfare of Livestock (Prohibited Operations) Regulations 1982;
- The Welfare of Livestock Regulations 1994;
- The Welfare of Farmed Animals (England) Regulations 2000;
- Welfare of Farmed Animals (England) (Amendment) Regulations 2002;
- Animal Welfare Act 2006;
- Welfare of Farmed Animals (England) Regulations 2007.

The legal provisions have progressed from preventing offences such as: to cause or allow livestock on agricultural land (including intensive and 'back yard' poultry units) to suffer unnecessary pain or distress; prohibiting the devoicing of cockerels; the castration of a male bird by a method involving surgery, or any operation on a bird with the object or effect of impeding its flight, other than feather clipping. From 1994, legislation focused on cage construction (openings), dimensions and, in particular, space allocation per bird, currently standing at 550 cm^2 per bird but increasing in 2012 when enriched cages are introduced. General flock management (food and water provision), bird inspection and system checks are also included. In 2002 legislation encompassed the permitted stocking and management of non-caged systems, again focusing on 2012 as the target date for full compliance.

The more recent UK legislation for animal welfare (for farmed species *and* for animals in zoos) relies heavily on the provisions outlined in the FAWC's 'five freedoms' for good welfare. However, I feel that in poultry production and management, the 'five freedoms' have been misinterpreted as goals or aims. These 'freedoms' are often seen as a welfare 'ceiling' rather than a legal minimum welfare standard or 'floor'. Also, the concept of birds' 'freedoms' does not really reinforce the responsibility of the human keeper or carer of the animals. Freedoms (even in human societies) are often abused and neglected. Increasingly, I am 'rebadging' the 'five freedoms' as the five 'minimum musts' (Table 7.10).

I concede that this is little more than a rewording of the five freedoms and I would not wish to be accused of criticising such an august body as the FAWC. However, these 'MUSTS' represent a change in emphasis and plant the responsibility for welfare of the animals firmly in the hands of the keeper or carer. A slight modification also changes the freedom to perform normal behaviours to 'socially acceptable' behaviour patterns, ruling out behaviours such as cannibalism in poultry. The means by which these 'musts' are provided remain the same as the FAWC recommendations, since they represent the most appropriate methods (Table 7.10).

An interesting development in the assessment of welfare are the 'Five Domains Model' (1994) and 'Five Provisions/Welfare Aims' paradigm, which can match the provisions against the FAWC 'Five Freedoms'. These also consider the physical and mental well-being of the individual and provide frameworks for 'structured, systematic, comprehensive and coherent animal welfare assessments' (Mellor 2017).

Table 7.10 The 'minimum musts' for animal welfare (adapted from the Farm Animal Welfare Council's 'five freedoms').

1. The keeper/carer MUST prevent hunger and thirst...	...by providing ready access to fresh water and a diet to maintain full health and vigour
2. The keeper/carer MUST prevent discomfort...	...by providing an appropriate environment including shelter and a comfortable resting area
3. The keeper/carer MUST prevent pain, injury or disease...	...by prevention or rapid diagnosis and treatment
4. The keeper/carer MUST allow expression of socially acceptable behaviour patterns...	...by providing sufficient space, proper facilities and company of the animal's own kind
5. The keeper/carer MUST prevent fear and distress...	...by ensuring conditions and treatment which avoid mental suffering

7.6.3 Egg Quality Assurance and Welfare Enhancement

In the 1960s the Egg Marketing Board introduced a lion logo on eggs and slogans such as 'Go to work on an egg!' and 'Happiness is egg-shaped', using comedic actors of the day in advertisements on television. This was a particularly successful campaign. Following declining egg sales, resulting from the proposed potential health risk of heart disease associated with cholesterol levels in eggs and the impact of the 'Salmonella in eggs' scare in the 1980s, the industry relaunched the lion emblem to encourage egg sales. Unfortunately, the new generation did not readily embrace the image (its impact had been lost with time). The Lion Quality Code was launched and now represents a mark of quality control. The RSPCA have also launched a marketing tool (Freedom Foods) which is an assurance scheme that the flock management and systems used for egg production meet the required welfare standards. The Freedom Foods scheme cannot be applied to caged systems (since the RSPCA believes that cages are intrinsically cruel). This is not so for the Lion Scheme, introduced by the British Egg Industry Council.

7.6.3.1 The Lion Code

The Lion Code of Practice sets out procedures and inspections to maintain bird health and welfare and control egg handling and quality. The following is a short summary of some of the key points. Lion Quality eggs, carrying the little red lion on the shell, have a 'best before' date ink-jet printed (using food quality dye) on the shell and on the pack. For Lion eggs, the 'best before' date is up to 25 days from pack (or for inline operations up to 27 days from pack). Since the legally defined 'best before' date is 28 days from lay, eggs in the scheme must be sold sooner than the legal requirement. Most Lion Quality eggs are packed within 48 hours of lay.

The Lion Code was developed to establish quality standards for eggs fit for human consumption. The Codes of Practice address quality and bird welfare and apply to:

- breeding flocks and hatcheries;
- pullet rearing;
- laying birds;
- production practices (including health hygiene and welfare).

Along with bird management, the quality of the product is considered with reference to on-farm handling of eggs; distribution of eggs from farm; feed; hen disposal; packing centre procedures; advice to retailers, consumers and caterers; environmental policy and enforcement. All farms involved in breeding, rearing (to point of lay) and production, egg packing centres and feed mills in this scheme have to be approved by independent inspectors. All flocks have a passport certificate which contains the history and treatments associated with the flock. All egg movements require sufficient documentation to enable traceability. All hatcheries and breeding flock accommodation (and birds) are subject to regular microbiological monitoring, with the necessary slaughter of any *Salmonella*-positive flocks, and heat/acid treatment of feed.

As part of the scheme, all egg-producing flocks are vaccinated during rearing (as part of the standard vaccination program) against *Salmonella enteritidis* using an approved vaccine. Pullet rearers are also required to undertake a hygiene monitoring program before birds are taken onto the farm. These flocks are tested for *Salmonella*, with a disinfection program for all bird transport systems. Records kept on the passport include:

- bird movements;
- testing for *Salmonella*;
- wild birds and rodent control measures.

For farms accommodating laying birds there are strict rules concerning:

- farm disinfection between flocks;
- prevention of cross-infection between birds on farms and between successive flocks;
- testing for *Salmonella*;
- wild bird and rodent control measures;
- record keeping.

The animal welfare requirements of the Lion Code exceed the legal requirements. These include:

- the banning of induced moulting;
- additional staff training procedures for the handling of end-of-lay hens;
- the Code mirrors the RSPCA's Freedom Food standards for free-range and barn egg production.

7.6.3.2 RSPCA Assured (Previously Known as Freedom Foods)

The RSPCA has established a quality control system based almost entirely on bird welfare. Since the organization considers cages to be intrinsically cruel the society will only give accreditation to barn and free-range systems. The scheme is based around the FAWC's 'five freedoms' (reflected in the name of the scheme). Subscribers to the scheme pay a levy and are inspected by representatives of the scheme. If proven satisfactory, the producer can use the RSPCA Assured logo on the packaging. The main points of the scheme include the following.

Chickens must be fed a wholesome diet which:

- is appropriate to their species (meeting nutritional needs for good health);
- is available to them at all times (unless authorized by a veterinary surgeon);
- of known nutrient content with no mammal or bird protein;
- contains no antibiotic (except for therapeutic reasons);
- birds must be fed insoluble grit at least once per week;
- continuous access to an adequate supply of clean, fresh water (unless under the instruction of a veterinarian).

The environment in which birds are kept must:

- be designed to protect them from physical and thermal discomfort, fear and distress (coping with local weather conditions);
- a sign must be prominently displayed at or near the building entrance with the following information:
- total floor area available to the birds;
- total number of birds and stocking density;
- total number of drinkers and feeders;
- target air quality parameters;
- lighting levels and regimes;
- emergency procedures, i.e. actions in the case of fire, flood, etc.;
- nest box area per bird;
- lighting in the sheds should meet the welfare needs of the birds (including resting time) and be recorded.

It is not compulsory for laying hens in the Freedom Foods scheme to have free range. Barn systems can be accredited with a maximum flock size of 32000 birds and free range systems are permitted a maximum flock size of 16000 birds (both subdivided in to colonies of 4000 birds). In free range systems there are further requirements within the scheme, such as continuous access to the range during daylight hours. The RSPCA only allow 2000 birds per hectare (compared to the maximum permitted 2500 for general free range units). For the RSPCA the maximum perimeter of range is 350 m from the house. Land use rotation must occur if there is a risk of accumulation of parasites (fowl sick land).

The scheme also includes the roles of managers and stock-keepers, bird inspection, health plans, and so on, along with requirements for transport and slaughter of the birds, but since these are not part of the bird environmental requirements, these will not be considered here.

7.6.3.3 Other Schemes

Other marketing, quality and welfare assurance schemes exist within the UK. For example, for eggs to be sold as 'organically produced', the production methods must meet the legal requirements. The Soil Association is a subgroup within organic production. The Soil Association adds further requirements for organic production and its members can market the product under the Soil Association banner as a mark of distinction.

Supermarkets are also using eggs in advertising campaigns, attempting to use the perceived welfare concerns of society as marketing tools. For example, some major retail chain stores (claiming to take advice from the RSPCA) have committed to phase out sales of eggs from caged hens, and a well-known manufacturer of mayonnaise has recently stated that their product will only use eggs from the free-range egg sector.

7.6.4 Welfare Monitoring Protocols

In the past it was the responsibility of the State Veterinary Service to monitor egg production sites to ensure compliance with current, relevant UK legislation concerning general management, cage sizes, stocking densities, and so on. Inspectors could visit sites and make recommendations to the producer, or have the authority to close the unit if there was gross non-compliance. This caused some resentment among some producers who felt that, where EU legislation applied, other member states were not being as closely monitored, or the legislation as strictly upheld. In 2007 the State Veterinary Service merged with other groups, including the Egg Marketing Inspectorate. The Egg Marketing Inspectorate had the authority to inspect egg production sites and packing stations, etc., mainly to ensure compliance with legislation associated with hygiene, marketing standards, labelling and egg handling and storage sites, etc., rather than dealing with bird welfare per se. The Welfare of Farmed Animals (England) (Amendment) Regulations 2002 was one of the first pieces of legislation associated with egg production which made provision for inspection to be carried out by inspectors from other EU member states.

The RSPCA uses inspectors to assess the welfare of laying hens for farms included in the RSPCA Assured scheme. These inspectors make farm visits and check bird welfare and ensure that all of the scheme's requirements are in place. This can be as simple as a tick-box check ensuring that requirements are in place, an examination of records and an assessment of the current flocks. Similarly assessors of the Lion scheme carry out farm assessments to ensure that all of the requirements of the scheme have been met.

There are other individuals and groups that are associated with the welfare of laying hens. Some research groups (e.g. the Roslin Institute in the past) and universities (e.g. Oxford, Cambridge and Bristol) have been particularly involved in research into animal welfare (including laying hens). Several welfare groups, such as Chickens' Lib and Compassion in World Farming, are also involved in promoting the welfare of laying hens. These have many publicity campaigns and lobby Parliament and the larger retailers to criticize cages and to promote higher welfare standards for farmed animals.

7.7   Conclusions: The Way Ahead

Eggs are a relatively cheap, highly nutritious food item or ingredient for other food products. As the human population continues to expand, the global demand for eggs will increase. It can be no surprise that the major egg producers of today are countries of high population (and rapidly developing economies). In fact, history may be repeating itself, as it was in Britain that areas of rapid growth in the poultry industry coincided with rapidly growing population densities and industrial development (requiring cheap food for factory workers).

Optimistically, one would hope that consumers' concerns for the welfare of animals in society, and in particular farmed species, will continue to grow. Also, if this is a real concern, consumers may be more willing to pay the higher prices to meet the corresponding higher costs of production. Certainly, in the UK and in the EU, legislation increasingly seeks to safeguard the welfare of farm animals. The pressures from the UK's larger retailers on the nation's major egg producers may also bring about changes in the methods of production.

In times of economic crisis consumers' concerns for welfare may be diminished. The dichotomy between consumers' concerns for bird welfare and purchasing patterns is well documented. As consumers in the UK change their purchasing habits, egg sales from the less prestigious retailers may increase.

Welfare concerns may not be considered as important in developing economies. As the influence of Asian economies increases in global trading, the association between production and the welfare concerns for the animals may become secondary. The EU has stated that it will not trade with any third country that does not produce eggs with the same standards of welfare for the birds. Such threats may be interpreted as protectionist trading, possibly leading to some form of global trade war.

Notwithstanding these political issues, one might hope that concerns will continue to grow and develop for the needs of animals used in agriculture. It is also essential that this increased awareness and concern should lead to real improvements in farm animal welfare and protection. This will require continuing research to more fully understand the needs, and the limits, of the birds that are used for egg production. Humans have an important responsibility to look after the birds that are used for egg production. Let us hope that we take this responsibility seriously and provide the birds with a safe environment that protects their welfare.

7.7.1   Chick Sexing

A major, but seldom considered, controversy of poultry egg production is the fate of the male birds. Since the males are not egg producers, and the eggs that we eat are not fertile, there is no direct role for male chicks in the egg industry. Currently male chicks cannot be identified until hatch. In some cases (particularly where brown feathered females are used) male chicks can be identified easily by down colour since it is obviously different to the female chick counterparts. In other cases 'chick sexers' are required. These are highly trained individuals who are able to determine the sex of the newly hatched chick by eye when examining the cloacal area of the chicks. Unfortunately, it is at this point that the male chicks' fates are sealed. In commercial production 50% of the total hatch are males and (bearing in mind that there are 40 million laying hens in the UK (AHDB 2018) this represents a substantial number. These birds are not suitable for growth for meat production. As a result, they are gassed at the hatchery. They are then frozen and are used as food for zoo animals and in 'birds of prey centres'. Some smaller-scale producers and breeders are selecting different parent stock, relaxing the selection for egg production and then using the surplus males for meat production (though this would never compete for food efficiency and growth compared to the commercial broiler stock). This 'open sourcing' (McKenna 2014) may be of greater impact in countries where systems other than western intensive systems are more common.

A more important development is the ability to sex the chick in ovo. This can be done as early as three to four days of incubation, with an accuracy of over 90% (Galli et al. 2016, 2017). This is close to being commercially available in hatcheries (Poultry World 2018). This means that eggs containing males can be removed and destroyed before there is any sensitivity in the developing embryo. It could be argued that this is a welfare improvement rather than waiting for full chick development before destruction, since the embryo is not sentient.

7.7.2 Consumer Pressure

A number of UK supermarkets no longer sell eggs from caged birds. Following a petition by a teenager in 2016 (The Guardian, 2016) Tesco has joined other supermarkets such as Sainsburys, Marks and Spencer, the Co-Op, Aldi, ASDA, Lidl and Morrisons in declaring that they will no longer source eggs from caged hens. It is likely that eggs from barn systems will replace those from caged systems. Currently eggs from barn systems account for less than 10% of UK sales. The move is supposedly based on the levels of welfare available in cages and any improvement in welfare must be welcomed. However, the suggestion that cages provide poor welfare whilst other systems automatically improve welfare is too simplistic. Table 7.5 has already demonstrated that some of the aspects of non-caged systems offer poorer welfare for the birds than their caged counterparts. It is well-documented that birds in barn (non-caged) systems suffer from broken bones during the production period, mainly caused by falls and collision with the structures in the barn (e.g. Gregory and Wilkins 1989; Knowles and Wilkins 1998). Smothering of birds, where birds pile on each other, causing suffocation, is also an important issue in the non-cage systems (Bright and Johnson 2011). Nigel Gibbens (the UK Government's Chief Veterinary Office) has called the decision to stop selling eggs from caged systems 'regrettable' mainly due to the risks from bird 'flu (Agerholm 2017). However, if it is possible to overcome the problems and issues associated with the change there could be an improvement in welfare.

7.7.3 Precision Agriculture

Precision agriculture is often promoted as an exciting, innovative approach to maximize outputs and efficiencies in modern agriculture. In truth, 'precision agriculture' has been applied in poultry production for decades. The motivational forces have been: reduction in manual labour; improved efficiencies, both in the production methods and the birds; attention to detail, especially at critical control points in, for example, biosecurity; excellent record keeping of flock performance and issues and the use of computer systems to provide for the needs of the birds. In so doing, the egg industry has worked to promote and maintain the health and welfare of the birds. The Lion Code Scheme's efforts were rewarded in 2017 when the Food Standards Agency declared that eggs from this scheme were effectively Salmonella-free (Hughes 2017). This also means that the birds are at a lesser risk, enhancing their welfare.

7.7.4   International Trade

At the time of writing, one of the greatest causes for political and economic debates is that concerning Brexit (the potential withdrawal of the UK from the European Union). Changes that occur to the UK egg industry as a result are currently, at best, speculative. Any implications of Brexit have concentrated mainly on economic performance, risks from controlled labour supply, changes in market share with imported eggs and food prices. Similarly, any effects on the welfare of the birds are also not known but impacts may result from issues such as movement of breeding stock (including any potential extra time to move through customs at borders), potential availability of medication if these are brought from Europe, potential erosion of on-farm welfare (in response to imports from other countries with lower welfare standards) or alignment with countries, such as the USA, as part of trading agreements. As the UK legislation replaces EU law, there is the possibility that welfare legislation may affect laying hen welfare, either positively or negatively. At the moment we simply do not know

References and Further Reading

ADAS. (undated). *Poultry technical note*. Agricultural Development Advisory Service.

Agerholm, H. (2017). Government's chief vet says supermarket plan to stop selling non-free range eggs "regrettable". The Independent. https://www.independent.co.uk/news/uk/home-news/free-range-eggs-caged-enriched-supermarket-tesco-morrisons-asda-nigel-gibbens-a8088301.html (accessed 18 April 2019).

Agriculture and Horticulture development Board (AHDB). (2018). *Poultry pocketbook*. AHDB Kennilworth.

Appleby, M.C., Mench, J.A., and Hughes, B.O. (2004). *Poultry Behaviour and Welfare*. Wallingford: CABI Publishing.

Brambell, F.W.R. (1965). *Report of the Technical Committee to Inquire into the Welfare of Animals Kept under Intensive Livestock Husbandry Systems*. London: HMSO.

Bright, A. and Johnson, E.A. (2011). Smothering in commercial free-range laying hens: a preliminary investigation. Vet. Rec. 168 (19) Short Communication. https://veterinaryrecord.bmj.com/content/168/19/512.1 (accessed 18 April 2019).

Council of the European Union. (1999). *Laying down the minimum standard for the protection of laying hens*. Council Directive 1999/74/EC, 19 July 1999.

Department for Environment, Food and Rural Affairs. (2002). *Laying Hens: Code of Recommendations for the Welfare of Livestock*. London: DEFRA.

Department for Environment, Food and Rural Affairs. (2006). *Compendium of UK Organic Standards*. London: DEFRA.

Department for Environment, Food and Rural Affairs. (2007). *Guidance on Legislation Covering the Marketing of Eggs*. London: DEFRA.

Department for Environment, Food and Rural Affairs. *Animal welfare: welfare of laying hens*. http://www.defra.gov.uk/animalh/welfare/farmed/layers (accessed 1 September 2009).

European Food Safety, Authority. (2005). Welfare aspects of various systems for keeping laying hens. Annex to *EFSA Journal* 197: 1–23.

FAWC. (1986). *An Assessment of Egg Production Systems*. Surbiton, UK: Farm Animal Welfare Council.

FAWC. (1991). *Report on the Welfare of Laying Hens in Colony Systems: PB 0734*. Surbiton, UK: Farm Animal Welfare Council.

FAWC. (1997). *Report on the welfare of laying hens*. http://www.fawc.org.uk/reports.htm (accessed 1 September 2009).

FAWC. (2009). *What is the Farm Animal Welfare Council?* http://www.fawc.org.uk (accessed 1 September 2009).

FAWC, (Farm Animal Welfare Council). (1982). *Report on the Welfare of Poultry at the Time of Slaughter*. Surbiton, UK: Farm Animal Welfare Council.

Galli, R., Kock, E., Preusse, G., Schnabel, C., Bartels, T., Krautwald-Junghanns, E., and Steiner, G. (2017). Contactless in ovo sex determination of chicken eggs. *Current Directions in Biomedical Engineering* 3 (2): 131–134.

Galli, R., Preusse, G., Uckermann, O., Bartels, T., Krautwald-Junghanns, M., Koch, E., and Steiner, G. (2016). In ovo sexing of domestic chicken eggs by Raman spectroscopy. *Analytical Chemistry* 88 (17): 8657–8663.

Gentle, M.J., Waddington, D., Hunter, L.N., and Jones, B. (1990). Behavioural evidence for persistent pain following partial beak amputation in chicken. *Applied Animal Behaviour Science* 27: 149–157.

Gregory, N.J. and Wilkins, L.J. (1989). Broken bones in domestic fowl: handling and processing damage in end-of-lay battery hens. *British Poultry Science* 3 (3): 555–562.

Harrison, R. (1964). *Animal Machines: The New Factory Farming Industry*. London: Vincent Stuart Ltd.

Hughes, D. (2017). UK eggs declared safe 30 years after salmonella scare. BBC news. https://www.bbc.co.uk/news/health-41568998 (accessed 18 April 2019).

ISA. (2009–10). General Management Guide: Commercials. Institut de Sélection Animale BV. http://www.isapoultry.com

Knowles, T.G. and Wilkins, L.J. (1998). The problem of broken bones during the handling of laying hens—a review. *Poultry Science* 77: 1798–1802.

LayWel Project. (2006). *Welfare implications of changes in production systems for laying hens*. http://www.laywel.eu (accessed 1 September 2009).

McKenna, M. (2014). Open-sourcing chicken: breaking free from corporate genetics. National Geographic. https://www.nationalgeographic.com/people-and-culture/food/the-plate/2014/08/29/open-sourcing-chicken-breaking-free-from-corporate-genetics (accessed 27 March 2015).

Mellor, D.J. (2017). Operational details of the five domains model and its key applications to the assessment and management of animal welfare. *Animals* 7: 60. https://www.ncbi.nlm.nih.gov/pmc/articles/PMC5575572 (accessed 16 April 2019).

Meunier, R.A. and Latour, M.A. (undated). *Commercial egg production and processing.* http://ag.ansc.purdue.edu/poultry/publication/commegg (accessed 1 September 2009).

Poultry World. (2018). Egg sexing close to market. https://www.poultryworld.net/Eggs/Articles/2018/6/Egg-sexing-close-to-market-301797E (accessed 18 April 2019).

Reece, W.O. (2009). *Functional Anatomy and Physiology of Domestic Animals*, 4e. Ames, IA: Wiley-Blackwell.

RSPCA, (Royal Society for the Protection of Animals). (2017). *RSPCA welfare standards for laying hens.* RSPCA, Horsham, UK. https://www.berspcaassured.org.uk/media/1244/rspca-welfare-standards-for-laying-hens-august-2017.pdf (accessed 16 April 2019).

RSPCA, (Royal Society for the Protection of Animals). (2018). *RSPCA welfare standards for pullets (laying hens).* RSPCA, Horsham, UK. https://science.rspca.org.uk/sciencegroup/farmanimals/standards/pullets (accessed 16 April 2019).

RUMA (Responsible use of Medicines in Agriculture Alliance). (2017). *Targets task force report 2017* http://www.ruma.org.uk/wp-content/uploads/2017/10/RUMA-Targets-Task-Force-Report-2017-FINAL.pdf (accessed 15 April 2019).

United Kingdom Register of Organic Food Standards (UKROFS). (2003). *UKROFS standards for organic food production.* http://www.defra.gov.uk.

Windhorst, H.W. (2007). Changes in the structure of global egg production. *World Poultry* 23 (6): 24–25.

8

Broiler Chickens

Andy Butterworth

Management and Welfare of Farm Animals: The UFAW Farm Handbook, Sixth Edition.
Edited by John Webster and Jean Margerison.
© Universities Federation for Animal Welfare 2022. Published 2022 by John Wiley & Sons Ltd.

8.1 The Industry

Broiler chickens are the most numerous of all farm terrestrial animals (with about 70 billion broilers being produced each year Worldwide, 8 billion in Europe). Poultry meat production has grown rapidly during the last 40 years (by a factor of 7 compared to a factor of 2–4 for other livestock production) and growth is expected to continue. Broiler chickens provide humans with a relatively inexpensive source of high-quality protein, which can be grown rapidly, with high food conversion efficiency and relatively low wastage through mortality. Husbandry systems have been developed over the last 50 years, which produce high quantities of meat product per unit of and in production. Broiler chicken meat is acceptable to all religious groups, other than those requiring members to be vegetarian or vegan and is included in the diet of most countries worldwide. Broiler chickens may be readily produced on an industrial scale but are also equally suitable for small, low capital investment domestic production.

The international broiler industry consists, for the most part, of large integrated businesses with the company supplying day-old chicks from a central hatchery, feed from centralized feed mills, and the birds receive medication and vaccination to company specifications. The integrated company may own the farms or may contract the growth of the birds from privately owned farms. The integrated company often trains, manages and employs, or contracts catching teams to depopulate houses and provides transport crates and transport vehicles to take birds to a central processing plant, or plants, for slaughter. It is common for the company to also be involved in further processing of the poultry meat into products for retail markets.

The typical, intensively produced broiler bird is slaughtered at between 36 and 54 days of age at a weight of between 1.7 kg and 3.5 kg Most broiler chickens are kept in enclosed, artificially lit and mechanically ventilated sheds (Figure 8.1), on a litter substrate on a flat floor

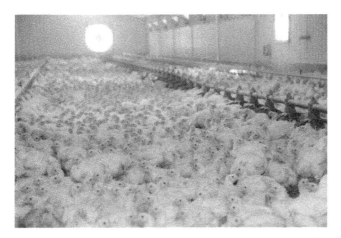

Figure 8.1 Chickens in a tunnel ventilated house (A Butterworth).

(not on slats or wire in the majority of the world, although in some countries litter is being replaced by mesh or slats) and fed either as 'meals', or with feed continuously available *ad libitum*. Stocking density in conventional intensive units is likely to range from about 17 to 22 birds/m^2 (600–450 cm^2 per bird) as birds approach slaughter weight. Productivity is measured in terms of food conversion ratio (FCR, kg feed/kg live-weight gain) or food conversion efficiency (FCE, kg live-weight gain/kg feed, see Chapter 1), or as slightly more complex metrics of performance such as the European Broiler Index (EBI) or European Production Efficiency Factor (EPEF) which take into account feed conversion, mortality and daily gain.

EPEF = (average grams gained/day × % survival rate)/Feed Conversion × 10

For example, an average growth of 61 g/day (for instance an end weight of 2,257 kg in 37 days), survival rate of 96% (100 – 4% mortality) and feed conversion of 1.62, would give a score of (61 × 96)/(1.62 × 10) = 361.5

Space allowance for broilers is conventionally described by stocking density (kg/m^2), rather than birds/m^2. The rationale for using stocking density in kg/m^2 is that this measure allows variable numbers of birds (lots of small birds, or fewer larger birds) in a given space and thus allows a degree of maximization of space usage, which 'birds per m$^{2'}$ would not.

By these measures of growth and efficiency, productivity has improved over the last 50 years by increasing the permitted (and technically possible) stocking density in sheds, and by genetic selection of birds for fast growth rate, improved FCE and higher breast yield as a percentage of the whole bird weight. A modern intensive unit operating with a fast-growing strain of bird would have a target FCR below 1.8, or an EPEF of 400. In fact, EPEF has become a marker of success, with, for example the Ross 400 club, to recognising producers who are achieve a European Production Efficiency Factor of over 400, and with some producers topping 450.

There has been an increase in public concern relating to the welfare of broiler chickens and to the use of antibiotics to control infection in broiler farming. Genetic selection for high growth rate, breast meat yield and low FCR has undoubtedly led to high potential for disease states linked with rapid skeletal, muscular system and cardiovascular system growth rates and compromised immunity (lameness, ascites, necrotic muscle disease and respiratory disease). In addition, deterioration in housing conditions as a result of high biological loading (high stocking density) can lead to high prevalence of skin diseases such as foot pad dermatitis, cellulitis, hock and breast burn and other welfare problems. This has been one of the motivations for consumers, especially in developed, more affluent societies, to choose broilers reared under alternative systems, for example, involving slower-growing strains of bird, lower stocking densities, and free-range, organic and other systems that may be able to provide higher welfare standards.

8.2 Production Systems

8.2.1 Chick Production

Most broiler chickens in intensive units originate from two international breeding companies; Aviagen (with the Ross, Hubbard, Arbor Acres, Indian River and Peterson brands) and

Cobb-Vantress (with the Cobb, Avian, Sasso and Hybro brands). Both of these companies produce several genotypes/strains of bird with specific characteristics, which differ slightly in terms of breast yield, growth rate, FCE and other characteristics. The commercial and biological rationale for these different strains is to produce a variety of strains best suited for different husbandry systems or geographical regions. The process by which the genetic merit of the parent pedigree stock is carried to the millions of final stage production birds involves a 'multiplication pyramid'. At each tier in the pyramid, fertile eggs are created, by mating hen and cock, and these eggs are hatched in a semi-automated process within a building known as a hatchery. Hatcheries receive fertilized eggs, incubate them, then distribute day-old broiler chicks to the production farms. Hatcheries have become very large, with single hatcheries capable of producing over a million chicks per week. To enable this, the process has become highly automated with chicks being handled in large numbers, and in some countries and some companies, at high speed. Fertile eggs arrive from the breeder farms where the males and females have been kept and mated to produce fertile eggs. The 'quality' of the fertile eggs – their cleanliness, the absence of deformed, broken or cracked eggs, and the care with which they have been stored and transported – affects the hatching outcomes. Typical hatchability rates are in the range 82 to 90%, i.e. between 10% and % of eggs were either not fertile or did not develop into a viable chick.

A relatively recent move in egg and chick handling is the process whereby eggs are hatched 'in the house'. Fertilized eggs at about 18 days of development are taken from the incubators at the hatchery and placed on trays in the shed. The house temperature and humidity are set up to suit chick hatching, and biosecurity arrangements must be in place to protect from early-onset disease. The chicks hatch out in the trays on the floor or on a tracked system in the house and can find food and water within a short time. Potential welfare concerns with this are that compromised chicks, which would have been humanely destroyed in the hatchery, must similarly be handled and destroyed humanely on farm. Additionally, farm staff must take on a new set of skills – namely careful house temperature and humidity control during the hatch period, and observation and humane handling of chicks immediately after hatch.

After hatching, chicks are vaccinated against various diseases, depending on local disease status. This usually involves release of an aerosol so that the chicks receive their vaccine through inhalation of droplets. Some vaccines (e.g. for Marek's disease) may be injected into the egg. Birds may then be individually sexed by trained operatives, although the majority of broiler flocks are mixed-sex ('as hatched', approximately 50/50 male to female ratio). A minority of producers raise male and female birds separately because of their differing growth characteristics. Most modern strains of broiler chicks can now be sexed according to feather appearance: day-old females have longer primary wing feathers than males. In high-throughput hatcheries, chicks are handled using mechanical systems, including high-speed conveyors. After grading, and vaccination, the chicks are placed in transport trays, and loaded into environmentally controlled vehicles and transported to growing houses.

8.2.2 Intensive Rearing Systems

Standards required for different housed systems for broiler chicken production are summarised in Box 1. Day-old chicks require house temperatures of approximately 32°C at placement. This high initial temperature is gradually reduced throughout the flock cycle, according to a pre-planned programme, to about 21–23°C when the birds are 5 weeks of age. House temperatures throughout the flock cycle are controlled by the use of in-house heating, which may be through gas or oil combustion in the house, through external boilers, or most recently, through biomass energy systems which burn wood or plant material outside of the house and transmit the heat into the house through water heat exchange systems. In some countries, under-floor heating is becoming increasingly common in new poultry house builds. Temperature and air flow are adjusted by changing the rate of flow of fans, by altering the number of fans operating, by use of evaporative cooling systems (very common in hot and tropical countries), and by altering the number and opening of air inlets. Management of house temperature and ventilation is, in the majority of farms, controlled semi automatically, and sensors in the house interact with the control computer, which is fed information on house temperature & humidity, and sometimes CO_2, CO, and ammonia levels, and also, in

---

Box 8.1 Comparison between standards required for different housed systems for broiler chicken production. (For further explanation see text.)

European Union (from 2010)
  Maximum stocking density 42 mg/m^2
  Minimum light level 20 lux
  Required dark period 6 hours
  Environmental enrichment: not specified
Red Tractor Farm Assured (UK)
  Maximum stocking density: broilers 38 kg/m^2, poussin 30 kg/m^2
  Minimum light level 20 lux
  Required dark period 6 hours
  Environmental enrichment: bales/boxes, at least one wrapped or treated bale/1000
    birds evenly spaced throughout the house.
Perches/platforms, not more than 15 cm above the ground, 2 linear metres of perches
  or 0.3 m^2 platform per 1000 birds
Pecking objects: at least one per 1000 birds
RSPCA Assured
  Maximum stocking density 30 mg/m^2
  Light level: Natural daylight must be provided: at all times during the natural day-
    light period through all the required openings. No area of the house must be lit at
    less than 20 lux.
Required dark period 6 hours
  Environmental enrichment: not specified

some systems, information on external climate conditions (wind, humidity, temperature) from weather sensors on the farm. Many integrated house control systems can signal status and alarms to the producer remotely, and the data from the house control system can be viewed remotely from the farm or the company office.

8.2.2.1 Brooding

Day-old chicks may be reared under brooders (gas-fired heaters) for the first few days of the flock cycle in order to prevent chilling, and to give them local temperature 'choice'. Alternatively, the entire house may be heated ('whole-house brooding'). Feed crumbs may be initially provided on paper placed on the house floor to encourage pecking and early feeding, as chicks are keen to peck small particles but do not initially distinguish between food and non-food items. Meat chicks may be further vaccinated during the flock cycle, delivered by aerosol or in the drinking water. Diseases controlled by vaccination include infectious bronchitis, infectious bursal disease (Gumboro disease), Newcastle disease and Marek's disease. Coccidiosis, a disease of the intestines caused by microscopic, spore-forming, single-celled intracellular parasites, may be controlled by vaccination or the inclusion of anticoccidial agents in the feed, however, use of any antimicrobial agents is increasingly under scrutiny as a result of increasing concern over antimicrobial resistance (AMR). Ionophores used to control coccidiosis in broilers are animal-only antimicrobials and are classified as feed additives by the UK Government's Veterinary Medicines Directorate.

8.2.2.2 Feeding

Feed is provided by two types of system; circular pan feeders fed by a long screw auger, or a continuous track feeder, which is open on its top surface and feed is pulled along its length by a chain. Broiler rations are based on cereals, together with supplements formulated to provide a balanced supply of metabolizable energy, amino acids, minerals and vitamins at different stages of growth. It should be noted that birds at five weeks of age (35 days), which would be a common age at slaughter, are still very immature, with only partly complete skeletal development, and not having reached sexual maturity. This impacts on nutritional requirements in that broiler birds are still very much in the 'growth' phase of early life. The starter ration containing 22–23% protein is usually fed as a crumb. After 3 weeks the feed will usually be pelleted and contain about 21% protein. Water may be provided in circular bell feeders or by rows of nipples, which may be fitted with drip trays or 'cups', which reduce leakage and so tend to improve litter quality by reducing litter moisture. The ratio of bird drinkers or drinker space per bird and the overall length of track available per bird are critical to prevent competition for feed and water between birds. Feed and water are usually provided constantly, i.e. *ad libitum*, throughout the flock cycle. Water may be treated with peroxide or chlorine products to reduce bacterial contamination. Several successive diets, the composition of which are suited to the different stages of growth, are usually fed, with the final 'withdrawal diet' provided for the last five to seven days containing no coccidiostat, to prevent residues of these agents entering the food chain.

8.2.2.3 Lighting

Lighting programmes are usually 24 hours of light during the first week of the cycle, to encourage young chicks to feed, and then again during the last week of the cycle to reduce 'flightiness' and the risk of damage to birds when sheds are depopulated. However, light intensity is usually low (10–20 lux; see Table 8.1). The EU Broiler Directive (2007), which came into force in 2010, for birds of 1 week of age and over, requires a continuous dark period of at least 4 hours in every 24 hours, and six hours of darkness in total in a 24-hour period. Birds given significant dark periods of over approximately 4 hours do not feed during dark periods but fill their crops ('crop up') immediately prior to the dark period and then feed again immediately after the lights come on. Lights may be controlled by a dimmer switch, which allows a gradual reduction and increase in light levels at the beginning (dusk) and the end (dawn) of the dark period: this is known as dawn/dusk dimming.

8.2.2.4 Litter Management

Broiler chickens are usually housed on litter material, usually initially of depth about 5 cm, although litter may be shallow in some systems. Litter materials include long or chopped straw, wood shavings or chips (Figure 8.2), sawdust, straw/wood shaving combinations,

Table 8.1 Prevalence of contact dermatitis in UK broiler flocks.

	Mean %	Range %
Foot pad dermatitis	11	0–76
Hock-burn	1.3	0–33
Breast-burn	<0.01	0–0.12

Source: Haslam et al. (2007).

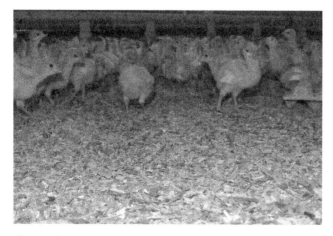

Figure 8.2 Wood shaving litter material (A Butterworth).

paper products, hemp, rice hulls, peat or earth. Litter may be replenished during the flock cycle if it becomes wet or greasy, but this is not always the case as introduction of litter into the house in quantity once the birds are partially grown is difficult and disturbing to the birds. In most European countries, it is routine to dispatch birds from all houses on the unit within a few days, remove all the litter and clean and disinfect and/or fumigate all houses, including feeder and drinker systems, before the next batch of chicks arrives. Swabs may be taken from house walls and equipment for bacteriology after cleaning and disinfection to check that these procedures have been effective, including sampling for *Salmonella*. In other countries, such as the USA, houses may not be completely cleared between flocks: new litter is placed onto that already in the house.

8.2.2.5 Stocking Densities

The stocking rate at which the birds are placed in traditional, intensive commercial houses varies between different areas of the world. In the most intensive housing systems it may exceed 45 kg/m^2 (i.e. provide an area of less than 500 cm^2/bird). EU and UK Codes of Welfare recommend that stocking rates should not exceed 42 kg/m^2 (Table 8.1). In practice many companies set maximum stocking densities below the theoretical legal maximum, for example, in the UK the AFS/Red Tractor (Red Tractor AFS 2018) specifies a maximum of 38 kg/m^2, and RSPCA Assured (RSPCA 2017) a maximum of 30 kg/m^2. In hot countries, the practical maximum stocking density may be in the region of 30 kg/m^2 in order to prevent potentially lethal conditions of temperature and humidity within the house when outside temperatures are high. Many companies have a policy of placing birds initially at high stocking rates, then later taking part of the flock out during the flock cycle in order to make more efficient use of the floor area. This practice is known as 'thinning' and may be carried out several times (often twice) during one flock cycle. Thinning is known to cause stress to both the birds removed and those remaining in the house. Many flocks tested negative for the food poisoning organism *Campylobacter* have been shown to become positive after thinning: thus thinning may represent a risk to human health as well as a compromise to bird welfare.

8.2.3 Less Intensive Indoor Systems

Less intensive indoor systems typically stock at up to 30 or 34 kg/m^2 as birds approach slaughter weight (600 to 650 cm^2/bird) and may have other modifications aimed at improving bird welfare. Some use slower-growing bird genotypes and/or restrict feed in order to reduce growth rate, and the broiler genetics companies can supply slow(er) growing strains such as Ranger Gold (Aviagen). There are various environmental enrichments which are compulsory in some poultry standards, such as windows in the shed, toys, perches, platforms and/or straw bales. There may also be a policy of not thinning for some 'higher welfare' schemes. In Europe, some large retailers incorporate these higher environmental standards into their producer requirements as part of their ethical sourcing policy. The RSPCA farm assurance scheme, 'RSPCA Assured' has articulated the following view on growth rate:

The RSPCA is concerned about the practice of deliberately slowing the growth rate of fast-growing broilers by adjusting either the quality or quantity of their feed to delay the time taken to reach slaughter weight, as can be the case when rearing fast-growing broilers in free-range systems: for example slowing the growth rate of a fast-growing broiler to reach typical slaughter weight at 81 instead of 49 days of age.

Broilers should be fed a diet that allows them to achieve their genetic growth rate potential. Therefore, when selecting broilers, their genetic growth rate potential should be as closely matched as possible to the time required to reach the desired weight at the time of slaughter.

(RSPCA Assured 2017)

The RSPCA Assured Scheme also prohibits thinning and requires environmental enrichment. These quality assurance schemes usually include regular audits to ensure that standards are being maintained (see Chapter 18). Birds from low-intensity, indoor systems cost more to produce than a traditional intensive bird but can sell at a premium price.

8.2.4 Free-range Systems

Free-range birds are housed in littered sheds, but have daytime access to a ranging area, through popholes (doors of a specified size) fitted at ground level in the walls of the shed. Free range systems have developed to meet a demand from consumers who consider that free-range birds experience a higher level of welfare than intensively reared birds and that the meat quality and taste are better. Free-range birds sell at a higher price than low-intensity indoor birds. Slower growth rates and greater age at slaughter may contribute to improved meat quality and will certainly reduce the prevalence of leg problems, and there is potential for these birds to experience a 'richer' life, with opportunities for behaviours not possible indoors such as dustbathing in soil, foraging, eating grass, 'sun-bathing', exposure to sun, wind, rain, and space to allow full expression of their behavioural range. However, problems can arise if the quality of husbandry is inadequate. Poor cover on range or inadequate perimeter fencing may increase the actual risk of predation, or the fear of predation. Poor litter and fouled ground around popholes may increase the incidence of contact dermatitis on the feet, termed 'foot pad dermatitis', especially if stocking density in the shed is high. The provision of environmental enrichment, bird protection measures and contact dermatitis are discussed in more detail later in this chapter.

There is also a market in some countries for organically produced broiler chickens. The specific requirements of different certification bodies vary but all organic schemes require birds to be fed on organically produced food, have access to range, to be slaughtered at older ages than conventionally reared birds, and to receive pharmacological products, such as antibiotics, only when they are essential to treat clinical disease. In the EU, the precise requirements for husbandry systems, which label birds as 'free range' and 'traditional free range', are laid down in the Poultry Marketing Directive.

8.2.5 Village Chicken Production

Chickens are a valuable source of high-quality protein in many rural areas in Africa and Asia. The FAO provides guidance and data on village chicken production (FAO 1998, 2014, 2019). Typical flock sizes vary from less than 10 up to around 100 birds, use indigenous, unimproved genotypes and birds are not segregated by age or gender. Smaller flocks are usually unhoused and receive little or no supplemental feeding; they are expected to scavenge for themselves. Birds are kept for eggs and meat. Approximately 20% of mature birds are likely to be in lay at any time. Birds eaten for meat are mature birds, as opposed to young birds in large scale commercial production, including non-laying hens. The productivity of the birds is extremely low in comparison with large intensive units and characterized by low hatchability and high mortality due to disease and predation, especially of chicks.

One aspect of the FAO reports is that they outline potential improvements for village chicken production, based on producer participation and aimed at increasing management skills, improving the way the final product is used and the use of marketing strategies. The recommendation is that the initial step in any programme aimed at improving bird productivity should be to identify and direct resources at the major problems occurring at village level. These are most commonly attributed to predators or infectious disease, especially Newcastle disease (ND). Locally run vaccination programmes for control of ND have allowed many families to expand their flocks without necessarily having to spend money on purchasing more feed. The FAO also recommend the introduction of 'improved genotypes': birds with higher-yielding traits. The potential for this is obvious provided there is sufficient food for both humans and chickens.

8.3 Health and Welfare Problems in the Production Unit

8.3.1 Mortality

Mortality in broilers may be caused by infectious and non-infectious conditions, including heat stress, and pulmonary hypertension syndrome (PHS) or 'flip-over', which is due to right-sided heart failure.

8.3.1.1 Using Mortality as a Welfare Assessment Measure

Levels of mortality in groups of animals may be used as a welfare assessment measure, however, 'being found dead' (i.e. a bird which was not detected to be sick and died) is a very blunt indicator of welfare – as it is the process of dying. For this reason, information on culling (see section below) is also important when using 'dead birds – culled and mortality' as a measure of welfare. The EU Broiler Directive (EC, 2007) requires farm mortality levels to be recorded. In studies of broiler chicken farms in the UK, the mean mortality level on farm was 4.1% (range 1.4% to 14.7%; Dawkins et al. 2004). However, it should be noted that a farm with 14.7% mortality would be in economic as well as health and welfare difficulties. For these reasons, 'mortality figures' for broiler flocks should be interpreted with caution when used as a welfare assessment measure, since they are likely to include in the same figure birds which have died or been culled both for reasons of sickness and injuries such as lameness. Where a farmer is rapidly and effectively identifying diseased or injured birds and humanely killing them, the overall welfare state of the birds on the farm may be good. Where culled birds are included in the mortality figure, a farmer may be tempted not to cull lame or diseased birds, with the hope that they will live long enough to be loaded for transport to the slaughter plant. The suffering of these diseased birds will be prolonged, and they are more likely to die due to stresses of handling and transportation, so increasing the number of birds found 'dead on arrival' at the slaughter plant.

8.3.1.2 Culling

When it is necessary to cull birds on farm, they are customarily killed by 'neck-pulling', which disarticulates the spinal column and breaks the spinal cord. However, disruption of the spinal cord without rupture of the carotid arteries in the neck, which supply blood to the brain, simply stops respiratory movement: there is evidence that birds killed by this method may be conscious for several minutes prior to brain death. Portable percussion stunner devices are commercially available (Figure 8.3) for bird euthanasia on-farm, and these can cause instant loss of consciousness. Currently percussive stunning is more commonly used for turkeys, but it is also effective for broiler chicken euthanasia, so long as the bird can be restrained to allow accurate placement of the stunning device.

8.3.2 Lameness

Studies in the UK found that a significant number of conventionally produced intensive birds are lame in the week before they are slaughtered (Knowles et al. 2008). One method for describing the walking ability of a bird is the 'Bristol Gait Score' (Kestin et al. 1992), which has a scale from 0, walking normally (e.g. a healthy free-range laying hen), to 5, completely

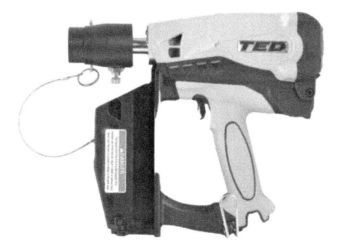

Figure 8.3 A percussive stunner for emergency slaughter of poultry (Bock 2019).

unable to walk. Birds at gait score 3 are obviously lame, their movement is greatly restricted and this reduces their frequency of visits to feeders and drinkers. Other lameness scoring assessment scales exist – including those of Aydin et al. (2010), Corr et al. (2007) and Garner et al. (2002). The overall activity of birds of higher gait scores using the Bristol score (Kestin et al. 1992) is reduced, and they are reluctant to remain standing. A number of farm assurance schemes require birds with a gait score of 3 or above to be culled on humane grounds: e.g. the RSPCA Assured Standard (RSPCA 2017) which states: *'There must not be any overtly lame birds (Bristol gait score 4 or above').*

Most lameness in broiler chickens is due to developmental abnormalities of the leg bones and joints. Lameness can also occur because of joint infections caused by bacteria such as *Staphylococcus aureus* and *Enterococcus caecorum* (IVH 2019), and it is possible that infectious causes of lameness are exacerbated by rapid growth in the broiler. The main causal factor would appear to be damage to growth plates, the rapidly growing end of the bone, when the bones are very soft. It has been shown that the prevalence of lameness in broiler chickens may be reduced by using slower-growing genotypes or by restricted feeding during the first weeks of growth, e.g. by feeding in meals, rather than *ad libitum*, by providing feed which has a lower nutritional density or by increasing the duration of the dark period, during which birds do not eat (Knowles et al. 2008).

8.3.3 Contact Dermatitis

Higher stocking densities tend to cause increased litter moisture and ammonia, which may result in contact dermatitis, a condition where the skin is altered by contact, turning it black. Lesions of contact dermatitis are commonly found on the foot pads (foot pad dermatitis, FPD, Figure 8.4), hock (hock-burn) and breast (breast-burn). Severe contact dermatitis lesions may penetrate the dermis, which is innervated, and are therefore likely to be painful. A high incidence of contact dermatitis in a flock usually indicates that the birds have experienced poor litter and air quality during the flock cycle. Birds from houses with poor litter quality but with good leg health tend to have high prevalence of FPD alone, whereas birds from houses with poor litter quality and also with poor leg health tend to have a higher prevalence of hock and breast burn, as they tend to spend longer periods of time with the hock and breast in contact with the litter.

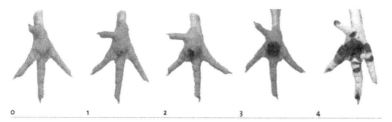

Figure 8.4 Foot pad dermatitis: examples of severity scored on a scale of 0 to 4 (WelfareQuality®, A Butterworth).

The prevalence of contact dermatitis may be reduced by use of wood shavings rather than straw as a litter material where this is a common substrate used, by adding additional litter during the flock cycle, by using nipples with cups rather than bell drinkers (the use of bell drinkers for broilers is becoming increasingly rare in broiler units, but still in common use for turkeys), by preventing drinker leaks, by reducing water pressure to the drinkers to reduce wastage of water, and by adjusting the ventilation to reduce humidity. Additionally, improved skin and footpad health is influenced by using less susceptible genotypes of birds, and by insulating pipes and water tanks, which may cause condensation, or relocating water tanks out of the area occupied by the birds. Litter may also be improved by increasing overall ventilation rates and, in cooler climates, through provision of under-floor heating, or heating which does not combust fuel in the house – as combustion creates water vapour, which adds to house humidity and therefore to litter moisture content.

8.3.4 Infectious Disease

An outbreak of infectious disease on an intensive commercial unit containing many thousands of birds can be very economically costly for the producer and may present a severe cost to bird welfare. The overall effect on welfare of any disease may be described by a combination of the variables; number of birds affected (morbidity), the number dying (mortality), and the severity (pain and malaise), and duration of suffering. Most of the major infectious diseases in poultry can be controlled through vaccination, However, antimicrobial and anticoccidial drugs can still play a role in the control of infectious disease in poultry houses, and their careful use has a very important potential role in protecting bird welfare in the face of a disease challenge. However, it is well recognized in the poultry business in the developed world that avoidance of the use of antimicrobials, unless clearly indicated to protect bird health and welfare is critical to protect the efficacy of existing antimicrobials.

8.3.4.1 Biosecurity

Biosecurity is an essential element of disease control on intensive poultry units. Unnecessary visitors should be discouraged and essential visitors should either be required to leave vehicles outside the farm or use a wheel wash or even car wash installed at the farm entrance. Visitors should be required to wear disposable, house-specific protective clothing and boots and use disinfectant footbaths and hand washes. Some farms use a barrier system at the entrance to each house, where people entering the house are required to put on house-specific clothing and boots which are kept on the house side of the barrier, leaving their own boots on the outside. In some countries, for example Thailand and Chile, for very large farms and for very high-value birds, extreme biosecurity measures are taken, which may include one or more showers and complete changes of clothes, disinfection of the interior of vehicles and fumigation, or ultraviolet light treatment, of any equipment taken onto the farm. For large commercial farms worldwide, records of previous sites visited by people or vehicles are usually kept in order to help enable the tracking of disease should it be found to be moving between sites.

8.3.5 Heat Stress

High levels of mortality may occur in broilers due to heat stress (high temperature and humidity) if mechanical ventilation systems fail. Almost all large commercial houses rely on electric fans. Because of the reliance on the electrical supply to provide ventilation, most farm assurance schemes demand installation of high temperature alarms, which sound in the house and, usually automatically, call a pager or telephone a stockperson to alert him/her if the power, ventilation or water fail. For the same reasons, back-up generators are also usually required by farm assurance standards, which can be started automatically in case of mains electricity supply failure and should incorporate an alarm if the auto-start fails.

Birds regulate temperature by panting and changed behaviour (aligning with air flow, reduced feed intake and reduced activity) if the environmental temperature is high, and by huddling and increased feed intake if the house temperature is low. The producer will observe bird behaviour and use this as part of the adjustment process for house ventilation and humidity control. When external air temperature exceeds 30°C, heat stress in poultry will be likely to occur in houses with mechanical ventilation alone. Beyond about 30°C the forced air may be cooled through the latent heat of evaporation of water. Evaporative 'cooling pad' systems are a part of the house/ventilation system design in hot countries, and these can enable air temperatures within the house to be reduced to levels within the thermo-tolerant zone of the birds. Misting systems and evaporative cooling systems need to be used with care to ensure that they do not create excessive humidity in the house. The relationship between safe temperature and safe humidity for broiler chickens is shown in Figure 8.5. This illustrates that it is the combination of air temperature and relative humidity (RH) which are important – and the interactions of temperature and humidity are what may put birds are at

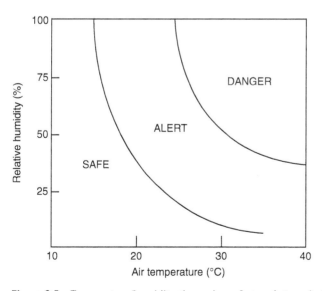

Figure 8.5 Temperature/humidity, thermal comfort and stress index. Reproduced from 'The Welfare of Poultry at Slaughter or Killing' © Crown copyright 2007.

risk. For example, a combination of an air temperature of 30°C and a RH of 60% would just put birds into the danger zone, whilst a temperature of 28°C and 90% humidity will also put birds at risk. This chart can be applied not only in the poultry house, but also in transport – where temperatures and humidity may rise due to high stocking density of birds in transport modules, and in the lairage where birds are waiting for slaughter, sometimes with poor air flow because the modules are no longer moving on the back of the truck but are static. In all systems, including backyard and hobby flocks, the effects of heat stress on birds may be reduced by maximizing the balance of ventilation and humidity through cooling systems, by reducing or withholding feed, which lowers metabolic rate and so reduces heat production by birds, and by reduction in bird numbers or stocking density (when prolonged high temperatures are anticipated) to reduce the amount of heat generated within the building. One broiler produces about 12 watts, so the heat generated within a house containing 30,000 birds would be about 35 kW.

In emergency it is possible to temporarily reduce house temperatures with sprinkler systems, which operate sporadically to produce a very fine mist or fog, which evaporates before hitting the litter. However, by raising the humidity, the overall impact on bird capacity to regulate temperature can be impacted if the humidity becomes too high, for too (Figure 8.5) and so sprinkler systems are not for continuous use, but for infrequent use.

8.3.5.1 Risks in Naturally Ventilated and Free-range Systems

Free-range and organic production systems operating in temperate climates do not usually have electrically controlled ventilation with fitted alarm systems. However, birds in some large, more densely stocked, naturally ventilated houses, with no access to range, are at risk of death due to heat stress in hot weather. These types of house should therefore be fitted with high temperature alarms and provision to increase air movement by mechanical ventilation when necessary. Birds with access to range may be able to escape the problem of heat stress in densely stocked buildings (provided they choose to go outside), and this is assisted if the birds out of doors have cover from direct sunlight (trees, shade shelters). Provision of overhead cover on the range will encourage birds to use the range. It provides protection from direct sunlight and some shelter from wind. It provides real protection from overhead predators and, more importantly in most circumstances, it provides birds with a sense of security since it reduces the perceived threat of predation. Cover may include shrubs, trees, long grass, biomass vegetation, netting, or low plastic tables and should cover as much of the range area as possible. Where separate shelters are provided, they should be sited close together to ensure that birds are not in the open for long periods when moving from one covered area to another.

The range area for free range birds should be designed and maintained to minimize both the real risk and the birds' perceived risk of predation, both from the air (birds of prey) and the ground (foxes, coyotes, cats). The farmer must then ensure that the perimeter fences surrounding the ranging area are constructed to exclude predators, either by height (for those that can jump), through the use of barbed wire or electrical fencing. In some areas it may be necessary to bury the fence below the ground to exclude burrowing predators. Perimeter fences should be regularly checked for integrity and well maintained. Electrical fences should be checked more frequently and kept free of vegetation to prevent shorting out the fence. Consideration should be given to installing electrical failure alarms and having a back-up electrical supply for the fence to provide power in case of failure.

8.3.6 Pulmonary Hypertension Syndrome

Pulmonary hypertension syndrome (PHS) may cause mortality or poor welfare due to right-sided heart failure. The prevalence is greater in some genotypes of birds, on farms with low temperatures, and at high altitudes. PHS can also be precipitated by acute stress, such as unexpected changes in light or sound in the house, moving birds, or thinning, and may be reduced by selection of less susceptible bird genotypes and careful control of house temperatures. It can also be reduced through the practice of dawn/dusk dimming, gradual rather than sudden switching between light and dark.

8.3.7 Environmental Enrichment

Bird welfare is thought to be improved by the provision of environmental enrichment, which is why some higher welfare accreditation schemes require such enrichments to be provided. For example the Red Tractor AFS scheme currently requires the following: (Red Tractor AFS 2018 *at least 1 bale/ box per 1000 birds used throughout the bird's life; 2 linear metres of perches per 1000 bird; 0.3 m^2 of platform per 1000 birds; at least 1 pecking object per 1000 birds.*

From October 2020, all Red Tractor AFS assured poultry houses in the UK will have windows to let in natural daylight.

Scientific evidence suggests that only enrichments that encourage natural exploration and foraging behaviour, such as the provision of straw bales, have a genuine effect in improving welfare. Access to range for chickens allows exploratory and ground-pecking behaviour, directed at different plants and invertebrates. Toys, compact discs, pecker blocks or balls are sometimes provided to encourage exploration, although birds rapidly habituate to these so that, although initially attractive, they may soon be ignored. Ground pecking on the soil or vegetation on the range is rewarding since it persists throughout the bird's life. Access to dry friable litter allows dust-bathing behaviour, but birds will not dust bathe in dirty, compacted or wet litter, and so it is not common to see reduced dust bathing in birds once litter has become dirty. Increased space allowance, in either indoor systems or those with range access, allows walking and running, dashing and sparring and wing flapping behaviour, which may not be possible in heavily stocked conventional houses, where there may be 15 birds in each m^2. Misting systems can encourage bathing and preening behaviour and perches may allow normal perching and roosting behaviour. However, although younger birds tend to use perches, fast-growing strains of birds in intensive systems tend not to use perches. Probable reasons for this include discomfort caused by leg disorders, difficulty in maintaining balance in birds with pronounced anatomical development of the breast muscle and difficulty in jumping up onto elongate perches once the birds reach higher body weights.

Birds kept in environments with a significant dark period of more than 4 continuous hours in a 24-hour cycle are generally more active and more reactive to stimuli than birds with less than 4 hours or no dark period. In the EU, and in many countries, birds must now be given a total of 6 hours of darkness in every 24 hours. Birds given significant dark periods throughout the flock cycle tend to have better leg health than those with short dark periods. However, there is evidence that birds which have had longer dark periods sustain more damage at depopulation than birds which have had shorter periods. This is presumably because more active birds are more difficult to catch. This problem can be reduced, by shortening the dark period during the last 3 to 7 days before catching.

8.4 Depopulation, Transport and Lairage

In very small systems, chickens may be killed for human consumption by neck dislocation, handheld electrical stunner system followed by exsanguination (or less commonly, using a percussive stunner, Figure 8.3) on the farm at the end of the flock cycle: this obviates the need for loading onto a transport vehicle, transportation and live shackling or gas stunning. However, nearly all birds from nearly all systems are caught and then transported in crates or modules on a transporter lorry to centralized slaughtering plants.

8.4.1 Depopulation

The best technique for collecting birds for slaughter would be to lift them individually, with both hands placed around the body to prevent wing flapping, so reducing bird stress and injury. Such best practice is followed in some Scandinavian countries, and in some Asian countries, that have well-enforced legislation to protect bird welfare, or where the value of birds is high, relative to labour costs, and so the number of catching personnel can be high, as in some South American & Asian countries. Houses may be depopulated at night to reduce the risk of heat stress. Many large commercial broiler chicken producers run training courses in bird handling in order to reduce injury and stress to birds and reduce carcass damage due to handling: such courses may include a visit to the slaughter plant to view carcass damage to birds on the line. Routine monitoring of carcass damage, feedback of levels of carcass damage to catchers and their managers, and bonus payment schemes for low carcass damage all contribute to reducing stress and damage at depopulation.

There is nevertheless evidence that house depopulation procedures may often cause very poor bird welfare, especially where labour costs are high and broiler meat relatively inexpensive since this encourages very rapid loading, low numbers of catching operatives, and increases the occurrence of injury to birds. Up to five or six birds may be carried by the legs, five in each hand, causing problems including hip dislocation (Gregory and Austin 1992), bruising and fractures. Many companies now use modular systems with drawers, which can be taken into the house, using a forklift truck, or rolled into the house on temporary roller track-ways, to limit the distance over which the birds have to be carried inverted from catching to placement in the modules. How the birds are placed in the module – carefully, or roughly, makes a significant difference to both the birds' welfare and to the quality of the carcass.

Poor bird welfare and carcass damage at depopulation may also be influenced by the use of mechanical depopulation, using one of the various commercially available 'harvesting' machines. Birds appear to show less fear response when catching machines approach, in comparison to human catchers, and may sustain less injury than with conventional methods of manual catching because they are not inverted or carried by their legs. However, 'harvesting' machines are expensive, are only economically viable for large broiler production companies and must be carefully controlled, set up and operated to ensure that birds are not injured. They can only be used in larger open-span houses, where there are no roof supports in the body of the house. They are complex machines, and if unreliable, can result in catching problems for the birds.

8.4.2 Transport

Levels of mortality due to heat stress may be high during transport of birds to the slaughter plant, or when held in lairage when ambient temperatures and humidity within the modules are high. Birds are at a greater risk of suffering from heat stress when there is a breakdown of transporter vehicles or delays at the slaughter plant due to line breakdown. Consequently, in countries with seasonal differences in ambient temperatures and relative humidity, the prevalence of birds found dead on arrival (DoAs) is usually considerably higher during summer, rather than winter months. Losses due to heat stress may be reduced by careful programming of catching and killing, to reduce waiting times in the lairage, by reducing stocking levels in transport crates, separating crates in the lairage to improve air circulation between crates, providing covered lairages (to keep birds out of direct sunlight) and providing an adequate number of fans, sometimes with misting systems, to cool birds by increasing air movement and reducing temperature.

In countries where daytime temperatures are usually high, such as in southern Europe or in Asia, birds are always collected and slaughtered at night and bird transporters are built with an air gap running longitudinally down the centre of the lorry trailer, between stacks of crates, to improve airflow around the birds. In hot climates, bird transporter vehicles may be placed under a shelter surrounded by 'curtains' of circulating air to keep temperatures low. The risk of heat stress in lorries and lairages may be monitored by routine recording of air temperature and humidity at bird level. Some companies monitor both lorry movement by GPS, and local bird temperatures during transport using dataloggers. Heat stress can be assessed by observation of the birds themselves; especially the proportion of birds panting (mouth-breathing) with beak open. If over 50% of birds are panting, and panting for more than a few minutes, then immediate action is required to reduce the risk of high mortality due to heat stress.

8.4.3 Stunning and Slaughter

The methods for stunning and killing poultry permitted by Regulation EC 1099/2009 in the EU are:

- *Electrical water bath stunning (about 80% of broilers [EC 2012]) – the birds move through a water bath suspended by the legs on a shackle, and their heads are immersed in water which*

> *carries the stunning current from the head through the body to the electrical contact in the shackle.*
> - *Gas stunning (about 20% of broilers) – usually progressing to gas killing through hypoxia – use of gases, commonly carbon dioxide, or carbon dioxide in association with inert gases such as Nitrogen, Argon, or inert gases only.*
> - *Head-only electrical stunning (very small numbers) – the use of manually operated 'tongs' which produce current flow across the head, and are most commonly used in turkeys, ducks and breeder poultry.*
> - *Penetrating and non-penetrating captive bolt, firearms (casualty animals on farm,* Figure 8.3*) – used for emergency on farm or casualty killing of birds on farm, and sometimes used for killing of larger birds including turkeys and ostrich.*
> - *Head-to-body electrical stunning (almost no birds killed in this way) – theoretically possible for use on poultry, applying the current from the head to electrodes on the body and inducing both a stunned state and cardiac arrest – predominately used in sheep, cattle and pigs.*

Currently almost all broiler chickens in the EU are slaughtered either by the electrical water bath (approximately 80%) or by gas stunning (approximately 20%).

If birds are stunned or killed using electrical stunning, or in a controlled-atmosphere chamber, they are then slaughtered and bled by a neck cut that severs the carotid arteries. Both stunning and neck cutting are automated but there should always be a human manual back-up neck cutter, to check that birds have been effectively stunned and neck cut, and this person needs to be replaced every 20 to 30 minutes, to prevent fatigue. EFSA (2014a, 2014b) has recommended that alternatives to water-bath stunning should be developed, as water baths in practical use may not ensure humane killing and hence not be capable of ensuring good animal welfare.

8.4.3.1 Electrical Stunning

For electrical stunning, birds are inverted onto a 'shackle line', a moving chain from which hang curved, metal shackles into which the legs of the birds are placed. Inversion of birds for shackling is stressful and birds with leg pathology experience pain when placed firmly into shackles, especially at high line speeds of up to 200 birds per minute in large plants, when the procedure must be performed very quickly. Bird stress at shackling may be reduced by providing a darkened, noise-free environment, by ensuring that shackle size is appropriate for the size of bird being killed, and by training operators to shackle birds in a two-stage process: the first person places the bird loosely in the shackle, reducing pressure on the legs, the second then pulls each loosely hung bird firmly into the shackle. Bird stress at shackling points and in areas through which the live bird line passes may be reduced by providing blue, or reduced intensity, lighting. 'Breast comforters', which consist of rubber strips placed in parallel with the bird line and along which the birds rub, can reduce activity levels and wing flapping. Live bird shackle lines should be straight, without bends, jolts or abrupt changes in height, and the line between hanging and stunning should be as short as is practical, with the bird being suspended for just long enough to settle after hanging, approximately 10 to 12 seconds before they are stunned. The effectiveness of measures taken to reduce bird stress can be monitored by recording the number of birds flapping on the live bird line, which should, in the best circumstances, be zero.

For electrical stunning, the head of the bird is immersed in a water bath and an electric current passed between the shackle line, through the body and head of the bird, into the water. Entrance ramps to electric stun baths should be constructed to provide a shallow incline to a sudden drop, thus ensuring that the head of the bird enters the bath suddenly. If the bird makes contact with electrified water before it is able to have its head immersed, then the wing, beak or neck will receive a non-stun 'shock' known as a pre-stun shock, and the bird will flap, pull away, vocalize and so indicate that it has been shocked but not stunned. Pre stun shocks are likely to be extremely painful. The adequacy of the entrance ramp to an electric stun bath may be monitored by recording the number of birds receiving a pre-stun shock in a given time period. Birds receiving an effective single stun display a single, immediate stiffening with their head properly immersed in the water, and a rapid single wing movement, to bring the wings sharply against the body. Birds receiving pre-stun shocks show multiple wing flaps and sometimes vocalization, and may attempt to 'fly the stunner', i.e. keep their heads out of the water bath by violent wing flapping.

The factors that determine the efficacy of electrical stunning are complex (see, for example, EFSA 2004, 2013, 2014a, 2014b). Many abattoirs use low-frequency stunning (50 Hz AC) and a current of over 105 milliamps per bird to ensure an adequate stun. Effectively stunned birds will not react to neck cutting, will show no rhythmic respiratory movement, no righting reflex (attempt to assume an upright position) or corneal reflex (i.e. they should not blink when the front of the eye is touched). The neck cut should be made as close as possible to the exit of the stunner. Effectiveness of stunning should be monitored by a manual operator standing immediately downline from the automated neck cutter. Birds may appear to be adequately stunned at the exit to the stunner but may recover consciousness on the bleed rail if the cut is inadequate for the bird to bleed to death before it recovers from the stun. Birds that are conscious when they enter the automated feather plucker because they have not been cut or have been cut inadequately constitute a very serious welfare problem. Uncut, and therefore unbled, birds are obvious as they appear as dark red carcasses on the line after exit from the plucker.

8.4.3.2 Stunning/Killing in a Controlled Atmosphere

The use of controlled atmosphere systems (CAS), for the killing of poultry, has become increasingly popular in the UK over recent years (CIWF 2018). In 2013, the Food Standards Agency's Animal Welfare Survey indicated that CAS accounted for 71% of poultry slaughtered in Great Britain (FSA 2013). The birds are 'introduced' to the gas by three possible means – by being passed though a gas filled tunnel, lowered in the module into a gas filled pit, or placed in the module in closed cabinets. The birds remain in their transport module throughout the killing process, and this can be beneficial from a welfare perspective, as this reduces the handling of the birds. Some systems do tip the birds from their modules before CAS stunning, and there are concerns over the impact on the birds of this. There is a potential problem in identifying birds which died in transport if the birds are killed in the CAS system without first being inspected. However, birds, which were dead on arrival at the plant should be distinguished from birds killed in the chamber by their bright red discolouration.

Most controlled-atmosphere stunning machines use high concentrations of carbon dioxide. However, inhalation of carbon dioxide at high concentration causes some distress, and so, in some systems currently in use in Europe, a two-stage process is used. Birds are first exposed to a low-concentration 'stunning' exposure, followed by a high-concentration killing exposure. This may reduce the intensity of distress but prolongs the time to loss of consciousness. In recent years, alternative methods using less aversive gases and gas mixtures have been developed and trialled for their effectiveness in stunning/killing, and their potential effects on bird welfare and carcass quality. Argon, for example, has been shown to be undetectable to birds, thus much less stressful than carbon dioxide. It is, however, much more expensive than carbon dioxide and it use can give rise to skin haemorrhages and so impair carcass quality.

A recent development in atmospheric stunning/killing systems is LAPS (Low Atmospheric Pressure Stunning/Killing) – in which gradual removal of air by pumps from a sealed chamber results in low oxygen tension, and induction of progressive hypoxia. In the available commercial systems, the time taken to create the low pressure is around 30 seconds. The LAPS system has recently been approved for use in broilers in the EU (EFSA 2014a, 2017).

8.5 Broiler Breeders: Parent, Grandparent and Great-Grandparent Flocks

Broiler chickens reared for meat production are sourced from flocks of parent birds, known as broiler breeders, which are in turn sourced from grandparent and great-grandparent flocks. Broiler breeders produce between 120 and 180 eggs in a laying cycle of approximately 47 weeks, depending on genotype. The birds are usually housed in climate-controlled, deep litter systems similar to meat birds but with rows of nest boxes, usually placed centrally along the longitudinal axis of the house on a raised, slatted area which constitutes approximately one-third of the house. Males and females are housed together throughout the flock cycle. Initially, the ratio of females to males is approximately 9:1. Broiler breeders are less heavily stocked than meat birds, at approximately 25 birds per square metre, including both male and female birds.

8.5.1 Welfare Problems for Broiler Breeders

8.5.1.1 Hunger

Broiler breeders are exposed to most of the same potential stresses as meat birds but also have additional, specific problems. The most significant of these, in terms of duration and severity, is hunger. One aspect of the genetic selection of broilers has been for very fast growth rates, and high muscle gain; with growth rates of over 100 g per day for some strains. If fed *ad libitum* broiler breeders would become very heavy; mortality rates would increase, and many birds would experience lameness problems before reaching sexual maturity at between 16 and 21 weeks of age, and mating, and so fertility, would be impaired by the high body weight of the birds. To prevent these issues, the growth rate of juvenile broiler breeder birds is controlled by restriction of feed, in terms of both nutrient density and volume. Adult male broiler breeders must be more feed restricted than females, as females require additional resources for egg production. This restriction is usually achieved by positioning metal wire racks over some of the feeders (Figure 8.6) which are separated into individual feeding places. The dimensions of the feeding places and the metal wire racks are designed so that they are too narrow for the head of cockerels, while permitting access to hens. This food restriction can create severe hunger, especially in male birds, which manifests itself as increased drinking and feeder-directed stereotypical pecking behaviours. Increase in drinking due to hunger can cause reduced litter quality, and this can be linked to contact dermatitis lesions. Competition between birds for food can lead to uneven growth in female flocks, which is very carefully managed by separating birds into groups by weight and moving individuals between the groups as they change between weight bands. Female juvenile broiler breeders are weighed frequently in order to control weight gain during growth (approximately 7% bodyweight gain per week) and weight control remains critical thereafter.

8.5.1.2 Injuries and Mutilations

Breeding hens may suffer from feather damage and skin wounds on the back due to mating. To help prevent this damage to hens during mating, the spur bud on the back of the leg of day-old male chicks is removed using a heated wire. Society is beginning to show significant concern for the welfare impacts of 'mutilations' – other mutilations in broiler breeders can include beak trimming/beak tipping, and removal of a specific toe at the first joint for the purpose of identification of pedigree birds, a practice which is distinct from de-clawing for

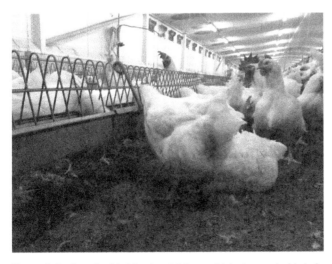

Figure 8.6 Breeder bird feed restrictors, which stop male birds from feeding from the female feed track (A Butterworth).

protection of females during mating and no longer considered as ethically justifiable. The dew claw and pivot claws of male broiler breeders may also be removed at this time using scissors, although genetic selection for birds with short, blunt spurs has made this unnecessary in some genotypes. In some countries, local legislation is beginning to cause a change away from mutilations. Damage to hens may also be reduced by progressively removing cockerels from the flock throughout the egg-laying cycle, to reduce the ratio of cockerels to hens.

Broiler breeders, and especially male birds, may be beak-trimmed to prevent injury due to feather pecking and cannibalism. Beak trimming can cause severe, lasting pain. The welfare consequences of beak trimming are reduced if carried out in young chicks, most particularly in the hatchery at 1 day of age, and if only the tip of the beak, which is not innervated, is removed. In many companies and for a number of standards, only infra-red beak tipping is permitted, and mechanical cutting of beaks is no longer permitted. Outbreaks of feather pecking and cannibalism can occur in broiler breeders. Feather pecking outbreaks are usually managed by reducing light intensity in the house but may be further reduced by the use of appropriate environmental enrichment, or use of divider boards in the breeder house to break up the house into more discrete areas. The combs of birds may be removed in some countries, at age 1 day-old, using sharp scissors, a practice known as 'dubbing', ostensibly to prevent comb damage. This practice is unnecessary in modern production systems.

8.5.2 Disease Control

Broiler breeders are economically valuable birds so often receive additional disease and biosecurity protection in comparison to meat birds. Biosecurity measures in place at broiler breeder farms tend to be stricter than those in place at final production meat bird farms; birds tend to receive additional vaccinations, both at the hatchery and on farm and are likely to be vaccinated for protection against coccidiosis rather than have coccidiostats in feed. Birds may be treated for ascaris worms at transfer to the laying house at approximately 18 weeks of age. Additional precautions to ensure that water is bacteriologically clean may be taken, such as ultraviolet-light treatment of water supplied to the birds. Daily water consumption may be monitored routinely, as sudden changes in water consumption can act as an early warning of a disease outbreak. Broiler breeders are at risk of red mite (*Dermanyssus gallinae*), a parasite which lives on the bird and in the house and feeds off birds' blood, usually at night. Birds may become anaemic and may even die in cases of severe infestation. Thorough cleaning of housing and equipment in the house, and the use of appropriate parasiticides are required to control this external parasite.

8.6 Broilers and Human Health

The principal risks to human health from broiler chickens are avian influenza, *Salmonella* and *Campylobacter*.

8.6.1 Avian Influenza

Avian influenza is a zoonosis, a disease which may pass between birds and humans, but which primarily infects domestic poultry but can be passed to humans, causing severe flu-like symptoms. Some strains of avian influenza virus can lead to death in approximately half of recognized human cases. All strains of avian influenza are carried by wild birds, which rarely show clinical signs of disease. Human cases of avian influenza have been linked to strains of five subtypes; H5N1, H7N3, H7N7, H7N9 and H9N2. These usually occur where there is very close contact between people and birds, such as for keepers of small flocks in rural locations, where birds are still traded individually at markets. Not all strains of avian influenza are pathogenic to humans. The H5N1 strain is highly pathogenic for poultry, transmissible from poultry to humans and has been recorded as passing *between* humans in very isolated cases. Since strains of influenza virus have a tendency to mutate there is a risk that the ability of the virus to pass between people may be enhanced. A vaccine has been developed to protect people against H5N1 and this and related vaccines have been available since 2008. The use of routine hygiene precautions, particularly if handling birds, including effective washing of hands and equipment, and adequate cooking of poultry products is recommended to reduce the risk of infection.

8.6.2 Salmonella

Salmonella bacteria are the most frequent causes of food poisoning in humans. There are many types and strains of *Salmonella*, some specific to poultry and some affecting many animal species. *Salmonella* infection in humans usually causes a mild to severe gastroenteritis, which may include fever, abdominal pain, diarrhoea, vomiting, dehydration and can progress to death in immunocompromised or frail individuals, or infants. Birds are rarely clinically ill as a result of carrying *Salmonella*, with the result that the risk to human health when handling birds is not as clear as, for example, strains of avian influenza which are pathogenic to birds, where affected birds are obviously clinically ill. People usually become infected through eating undercooked poultry products which are contaminated with *Salmonella*, or with food which has come into contact with contaminated products. In the EU, there is a legal requirement for member states to have a surveillance system in place to identify poultry flocks infected by *Salmonella*. For flocks known to be infected, additional precautions can be taken during slaughter, such as killing suspect infected birds last in the slaughter programme to minimize the risks of cross-contamination to uninfected carcasses.

 Salmonella is transmitted via the egg from the parent to the chick, and for this reason most control strategies aim to ensure that broiler breeder flocks are *Salmonella*-free, either by slaughtering infected flocks, or by vaccination. The risk of infection from outside is reduced by strict biosecurity precautions, as discussed earlier in 8.3.4.1. Breeder birds should be tested *Salmonella*-free, eggs taken to the hatchery should be clean and disinfected or fumigated, water on the farm should be chlorinated, feed should be heat or acid treated and should not be allowed to be contaminated by wild bird or other animal droppings, and litter should be clean when sourced and not allowed to be contaminated with rodent or bird faeces.

8.6.3 Campylobacter

Campylobacter spp. bacteria commonly infect poultry and colonise the hindgut, particularly the caecae. *Campylobacter jejuni* is the most common species found in poultry. *Campylobacter jejuni* infection is not currently considered to be pathogenic, i.e. it does not cause clear signs of clinical disease in the live bird, although it may be linked to 'Vibrionic Hepatitis' in poultry. About 80% of cases of human *Campylobacter* food poisoning in the UK are derived from poultry. People can get, and spread, campylobacter through cross-contamination of other foods, or their hands, or cooking utensils, from raw chicken. Human infection with *Campylobacter* causes fever, abdominal pain and diarrhoea, which is usually self-limiting. However, in about one out of 1,000 cases, the infection is followed two to three weeks later by Guillain-Barre syndrome, a debilitating inflammatory polyneuritis characterized by fever, pain and weakness that progresses to paralysis, which may be fatal unless intensive care facilities are available.

It is not clear whether vertical transmission of *Campylobacter*, via the egg, is possible, but most infections in meat birds seem to occur after they arrive at the farm. *Campylobacter* is ubiquitous and birds are thought to be contaminated from the environment, with one study showing that 30% of European starlings sampled on farms in Oxfordshire, United Kingdom, were carriers of *C. jejuni* (Colles et al. 2011). All of the birds in a house tend to have the same *Campylobacter* status, i.e. they are either all negative or all positive, and there is evidence that common husbandry procedures such as the difficulty in completely disinfecting a house between flocks, contamination as chicks in the hatchery, risk of exposure from wild birds, and shared water, shared feed, and shared bedding on the production farm, may increase the probability that a flock is positive and also increase the burden of infection, which will add to levels of potential contamination and cross-contamination at the slaughter plant.

Control methods include chlorination or other treatment of drinking water, reduction of feed withdrawal periods prior to depopulation for slaughter, reduction or elimination of the practice of thinning, and, potentially, the use of probiotics (competing microbial populations) in newly hatched chicks. None of these methods is entirely effective and *Campylobacter* contamination of poultry meat remains a common problem in most countries.

8.7 Assessing Broiler Chicken Welfare

Demands by consumers and retailers for ethical standards and satisfactory attention to animal welfare in food production have led to the development of farm assurance schemes and retailer assurance schemes. There is an emerging trend to assess animal welfare using animal based (rather than resource based) output measures, such as the percentage of lame birds, the prevalence and severity of foot pad dermatitis and walking ability, which are increasingly seen as more valid measures of welfare than, for example, repetitive assessment of the farmhouse dimensions and the provision of feeders and drinkers (Weeks and Butterworth 2004). For example, the 2017 RSPCA standards in the UK, require 'animal based' measures (many of which are collected at slaughter) to be assessed. These include lameness, hock burn, foot pad burn, breast blisters, back scratches, dirty feathers, emaciation, ascites/oedema, leg damage (caused prior to slaughter), wing damage (caused prior to slaughter), dead on arrivals (DOAs), cellulitis and dermatitis, joint lesions, and septicaemia/respiratory conditions.

In 2007 new EU rules were agreed (Council Directive 2007/43/EC) for protecting the welfare of chickens kept for meat production, and this 'Broiler Directive' came into force in the UK on 30 June 2010. The Directive requires the collection and monitoring of post-mortem condition data ('trigger conditions') when the birds are slaughtered to help identify poor welfare on-farm. The Directive provides for variable levels of stocking density dependent on the performance of the farm. It states that the basic maximum stocking density should not at any time exceed 33 kg/m^2, however, derogations permit higher stocking densities if it can be shown from outcome-based measures that these do not compromise bird health and welfare. Almost all farms in the UK meet these derogation requirements and their stocking density can go up to 39 kg/m^2 (or 38 kg/m^2 for Red Tractor standard).

In line with the requirements of the Directive, a number of animal-based outcome parameters are used to identify possible on-farm welfare problems. Cumulative daily mortality rate and seven post-mortem conditions are monitored: (1) ascites/oedema, (2) cellulitis and dermatitis, (3) dead on arrival, (4) emaciation, (5) joint lesions/arthritis, (6) septicaemia/respiratory and (7) total rejections. A trigger level has also been set for foot pad dermatitis (FPD), and data are collected if foot pad lesions are noted at slaughter.

8.8 Ethical Considerations, Summary and Conclusions

The key current drivers for agricultural production are for more efficient production: more and cheaper food. More recently, there has been a greater consideration of the sustainability of systems, including food production systems, where 'development meets the needs of the present without compromising the ability of future generations to meet their own needs' (Brundtland Commission 1987). This definition implicitly argues that the rights of future generations to have access to both raw materials and vital ecosystems should be taken into account in contemporary decision-making. Many organizations have made policy statements about sustainability, but very few have linked animal welfare to sustainability issues. One is the FAWC (Farm Animal Welfare Committee) in the UK, who in their 2016 (FAWC 2016) report on Sustainable agriculture and farm animal welfare state the following principles;

i.   *Agriculture cannot be considered sustainable if it is achieved at an unacceptable cost to animal welfare.*
ii. *Sustainable agriculture must take account of the fact that farmed animals are sentient individuals.*
iii. *Sustainable agriculture must include a duty of care for the physical and mental needs and natures of farmed animals and should not depend on prolonged or routine use of pharmaceuticals, or on mutilations.*

These principles may have particular resonance for poultry, particularly the broiler production industry. With about 70 billion broilers produced a year in the world, minor changes in methods of production can have a major influence on the sustainability of food production systems.

The massive increase in supply of food (poultry meat) at a much lower cost to the consumer has been achieved through genetic selection of birds for faster growth rate and more breast muscle, increased feed efficiency, intensification within housing systems, and control of disease through biosecurity and the development of vaccines. Intensification of production has allowed more food to be produced from relatively less land and has made chicken meat affordable to a much wider population. However, a small, but significant, proportion of consumers in some developed countries are choosing to eat chickens produced in less intensive, free-range or organic systems. The reasons for this are complex; animal welfare is but one: However, the trend is significant and cannot be ignored by the poultry industry.

Some apparent problems arising from the intensification of broiler chicken production are poor bird welfare, amplified by the large numbers of animals, the development of antibiotic resistance, and the risk of contamination of poultry meat by food poisoning organisms and feed toxins. The most visible welfare problems occurring within intensive broiler chicken production systems are lameness, which is painful and affects the ability of birds to eat, drink and show most normal behaviour, and contact dermatitis, attributable to poor litter and air quality in bird houses. Elite and broiler breeder birds suffer from severe hunger and pain due to feather pecking and mutilations in male birds. In addition, fear, injury and distress are caused by intensive methods of depopulation and transport; live shackling; ineffective electrical stunning, and in some plants, the use of aversive gases with long induction periods for stunning and killing, in the name of carcass quality. The use of such intensive systems, where each individual bird is worth very little in economic terms and is treated with total indifference, clearly breaks the covenant of respect for animals slaughtered for human consumption which is basic in all religions that allow the consumption of meat.

While many communities in developing countries have a precarious food supply, and are regularly subject to food shortages and famine, the most serious health problems in the developed world are associated with the rapidly rising prevalence of obesity, including diabetes, stroke and cardiac disease. One of the main drivers of the obesity epidemic is the fact that food has become cheap, and broiler production is one of the most obvious examples of this fact. The challenge for the next 20 years is whether we can flex broiler chicken production in a direction which both improves bird welfare globally, while increasing food security in developing countries, and sustainability in developed ones. When we make decisions with respect to which systems we ought to use in the production of broiler chicken, we need to consider the interests of *all* stakeholders: people in developed and developing countries, generations yet to come, and, of course, the chickens.

Acknowledgement

This chapter owes much of its shape and form to its original author in Edition 1, the late Dr Sue Haslam. Much of the text is evolved from her original writing, for which we are grateful. We keep Sue in our minds.

References and Further Reading

Aydin, A., Cangar, O., Ozcan, S.E., Bahr, C., and Berckmans, D. (2010). Application of a fully automatic analysis tool to assess the activity of broiler chickens with different gait scores. *Computers and Electronics Agriculture* 73: 194–199.

Bock. (2019). TED Stunner. https://www.qcsupply.com/ted-captive-bolt-stunner.html (accessed 2 May 2019).

Bruntland Commission. (1987). United Nations 'Report of the World Commission on Environment and Development'. General Assembly Resolution 42/187. http://www.un.org/documents.

CIWF, Compassion in World Farming. (2018). Controlled atmosphere systems for broiler chickens (April 2018). https://www.compassioninfoodbusiness.com/media/7432907/controlled-atmosphere-systems-for-broiler-chickens.pdf (accessed 2 May 2019).

Colles, F.M., McCarthy, N.D., Howe, J.C., Devereux, C.L., Gosler, A.G., and Maiden, M.C.J. (2011). Dynamics of Campylobacter colonization of a natural host, *Sturnus vulgaris* (European Starling). *Enviroment Microbiology* 11 (1): 258–267. doi: 10.1111/j.1462-2920.2008.01773.x.

Corr, S.A., McCorquodale, C., McDonald, J., Gentle, M., and McGovern, R. (2007). A force plate study of avian gait. *Journal of Biomechanics* 40: 2037–2043.

Dawkins, M.S., Donnelly, C.A., and Jones, T.A. (2004). Chicken welfare is influenced more by housing conditions than by stocking density. *Nature* 427: 342–344.

EC Council Directive 2007/43/EC Laying down minimum rules for the protection of chickens kept for meat production.

EFSA. (2004). Welfare aspects of the main systems of stunning and killing the main commercial species of animals. *EFSA Journal* 45: 1–29.

EFSA. (2013). Guidance on the assessment criteria for studies evaluating the effectiveness of stunning interventions regarding animal protection at the time of killing. *EFSA Journal* 11 (12): 3486.

EFSA. (2014a). Scientific opinion on electrical requirements for poultry waterbath stunning equipment. *EFSA Journal* 12 (7): 3745.

EFSA. (2014b). Scientific opinion on the use of low atmosphere pressure system (LAPS) for stunning poultry. *EFSA Journal* 12 (1): 3488.

EFSA. (2017). Scientific Opinion on the low atmospheric pressure system for stunning broiler chickens. *EFSA Journal* 2017 15 (12): 5056, 86. doi: 10.2903/j.efsa.2017.5056.

European Food Safety Authority. (2004). Welfare aspects of animal stunning and killing methods. AHAW/04-027. http://www.efsa.eu.int/EFSA/Scientific_Opinion.

European Union. (2007). European Union Broiler Directive (2007). http://eurlex.europa.eu.

FAWC. (2016). Sustainable agriculture and farm animal welfare. Published by Defra, Farm Animal Welfare Committee Area 5B, Nobel House, 17 Smith Square, London SW1P 3JR, UK. https://assets.publishing.service.gov.uk/government/uploads/system/uploads/attachment_data/file/593479/Advice_about_sustainable_agriculture_and_farm_animal_welfare_-_final_2016.pdf (accessed 1 May 2019).

Food and Agriculture Organization. (1998). Village chicken production system in rural Africa – household food security and gender issues. FAO Animal Production and Health Papers 142: 81.

Food and Agriculture Organization. (2014). Decision Tools for Family Poultry Development. ISSN 1810-0708.

Food and Agriculture Organization. (2019). Overview of global meat market developments in 2018. http://www.fao.org/3/ca3880en/ca3880en.pdf (accessed 2 May 2019).

FSA, Food Standards Agency. (2013). Results of the 2013 animal welfare survey in Great Britain. https://www.food.gov.uk/sites/default/files/2013-animal-welfare-survey.pdf (accessed 6 October 2017).

Garner, J.P., Falcone, C., Wakenell, P., Martin, M., and Mench, J.A. (2002). Reliability and validity of a modified gait scoring system and its use in assessing tibial dyschondroplasia in broilers, British. *Poultry Science* 43 (3): 355–363. doi: 10.1080/00071660120103620.

Gregory, N.G. and Austin, S.D. (1992). Causes of trauma in broilers arriving dead at poultry processing plants. *Veterinary Record* 131: 501–503.

Haslam, S.M., Knowles, T.G., and Brown, S.N. (2007). Factors affecting the prevalence of foot pad dermatitis, hock burn and breast burn in broiler chicken. *British Poultry Science* 48: 264–275.

IVH. (2019). Enterococcus caecorum - *Enterococcus caecorum* pathogenesis. https://ivh.ku.dk/english/research/veterinary_clinical_microbiology/preventive_veterinary_microbiology/kyllinegprojekt Department of Veterinary and Animal Sciences University of Copenhagen (accessed 1 May 2019).

Kestin, S.C., Knowles, T.G., Tinch, A.E., and Gregory, N.G. (1992). Prevalence of leg weakness in broiler chickens and its relationship with genotype. *Veterinary Record* 131: 190–194.

Knowles, T.G., Kestin, S.C., Haslam, S.M., Brown, S.N., Green, L.E., Butterworth, A., Pope, S.J., Pfeiffer, D., and Nicol, C.J. (2008). Leg disorders in broiler chickens: prevalence, risk factors and prevention. *PLoS One* 3 (2): e1545.

Red Tractor Assures Food Standards, Chicken Standards: Broilers and Poussin. (updated 1st October 2018). Version 4.1. https://assurance.redtractor.org.uk/contentfiles/Farmers-6803.pdf?_=636790159730579749 (accessed 2 May 2019).

RSPCA. (2017). Welfare Standards for Chickens. https://science.rspca.org.uk/sciencegroup/farmanimals/standards/chickens (accessed 2 May 2019).

Weeks, C.A. and Butterworth, A. (eds.) (2004). *Measuring and Auditing Broiler Welfare*. Wallingford: CABI Publishing.

9

Goats

Alan Mowlem

KEY CONCEPTS

Management and Welfare of Farm Animals: The UFAW Farm Handbook, Sixth Edition.
Edited by John Webster and Jean Margerison.
© Universities Federation for Animal Welfare 2022. Published 2022 by John Wiley & Sons Ltd.

9.1 Introduction

Archaeological evidence confirms that the dog and the goat were the first animals to be domesticated. Remains from sites in Jericho show that the goat was kept by humans in settlements dating back some 8000 to 10000 years (Zeuner 1963). The domesticated goat (*Capra hircus*) is now found throughout the world and is absent only from areas of extreme cold near the polar regions. It almost certainly derives from the so-called Persian wild goat or bezoar (*Capra aegagrus*) found in Turkey, Iran and Western Afghanistan. The total world population of goats is estimated to be almost 500 million.

The difference between goats and sheep is often discussed. In spite of similarities between breeds of sheep and goats, hybrids do not naturally occur. Fertile matings between the species can sometimes occur, but when this happens the embryo is reabsorbed at around 15 weeks. The most obvious difference, though not visible, is that goats have 60 chromosomes, compared with 54 in sheep. Visible differences are not obvious. Usually with most breeds the tail of a goat is raised up, whereas that of a sheep hangs down. The male of both species smells, particularly in the breeding season, but the smell is quite characteristic of the species and would allow them to be identified even if they were not visible.

The most obvious difference between goats and any other farmed species is their behaviour. Goats are active and inquisitive. This can make them hard work until their habits and behaviour are understood. They seem unable to ignore anything they have not seen before and this inquisitiveness can lead to escapes from seemingly secure paddocks and buildings and the destruction of any fitting or equipment that has been fixed or left within their reach. An American author, Robert Wernick, wrote: 'Sheep are conformists: goats are unpredictable, flighty, capricious' – the word comes from the Latin *capra* meaning goat. In the words of a French goat breeder, they are capricious not lunatic. 'Sheep with their heads usually down, are in general quite unaware of and uninterested in the external world. If a sheep hears a low-flying plane, for example, it will become frightened and is likely to run, whereas a goat will often stand and watch. Despite their friskiness and unpredictability, goats are basically down-to-earth creatures, with a genius for making the best of any situation they may find themselves in. Centuries of co-habitation with mankind have put them in all kinds of situations: they have learned how to survive them all.'

It is almost a paradox that animals of such independent spirit take so well to the relatively intensive conditions found on most goat farms in the developed world, where they may be kept in straw-bedded yards all year round. This helps to control levels of internal parasites to which they are particularly susceptible. For large herds this can also make other aspects of their management easier, as will be explained later.

9.2 Farmed Goats

Particularly in the Western world, goats are unusual in that they are the only farm species kept in large numbers as a hobby by people with no commercial aspirations. The converse of this is the subsistence farmer in a developing country who only has a few goats but who depends on them for the livelihood of himself and his family. Goats may be farmed for their milk, meat or hair. The extremes of developed milk production can be found in the UK and some other European countries. Here herds of over 1000 milking goats may be found, and milking is often carried out using a sophisticated and complicated rotary milking parlour. Their lively and inquisitive nature is a real benefit when introducing goats to new and complex milking parlours. One farmer reported that using a new rotary parlour with no in parlour feeding for the first time increased the rate of milking from 100 goats per hour to 400 per hour. The standard of milk production and storage found in these establishments is as good as or even better than may be seen with dairy cow production. The processing of the milk for drinking or into other dairy products may be on the farm or, more typically, at a separate dairy. This may be independent of the production business or may be managed by a group of farmers within a cooperative (Mowlem 2002).

Milk production in the developing world is usually for direct consumption by small family units. If a surplus is produced, which is quite likely if improved goats are available, some may be sold or converted into other products such as cheese if local market opportunities exist. Throughout the world more goats are kept for their meat than for milk or fibre. Most of these will be kept extensively on improved pasture or, more likely, on scrubland considered unfit for other livestock. Improved dairy production in the developed world generates many surplus kids which are usually reared for meat for a growing restaurant market in Western countries. Goat meat is the preferred choice in the developing world.

9.3 Breeds

There are more than 200 identifiable breeds of goat in the world (Porter 1996). The principal dairy breeds in the UK originate from breeds from other countries. The Saanen and Toggenberg are from Switzerland and the British Saanen, British Toggenberg and British Alpine are derived from crossbreeding Swiss breeds. The Anglo-Nubian is the result of crossbreeding goats from the Middle and Far East with the indigenous English goat. These eastern goats were brought to the UK by ships returning from what was then the British Empire. They provided milk on the journey and when they eventually arrived in the UK there were always people keen to buy them. Two other minority UK breeds that are kept for milk are the Golden Guernsey and the Old English. Of all these dairy breeds the Saanen or Saanen type, with its impressive milk yield and relatively placid nature, is becoming the breed of choice for most large commercial dairy farms.

The increase in interest in the quality of goats and the development of specific breeds has led to the formation of breed societies with the registration of goats and the selection of specific traits being an important function. In the UK the British Goat Society was formed over 100 years ago and has been organizing breed shows since its formation.

Although more goats are kept throughout the world for their meat than for any other product, there are very few breeds that have been developed specifically for meat production. The best-known improved meat breed is the Boer from South Africa. This impressive breed has been selectively bred to improve carcass conformation and now good males can be seen in South Africa with live-weights exceeding 200 kg A few Boer goats are now to be found in some European countries including the UK.

There are two types of goat hair that are produced commercially. Mohair is produced by Angora goats which originate from Turkey but are now to be found in the largest numbers in South Africa, the USA, Australia and New Zealand. Some are also farmed, albeit in comparatively small numbers, in European countries including the UK. Although large numbers of goats are kept in some countries for the production of cashmere, there is not a specific cashmere breed. Cashmere is harvested, by combing, from a number of breeds that have been improved for cashmere production, notably in the People's Republic of China. Meat is essentially a secondary product from fibre-producing goats.

9.3.1   Breed Improvement

In many countries and in many cultures goats have not been part of mainstream agriculture and have never received the benefit of improvement programmes enjoyed by other species. France is one of the few countries where goat milk production is part of main-stream agriculture with a dairy goat population of more than 1 million. This large population has made the formation of an AI service, using frozen semen a commercial possibility with all of the benefits seen in the cattle sector. Although artificial insemination is possible it is not a technique that has been used extensively to speed up genetic improvement as has been the case with cattle. In the UK the improvement of dairy goat production is largely due to pedigree breeders who will be members of the 100-year-old British Goat Society and whose hobby is goat breeding and improvement through competition with others. Their efforts have not been without success. The world record for milk production comes from a British Saanen that produced over 3500 litres of milk in one lactation. This compares with undeveloped indigenous breeds in the developing world that would produce a few hundred litres per lactation. In some other countries improvement schemes developed by NGOs involving the use of indigenous goats crossed with improved European breeds, has doubled milk yields in some cases (Peacock 1996).

Selective breeding on farms has resulted in greatly increased mohair yields from Angora goats. For example, the average yield in South Africa is about five times greater than produced by the goats imported from Turkey more than 150 years ago. Over a shorter time span the South African breeders have transformed the performance and conformation of the indigenous Boer goat for meat production.

The interest in cashmere production, particularly in the UK, has focused attention on improving the yield of fibre. The labour-intensive methods of harvesting cashmere means that commercial production in countries such as the UK would only be possible if yields could be significantly improved.

9.4   Environmental Requirements

Goats are, by and large, tolerant and adaptable to a variety of environments. Kept extensively, the one thing they do not tolerate well is prolonged rain, particularly if it is cold. In such environments some form of shelter is a minimum requirement. As already mentioned, most dairy farms in Western countries do not allow their goats to graze. They are kept in large groups in covered yards. In these conditions a minimum floor area of 12 m^2 per goat should be provided. This should be increased when unfamiliar goats are put together such as when establishing a new herd. Goats in groups may fight to establish dominance and there will be a lot of stress at this time until they are used to each other. When available, straw makes a suitable bedding, and in warm dry environments slatted floors can be used. A good level of ventilation is necessary for all housed goats if respiratory problems are to be avoided. A reasonably high roof with air outlets and openings at goat level will allow air to circulate from floor level and out through the roof (Figure 9.1).

It is becoming conventional, with large numbers of milking goats, to house them in sheds with a central feed passage bordered by feed barriers through which the goats can feed on their daily forage ration. Goats seem to prefer to feed upwards, and if the floor of the feed passage between the feed barriers is at a higher level, this will allow this and will also reduce contamination of the forage with faeces (Figure 9.2).

Any goat building must be constructed with due consideration for their inquisitive behaviour. They can be quite agile and therefore anything that may be damaged by them must be at least 2 metres above the ground. They will also jump onto windowsills, feed racks, ledges and in fact almost any near horizontal surface. It is also important that electrical fittings, cables water pipes and taps are all out of reach. For those used to placid cows, goats can appear to be a nuisance but, if their behaviour is understood and buildings are provided that take this into account, most problems can be avoided. Goats are sociable animals and, once a hierarchy has been established, seem to be most content when housed together in groups. For those who just keep one pet goat, another animal will often provide sufficient companionship. Even chickens can fulfil this role. Without this, a single goat will always be calling for attention whenever it thinks anyone is about.

Non-dairy breeds are likely to be turned out to pasture as internal parasite infestations can be controlled by drenching with an anthelmintic without the problem of milk withdrawal. It will not be a great surprise to discover that fencing goats can be a problem. If sheep are turned into a fresh field or paddock they immediately start to graze. When goats are put into a fresh

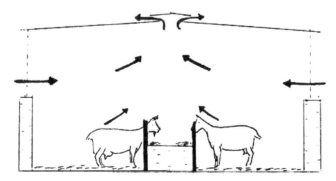

Figure 9.1 A simple naturally ventilated barn for dairy goats. Note the raised feed barrier.

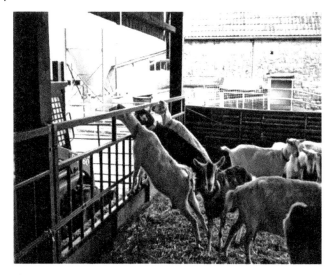

Figure 9.2 Feed barrier and restraining wall in a barn for agile, inquisitive goats.

field they will run all round the perimeter, clambering up any available fences to reach any tasty herbage on the other side. This behaviour results in them quickly finding weaknesses in the fence and if they do they will escape. In fencing terms there is no such thing as goat-proof, but there are systems that will confine goats quite satisfactorily if well maintained. Any form of wire mesh will eventually fail but the clambering habit can be discouraged if an offset or hotwire is fixed. This is an electrified wire fixed just below the top of the wire mesh by supports that hold it 15 to 30 cm from the fence. Much the same result can be achieved if the offset is fixed at the bottom of the fence (Mowlem 2001). Electrified high-tensile wire fences are effective, but it is necessary to have at least five wires to prevent the goats escaping. Unlike sheep they learn very quickly if the electric fence unit is not working and, when they do, they will escape. It is important that any electrified system is checked regularly.

Tethering is sometimes used as a simple alternative to fences. It should be considered only as a last resort. While undoubtedly it saves a lot of elaborate and expensive fencing there are many potential problems. As has already been described, goats are very active animals and there is a real risk of them becoming entangled in the tether. There have been cases when this has been fatal. If a tether is the only option then it should be made of lightweight chain rather than rope. There should be a swivel at each end and one in the middle. There should be no nearby bushes or trees on which the chain could be caught. The goat will need access to a shelter and care must be taken to ensure it cannot become caught on any part of it. In addition to the problems of being caught up, a goat on a tether will be vulnerable to dog worrying, vandalism and bad weather. All this suggests that if a goat must be tethered it should at be checked a minimum of twice a day.

9.5 Nutrition and Feeding Systems

Goats are ruminants and as such have much in common with sheep and cattle. However, their choice of feedstuffs and their feeding behaviour is different from these two species. Goats are browsers and generally feed at a higher level from the ground than sheep. They prefer shrubs, tree leaves and woody material. Many so-called weeds have a reasonably high nutritional value. Given the opportunity, goats are capable of selecting nutritious material so that selection of so-called weeds will go towards improving the nutritional value of their feed. This food selection can be useful in improving rough grazing, while improving the nutritive value of the overall diet. In sown pastures they eat grass-inhibiting weeds and do not eat much clover and thus they can be very beneficial when grazed before or with sheep. In terms of nutrient requirements the dairy goat is very similar to the dairy cow and the requirement for energy to produce a litre of milk from a given weight of animal is virtually the same for the two species (Agricultural and Food Research Council 1998, Oldham and Mowlem 1981). The values for a dairy goat's energy needs are shown in Table 9.1. These are only a guide because various factors will affect the requirement for energy. If a goat is outside grazing it will need more energy than a housed goat that has its food brought to it. Milk quality also influences the energy needs; goats producing particularly rich milk with a high fat content will require a higher energy intake.

When free to graze, goats tend to select plants that are often the most nutritious in terms of protein and trace element content. Metabolic problems are rare in goats that have free access to natural grazing and browse material. This ability to select can be used in an intensive farming system. It has been shown that goats fed poor-quality forage at amounts equivalent to 50% more than appetite do better than sheep in similar conditions. It is interesting to note that when maize silage is fed to dairy goats the make-up of the silage changes as the day progresses. They initially select the parts of the maize they prefer and will only eat all of it if they are not offered any more silage or other material. Goat farmers who keep cattle may feed the silage refusals collected from the goats in the afternoon to their cattle and will then give the goats some fresh silage. Apart from this helping towards the quality of the goats' intake of nutrients the new silage will encourage them to eat more, thus increasing their dry matter intake (DMI). The greater the DMI the greater the potential for maximizing performance in terms of milk yield.

Dairy goat farmers, like their cattle counterparts, have the same aim, i.e. to feed their goats enough nutrients for them to be able to perform to their full genetic potential. It is not possible to achieve this with forage alone. High-yielding dairy goats will be fed up to 2 kg/day of concentrate feed containing about 18% protein. Daily feed intake, best described according to DMI, will be between 3.5% and 5% of their live-weight. Breeders of high-yielding pedigree

Table 9.1 Daily energy requirements for dairy goats.

Maintenance 0.5 MJ ME/kg of metabolic bodyweight ($kg^{0.75}$)

Pregnancy 0.5 MJ ME/$kg^{0.75}$ rising to 0.7 MJ ME/kg $^{0.75}$ for the last month

Lactation maintenance needs + 5 MJ ME per kg of milk produced goats sometimes achieve DMIs as high as 7% live-weight/day by feeding their goats often throughout the day and by introducing different feeds. While this level of feeding would not be realistic in a conventional farming situation, the achievements of these breeders do show what the genetic potential of goats can be.

The principles for increasing or optimizing production are the same for goats in any environment. Even in poorer countries much can be done by selecting the best goats and then doing all that is realistically possible to increase their intake of nutrients. This may create a slight conflict of considerations with some fibre-producing goats. These also need a reasonably high plane of nutrition if they are to perform well. However, particularly with Angora goats, there is some evidence to suggest that if the quality of their feed is too good the fibre will be coarser and thus less valuable. It should be borne in mind that the return from these animals is dependent on the weight of mohair produced as well as the quality, and thus the right balance must be achieved if they are to be profitable. The level of nutrition and feeding is not only related to productivity. For goats to remain healthy a good supply of all essential nutrients is necessary. Water must be available at all times. Dairy goats in particular must have a good supply if they are to be able to maintain a high milk yield. They need to drink about 1.5 litres of water per day for each litre of milk produced.

9.6 Reproduction and Breeding

Goats are seasonally polyoestrous, with females coming into heat or oestrus at regular intervals during the breeding season which, in the northern hemisphere, extends from about August to February. However, it is not safe to assume that females will not exhibit oestrus or conceive at other times of the year. Males are generally capable of breeding throughout the year but libido and sperm production are likely to be poorer during the spring and early summer. Female kids become sexually mature and show oestrus for the first time at about 6 months of age. Male kids are usually reported to be sexually mature at 6 months but in fact fertile matings can occur as early as 3 months of age. If entire kids are kept it is important to separate them before unplanned matings occur. Hobbyist goat breeders often do not mate their young females until they are 18 months of age. Most commercial farmers would consider this wasteful and would normally expect to mate their goats when they have reached about 75% of their expected mature bodyweight. In practice this means spring-born kids that have grown well should be fit for mating by the end of the year in which they were born.

The length of the oestrous cycle is about 21 days and oestrus generally lasts for 2 to 3 days. Sometimes, particularly with females kept separately from others, oestrous activity may be delayed. The smell of a male may often stimulate the onset of oestrous cycling. If a male is not available a rag that has been rubbed over a male may have the same effect. Oestrus is readily detected by a range of behavioural changes including bleating, tail wagging, and staring in the direction of a male if there is one nearby. Often the vulva may be swollen and reddened. Where males are run with a herd of females one male can be expected to serve at least 40 females. However, it is common practice on large dairy farms to run one male with groups of several hundred females and he would be expected to mate with most of them over a period of two to three months. If he seemed to be working particularly hard and losing condition he would be rested while another male was used.

Artificial insemination can be used with goats (Mowlem 1983). Goat semen freezes as well as cattle semen although the processing method is more difficult. The technique used to inseminate goats is similar to that used with sheep. It is important to hold the female goat in a head-down, rump-up position. This is achieved by the handler straddling the goat's neck and then lifting her by her folded-back legs to present her rear to the inseminating technician (Figure 9.3). A duck-billed speculum, equipped with a light probe, is used to look into the vagina to locate the cervix. The appearance of the cervix indicates at what stage of oestrus the goat is, and this plus all the other behavioural signs helps to ensure the goat is inseminated at the correct time. The semen is deposited into and sometimes through the cervix. An experienced inseminator would expect to achieve a 60 to 70% conception rate for the first insemination.

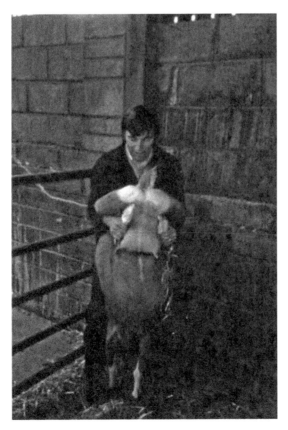

Figure 9.3 Restraining a nanny goat for artificial insemination.

Gestation lasts 146 to 156 days with an average of 150 days. Most females are bred annually although it is possible to achieve two kiddings per year. Dairy goats can have a prolonged lactation lasting 18 months and may be mated only once in two years. Some will even lactate without kidding and are referred to as maiden milkers. The number of kids produced varies with age and breed. Generally unimproved goats such as ferals average only one kid whereas more improved dairy goats will often produce 2 or 3

Pseudo-pregnancy, false pregnancy or 'cloudburst', in which the female shows all the external and behavioural signs of pregnancy, without actually being so, can occur. This condition may last for the full term or longer and will end in a large release of fluid but no kid. Sometimes lactation will follow or sometimes it will be delayed with the goat coming into milk some months after the pseudo-pregnancy has ended. Ultrasonic scanning can be used to detect pregnancy and it should be possible to determine the number of kids or whether it is a false pregnancy.

9.6.1 Management of Breeding Males

Considering their importance, male goats often do not get the same level of care as breeding females. They have a very strong smell, especially during the breeding season, which means they tend to be kept away from, and out of sight of, the other goats. Even though they are rarely aggressive they will be much more amenable if they can be kept as part of, and with, the rest of the herd. They can work very hard for several months during the mating season and they often seem to lose interest in food. It is therefore important that they are allowed to improve their body condition by increasing their food ration before the start of the breeding season. The other aspect of male care that justifies special attention is housing. They require a dry, airy shed with adequate room for them to move around and it must be strongly constructed as they can sometimes be destructive for no obvious reason. This is also the case with fittings and fitments. The males can be just as inquisitive as the females but they are of course much stronger and when standing up on their hind legs can reach further.

9.6.2 Management of Breeding Females

Females in dairy herds should be so well cared for, to optimize milk production, that they are unlikely to need any special care for breeding. One possible problem may be a tendency towards fatness. When goats do get fat, most is deposited in the abdomen rather than subcutaneously or intramuscularly. For breeding females this may affect fertility and may cause problems at parturition. It is unlikely that a healthy farmed goat would ever be undernourished to a level that would affect its breeding performance.

Many European dairy farmers will be interested in controlling the breeding season in order to stimulate their goats into breeding all the year round to eliminate the problems of seasonal milk production. The two methods used most in a practical farm environment are intravaginal hormonal sponges or artificial lighting regimes. The sponge method involves implanting a sponge impregnated with the hormone progesterone, into the vagina, which remains in place for 11 days. Two days before it is withdrawn the goat is injected with pregnant mares' serum gonadotrophin (PMSG) and prostaglandin. The PMSG is a convenient source of follicle-stimulating hormone (FSH) and luteinizing hormone and the prostaglandin is given to cause regression of any corpus luteum that may be present, thus removing any source of endogenous progesterone. The goats will usually come into oestrus within 1 to 2 days of sponge removal. If artificial insemination is used, the goats will be inseminated 42 to 44 hours after sponge removal.

In temperate countries, such as the UK, the decreasing daylight and increasing dark period after the mid summer day triggers breeding activity in goats. The lengthening nights cause the release of the hormone melatonin which in turn triggers the release of the hormones which stimulate the ovaries to produce a follicle from which an ovum will be released. The onset of this sequence of events gives rise to oestrous behaviour, or heat, in the goat and the whole cycle of events is called the oestrous cycle. It is possible to mimic this effect by subjecting the goats to prolonged periods of light during the winter and then reverting to periods of increased darkness. Ashbrook (1982) has recommended an extended light regime, in which goats are exposed to 20 hours of light for 60 consecutive days during the period January to March. Oestrus will occur approximately 10 weeks after the return to ambient lighting. Melatonin implants are also used, in some cases in conjunction with an extended light regime. Such methods of controlling the breeding season are only really possible with housed goats and therefore are used mainly with dairy animals where the need for all-year-round breeding is greatest.

9.6.3 Mating

Most goats are mated naturally, although artificial insemination is possible and in some of the major European goat farming countries is becoming more widely used. Where small numbers are kept, it is not always appropriate for the goat-keeper or farmer to keep a male. In these cases, a female will be taken to the nearest male of the correct type, when oestrous behaviour is observed. On large farms several males will be kept and one may be run with a large group. A male can successfully mate more than 100 females over a period of two to three months. If concentrated mating is required the male may be changed weekly. Sheep raddle harnesses may be used to time matings, although there have been instances of the female goats chewing the crayon to complete destruction! Regular ultrasonic scanning is often used in large herds to check on state and stage of pregnancy. Goat breeders with small numbers of goats may wish to take a female to a male some distance away. Unfortunately, the journey could well be a factor in the female not being in what is called standing heat when presented to the male, or it may simply be a case of the wrong time where the owner has not recognized the signs of heat or oestrus.

Artificial insemination, using either fresh or frozen semen, presents opportunities for extending the use of superior males. There are other advantages to artificial insemination even though it is not used widely in many countries. It reduces the risk of infection because it does not involve direct contact between the male and female goat. When goats are kept in small numbers it is hard to justify keeping a stud male, given all the problems associated with them, such as their strong smell and their superior strength. With small numbers there is always the problem of inbreeding, i.e. a male mating his own daughters. In some countries breeding groups have been set up where a high-quality male is shared by a number of goat-keepers, often by bringing their goats to him. There is also the possibility of semen being collected and diluted and used fresh. If kept cool this should allow use within 24 hours of collection and would be useful where it is difficult to move females to the male.

9.6.4   Feeding Pregnant Females

Whatever the goats are being farmed for, they will need good input of nutrients if they are to be fit for pregnancy and parturition. If they are dairy goats they will require feed to support milk production which will probably continue for the first three months of gestation. Whatever the type of goat, it is generally recommended that the energy and protein intake should be increased during the last month of gestation. Also goats that are encouraged to eat a high level of forage during gestation will be conditioned for a high forage intake during lactation as this will benefit milk yield and quality. Conversely goats with a poor forage intake during gestation will have a lower intake during lactation even if the quantity and quality of the forage is increased. As a rough guide, an average dairy goat of around 65 kg live-weight should be offered a good-quality forage *ad libitum*, and, two months before parturition, 250 g of a dairy concentrate feed per day which should be increased to 450 g per day one month before parturition is due. Goats that are not kept for milk production will not require such a high plane of nutrition but they will require more than just forage in late gestation and early lactation. Goats require access to drinking water at all times but it is particularly important that they have a good clean supply during gestation and at parturition.

9.6.5   Housing Pregnant Females

The abdomen of pregnant goats can become very large as multiple kids are quite common. Also, the udder on a high-yielding female can become very swollen and sometimes pendulous to a point where it may drag on the ground (Figure 9.4). Goats in this condition require an unchallenging environment in which there is no risk of injury. All projections on which they could become caught must be removed or made safe. Goats with horns should not be housed with hornless ones. Even if they do not cause any injuries they will certainly dominate any feed racks or troughs, thus depriving some of their correct feed intake.

9.6.6   Parturition and Suckling

The ideal environment for a goat about to give birth is a separate, freshly bedded pen, possibly constructed at the end of the pen in which the rest of the herd is housed. This is not always possible and a compromise is to house those goats that are close to parturition together, separate from the main herd. The reasons for housing the goats in separate pens is to ensure the mother-to-kid bond is well established and to make sure the kid gets a good chance to suck

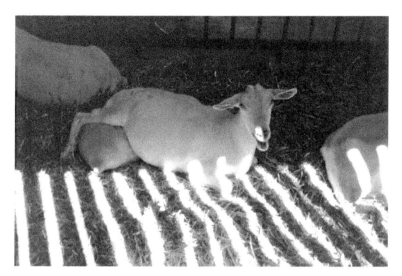

Figure 9.4 A nanny goat with a pendulous udder. These animals require special attention to housing and bedding.

its mother's udder. It is most important that newborn kids feed from their mother within a few hours of parturition.

When a female is close to parturition she will become restless, sometimes scratching the ground, and will usually stand away from the rest of the group. A sure sign that parturition is imminent is discharge from the vagina as the foetal sac ruptures. If the goat appears to be straining for several hours without any obvious progress it is best to call the veterinarian or someone else experienced with kidding or lambing. The first sign of a correct presentation is the appearance of front feet followed by a nose. If these can be seen, the goat should be able to kid without assistance. If one or, at worst, two feet are pointing back and/or the head is back, manual assistance will probably be required but it should be remembered that any interference does present some risk. If there is any chance the female will kid by herself she should be left to do so. Once the kid or kids have been born it is important that the mother has the opportunity to lick them. This stimulates the kids, strengthens the mother–offspring bond and the mother will normally dry and clean the kids very effectively. Goats with very pendulous udders will have difficulty feeding their kids but if the kid can be helped to feed for the first 24 hours there is a good chance they will be strong enough to seek out and suck from even the most awkward teats. In all cases it is most important that the kids are fed on colostrum for at least the first 24 hours after birth. If the mother cannot do this then feeding the kid with a stomach tube may be the only option. These are available, often under the generic name of 'lamb reviver'. These are graduated plastic bottles of about 250 mL capacity with a small rubber stomach tube attached to a spout on the lid. With care, warm colostrum can be fed directly into the kid's stomach. This is a most effective way of reviving weak kids. Often a kid can be transformed from being too weak to stand to one that is running around looking for its next feed, after a single feed of warm colostrum.

9.6.7 Kid Rearing

Kids from dairy herds will be artificially reared so that the milk can be sold. Those from meat- or fibre-producing herds are more likely to be reared naturally by their mothers. Milk replacers formulated for calves are quite suitable for kid rearing. This is not surprising as the gross composition of goat milk is very similar to cow milk. Table 9.2 shows a regime for feeding milk replacer to kids for either six or eight weeks, and Table 9.3 shows an alternative regime for restricted quantities of milk replacer. Some goat-keepers rear their kids on sheep milk replacer. The high fat level in this replacer makes it an expensive and unnecessary luxury. The kids will grow well on such a product but it will not be a cost-effective method. The most cost-effective method uses a calf milk replacer which may be given initially *ad libitum* although a rationed system may be preferred and will certainly cost less (Mowlem 1984).

Kids do not grow as well as comparable lambs when kept out on pasture. This is probably due to heavy endoparasite infestations and also to kids' behaviour. Young lambs seem intent on feeding and growing. Goat kids seem more intent on having a good time and spend a lot of time playing and investigating their environment. When doing this they are not only using up more energy but also eating less.

Kids reared for the more intensive dairy systems should be disbudded within a few weeks of birth. The longer the horn buds are left, the more difficult disbudding will become. With goats this is a veterinary procedure. It is virtually impossible to anaesthetize the horn buds using a local anaesthetic and general anaesthesia is therefore necessary. It is particularly difficult to completely disbud entire male kids and most of these will have some horn or scurs when they reach maturity (Buttle et al. 1986). The main disadvantages of horns are the difficulty they present for goats going through a milking parlour and the injuries they can inflict on each other and their handlers. These will not be a problem where goats are kept extensively and go out to graze, and therefore it is unlikely the farmer will consider it necessary to go to the expense of having kids disbudded.

Table 9.2 Feeding regime for artificial rearing of goat kids. (Figures in parenthesis show ages for a later weaning system.)

Age	Milk feeds
Weeks 1–4 (1–6)	Supplied *ad libitum*
Weeks 5–7 (7)	Half amount consumed end of week 4 (6)
Week 6 (8)	Half amount consumed end of week 5 (7)

Table 9.3 A regime for feeding a rationed amount of milk replacer.

Weeks	Milk quantity	Number of feeds per day
1–7	1 litre/day	2
8	0.5 litres/day	1
9	No milk	

There are a number of ways of dispensing the milk feed. If relatively small numbers of kids are to be fed then bottles with teats placed in a rack are a labour-saving alternative to holding bottles while the kids feed. For large numbers of kids, as may be the case on large dairy farms, an automatic calf-feeding machine may be used. A more simple system is to use containers with a number of teats attached which allow several kids to feed at one time (these are often given the generic name of 'lambbar'). Open troughs can be used but they are best placed outside the pen with the kids putting their heads through a hole or slot to gain access to the milk. This prevents the kids climbing into the trough and fouling the milk.

9.6.8   Housing Kids

Kids are very adept at finding their way out of pens, and therefore solid partitions are preferable with sides about 1.2 m high. Approximately 0.5 m^2 of floor space should be provided per kid up to two months of age, increasing to 1.5 m^2 at six months of age. Care should be taken to ensure that there are no projections in the pens, or gaps where feet or legs may be trapped. Hay nets are not recommended because the kids will jump onto them and some will inevitably get their legs caught in the mesh.

Infection is likely to spread through groups of intensively reared kids and it is therefore important to maintain a high standard of hygiene and husbandry. Kids should be checked for signs of ill health and appropriate action should be taken if disease or infection is suspected.

9.7   Milk Production

9.7.1   Milking Systems

The choice of milking system depends largely on the scale of the enterprise and the environment in which the goats are kept. A complicated, highly mechanized system would not be appropriate in countries where, for example, a reliable electricity source or the infrastructure for servicing milking machinery was not available. In this situation hand milking would be the only practical method. If milking by machine is an option then the choice of system ranges from a simple, small-scale and, usually, portable bucket unit to large sophisticated rotary or static milking parlours (Figure 9.5). The principles of machine milking goats are the same as for cows. Apart from the difference in size and the fact that goats have only two teats, much of the equipment is the same or similar.

The vacuum level is set lower for goats than for cows and the pulsation is faster (Table 9.4). As with other aspects of goat husbandry the goats' speed of movement and ability to learn means they quickly adapt to new and relatively complicated milking systems. With practice one person could milk about 150 goats per hour in a well-designed static milking parlour, whereas one person could milk about 400 goats per hour with a rotary parlour. Although the latter is expensive it is the only layout that can cope with really large numbers that may now be seen on dairy goat farms in a number of European countries. The fact that, with machine

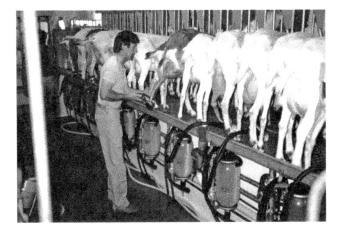

Figure 9.5 A large-scale milking unit on a commercial dairy goat farm.

Table 9.4 Mechanical settings for goat milking machines.

Vacuum	Pulsation rate	Pulsation ratio
37 kPa	70–90/min	50 : 50

milking, the milk travels through a closed pipe system means that there is less chance for it to be spoilt or contaminated if good hygiene is observed. It is advisable, immediately before milking, to wash goats' udders with an approved disinfectant and then dry each using a disposable paper towel. A poor washing routine such as washing with plain water and using the same cloth to dry more than one udder is likely to cause more problems than no washing at all. In Europe, legislation is in place to regulate the standard of goat milk production. In the UK, goat milk production is regulated by the Dairy Products (Hygiene) Regulations 1995.

Goats are clean animals and their milk should have a very low total bacteria count (TBC), which means even after storage in a refrigerated bulk tank for several days it is still likely to have a lower TBC than relatively fresh cow milk.

For milk production in less controlled environments, as may be found in a tropical country, little can be done to reduce contamination of the milk. It is likely in these circumstances that the goats will be hand milked and if so this should be carried out on a clean surface on which the goat will stand. This may be, for example, concrete, a smooth rock or a wooden platform. Care should be taken to remove any visible dirt or faeces from the udder so that it will not drop into the milking vessel. If water is available, udders should be washed with a sanitizing solution. Clean cloths or paper towel should be used to dry the udder. If udders are not dried there is a very good chance that along with the first drop of milk will be a drip of washing solution containing all the contaminants that were on the surface of the udder. Mastitis seems to be much less of a problem with goats than with cows in a comparable environment.

9.7.2 Handling Goat Milk

The most important aspect of handling goat milk is keeping it as cool as possible immediately after milking. There are several reasons for doing this: for example, contaminating micro-organisms will work much more slowly if the milk is cooled and therefore the time the milk can be kept will be extended. In good hygienic on-farm dairies, where the milk will be stored in a refrigerated bulk tank with a temperature of 4°C, it will remain in good usable condition for at least four days. When refrigeration is not available, standing the container of milk in cold water will be of some advantage. If the milk is not cooled immediately after milking, lipolytic enzymes break down the fat and fatty acids will be released. Two of these in goat milk, caproic and capriloic acid, will give the milk an unpleasant flavour which will taint any products made from it. This lipolysis can also be the result of too much agitation of the milk when the fatty acids will be released as a result of mechanical action. This may happen if the milk travels through a complicated pipe system, particularly if moved by centrifugal pumps. If goat milk is handled carefully and cooled quickly after milking it is difficult to differentiate it from cow milk by taste alone.

9.8 Fibre Production

Goats produce two types of hair. The primary hair follicles produce relatively coarse hairs which make up the main outer coat of most goats. Secondary follicles produce much finer hairs which usually grow as an undercoat beneath the outer hairs. This soft underhair is used commercially in the textile industry and is called cashmere. The Angora goat has evolved to produce its main coat from secondary follicles which, in the case of this breed, is soft and lustrous and any primary hairs in the fleece are regarded as a contaminant and are called kemp. The hair produced by Angora goats is called mohair. Mohair grows at about 2.5 cm a month and the ideal processing length is 12 to 14.5 cm. To achieve this, farmers shear their goats twice a year, ideally just before mating and before kidding. Good-quality Angoras may produce 10 kg of mohair per year, the most valuable being the very fine fleece produced by young goats. In the UK, farmers may add value to their mohair by processing it into fashion garments or they may sell it raw and in bulk to the processing mills, mainly in Yorkshire, which traditionally have been a world centre for processing animal fibres for hundreds of years. Mohair has many qualities that make it a valuable natural fibre. It is lustrous, hard-wearing and accepts and retains dyes, and, when used for garments such as suits or skirts, is extremely comfortable to wear. Its hard-wearing and non-fading qualities make it suitable for furnishing fabrics.

Cashmere is fine hair grown as an insulating layer of fine hair under the main outer coat of a number of types and breeds of goat. There is not a cashmere breed but there are a number of types that are bred specifically for cashmere production. The main cashmere-producing countries are the People's Republic of China, the Mongolian People's Republic, Tibet and parts of Northern India. In these countries the fibre is harvested by hand combing the goats when they are close to moulting and also by collecting the hair after moulting. A maximum of about 250 g per annum would be produced by a good goat.

As with mohair, the United Kingdom is a major importing and processing country and this has generated an interest in home production. Feral goats from some of the more mountainous regions have been selected for this purpose and these have been crossed with improved cashmere-producing goats from other countries. Relatively poor yields and the costly labour-intensive harvesting methods have so far prevented profitable production in the UK, but small numbers of producers have been successful with small-scale added-value enterprises. Profitable fibre production is more likely if it can be underpinned by a good market for the meat. This is by no means the case throughout the UK.

9.9 Meat Production

Throughout the world more goats are kept for their meat than for any other product. However, there are very few developed meat breeds. One of the few breeds to have been improved for meat production is the Boer from South Africa. These have been selectively bred for carcass conformation and now some males have been produced with live-weights of well over 200 kg

In some countries such as the UK, cultural prejudices have been difficult to overcome to create a market for goat meat. In many other countries, however, the lean nature of the meat coupled with its unique flavour has pushed it to the top of the meat market. For meat production to be profitable, low-cost rearing systems are necessary which generally means kids are left to be reared by their mothers. In countries such as the UK it is difficult to achieve prices for the meat that will cover the cost of the artificial rearing of surplus dairy kids. As most developed breeds average at least two kids per year the large dairy herds that now exist generate large numbers of surplus kids which cannot be reared profitably, with the exception of the relatively small numbers reared for herd replacement.

Large numbers of surplus kids raise the question of euthanasia. Various methods are used and it is an aspect of goat farming that is under discussion. A light-weight captive-bolt humane killer or an overdose of barbiturates would be the preferred method at present although the latter may be considered too expensive for large numbers and of course would render the meat inedible.

9.10 General Care and Handling

In general the care of goats is similar to that of other farmed ruminants. Their independent and inquisitive nature, however, is different from other livestock and it is only after much experience that the understanding necessary for successful management is acquired. Anyone contemplating starting a goat enterprise, however small, is advised to visit other farms and even to arrange for a few weeks' working experience to help understand what is required to farm them successfully.

9.10.1   Handling and Restraint

Most dairy goats will have been artificially reared and therefore will have grown up used to a lot of human contact. This means they will be confident and inquisitive and will generally crowd round their handler, seeking attention or, if on offer, food! This friendly behaviour makes them easy to catch and restrain because by and large they seem to enjoy it. However, they are intelligent and if they feel threatened they will become suspicious and uncooperative and will be difficult to catch. Once caught, they can be restrained by being gently but firmly held around the neck, just behind the ears. This is easier if the goat has a collar and if they need to be moved, they will usually walk on a lead. If a procedure such as an injection is necessary, the goat can be tied to a gate or hurdle by way of its collar. If another person is available, it can be gently but firmly held.

Unlike sheep, groups of dairy goats are not easy to drive and are more easily moved by being led, particularly if the person in front is carrying a bag or bucket of food. It is advisable to have a second person walking behind the group to move along those stopping to investigate points of interest. Goats that have been used to a fair degree of freedom and little human contact, such as ferals, are a much more difficult proposition. They will be faster and more agile than sheep and will jump out of most sheep-handling systems, which therefore need to be higher and with no surfaces on to which the goats can jump. They do not usually respect a trained dog and in fact will often face up to one, which may create a difficult situation for both goat and dog. A little time spent on training goats to recognize a bag or bucket of food will be time well spent. Once kept in more confined conditions, they will settle down and kids that are hand reared will be as tractable as adult dairy goats.

9.10.2   Routine Procedures

Goats, like sheep, need their hooves to be regularly trimmed. They do not seem to suffer from foot rot nearly as much as sheep but occasional chronic infection may occur, with some animals not responding to treatment. Overgrown hooves can be the cause of severe lameness. Ideally, they should be trimmed three or four time a year unless, as in some countries, they are constantly out on hard dry ground. It is important to make sure the feet of heavily pregnant goats do not need trimming.

With the exception of Angora goats, foot trimming is carried out with the goat in a standing position tethered to a convenient fence or hurdle. With their thick fleece and rounder conformation Angoras can be cast and all four feet trimmed with the goat restrained between the handler's legs. Handling crates, in which a goat can be restrained and raised up on its side, are available for foot trimming and these can speed up the procedure and reduce back strain for the operator.

If housed on clean dry straw or other dry bedding material goats have less problems than sheep with foot infections However it is not unusual to have individual cases of foot rot and other lesions where the nail becomes soft and rotten and may come away from the hoof. A copper sulphate foot bath often proves efficacious both as a preventative and a treatment.

Male kids to be kept for reasons other than breeding should be castrated, and the simplest way is to use the rubber rings available for castrating lambs. This procedure must be carried out within one week of birth. The problems of disbudding have been mentioned earlier in the chapter (Section 9.6.7) but it is perhaps appropriate to reiterate that the earlier this is carried out the easier it is. De-horning mature goats is a difficult and unpleasant procedure that is very traumatic for the goat and should only be carried out as a last resort.

In the UK it is now a requirement by law that goats are tagged for identification in both ears. The tags need to identify the animal by number and they must show the herd number and an identification code to show the farm of origin. Pedigree goats registered with a breed society are normally tattooed and it is possible this may eliminate the need for tags as long as the correct information can be seen. A number of marking systems are available for the farmer to identify individual goats. Numbered collars are useful and have the added advantage of being something to hold on to when restraining or leading goats. Leg bands are available for identifying goats from the rear, which is useful in many types of milking parlour.

Oral drenching of goats is the same as for sheep and the same equipment can be used. Vaccinations are relatively straightforward because of the very small subcutaneous fat deposits on a goat. The jugular vein is particularly easy to locate compared with a sheep. It is, however, quite difficult to find in very young kids.

Goats are able to reach almost all parts of their body with their mouths and it is difficult to apply dressings in such a way that they will not be pulled off. The only way this can be avoided is to restrain the goat so that it cannot turn round. This can be achieved by short tying the goat using a halter or by confining it in a narrow pen which restricts movement.

9.10.3 Transport

If goats have to be moved long distances a suitable vehicle should be used. Goats generally travel well, being able to maintain their balance easily, provided they do not slip on the floor. The ideal floor covering for a truck or van is a rubber mat covered with a thin layer of straw. Space should be adequate but not excessive; otherwise, they may fall when the vehicle turns or brakes sharply. In the interest of safety, a partition should separate the driver from the area occupied by the goats.

9.11 Health and Disease

The maintenance of a healthy herd in any environment demands a high standard of stockmanship and the ability to recognize diseases and disorders in the early stages so that proper attention and treatment can be given promptly.

9.11.1 Parasites

Whatever environment the goats are in, internal parasites will be a major issue. Goats are particularly susceptible to intestinal parasites (generically called worms). They do not build up the same level of resistance as sheep and, although they may not show obvious signs of infestation, if this is uncontrolled it is likely that production performance will be considerably reduced. One possible explanation for the different susceptibility of sheep and goats is that sheep graze close to the ground whereas goats feed on shrubs and tree leaves (browse). These different feeding habits mean that sheep have always ingested worm larvae whereas goats have not. This has possibly resulted in sheep evolving with a greater resistance or tolerance. This problem of high worm burdens is the main reason why dairy goats in many countries are permanently housed. If they do not graze, they will not ingest worm larvae and therefore with suitable medication can be cleared of internal parasites. It has been estimated that heavy worm infestations can reduce milk yield by as much as 18% (Lloyd 1982).

Parasite infestations can be controlled by regular oral drenching with an anthelmintic, in severe cases as often as every three weeks, but this will mean milk withdrawal for up to three days each time and therefore will not be used in large dairy herds. This is not a problem with goats kept for meat or fibre and consequently these goats will be turned out to graze during spring through to autumn in the northern hemisphere and anthelmintics will be used to reduce the worm burden. Parasite resistance is an increasing problem and it is vital that the correct dose of anthelmintic is given; it is recommended to change the drug on a rotational basis.

Goats, like most animals, can be infested with external parasites. Lice are common; goats can also be infested with various types of mange mites. The ivermectin group of drugs are effective against both ecto- and endoparasites but, again, there will be the problem of milk withdrawal in dairy herds. It should be noted that in the UK very few veterinary products are licensed for use with goats. If unlicensed products are used it is a statutory requirement that milk should be withdrawn from sale for human consumption for 21 days.

9.11.2 Bacterial and Viral Diseases

The *Clostridium* bacteria are a group which thrive in anaerobic conditions. They produce powerful toxins. The diseases they cause include tetanus, botulism and gangrene. In ruminants, specific types exist in the gut and normally do not cause problems. However, if conditions are favourable they multiply and the toxin they produce will be fatal. The clostridial diseases most commonly seen in goats, caused by *Clostridium perfrigens* type D, are enterotoxaemia in adults and pulpy kidney disease in kids. These are most usually seen after an abrupt change in diet which often results in a period of incomplete digestion and when conditions in the gut encourage the bacteria to multiply. Goats are particularly at risk when turned out to grass after being housed through the winter months. It is possible to vaccinate goats to protect them from these diseases. Many vaccines are available which give immunity to a wide range of *Clostridium* species but it is recommended that those that are most effective are those that protect against the specific types that affect goats. Adult goats should be vaccinated twice a year, not once yearly as with sheep, and if one vaccination takes place during late pregnancy some immunity will be passed to the kids. Kids from vaccinated mothers should be vaccinated at eight weeks of age and those from unvaccinated mothers at three to four weeks of age. In both cases they should receive a booster vaccination 4 to 6 weeks later.

9.11.2.1 Johne's Disease

Johne's disease, otherwise known as paratuberculosis, is caused by the bacterium *Mycobacterium avium* ssp. *paratuberculosis* and can be a problem in all ruminants. In goats, clinical disease seems to be seen more often in large commercial herds and is thought to be initiated by low levels of stress. Typical signs are a short period of diarrhoea followed by a rapid loss of condition and, in the case of dairy animals, loss of milk. There is no cure or treatment and, if left, the infected goats will usually die two to three months after the first clinical signs. To control the disease it is necessary to eliminate all those animals showing signs and to vaccinate all kids within one month of birth. It is possible to test for the organism in blood and faeces and a skin test is also possible. None are 100% reliable as false-negatives can occur with all three tests. However, if all are positive, it is highly likely that the mycobacterium is present.

9.11.2.2 Caprine Arthritis and Encephalitis

Another disease that has become economically important is caprine arthritis and encephalitis (CAE). This disease is cased by a lentivirus closely related to the one which causes Maedi-visna in sheep. The signs of the disease are varied, with adult goats usually showing signs of arthritis with inflamed and swollen knee joints which will make walking painful. There will be loss of condition with extreme cases becoming emaciated and very weak. There is no cure and, if a high incidence is to be avoided, it is important to test goats regularly and to cull any positive reactors. In some European countries, the USA and Australia around 80% of goats tested are reactors. In the UK, an effective testing and culling scheme has resulted in an incidence of around 2%.

9.11.2.3 Mastitis

The prevention and treatment of mastitis is a major issue with dairy cow farmers. The importance of this disease has generated a lot of good advice, and a wide array of treatment and preventive drugs are available for the dairy cattle industry. As mentioned earlier (Section 9.11.1) there is a problem with so few drugs licensed for use with goats, and if unlicensed products are used farmers in the UK are faced with a 21-day milk withdrawal period. However, mastitis is much less of a problem with goats. One factor may be the fact that a goat's udder is rarely dirty and because of their dry faeces the milking parlour is much less dirty and wet than would be the case with cows. If sensible precautions are taken, such as teat dipping with an approved bactericidal dip and if a clean environment for milking can be created, mastitis should not be a problem. It is worth noting that goat's milk contains a high level of cellular debris that may have nothing to do with infection. It has been shown that 65% of goat milk samples will have a somatic cell count greater than 106 cells/mL. In the case of cow's milk this would be indicative of mastitis. To get a more accurate picture it is necessary to do a much more specific differential cell count.

9.11.2.4 Listeriosis

A disease that is becoming more prevalent, particularly on large dairy farms, is listeriosis. It is caused by the soil-borne bacterium, *Listeria monocytogenes*, which can occur almost anywhere. The main reason for its increase in larger dairy herds is because of the increased feeding of silage. It has been alleged that *Listeria* bacteria are not able to survive when the pH is below 4, yet the disease can occur in goats fed on maize silage at pH values less than 4. As with any other silage it is assumed the bacteria survive in pockets of the material where fermentation is not so good, in some cases because there is contact with air. This is more likely with bagged or wrapped silage where damage to the wrapping can occur. This is such a problem with goats that it is probably appropriate to advise that they should never be fed wrapped or bagged silage.

9.11.3 Metabolic Diseases

Goats rarely suffer from metabolic diseases. This is surprising in the case of the high-yielding dairy goat which, as already mentioned, on a live-weight (or metabolic bodyweight, $kg^{0.75}$) basis produces as much milk as a high genetic-merit Holstein cow. Milk fever (hypocalcaemia) and grass staggers (hypomagnesaemia) are rarely seen. The one metabolic disease that is seen in dairy goats is ketosis or acetonaemia. When a goat becomes fat most of the fat is deposited in the abdomen; if the goat is pregnant at the same time, bearing in mind that she could be carrying three or four kids, there will not be much space for normal digestion. In this situation it is necessary for the goat to have frequent small meals; if not, the goat may draw on its own fat reserves to get enough energy. When this happens chemicals called ketone bodies are produced and these can poison the system, giving rise to the disease ketosis or acetonaemia. A goat suffering from this disease will be listless and will not be interested in its food and its breath may smell like 'pear drops', or acetone. Treatment is difficult; an injection of corticosteroids and a multivitamin preparation may restore normal metabolism in about 30% of cases. This is a very good example of prevention being the best solution. Goats should not be allowed to get fat, particularly when pregnant, and at this time they should be given at least four feeds a day so that they are able to obtain enough energy from their feed. Exercise also helps so they should be turned out into a yard or paddock where they can run around.

9.11.4 Zoonotic Diseases

All people working with goats, particularly veterinarians, should be aware there are some diseases that can be transmitted to humans. These include enzootic abortion, toxoplasmosis, ringworm, orf (contagious pustular dermatitis), anthrax, listeriosis, louping ill, pox virus, brucellosis and leptospirosis. Precautions against some of these can have a serious affect on work routines; for example, it is generally advised that women of child-bearing age and certainly women who are pregnant should not work with kidding goats. Some of the diseases that cause abortion can have teratogenic effects on unborn children.

As with any animal, there are many diseases that can affect goats, but a large number are only seen rarely; therefore only the more common diseases have been included in this chapter. More information can be found in the publications listed at the end of the chapter.

References and Further Reading

Agricultural and Food Research Council (Great Britain). (1998). *The Nutrition of Goats*. ARC Technical Committee on Response to Nutrients. Report No 10. Wallingford: CABI Publishing.

Ashbrook, P.F. (1982). Year-round breeding for uniform milk production. In: *Proceedings of 3rd International Conference on Goat Production*, 153–154. Scottsdale, AZ: Dairy Goat Journal.

Buttle, H., Mowlem, A., and Mews, A. (1986). Disbudding and dehorning goats. *In Practice* 8: 63–65.

Lloyd, S. (1982). Parasite control. *Goat Veterinary Journal* 3 (1): 91.

Mowlem, A. (1983). *The Development of Goat Artificial Insemination in the United Kingdom*. Newton Abbot, UK: *British Goat Society Yearbook*. British Goat Society.

Mowlem, A. (1984). Artificial rearing of kids. *Goat Veterinary Journal* 5 (2): 246.

Mowlem, A. (2001). *Practical Goat Keeping*. Marlborough, UK: Crowood Press.

Mowlem, A. (2002). Current state and future prospects for dairy goats in England. *Journal of the Royal Agricultural Society* 163: 132–140.

Oldham, J.D.A. and Mowlem, A. (1981). Feeding goats for milk production. *Goat Veterinary Journal* 2 (1): 97.

Peacock, C. (1996). *Improving Goat Production in the Tropics*. Oxford: Oxfam-Farm Africa.

Porter, V. (1996). *Goats of the World*. Ipswich: Farming Press.

Zeuner, F.E. (1963) *A History of Domesticated Animals*. London: Hutchinson.

General reading

Department for Environment Food and Rural Affairs. (1989). Codes of Recommendations for Welfare of Livestock: Goats.

Dunn, P. (1994). *The Goatkeeper's Veterinary Book*. Ipswich: Farming Press.

Matthews, J. (1999). *Diseases of the Goat*. Oxford: Blackwell Scientific Publications.

Mackenzie, D. (1993). *Goat Husbandry*. London: Faber & Faber.

Mowlem, A. (1992). *Goat Farming*. Ipswich: Farming Press.

Mowlem, A. (2001). *Practical Goat Keeping*. Marlborough, UK: Crowood Press.

Porter, V. (1996). *Goats of the World*. Ipswich: Farming Press.

10

Red Deer

Alison Hanlon and Laura Griffin

KEY CONCEPTS

Management and Welfare of Farm Animals: The UFAW Farm Handbook, Sixth Edition.
Edited by John Webster and Jean Margerison.
© Universities Federation for Animal Welfare 2022. Published 2022 by John Wiley & Sons Ltd.

10.1   Introduction

Parkland deer have been kept for centuries for venison production. In contrast, venison production from farming deer only started in the UK and New Zealand in the 1970s. One of the main objectives of the deer farming initiative was to find an alternative land use for poor quality hill pasture and to exploit the large populations of wild red deer. Deer farming has progressed for over 40 years and adopted semi-extensive management systems. Red deer (*Cervus elaphus*) and fallow deer (*Dama dama*) are the most common species farmed in England, Scotland, Wales and Ireland. Other species of deer are farmed worldwide including sika deer (*Cervus nippon*) and rusa deer (*Cervus timorensis russa*). This chapter will focus on farmed red deer.

In Europe, red deer are farmed for venison, elsewhere in the world, antler velvet is also harvested by removing the antlers whilst still 'in velvet', which is a practice that is prohibited in the UK and the European Union. The main supply of venison comes from wild populations, however, as demand continues to rise, red deer farming is being encouraged in order to reduce reliance upon these wild populations. This is evident from Scotland's strategy to develop the farmed venison sector, which aims to produce an additional 750 tonnes of farmed venison per annum by 2030 (Scotland Food and Drink, 2018). DEFRA's farming statistics for the UK (excluding Wales) indicate that there were 37000 farmed deer in 2020 (DEFRA 2020).

There are two systems for venison production:

1) Deer Farms: Deer are managed in artificial groups, enclosed in fenced paddocks. Some stock, especially calves may be housed over-winter. The management of deer farming involves the management of breeding and weaning, administration of routine veterinary treatments, supplementary feeding and some husbandry procedures that optimize productivity.
2) Deer Parks: These present a more extensive form of deer management and involve less direct human contact and intervention. In contrast to a deer farm, park deer form natural social groupings throughout the year. The management of deer parks may involve providing supplementary feed and organized culling during set seasons. The removal of sick or injured individuals is common practice and permitted outside of the set culling seasons.

In the assessment of animal welfare, it is useful to consider a framework such as the Five Freedoms and/or Welfare Quality's four principles of Good Feeding, Good Housing, Good Health and Appropriate Behaviour (Botreau et al. 2009). The application of these criteria will vary depending on the deer farming calendar, e.g. some periods or events may pose a greater risk to deer welfare than others, equally the age and previous experience of the deer will influence the welfare outcomes.

10.2   Structure of the Industry

Deer farming can be divided into three husbandry systems:

1) Calf rearers
2) Calf finishers
3) Breeder, finishers

The choice of system generally depends on the location of the farm, the type of land and suitability (Venison Advisory Services Ltd., 2016). Lowland farms are likely to have better grass growth than upland areas and can support breeding, rearing and finishing calves. Whereas upland farms may be more suitable for breeding and selling weaned calves for finishing.

10.3   Natural History and Behaviour of Wild Red Deer

Red deer evolved as forest dwellers inhabiting open woodland and forest margins and adapted to survive on moorland. As a prey species, they are vigilant and agile animals, which are easy to excite and/or frighten. During the majority of the year wild red deer form single-sex groups, only coming together during the mating (rutting) season. The adult females (hinds) form family groups comprising related adult hinds and their offspring from the current and previous years. The group size varies, depending on habitat and season, and may range from 2 to more than 50 individuals per group. Stags form exclusively male 'bachelor' herds, which are smaller and less stable than the female herd, comprising adult and juvenile stags.

10.3.1   Feeding

In temperate climates red deer show seasonal variations in feeding behaviour. Photoperiod and the quantity and quality of food available determine seasonal feeding activity. Under natural conditions, red deer undertake 5 to 11 grazing bouts per day, the majority of which occur during daylight, with peaks in activity at dawn and dusk. The feeding behaviour varies with sex; hinds tend to select areas with higher quality forage than stags. In addition, both stags and hinds modify their feeding strategy to optimize their nutrient intake. Stags and hinds on poor quality grazing will extend their feeding time to increase nutrient intake, while hinds will also increase food intake prior to parturition, due to the nutritional demands of lactation, and stags will increase food intake prior to the breeding season.

10.3.2   Life Cycles: The Rut

The annual breeding period, known as the rut or rutting, occurs in the autumn. (Asher2011) Alterations in behavioural patterns are evident in stags in the late summer, as they start to compete for hierarchical status, territories and access to females. The initiation of aggressive behaviour in males during the pre-rut period corresponds to increasing levels of testosterone. During this period, stags perform dominance displays to establish and/or reinforce their position in the hierarchy. Some typical behaviours include roaring, sparring (frontal fighting) with interlocking antlers and scent marking. The mating strategies differ between different species of deer. Red deer stags commonly compete for a territory, for example, the area surrounding an oak tree, providing food sources such as acorns or browse to attract hinds. Stags in possession of a territory are extremely aggressive, instigating fights against trespassing stags and stags on neighbouring sites.

After establishing a territory, stags then focus on attracting hinds and gathering a 'harem' onto their territory. Apart from mating, stags have no other investment in their offspring, thus, to maximize their reproductive success it is important for each stag to mate with as many hinds as possible. Stags therefore devote most of their time and energy to defending territory, attracting, guarding and mating with hinds. As a consequence, stags spend significantly less time feeding, losing up to 20% in live weight and 80% of their fat reserves. Under natural conditions, stags maintain their harems for approximately three weeks, abruptly terminating rutting behaviour once a critical lower live weight is reached.

Sexual behaviour manifests in early October, coinciding with the onset of oestrous in hinds. Mounting by hinds is indicative of oestrous behaviour. To assess oestrous and sexual receptivity, stags periodically sniff and lick the anogenital area of hinds. Stags also chase and attempt to mount hinds but, unless the hind is sexually receptive, she will not stand for the stag. Standing immobility in response to tactile stimulation by the stag is a key sign that a hind is ready to be mated. Copulation consists of a true mount, with simultaneous intromission, and a single ejaculatory thrust. The stag dismounts and enters a brief rest period before resuming guarding and mating of his harem. In the wild, normally only adult stags are strong enough to compete for territories and harems, precluding younger juvenile stags from mating. However, observations have shown that young stags may mate with hinds when the territory holder is distracted or otherwise engaged.

10.3.3 Calving

Red deer produce singleton calves, although twins have occasionally been reported. The gestation length in wild adult hinds ranges from 228 to 249 days. Calving normally starts in May and continues until the end of June. Swelling and reddening of the udder occurs 1 to 2 days prior to parturition. Shortly before calving, hinds move away from the herd to give birth in isolation. The stages of parturition are not well defined in red deer. The perineal area typically begins to swell and redden several hours before birth. The onset of parturition and uterine contractions often manifest as restless behaviour, characterized by the hinds repeatedly touching and grooming their flanks, running in a high step gait with the neck outstretched, and fence pacing. As parturition progresses, hinds become increasingly restless, alternating between lying and standing. Hinds typically stand as the calf is delivered to ease the calf's delivery and most likely to facilitate the severing of the umbilical cord. Calves are normally born in the anterior-dorsal position, although breech births may also occur. The duration of calving varies from 30 to 120 minutes depending on factors such as the size of the calf and the ease with which the calf passes through the pelvis.

10.3.3.1 Mother–infant Interactions

Following parturition, the hind consumes all traces of the foetal membranes from the calf and the birth site. In farmed red deer, new-born calves normally stand within 30 minutes and suckle within 40 minutes. After the hind has nursed the calf, she moves away from the birth site followed by the calf. At this stage the neonatal calf is not strong enough to run with the maternal herd, so after a short distance it lies down and remains at this location until the hind returns to nurse it. In terms of behavioural development, although calves are precocious, i.e. born in an advanced neural and motor state, they are considered a 'hider' species. Neonatal calves remain hidden for up to one week postpartum and are periodically nursed by their dam in the hide-out.

Hinds nurse their calves for the first few days at 2 to 3-hour intervals. As the calf suckles, the hind licks the calf's anogenital area to stimulate defaecation and urination, which is involuntary in neonatal calves. The hind ingests the meconium (first faeces) to remove all traces of the presence of the neonatal calf. Peak lactation occurs at approximately 40 days postpartum. Under natural conditions, weaning is a gradual process. Suckling bouts decrease as lactation progresses and by three months of age calves suckle on average three to four times a day. The hind rejects up to 50% of suckling attempts by the time calves are six months old. At this stage the suckling bout lasts for approximately 30 seconds. The timing of weaning depends on the reproductive state of the hind. Pregnant hinds will gradually stop lactating in the winter, although barren hinds may continue to nurse their young until the following summer.

10.3.4 Life Cycles: Breeding

Red deer are seasonal 'short day' breeders such that breeding occurs during the autumn corresponding to shorter day length. Body weight largely determines the onset of puberty in both hinds and stags. Stags normally reach puberty at approximately 16 months old. However, the presence of mature stags will preclude yearlings from mating. Thus, stags do not successfully mate until they are able to compete for territories and gain access to hinds. In the wild, red hinds reach puberty at two to three years of age. Red deer are seasonally polyoestrous and come into oestrous every 18 to 20 days for 12 to 24 hours until they have successfully mated and conceived. Wild hinds have a lower live weight and reproductive success than their farmed counterparts corresponding to the poorer quality of forage and the lack of shelter.

10.3.4.1 Antler Development

Antlers are a unique anatomical structure and are not equivalent to horns of other ungulates. Horns are permanent with growth developing from the base of the horn. In contrast, antlers are grown and shed annually by red deer stags (antlers develop in both sexes in some species of deer, e.g. reindeer). Antlers grow from the tip and form new branches after the first year of growth. Stag calves develop pedicles (circular bony 'stalks') on frontal lobes of the skull, which later act as a platform for antlers. The antler growth cycle begins in Spring, between April and May, and is completed by August. Growing antlers are covered with a thick skin, called "velvet", which contains a network of blood vessels and nerve endings. In the final stages of growth, a ring, the coronet, forms around the antler base, constricting blood and nutrient supply to the antlers. Therefore, the velvet starts to shrivel and peel off, assisted by stag actively rubbing the antlers against trees and bushes. At this stage strips of velvet hang from the antlers, exposing the hard-calcified bone of the antler. This process is referred to as antler cleaning and is associated with an increase in testosterone levels. Once the velvet has been shed, the stag remains in hard antlers during the rut and over winter. Antlers are cast in early spring, which coincides with a decline in circulating testosterone concentrations. Before casting, stags typically leave the herd and each antler is cast separately within a day or two. New antler growth begins shortly after casting, thus completing the cycle. The complexity of antler architecture increases with age and the number of points (tines) on an antler is related to the age of the stag. For example, the antlers of yearling stags are simple spikes. However aged stags (>12 years old) undergo a gradual decrease in overall antler size and tine number.

10.4   Management of Farmed Red Deer

Deer farming is seasonal. Unlike other livestock species, seasonal cycles such as breeding and calving are not easily manipulated. There are three key events in the management calendar that influence social groupings and normal patterns of behaviour: breeding, calving, and weaning (Figure 10.1).

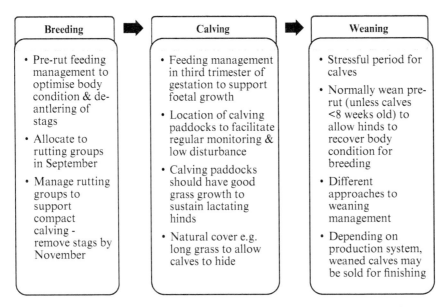

Breeding	Calving	Weaning
• Pre-rut feeding management to optimise body condition & de-antlering of stags • Allocate to rutting groups in September • Manage rutting groups to support compact calving - remove stags by November	• Feeding management in third trimester of gestation to support foetal growth • Location of calving paddocks to facilitate regular monitoring & low disturbance • Calving paddocks should have good grass growth to sustain lactating hinds • Natural cover e.g. long grass to allow calves to hide	• Stressful period for calves • Normally wean pre-rut (unless calves <8 weeks old) to allow hinds to recover body condition for breeding • Different approaches to weaning management • Depending on production system, weaned calves may be sold for finishing

Figure 10.1   Key events in the deer farming calendar: breeding, calving and weaning.

10.4.1 Breeding

The deer farming year begins in the early autumn, with preparations for the rut. One month before the rut, stags are routinely de-antlered as a safety measure, weighed and prophylactic treatments such as anthelmintics may be administered. From a management perspective, the main objectives are to achieve a high conception rate and manage groups to ensure early and compact calving. To achieve the first objective, both stags and hinds must enter the rut in good body condition. Stags are allocated to rutting groups in mid to late September or immediately following weaning. Research has shown that it is beneficial to form rutting groups in advance of the mating season, because the presence of a sexually mature male can stimulate the onset of oestrous by several days.

Deer farms commonly adopt single sire mating systems – allocating one stag to a group of hinds. This system guarantees the paternity of the offspring, but reproductive performance is largely dependent on the libido of an individual stag and monitoring of stag behaviour is important (British Deer Farms and Parks Association 2018). Multi-sire mating systems can be successfully managed, provided that stags have sufficient space to establish a territory (British Deer Farms and Parks Association 2018). The stag to hind ratio depends on the age of the stag (Table 10.1). Yearling stags are not commonly used for breeding because they have a lower fertility and are inexperienced compared with adults. In addition, the presence of adult stags can suppress the libido of yearling stags and, therefore, it is advisable to ensure that when yearling stags are not situated in close proximity to adult stags if they are allocated to rutting groups. Stags are removed from the rutting group after 1 to 2 oestrus cycles (the equivalent of 20 to 40 days) and commonly replaced by a 'chaser' or 'sweeper' stag, to ensure that all hinds have been mated (British Deer Farms and Parks Association 2018). It is recommended that all stags are removed by November, to avoid late calving, which is associated with lower calf survival rates and lower conception rates.

Approximately 85% of farmed hinds normally conceive in their first oestrous cycle, the remainder will continue to cycle two or three times before conceiving. Large scale studies on the reproductive performance of farmed red deer yearlings and hinds have been conducted in New Zealand (Audigé et al. 1999a,b) and identified a number of risk factors influencing reproductive success (Figure 10.2). As expected, body condition score (BCS) is important, together with achieving a certain weight threshold. The nutritional demands of lactation

Table 10.1 Stag to hind ratios for breeding.

Age of stag	Number of hinds
16 months	10 to 20
2 years	25 to 30
3 years	30 to 50
4 to 8 years	40 to 60
> 9 years	< 50

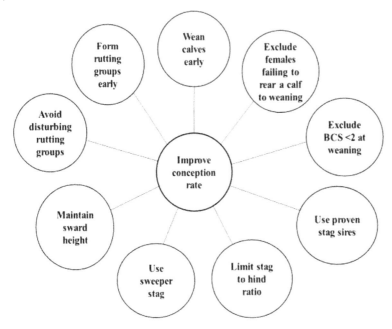

Figure 10.2 Risks factors affecting conception rate in farmed Red Deer Hinds (Audigé et al. 1999b).

have a direct impact on BCS and thus reproductive success, especially on yearlings. Hinds should have a minimum BCS of 2 and the odds of conception are further increased for hinds with a BCS 2.5. Therefore, it is important to ensure rutting groups are kept on good pasture. It is also recommended that supplementary feed is provided before the end of the rut. However, overfeeding is discouraged as hinds with a BCS of > 3.5 have been shown to experience difficulties during calving (Audigé et al. 2001). Yearling hinds have a lower body weight and consequently a longer latency to their first oestrous than adult hinds and thus yearlings should be managed in a separate group from adult hinds. Another important factor reported to affect reproductive performance is the risk of abortion, which is higher in yearling than adult hinds. The longevity of breeding stock varies from 15 to 17 years for hinds (FAS 2021) and 6 years for stags (Beattie and SAC Consulting 2021).

10.4.2 Calving

Calving normally starts in mid-May and continues until late June. As already stated, the mating period should be designed to support compact calving. Research has shown that calves born early in the calving season have higher weight gains than later born. In addition, late born calves have a higher risk of contracting bacterial diseases in the immediate postnatal period.

The adult and yearling hinds are allocated to calving groups in early May. Stocking densities of 4 to 8 hinds per ha are recommended to reduce the risk of competition. Most hinds calve unassisted. As previously mentioned, hinds tend to move away from the herd shortly before calving. They show a number of characteristic behaviours at this time including restlessness, increased walking activity, alternating between lying and standing; touching, sniffing and grooming their flanks and anogenital area; running in a high-stepping gait with neck out-stretched and fence-pacing. Fence-pacing is indicative of a sub-optimal calving environment and may be linked to increased calf mortality. Calving paddocks should provide adequate space, and low scrubby cover to facilitate normal calving behaviour. The duration of calving, from the appearance of the foetal sac to the expulsion of the calf, takes 20 to 120 minutes. Calving difficulty can be identified in hinds by observing the behaviour and the relative duration of calving. However, disturbance should be kept to a minimum to avoid causing stress to hinds and observations conducted from a vehicle or at a discrete distance.

Immediately following parturition, the dam normally initiates grooming, removing the foetal fluids from the calf. Thereafter the calf attempts to stand and teat seek. Calves are able to stand within an hour postpartum and suckle within 30 to 40 minutes of birth (Clutton Brock et al. 1982; Ekesbo and Gunnarsson 2018). The latency to suckle was reported to take longer for calves born to yearling than adult hinds. Whilst some farmers may tag and weigh calves from 12 to 48 hours after birth, because calves are easy to catch, handling neonatal calves within 12 hours of birth increases the risk of abandonment and mismothering. Furthermore, the stockperson should be aware that hinds can become aggressive at this time. Instead tagging and weighing can be conducted at weaning. Notably, tagging or identification must be performed before deer are moved from the premises. When moving hinds and their calves to grazing pastures for the first time, it is important to apply measures to prevent stampeding or injury. It is, therefore, recommended that feed be offered at the opposite end of the enclosure as a distraction while the gateway is opened. Ensure that no calves have been left behind prior to closing the gateway.

10.4.3 Weaning

As with other farmed species, weaning is associated with a series of potential stressors such as changes in the social and physical environment, handling and restraint for routine herd health procedures such as weighing, vaccination and worming. Calves can be weaned either before or after the rutting season. There are advantages and disadvantages associated with both time periods. Commonly weaning takes place before hinds are allocated to rutting groups in September when calves are approximately 100 days old. The main advantage is that this enables hinds to recover body condition before the breeding season, influencing the onset of oestrous and improving the conception rate. However, it may impede calf growth rate and increase the risk of stress-related disease of weaned calves in the short term. Younger calves, that are less than eight weeks old in September, should be weaned after the rut (FAWC 2013). Late weaning delays oestrous and recovery of BCS in breeding hinds before the rut.

At weaning calves are weighed and allocated to groups. Worming, vaccination against clostridial diseases and other treatments may also be administered (e.g. copper boluses if there is evidence of copper deficiency). Routine worming is repeated during housing, turn out, and during the second summer, up until the individual is 18 months old. Weaned calves are moved to an enclosure or housed, depending on the time of weaning and the climatic conditions. There are two schools of thought regarding the location of the paddock, whether it should be adjacent to or away from the maternal herd. The rationale for locating weaned calves within sight and scent of their maternal herd is to reduce stress. Inclusion of at least two dry hinds with weaned calves has been reported to assist in the overall settling of calves, as well as improve ease of movement during handling. Due to the potential for impeded growth and increased stress, it is recommended that weaning occur in good weather, keeping calves in stable groups and providing with high-quality feed and shelter when kept outdoors at weaning. As weaning progresses, feed should be monitored to prevent the risk of acidosis.

10.5 Environment and Housing

As a semi-extensive production system, farmed deer are kept on pasture for all or most of the year. Weaned calves and hinds may be housed overwinter to prevent poaching of pasture and protect against extreme weather. Calves are typically housed between November and April. While hinds are housed in lowland farming systems between January and April whereas those in upland farming systems may be out-wintered in a paddock with sheltered areas. Stags over three years of age in antler, if housed should be kept in individual pens (DEFRA 2015b).

10.5.1 At Pasture

The number of paddocks depends on the production system. Location, access to paddocks and integrated raceways to handling facilities are important considerations especially during calving. Calving paddocks are often situated close to the farm, to enable farmers to monitor calving without disturbing the deer. Trees provide natural shelter, although not essential, create a more naturalistic environment and help to improve calving success. Similarly, having areas of cover in calving paddocks, such as long grass or nettles facilitates hiding of neonatal calves. The calving paddocks should have good grass cover and sufficient growth to sustain lactating hinds during this period. The stocking rate depends on the type of land and quality of grazing (Table 10.2). Deer should be stocked at a rate that maintains an adequate body condition during winter; otherwise, supplementary feeding will be necessary. Overstocking during calving can lead to undesirable behaviour in hinds such as aggression towards calves.

10.5.2 Housing

Good housing is a benchmark of animal welfare. It should provide thermal and physical comfort as well as ease of movement. In temperate climates producers usually house weaned

Table 10.2 Stocking densities associated with different pasture-types.

Land type	Hinds (with calves) per ha	Yearling stags per ha
Arable lowland pastures	10 to 12	15 to 20
Upland sown pastures	8 to 10	12 to 15
Rough grazing (with forage provision)	1	NA

Source: Venison Advisory Services Ltd. 2016.

Table 10.3 Recommended feeding space (cm) for farmed red deer during housing according to age and live weight (kg).

Category of Stock	Live weight (kg)	Feeding Space (cm)	
		Ad libitum	Restricted
Weaned calves	25 to 40	15	25
	40 to 90	20	30
Yearlings & Adults[1]	75	40	50

[1] Additional feeding space will be required for yearlings and stags with antlers.

calves in groups over winter, because they possess proportionally less body fat than adults and are therefore less able to cope with climatic stress. Some producers also house breeding hinds and yearlings over winter to prevent poaching of grassland. However, confinement in housing increases the risk of aggression and damage to the skin of animals.

Whilst research has supported managing housed deer in small groups balanced for size and weight, FAWC reported that larger groups of up to 75 deer can also be successfully managed (FAWC 2013). Deer are housed in pens with deep bedded straw. The space allowance depends on the age and live weight (LW) and should be adjusted should bullying occur. Weaned calves (25 to 40 kg LW) should have a minimum space allowance of 2 $m^{2/}$head at weaning. Older calves (5 to 10 months old; 40 to 90 kg LW) require additional space of at least 2.5 $m^{2/}$head, while hinds and yearlings (>75 kg LW) require a minimum 3 $m^{2/}$head (SAI Global 2017). Bullying may occur during housing and can be reduced by providing adequate trough space (Table 10.3) to reduce competition for access to feed and environmental enrichment such as placing a round bale of straw in the pen. Stags are normally overwintered outdoors, however in cases where they are housed, males > 3 years old and in antler must be individually penned and stags with a live weight greater than 130 kg should have a space allowance of 5 m^2 (SAI Global 2017).

The main principles of animal housing apply to deer as other farmed livestock, which includes adequate ventilation and lighting, and dry bedding. Pens should be constructed with non-harmful material that can be disinfected between groups when the animals are turned out. The pen walls should be at least 2 m high, to discourage deer escaping.

10.5.3 Handling

Good stockperson-ship is a benchmark of animal welfare and is provided by calm and positive interactions with farmed deer. Overall the agility of deer and infrequency of handling can combine to elicit fear related behaviours. Depending of the type of production system, farmed deer may be handled up to five times a year or more if veterinary treatments are required. The age and experience of the deer, as well as the experience and skill of the stockperson along with the type of handling facilities available determine the ease of handling. Novice stock and calves at weaning are generally more difficult to handle because they are unfamiliar with the stockperson, being handled and the layout of the handling facilities. At weaning calves may attempt to escape through fencing and/or underneath gates. Including a tame hind in the weaning group can reduce panic among calves. The same principle applies to novice stock and locating novice and young stock closer to areas of human activity may also help to habituate animals to the noise and presence of humans. The habituation of animals to noise coupled with early handling may reduce stress at handling later in life. Regular movement of stock through corridors and handling facilities may also help to reduce stress when handling is required.

It is better to gather or muster deer as a group, with the exception of stags during the rut. If an individual becomes separated from the group, it may panic and try to escape. In this situation it is easier to allow the separated animal to re-join the group by moving a small group towards the separated animal. Loud noises including shouting should be avoided. Positive reinforcement to train young deer to respond to a particular call using a food reward, can help to reduce stress and improve ease of handling.

Stags during the rut and, to a lesser degree, hinds during calving may behave aggressively towards the stockperson. In addition, individual deer may respond aggressively to stockpersons during handling and even routine feeding. It is therefore important to be able to recognize threatening behaviour that precedes an attack, such as prolonged eye contact, ears flattened back, grinding teeth, stamping and snorting. The handling of stags during the rut should ideally be avoided. However, if it is necessary, for example moving a stag into a new rutting group, special precautions should be taken. Stags during this time should be handled individually and not in a group, because of the risk of fighting and associated injury, especially if they have not been de-antlered. Notably, movement of hinds in an advanced state of pregnancy or during the calving season should be avoided as this has been linked to an increased risk of calf mortality and calf rejection, respectively. However, if handling is unavoidable during these periods it should be conducted by a stockperson who is familiar with the animals.

10.5.3.1 Handling Facilities

In addition to good stockperson-ship it is possible to reduce stress during handling by incorporating specific features into the design and layout of handling facilities. The system should enable animals to move continuously from the home paddock or pen through the raceway(s) to the handling area with minimum stress and risk of injury.

The design of paddocks and access to handling facilities are important considerations. Some farms have an integrated system of raceways linking paddocks with the handling facilities. Where this is not possible, paddocks should be long and narrow or tapered towards the gate. Deer like other livestock move faster along curved raceways. Walls in the handling facility and fences should be sufficiently high, to prevent deer from attempting to jump over them and escape. Depending on the topography of the farm, it is recommended that paddocks are downhill from the yard, to help reduce the speed of movement and potential risk of injury during mustering (Venison Advisory Services Ltd. 2016). Inclusion of a holding area, prior to the yard, will allow the deer to settle before entering the handling facilities. Corners should be avoided, to prevent deer from clustering when yarded.

All deer farms should have handling facilities so that deer can be restrained for veterinary treatments. The most important requirements are a drop floor or pneumatic crush, weighing crate and at least one holding pen, but ideally several holding pens of different sizes. Some procedures such as body condition scoring and administration of anthelmintic treatments can be conducted in holding pens, when animals are grouped (Table 10.4). In contrast, de-antlering will require physical restraint in a drop-floor crush, short-term sedation or anaesthesia. Most accidents occur between the home paddock and handling facilities. Deer should be gathered and moved in a group at a walking pace. Raceways need to be sufficiently wide to enable group movement and raceway walls should be clearly visible to prevent the deer from jumping against them.

10.5.4 Fencing

Deer farmers use three main types of fencing: strained wire (horizontal wires), mesh and wire and baton. While electric fencing is used for controlling grazing, e.g. strip grazing of crops. The fencing requirements differ for perimeter and internal use, with perimeter fences

Table 10.4 Considerations for yard design and handling facilities.

Yard Location	Activities requiring handling facilities
Access for vehicles	Separating calves from hinds
Water and electricity supply	Splitting groups into smaller subgroups
Adjacent sheds for winter housing	Ear tagging
Uphill from paddocks and fields, roof optional	Antler removal
Under a roof is optional	Worming and supplement provision
	Weighing
	Loading into livestock trucks/ trailers

Source: Venison Advisory Services Ltd. 2016.

needing to be approximately 2 m high to prevent deer from escaping and other wildlife entering. In some areas of internal fencing such as raceways, need to be stronger, as they will be under greater pressure. At pressure points, fencing needs to prevent livestock from escape, entanglement and injury and be visible to livestock, to prevent deer, especially weaned calves and new stock, from accidentally running into it.

To prevent entanglement and injury, wire spacing needs to be sufficiently small to prevent deer from pushing their heads through; otherwise, it can lead to damage to antler buds and ears, as tags are pulled out. The wire spacing vary depending on enclosure type i.e. closer together for handling enclosures than for pasture paddocks. The calves are most at risk from entanglement in fencing, this can be minimized by using small mesh netting on the lower portion of fence. It is inadvisable to use electric fencing in calving paddocks, because of an obvious risk of the electrocution of calves.

10.6 Nutrition

Good feeding and nutrition support the health and fitness of deer, including optimum reproductive performance. Farms should have a feed plan, providing the dietary requirements according to age, stage of growth, season, feed quality and pasture management (SAI Global 2017). Feed intake for red deer is lower during the winter and the rut compared with during the summer, which is referred to as seasonal inappetence. Special attention should be given to minimize loss of body condition during this period, especially in stags kept at pasture overwinter. An increase in weight gain occurs during spring, with up to 40% of annual growth occurring in this period, and it is important that farmed deer be provided with high-quality feed or pasture during spring. All deer should always have access to fresh clean water, at all times.

Deer farming in the UK is predominantly a pasture-based system. Grass quality and sward height are key determinants of feed intake and live-weight gain, especially during spring and summer. High-quality short pasture (13 MJ ME/kg DM) is important in spring to optimize herd performance (Sneddon 2015). Farmed red deer have a higher basal metabolic rate than sheep and require approximately one third more energy. The digestion is like that of traditional ruminant livestock given a similar diet and, as with other similar livestock, changes in diet, such as supplementation with brassica crops, need to be gradually introduced over two to three weeks.

10.6.1 Nutrition of Breeding Hinds

Nutrition and corresponding live weight and body condition can dramatically increase the reproductive success of red deer hinds by:

- Reducing the age of first calving
- Increasing the rate of conception
- Increasing calf survival

Live weight is an important determinant of the age at first calving. Improvements in the nutrition of red deer hinds have allowed producers to hasten the onset of puberty, reducing the age to 16 months in farmed deer, compared with 24 to 36 months in their wild counterparts. In addition, adequate body condition and, as such live weight, also influences the subsequent reproductive success of hinds. In the wild, lactating hinds have a 50% chance of calving in the following season. The conception rate of hinds is positively correlated with the pre-rut live weight of hinds, with hinds > 70 kg having a conception rate of 90 % compared with 50% for hinds < 65 kg (Hamilton and Blaxter 1980).

The energy requirements for adult hinds vary according to, live weight, season and reproductive status. The dry matter intake (DMI) required by hinds increases from mid-pregnancy to before parturition, while the hinds' energy requirements continue to increase during lactation. The provision of adequate forage for grazing hinds during lactation, can be achieved by farmers providing young leafy grass and by maintaining sward heights between 8 and 12 cm (Sneddon 2015). Annual stocking rates depend on pasture quality and growth rate; e.g. poor quality pasture such as heather moorland can only maintain a maximum of 1 hind per hectare, while in contrast cultivated upland and lowland pasture can support 8 to 10 and 10 to 12 hinds per hectare, respectively (Table 10.2).

Maintaining an adequate body condition during pregnancy is critical in ensuring high rates of prenatal development and neonatal survival. As with other livestock species, poor nutrition during gestation, especially the third trimester, influences the birth weight of calves, thereby increasing the risk of calf mortality. Furthermore, gestation length is extended in underfed hinds, conflicting with management goals for an early and compact calving season. In contrast over-feeding is equally undesirable because of the increased risks of dystocia. The constant provision of supplementary feed has been reported to lower the muscle tone and fitness of hinds, due to lack of exercise associated with the reduced need for foraging activity.

10.6.2 Nutrition of Calves

The weight and body condition of hinds during gestation, especially during the third trimester, determines the birth weight of calves and influences subsequent growth rate. Optimum feeding of farmed hinds can achieve an average calf birth weight of 9.5 kg (Sneddon 2015). Calves are dependent on milk for their energy requirements during the first 30 days of life, consuming between 200 and 600 g of milk per suckling bout and a maximum intake of 2.0 kg/day (Arman et al. 1974). Male calves show higher growth rates than female calves. As lactation progresses the dependency on milk gradually decreases and by the time calves are approximately three months old, milk accounts for only 10 to 20% of the total daily energy intake. During this time, suboptimal nutrition in lactating hinds can result in substantially lower calf live weights, requiring increased supplementary feeding of calves to promote higher growth rates.

High-quality pasture during the summer, with 40 to 80% green leaf, can support calf weight gains of between 250 and 500 g/d (Sneddon 2015). However, calf live-weight gain falls as the quality of pasture decreases during late summer. The provision of concentrate feed supplements to calves for approximately 10 days pre-weaning is good practice. The average live weight of calves at weaning depends on the production system, but well-managed farms, with calves born at the end of May, can achieve an average weaning weight of 50 kg in late September (Sneddon 2015). Over the winter, seasonal inappetance greatly affects live-weight gain, although skeletal growth continues at a slower rate. In many circumstances, particularly on hill and upland farms, supplementary feeding and housing may be necessary to achieve target live weights at 15 months of age. Weaned calves that are housed and offered maintenance rations over winter have a lower live-weight gain than those on *ad libitum* diets. However, the rapid growth of calves following turnout on pasture in late spring partly compensates for this differential growth.

10.6.3 Nutrition of Stags

During the rut, stags may lose up to 30% of their live weight due to spending a large proportion of the time guarding, mating and/or competing for hinds, and spending a correspondingly decreased amount of time spent feeding (British Deer Farms and Parks Association 2018). At the end of the rut, stags can typically be in poor body condition and this problem can be compounded by the onset of seasonal inappetance. It is therefore important to ensure that stags enter the rut in good body condition and are removed after a four to six-week period to reduce the detrimental impact of rutting on body condition before the onset of winter. Over winter, stags should be kept in a sheltered paddock and provided with supplementary concentrate feed to minimize further loss in body condition (Sneddon 2015).

10.6.4 Mineral Requirements

Calcium, phosphorous and magnesium are essential components in the diet. Deer can, to some extent, counteract short-term dietary deficiency in the major minerals by mobilizing body reserves, although this may impair skeletal growth and development of calves. Mineral requirements are normally higher during growth and lactation with hinds losing approximately 2.2 g calcium and 1.9 g phosphorous per kg milk (Alexander and Buxton 1994). Phosphorus deficiency may reduce fertility. Deer require other minerals such as copper, cobalt, selenium and iodine in trace quantities. Deficiency in all except iodine can cause subclinical problems; clinical signs may become evident only when compounded by other factors.

10.6.5 Body Condition Scoring

The assessment of body condition score (BCS) is an important management tool to ensuring that the nutritional intake of animals is enough to support good health and productivity, especially of breeding females. A scoring system is commonly used for farmed red deer hinds and yearlings, based on a scale of 1 (lean) to 5 (fat) with half unit increments (Table 10.5), which is very similar to body condition scoring of sheep. The animal assessment is based on

Table 10.5 Body condition scoring chart for farmed red hinds and yearlings.

Body condition	Wings of the pelvis	Spinous processes	Rump area
1: Very poor	Extremely prominent and sharp	Very sharp	Concave on palpation, little muscle or fat cover
2: Poor (lean)	Prominent, but rounded and easily felt by palpation with slight finger pressure	Slightly rounded and not prominent	Flat
3: Moderate	Prominent, but rounded and easily felt by palpation	Slightly rounded and not prominent	Flat
4: Good	Rounded and easily felt by palpation under a thin layer of fat	Rounded and felt by palpation only with firm pressure	Slightly convex
5: Very good (fat)	Concealed under a thick layer of fat and cannot be felt with firm pressure	Well-rounded and not felt on palpation	Convex

Source: Audigé et al. 1999b.

the muscle and fat coverage over three distinct areas: the wings of the pelvis, the tuber coxae and the spinous processes. A minimal or mild amount of animal restraint is required to assess BCS and, to achieve this, a group of deer should be moved into a small holding pen, which will allow the stockperson to move amongst the deer and gently palpate the pelvic area, spinous processes and rump.

10.7 Health and Disease

The Welfare Quality® principle of good health consists of absence of injury, absence of disease and absence of painful procedures (Figure 10.3) and apart from animal tagging for identification purposes, painful procedures such as castration are not undertaken. Any de-antlering that is performed is only undertaken for the future benefit of all animals concerned and is completed when the antlers are calcified and insensitive. The removal of antlers in velvet ('velvetting') is not permitted in the UK and EU.

A written herd health plan, prepared in consultation with a veterinarian, is the best practice approach to the prevention and absence of disease. The plan should include routine health monitoring such as checking for lameness (e.g. hoof overgrowth of housed animals before turnout in the spring), respiratory, digestive and/or nutritional disorders and parasite control, and provide a standard operating procedure for calving including the provision of colostrum (SAI Global 2017). Finally, biosecurity measures are also included, as these are key in preventing the introduction and spread of disease (FAWC 2013).

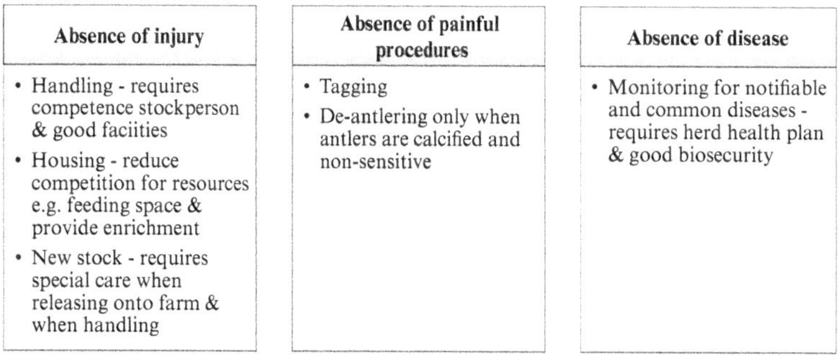

Absence of injury	Absence of painful procedures	Absence of disease
• Handling - requires competence stockperson & good faciities • Housing - reduce competition for resources e.g. feeding space & provide enrichment • New stock - requires special care when releasing onto farm & when handling	• Tagging • De-antlering only when antlers are calcified and non-sensitive	• Monitoring for notifiable and common diseases - requires herd health plan & good biosecurity

Figure 10.3 Outline of factors influencing the principles of good health in farmed red deer.

The Department for Environment, Food and Rural Affairs (DEFRA) in the UK and other competent authorities such as the world organization for animal health (OIE) and European Food Safety Authority (EFSA) provide information on current notifiable and emerging diseases. The notifiable diseases listed for farmed red deer include tuberculosis, bluetongue, epizootic haemorrhagic disease and foot and mouth. A brief description is provided of some of the common and notifiable diseases. A more comprehensive review of diseases in farmed deer is available in Alexander and Buxton (1994).

10.7.1 Tuberculosis

Tuberculosis (TB) in deer is a notifiable disease in the UK and is caused by infection with species within the *Mycobacterium tuberculosis complex*. The complex members include *M. tuberculosis*, *M. canetti*, *M. africanum*, *M. pinnipedii*, *M. microti*, *M. caprae*, *M. bovis* and the *Bacillus Calmette-Guerin* strain (BCG vaccine). The disease has a slow progression in deer and infected deer can appear to be clinically healthy, even in the advanced stages of the disease. Farmed deer are also susceptible to other Mycobacterial diseases such as Johne's disease (paratuberculosis) and avian tuberculosis. Some of the pathological lesions present in deer infected with the latter can be similar to those caused by *M. bovis*, thus confounding slaughterhouse surveillance of TB. A number of diagnostic tests are available to detect TB in deer; however, it is unlikely that all infected deer in a herd will be detected at the same time. Therefore, testing should be repeated in order to provide any degree of certainty regarding whether a herd is TB free.

10.7.2 Johne's Disease

Johne's disease or paratuberculosis, caused by *Mycobacterium avium sub spp. paratuberculosis* (MAP) is more commonly seen in young deer between the age of 8 and 15 months than in older livestock. It is transmissible in utero, in milk and via ingestion of pasture or drinking water contaminated by faeces of infected animals. The clinical signs include loss of condition, retention of the winter coat and as the disease progresses, diarrhoea. Enlarged lymph nodes and abscesses may also occur. Infected stock may show subclinical signs such as slow growth rates. There are no effective treatments available and death will occur in weeks or months. It is advisable to isolate and cull infected animals because of the poor prognosis and risk of disease transmission to the herd. A key risk factor is purchasing infected stock, while preventative strategies include keeping a 'closed herd' i.e. not buying in new stock or ensuring that new stock have been tested.

10.7.3 Yersiniosis

The bacterium *Yersinia pseudotuberculosis* causes yersiniosis. Both wild and domestic animals are carriers, and it can occur in the faeces of healthy deer. Infected deer shed large quantities of the organism in their faeces and so infection can rapidly spread within a group. Deer commonly encounter Yersinia in their first winter but may not show any clinical signs of infection. Clinical disease is triggered by stress such as weaning, under-feeding, overcrowding, rough handling and transportation. The clinical signs include weight loss, green diarrhoea, dehydration and prolonged inactivity before death. Yersiniosis can be successfully treated with antibiotics, combined with non-specific diarrhoea treatment and fluid replacement therapy. Some countries have a vaccine available for yersiniosis.

10.7.4 Clostridial Diseases

Species of *Clostridium* cause a variety of disease. For example, *C. perfringens* (also called *C. welchii*) causes enterotoxaemia. Clostridial infection can occur when the diet changes suddenly; affecting a change in the gut flora supporting clostridia growth, which produce a lethal toxin. Other examples include blackleg and malignant oedema, caused by infection of open wounds by Clostridial species and results in septicaemia. The condition is fatal unless diagnosed in time. Commencement of a vaccination programme (usually at weaning) followed by re-vaccination at yearly intervals using multivalent vaccines can reduce clostridial infections.

10.7.5 Bluetongue

Bluetongue (BT) is caused by a virus within the Orbivirus genus of the Reovirus family, it affects all ruminants, including deer. There are approximately 27 serotypes of the virus (BVT), and red deer are a reservoir host for BTV 1–24. The OIE reported clinical signs in sheep and some species of deer to include changes to the mucous linings of the mouth and nose and the coronary band of the foot. The disease is spread by the Culicoides family of biting midges. However, according to DEFRA the likelihood of mechanical transmission of the virus between herds/flocks and within a herd/flock by unhygienic practices (e.g. use of contaminated surgical equipment or hypodermic needles) cannot be excluded. A vaccine against BT serotype 8 is available but is not licensed for use in deer (though could be used under the cascade system in the UK). Culicoides are most common between March and September. In the UK and elsewhere it is a notifiable disease and therefore its occurrence should be reported to the competent authority, e.g. DEFRA in the UK.

10.7.6 Epizootic Haemorrhagic Disease

Epizootic haemorrhagic disease (EHD) is a notifiable disease and also stems from the Orbivirus genus. It occurs in wild ruminants, especially white-tailed deer in North America and causes high rates of morbidity and mortality. As with bluetongue, EHD is transmitted by biting midges from the Culicoides family. Infected deer can be virulent for up to two months. The symptoms and clinical signs in deer are similar to bluetongue and foot and mouth disease. The OIE provides clinical indicators for diagnosis of acute EHD in deer including fever, weakness, inappetence, excessive salivation, facial swelling, hyperaemia (increased blood supply) to conjunctiva and mucous membranes in the mouth. Chronic signs include ulceration of the mouth (the dental pad, hard palate and tongue), diarrhoea containing blood and dehydration. This disease has not been reported in wild or farmed red deer in the UK.

10.7.7 Chronic Wasting Disease

Several deer species are susceptible to this notifiable disease. Whilst there have been no reports of it in the UK, the first European case was reported in reindeer in Norway in 2016. Chronic wasting disease (CWD) is a transmissible spongiform encephalopathy (TSE), highly infectious and fatal. The disease can take 18 to 24 months to incubate, before clinical signs manifest. As the incubation period progresses, the risk of disease transmission increases. Clinical signs are characterized by changes in behaviour, posture and movement and include the following indicators:

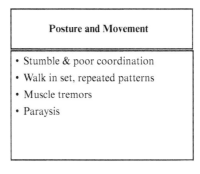

Behaviour	Posture and Movement
• Separation from the herd	• Stumble & poor coordination
• Lowering of head	• Walk in set, repeated patterns
• Difficulty swallowing	• Muscle tremors
• Increased thirst & urination	• Paraysis
• Salivation	
• Teeth grinding	
• Nervousness	

Figure 10.4 Characteristic behaviours indicating chronic wasting disease in red deer (DEFRA 2015a).

10.7.8 Malignant Catarrhal Fever

Malignant catarrhal fever (MCF) has been a major cause of mortality in farmed deer in New Zealand. It is caused by two viruses *Alcelaphine herpesvirus-1* (AHV-1) and *Ovine herpesvirous-2* (OHV-2). Wildebeest and sheep are hosts of AHV-1 and OHV-2, respectively. The viruses become pathogenic once they are transmitted to another species. Susceptibility to MCF varies with deer species and the disease can be fatal. Stress can trigger the onset of clinical disease in deer. Clinical signs include inappetance, dysentery, enlargement of lymph nodes, bilateral corneal opacity, mucosal secretions and skin ulcers. There are no vaccines available. As part of a herd health strategy it is important to reduce the risk of disease transmission by ensuring that farmed deer are not kept in close proximity to sheep and wildebeest. Biosecurity measures should be taken on farms containing both sheep and deer; for example, separate stockpersons should be responsible for managing each species.

10.7.9 Parasites

Farmed red deer are susceptible to gastrointestinal and thoracic parasites. Risks factors for infestation include age, e.g. young deer are more susceptible than adults during their first autumn and winter. Periods of stress including suboptimal nutrition increase the risk of infestation in adults. Furthermore, climatic conditions influence the life cycle of internal parasites with larvae development favoured during warm and humid weather.

Ostertagia species are the main gastro-intestinal parasites, although others may also be present in the gut, but at such low numbers that they are effectively non-pathogenic. Clinical infestation with *Ostertagia* causes the same symptoms as in other livestock, namely weight loss and poor coat condition, soft faeces and a soiled tail. Treatment depends on the degree and spread of infestation and grassland management. The most effect strategy is to combine anthelmintic treatment with pasture rotation.

Cryptosporidiosis caused by *Cryptosporidium parvum*, is a coccidial parasite that infects the small intestine. The disease is transmitted through ingestion of Cryptosporidium eggs shed in the faeces of infected animals. It is highly contagious and can spread rapidly in a group of young calves either at pasture or in a pen. Clinical signs occur within five to six days and include inappetance and diarrhoea. Infected animals should be immediately isolated to prevent further spread. Anticoccidial vaccines are ineffective and most farmers treat infected calves for dehydration. Cryptosporidium is also a zoonotic disease, causing acute gastroenteritis in humans.

Lungworm (*Dictyocaulus viviparous*) can have a significant impact on health, welfare and productivity of red deer. Calves are the most vulnerable age group, particularly in autumn. Clinical signs include inappetance, weight loss, poor coat condition, tachycardia and tachypnoea. Heavy infestations can lead to sudden death. Stressors such as high stocking densities, suboptimal nutrition and transport increase the risk of infection. The prepatent period (time between infection and detection) is from 20 to 24 days, and larvae are excreted for approximately 25 days. Faecal eggs counts should be part of a herd health strategy. Prophylactic treatment with anthelmintics should be considered for hinds on farms with a history of calves infected with lungworm.

Nasal bot flies (*Cephenemyia auribarbis*) may cause respiratory distress in red deer. From May to July female bot flies inject larvae into the nostrils of deer. Initial growth occurs in nasal cavities; by April or May the larvae migrate to the pharyngeal pockets until they develop fully. Before pupating, larvae drop out of the nose and onto the ground. Heavy infestation with bot fly larvae may cause suffocation or secondary infections at the site of attachments following inhalation of larvae. Warbles (*Hypoderma diana*) and headfly (*Hydrotaea irritans*) can also cause problems.

Liver fluke (*Fasciola hepatica*) infection in red deer commonly occurs at a sub-clinical level. However, it is an important cause of liver condemnation post-mortem. Treatment with fluki-cides is more effective for adult (90 to 100%) than immature fluke. To ensure effective treatment, application of flukicides should be repeated approximately one month after initial treatment.

10.7.10 Management-Related Problems

During the early years of deer farming, problems related to the stress associated with the capture and captivity of wild deer. Although farmed red deer may not yet be considered domesticated, selective breeding over the past 40 years is likely to have selected deer best suited to a farm environment. As with most livestock, stressors such as handling, housing and transportation have the potential to reduce the health and well-being of farmed red deer. Handling in particular needs to be performed by skilled stockpersons. The three Ts provide guidance on handling: training, taming and tempo (Haigh and Hudson 1993). Training and taming relate to habituating and the use of positive reinforcement to accustomize deer to the stockperson and handling system. Moving deer at a slow pace, the Tempo, is important to reduce the risk of injury.

Metabolic disorders such as acidosis may arise from inappropriate supplementary feeding. Excess lactic acid is produced during fermentation in the rumen, following the consumption of large quantities of concentrated feed. The consequent increase in acidity can destroy the tissue lining and microflora of the rumen. Once the lactic acid enters the circulation it can cause damage to other tissues and organs. Dominant animals are more likely to suffer from acidosis because they have priority of access to feed. The clinical signs include inappetance, increased inactivity eventually resulting in an inability to stand and in severe cases leading to death. The treatment for acidosis is to wash out the rumen, a procedure which must be conducted by a veterinary surgeon. The condition can be prevented by the gradual introduction of concentrate feed and spreading the distribution over a wide area to stop individuals from gorging.

An average of 92% of breeding hinds will successfully produce a live calf during the calving season. Of these approximately 85% are successfully reared to weaning, giving an average postpartum mortality rate of 15% (Beattie and SAC Consulting 2021). Management and environment play an important role in calf survival (Pollard and Stevens 2003). In particular, the environment should facilitate the behavioural ecology of red deer at calving; providing areas of cover that enable calves to hide, and minimizing disturbance, as described earlier.

10.8   Transportation

Farmed deer are mainly transported to supply breeding stock or weaned calves for finishing either directly to farms or to abattoirs for slaughter. The regulations on the welfare of animals in transport change over time. Updates are published on the DEFRA website (and national counterparts in the EU). Deer must be 'fit' for transport, unfit categories include:

- Injury, illness, fatigued or stressed
- Heavily pregnant females in the last month of gestation, and females that have given birth within 48 hours.
- Newborn calves with unhealed navels
- Stags in velvet and during the rut (males > 24 months)

Deer that become 'unfit', e.g. injured during the journey must be taken to the nearest suitable place. Exceptions to the 'fitness to travel' rule may be permitted in an emergency where transportation is not likely to cause additional unnecessary suffering, e.g. for veterinary treatment at a nearby destination, provided that it is in compliance with relevant local or national legislation. The transporter is responsible for monitoring animals during the journey. For stags in hard antler, it is advisable to de-antler several days before transportation. De-antlered stags should not be grouped with stags in antler, due to an increased risk of injury. In addition, groups of animals that have been housed or kept together should not be mixed with unfamiliar animals for transport (SAI Global 2017).

The vehicle, loading and unloading facilities should be designed and maintained to avoid injury and suffering to the animals. Loading ramp angle should be 20 (preferable) to 30 degrees (SAI Global 2017). The stocking density required during transport (Table 10.6) needs to be reduced to allow additional space during hot weather. Most notably, a height of 1.5 m is deemed adequate for red deer hinds, while stags require greater headroom due to their increased size. The provision of adequate ventilation is necessary for all journeys, while water and food requirements vary according to journey length.

Planning is important to minimize journey length and confinement in the vehicle. In addition to the above a number of technical rules involving authorization apply to journeys over 40 miles (equivalent to 65 km). The level of authorization depends on journey length and duration.

Table 10.6   Stocking density requirements for deer during transport.

Animal Size	Space allowance/head (m^2)
Adult stag (De-antlered)	0.8 to 1.0
Adult hind/Yearling stag	0.5 to 0.6
3-month-old calves – Yearling hinds	0.4 to 0.48

Source: Venison Advisory Services Ltd. 2016.

10.9   Slaughter

In contrast to other farmed livestock, deer can be humanely slaughtered either in an approved abattoir (which may be purpose-built) or by shooting by a licensed marksman (certified as competent) at the home farm (field slaughter). An ante mortem inspection by a veterinarian is required for all animals within 72 hours of slaughter. Field slaughter has the advantage of being conducted in a familiar environment with minimal stress. DEFRA provide a code of recommendation for field slaughter. Deer should be quiet and inactive at the time of field slaughter and this can be achieved by providing lines of concentrate feed for the deer. Tame or inactivate deer can be shot at close range (10 to 20 m) using a head shot. Less tame deer can be dispatched up to a range of 40 m using a high neck shot. Ranges beyond 40 m should only be undertaken by proven marksmen but should be unnecessary for farmed deer. In addition to the skill of the marksmen a suitable rifle and ammunition should be used.

Limitations to field slaughter include throughput, and human safety. In terms of throughput, only a limited number of deer can be shot at any one time, before the noise of the shooting starts to agitate other deer on the farm. Public safety is an issue for farms that adjoin areas accessible to the public. DEFRA recommend that farmers should:

- Walk the fence perimeter of the farm to check that there are no members of public in the vicinity
- Conduct field slaughter early in the morning
- Shoot away from roads, houses and gardens

Food hygiene regulations apply to field slaughter, requirements depend on whether the carcass is transported to an approved abattoir or processed on-farm in a licensed facility. Humane slaughter in an abattoir normally includes a series of potentially stressful events between unloading and slaughter. Competent handling and appropriately designed unloading, lairage and handling facilities in the abattoir are important to minimize stress to deer. Captive bolt stunning is used on farmed red deer and FAWC recommends pithing post-stunning to ensure insensibility to pain and reduce risk of injury to the slaughter person (FAWC 2013).

10.9.1   Meat Quality

Farmers produce prime venison from deer slaughtered at 1 to 2 years of age, at a maximum of 27 months. Venison has a reputation for being a low in fat, and cholesterol and has a higher lean to bone ratio in comparison with beef, lamb and chicken. The proportion of fat is higher in hinds than stags (except pre-rut) and in older animals. As with other livestock species, poor quality handling immediately pre-slaughter can have a detrimental effect on carcass quality.

10.10   The Way Ahead

The underlying ethos of deer farming has been to adapt management systems and environs to the nature of deer, facilitating normal patterns of behaviour such as rutting and calving. Consequently, it is more naturalistic. From an ethical perspective, it may be considered to be more acceptable than intensive livestock production systems, which are associated with production diseases, stereotypic and injurious behaviours, and other indicators of poor animal welfare. There are opportunities and threats to the welfare of farmed deer identified by FAWC (2013). Establishing a system for centralized data capture and utilization by competent authorities is important for biosecurity and herd health. As a small sector within animal agriculture, there is a lack of centralized data recording on farmed deer, such as industry demographics, disease surveillance and research. Research is important to identify and address emerging threats to herd health and support good farming practice.

The handling of farmed deer is a key risk of injury to the deer and stockpersons and the provision of appropriate on-farm facilities should be a requirement for all deer farms. The training and competence of personnel involved in deer farming including stockpersons and veterinary professionals are important to support best practice during handling and the provision of appropriate health care. Furthermore, there is an opportunity for industry, professional organizations and universities to develop continuing agricultural, animal science and veterinary education on deer farming.

Sustainability is a major driver in agriculture; in addition to economic and environmental pillars of this concept, it also includes social sustainability comprising farmer well-being and animal welfare. Whilst wild deer were used as breeding stock in the early years of deer farming, it posed a number of challenges to animal welfare. Returning to this practice is ethically problematic and at odds with the progressive nature of deer farming. It is important that deer farmers continue to demonstrate a good understanding for the behavioural and physical requirements of deer and to avoid the mistakes made by intensive agriculture.

References

Alexander, T.L. and Buxton, D. (eds.). (1994). *Management and Diseases of Deer: A Handbook for the Veterinary Surgeon*, 2nd edition. London, UK: Veterinary Deer Society: London, UK.

Arman, P., Kay, R.N.B., Goodall, E.D., and Sharman, G.A.M. (1974). The composition and yield of milk from captive red deer (Cervus elaphus L.). *Reproduction* 37 (1): 67–84.

Asher, G.W. (2011). Reproductive cycles of deer. *Animal Reproduction Science* 124: 170–175.

Audigé, L., Wilson, P.R., and Morris, R.S. (1999a). A body condition score for use in farmed red deer (Cervus elaphus). *New Zealand Journal of Agriculture Research* 41 (4): 545–553.

Audigé, L., Wilson, P.R., and Morris, R.S. (2001). Risk factors for dystocia in farmed red deer (Cervus elaphus). *Australian Veterinary Journal* 79 (5): 352–357.

Audigé, L.J.M., Wilson, P.R., Pfeiffer, D.U., and Morris, R.S. (1999b). Reproductive performance of farmed red deer (Cervus elaphus) in New Zealand: II. Risk factors for adult hind conception. *Preventive Veterinary Medicine* 40 (1): 33–51.

Beattie, A., and SAC Consulting. (2021). The Farm Management Handbook 2020/21. https://www.fas.scot/downloads/farm-management-handbook-2020-21 (accessed 09 September 2021).

Botreau, R., Veissier, I., and Perny, P. (2009). Overall assessment of animal welfare: Strategy adopted in Welfare Quality®. *Animal Welfare* 18 (4): 363–370.

British Deer Farms and Parks Association. (2018). Red Deer in a Farm System – Stags. http://www.bdfpa.org/deer-info/4590929468 (accessed 25 January 2019).

Clutton Brock, T.H., Guinness, F.E., and Albon, S.D. (1982). *Red Deer Behavior and Ecology of Two Sexes*. University of Chicago Press.

DEFRA. (2015a). Chronic wasting disease: How to spot and report the disease. https://www.gov.uk/guidance/chronic-wasting-disease (accessed 24 January 2019).

DEFRA. (2015b). Guidance caring for Deer. Published 15 October 2015. https://www.gov.uk/government/publications/deer-on-farm-welfare/caring-for-deer#housing-and-shelter (accessed 09 September 2021).

DEFRA. (2020). Farming Statistics- final crop areas, yields, livestock populations and agricultural workforce at 1 June 2020 United Kingdom. https://www.gov.uk/government/statistics/farming-statistics-final-crop-areas-yields-livestock-populations-and-agricultural-workforce-at-1-june-2020-uk (accessed 08 September 2021).

Ekesbo, I. and Gunnarsson, S. (2018). *Farm Animal Behaviour: Characteristics for Assessment of Health and Welfare*. CABI.

Farm Advisory Service. (2020). Alternative livestock factsheet. www.fas.scot (accessed 08 September 2021).

FAWC. (2013). FAWC Opinion on the Welfare of Farmed and Park Deer. https://www.gov.uk/government/publications/fawc-opinion-on-the-welfare-of-farmed-and-park-deer (accessed 12 November 2018).

Haigh, J.C. and Hudson, R.J. (1993). *Farming Wapiti and Red Deer*. Mosby.

Hamilton, W.J. and Blaxter, K.L. (1980). Reproduction in farmed red deer. 1. Hind and stag fertility. *The Journal of Agricultural Science* 95 (2): 261–273.

Mysterud, A., Meisingset, E., Langvatn, R., Yoccoz, N.G., and Stenseth, N.C. (2005). Climate-dependent allocation of resources to secondary sexual traits in red deer. *Oikos* 111 (2): 245–252.

Patel, K.K., Howe, L., Heuer, C., Asher, G.W., and Wilson, P.R. (2018). Pregnancy and mid-term abortion rates in farmed red deer in New Zealand. *Animal Reproduction Science* 193: 140–152.

Pollard, J.C. and Stevens, D.R. (2003). Some production outcomes when management practices and deer behaviour interact. *The Nutrition and Management of Deer on Grazing Systems. Grassland Research and Practice Series No 9*: 73–78.

SAI Global (2017). SAI Global Quality Assured Farm Venison Standard. Version 6 November 2017. www.bdfpa.org (accessed 09 September 2021).

Scotland Food & Drink. (2018). Beyond the Glen. A strategy for the Scottish venison sector to 2030. https://www.foodanddrink.scot/resources/sector-strategies/beyond-the-glen-a-strategy-for-the-scottish-venison-sector-to-2030 (accessed 08 September 2021).

Sneddon, A. (2015). Feeding Farmed Deer for Profitable Production. Presentation to the Deer Farm & Park Demonstration Project. https://deerfarmdemoproject.scottish-venison.info/wp-content/uploads/2015/11/Alan-Sneddon-Fife-20.11.15.pdf (accessed 13 February 2019).

Venison Advisory Services Ltd. (2016). A Starter Guide to Deer Farming and Park Deer Management. *The Deer Demonstration Project.* http://deerfarmdemoproject.scottish-venison.info/wp-content/uploads/2016/04/starter-guide-deer-farming-park-management.pdf (accessed 12 November 2018).

Further Reading

British Deer Farms and Parks Association publish a range of advisory fact sheets on deer farming. www.bdfpa.org.

DEFRA. (2011). Welfare of Animals during Transport. www.gov.uk/DEFRA.

DEFRA. (2015). Guidance: Caring for Deer. https://www.gov.uk/government/publications/deer-on-farm-welfare/caring-for-deer (accessed 28 January 2019).

Mackintosh, C., Haigh, J.C., and Griffin, F. (2002). Bacterial diseases of farmed deer and bison. *Revue scientifique et technique-office international des épizooties* 21 (1): 249–264.

Whitehead, G.K. (1993). *Whitehead Encyclopedia of Deer.* Voyageur Press.

11

Horses and Donkeys

Helen(Becky) Whay

KEY CONCEPTS

11.1 Introduction

11.1.1 The Domestication of Equids; Uses and Worldwide Distribution

The wild ancestors of today's horses and donkeys (equidae) had unique qualities which led to their domestication; indeed, it was the use of horses and donkeys, not wheels, which marked the first significant step in land-based transportation and trading over long distances. Their speed, strength, stamina and ability to cross difficult terrain while carrying loads or being ridden became pivotal in human evolution. They allowed travel over greater distances, more effective hunting, aiding warfare and trading, changing agricultural practices and social organization. In Central Asia there is a saying: 'the horse is the wings of the human being'. Horses and donkeys appear to have been amenable to domestication, prepared to live in close proximity to humans, showing a versatility and adaptability which probably underpins their unique position in human society today where they straddle the boundary between a working animal and a pet.

The process of domestication began with the use of both horses and donkeys for meat. It is likely that humans began capturing and breeding wild equidae so that their meat supply could

Management and Welfare of Farm Animals: The UFAW Farm Handbook, Sixth Edition.
Edited by John Webster and Jean Margerison.
© Universities Federation for Animal Welfare 2022. Published 2022 by John Wiley & Sons Ltd.

be farmed rather than chased. Although it is still not clear how the process of domestication took place, at some point their potential to help with work and transportation must have been recognized. There would have been a transition from capturing and keeping wild animals to selecting and breeding animals most suited to specific tasks such as carrying packs or being ridden. Recently, 5000-year-old ass skeletons were discovered in tombs adjacent to the mortuary complex of an early Egyptian king (Rossel et al. 2008). Archaeological evidence showed that, although the process of domestication began 6000 years ago, these ass skeletons still had many characteristics of the wild ass, from which modern donkeys are descended, but showed pathologies and skeletal wear consistent with load carrying. This implied that 1000 years on from the start of domestication, the selection strategies that led to the emergence of what we now recognize as the donkey were far from complete. It is also worth noting that these asses were buried near an Egyptian king. Archaeologists interpret this as an indication of the ass's importance and status in Egyptian society. The greatest density of archaeological evidence for the process of horse domestication comes from the Ukrainian steppes, again dating from 6000 years ago. Skeletal remains from as far back as the Copper Age have provided evidence of tooth wear in horses, indicative of the use of bits (Anthony and Brown 1991).

Domestication occurs when humans take control of animal breeding. Selective breeding describes the practice of identifying particular traits in individual animals which the breeder would like to keep and even enhance in future generations. These qualities might be physical attributes such as strength, height or colour or behavioural characteristics such as a quiet temperament, being amenable to human company, or competitiveness. Not all desirable traits are particularly heritable, and some may have negative relationships with other traits. For example, selecting a mare for good maternal ability might result in the diminution of another desirable trait in the offspring. Early attempts at selective breeding would have been carried out on a trial-and-error basis and learning by experience. However, it is possible to see the routes which have led to the huge diversity of breeds that we see today, with horses (especially) selected for many specific purposes; e.g. pulling, speed, stamina, manoeuvrability, agility and aesthetic appearance.

Figure 11.1 illustrates some of the different types of use to which modern equines are put. These range from leisure and sport, predominantly in developed countries, through to the military and traction work still widely relied on in the developing world. In 1998 the US Congress estimated that 75% of all traction energy in the developing world was provided by animals, rather than lorries, tractors and vans. In times of high global fuel price rises and restrictions on power generation capacity, dependence on animal power is likely to grow and horses are the fastest transporters available. Figure 11.1 also lists some more unusual and less widely recognized roles of the horse, such as antivenom production and the harvesting of horse hair for wig making.

The Food and Agriculture Organization (FAO) estimated that in 2005 there were over 112 million equids in the world, the vast majority of which are domesticated. Of these 112 million, nearly 95 million (85%) are to be found in the developing world. Their distribution throughout the world's continents is illustrated in Figure 11.2 where it can be seen that the greatest numbers (38.5 and 36 million) are in Central/South America and Asia, respectively, while the smallest numbers (0.4 and 7 million) are found on the continents of Oceania and

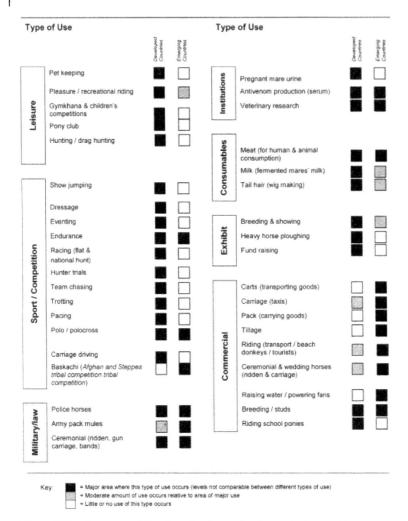

Figure 11.1 Summary of the diversity of uses for domesticated equidae.

Europe. Table 11.1 divides the count of equidae into horses, donkeys and mules and examines their distribution across continents.[1] From the table it is possible to see that different species predominate in different regions of the world. For example, in Africa there are more than twice as many donkeys as horses (15 million vs 4 million); donkeys being very well adapted to living in the arid environments of this region where water is scarce. In Central and South America 24 million horses predominate over roughly equal numbers of donkeys and mules (approx. 7 million of each). These figures clearly illustrate that equids are not only a feature

─────────

1 No count of mules was available for Oceania.

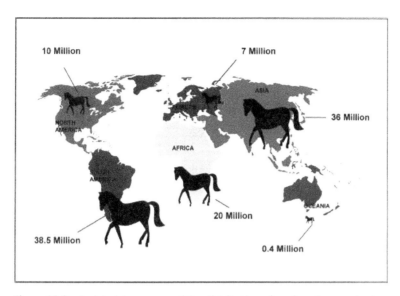

Figure 11.2   A pictorial summary of the distribution of equines (horses, donkeys and mules) across the world calculated from the 2005 Food and Agriculture Organization (FAO) statistics (courtesy of Dr Charlotte C. Burn).

Table 11.1   The numbers of horses, donkeys and mules in the world and their distribution between developed and developing regions in 2005.

	Horses	Donkeys	Mules
Oceania	374,657	9,000	–
Europe	6,298,202	653,244	228,503
North America	9,586,060	52,005	32,001
Africa	4,177,841	15,014,947	1,086,771
Central & South America[1]	24,112,558	7,769,956	6,596,912
Asia	14,234,985	17,455,571	4,501,463
World population	58,784,303	40,954,723	12,445,650

Source: FAO statistics (http://www.fao.org/corp/statistics/en).

[1] Central & South America data includes equids from the Caribbean.

of the developed world but are extremely important in the developing world. In developing countries the majority of horses, donkeys and mules are owned and worked by poor, marginalized and vulnerable people. The harsh position in which people find themselves means that they are often compelled to overwork their animals, leading to many animal welfare compromises and considerable suffering. However, the ways in which we use horses in the developed world can also present considerable challenges to their welfare. It is perhaps for horses in the developed world where there is the greatest opportunity for change and welfare improvement. Far more attention has been paid to the welfare of horses in developed countries compared to the developing world in terms of funded research, scientific publications and textbooks. Very few texts address the special problems in developing countries, still less the special problems of donkeys. This means that much of the information available refers to horses in the developed world. However, throughout this chapter equids from all around the world, performing all sorts of different types of work, will be considered as far as possible.

11.1.2 Equidae in the Wild: Reference Point for Considering Equine Welfare

In order to consider the welfare of domesticated equidae it is useful to understand something about the behaviours, social structures, feeding and breeding habits of their non-domesticated relatives. This allows us to infer something about how they have been adapted to meet the needs of humans through domestication. It can also highlight areas where the lives of modern domesticated equidae differ so dramatically from the lives of feral animals that we would want to consider what implications these changes might have for their welfare.

The success of horses and donkeys as domesticated animals and the methods by which humans carried out domestication mean that the majority of equine species we see today, with the possible exceptions of zebras, African and Asian asses and Przewalski horses, are descended from previously domesticated animals. The obvious limitation of this is that the wild horses that we might use as our reference point for a 'natural animal' have themselves been modified in some way by domestication. However, observing modern-day herds of wild, feral and free-range horses does give us some insight into how, given some free choice, horses and donkeys might organize their social structures. We can see how they budget their time, protect themselves against predators, communicate with their peers and organize their breeding.

11.1.2.1 Social Organization

Horses are extremely social animals that organize themselves into herds, sometimes containing hundreds of individuals. Herds organize themselves into social subgroups known as 'bands' that allow for protection of the young and the breeding mares while ensuring a place within their society for groups of sexually mature males. There is a band which consists of one breeding stallion, some breeding mares and their young. This band used to be called the harem band, implying that the stallion was in total charge of the mares. More recently it has become understood that some mares within the group have leadership roles, so to recognize this sharing of responsibility these bands are now more commonly referred to as natal bands. The natal band is where the main reproductive activity of the herd takes place. The stallion and lead mares have an important protective role within the band, defending the remaining mares and their offspring against other stallions, bands or predators. The young stay within the natal band for between one and three years, during which time they participate in a considerable amount of play behaviour with their young relatives. As they grow older the young male and female horses begin to form affiliations with yearlings and 2-year-olds from other bands. Eventually, the young females will leave the natal band into which they were born to join or form new ones. This leaves considerable numbers of males outside these reproductive bands: these males form themselves into bachelor groups which stay on the margins of natal groups. Current wisdom within the domesticated horse world assumes that stallions cannot be kept within this type of social order without vicious conflicts occurring between the males. There are undoubtedly lots of agonistic and competitive interactions within the bachelor groups but serious injuries are uncommon. Indeed, there is evidence that within the bands, including the bachelor groups, individuals form close relationships with some of their peers, which may involve co-operation to control or manage resources.

The social structures of feral donkey groups are far less rigid and, while they can form family structures similar to those described for horses, if resources are limited then they are equally likely to break away and function as individuals.

11.1.2.2 Feeding and Drinking Behaviour

Horses and donkeys are by preference grazing animals but they do have the capacity to browse trees, shrubs and woody plants when grazing is sparse or unavailable. Free-ranging populations of horses typically spend between 16 and 17 hours a day grazing, but this may go above 19 hours when forage becomes scarce, and grazing activity occurs at night as well as during the day. In contrast to ruminants, horses can graze for long periods of time without stopping; they can exploit shorter grass than cattle and have also been shown to increase their bite rate when grazing material is in limited supply. Horses move continuously when grazing so that they take a few bites and then move forward to the next piece of sward. These grazing strategies reflect the anatomy of their digestive tract where most of the fermentation of fibre occurs in the hind gut. During grazing, horses are selective about what they eat; this is important for avoiding the accidental ingestion of contaminated or toxic plants. It also appears that in free-ranging herds of horses social facilitation, or eating in company at times determined by herd leaders, is a cue for eating to take place. The frequency and volume of water drunk by free-ranging horses is determined by the climate in which they are living, the distance between forage and water supply and the amount of work or exercise undertaken. Where water is easily accessible and freely available then horses will tend to drink once or twice a day. Where access and availability of water are limited then drinking bouts may become as far apart as three days. Drinking is again a social activity and is also a time when individuals are at high risk of predation. Donkeys are particularly efficient at drinking and then departing rapidly from the watering site.

11.1.2.3 Communication

Much of the communication that takes place among horses is subtle and non-vocal. This is a good strategy for predated animals where efficient passing of information is essential for protection but loud or obvious communications would either draw attention to the group or forewarn predators of their intentions. In addition, many of the behaviours of horses are highly coordinated. In observations of Przewalski horses the behaviour of the whole herd was synchronized up to 89% of the time (van Dierendonck et al. 1996). These subtle forms of communication are based around body language, olfaction, touch and posturing.

The ears and tails of horses appear to be very important for communication through body language but sounds made by the hooves, such as pawing and stamping, are also mediums for transferring information. Vocal communications such as neighs, grunts and snorts are also valuable tools, although, as previously highlighted, not always appropriate. Urinary and faecal marking are both used as a means of communication between horses and as a threat to potential predators. Males in particular devote considerable time to this form of communication and the way in which marking is carried out can have ritualized components. Both male horses and donkeys can build up large mounds of faeces as a means of marking territories. Touch between equids possibly serves multiple purposes; mutual nibbling, biting and swatting of flies serve a useful function but they may also communicate bonding and trust between adults or between a mare and foal. Finally, displays and posturing, and approaches and retreats allow hierarchies to be established within groups without resorting to fighting.

The large array of communication tools used by horses and donkeys highlights the social nature of these animals and the importance of communication within their social groupings. This may suggest how much communication domesticated equids offer to their owners who are then not able to respond in an appropriate way.

11.1.2.4 Reproduction

Mares have a gestation period of just over 11 months and in wild or free-range herds the time of foaling would usually coincide with the time of year when the best and most appropriate vegetation is available to support the new foal. Thus most foaling occurs in the spring time. A mare would normally have one foal a year so would come back into oestrus shortly after foaling and need to be pregnant again within 1 month. During oestrus the mare will offer an array of signals to the stallion, who will stay close by, to indicate that she is receptive to mating. Regular repeated mountings occur while the mare is in oestrus; each mounting would be unlikely to last for more than 1 minute and should be a relatively quiet event. In free-range groups parturition will be rapid and the mare will show few signs that she is preparing to give birth until just before delivery begins. Although a foaling mare is likely to be kept away from other herds she may well be attended by other members of her family or horses from her own natal band. Newborn foals quickly rise to their feet and are often ready to run with the herd within half an hour of being born. By the end of the first day of life the foal will already be performing many of the basic behaviours needed for successful integration and communication within a herd; grooming, foraging, vocalizing and playing.

What we see from observing free-ranging herds is that stallions retain involvement in the care and upbringing of foals they have sired. Mares do not necessarily give birth in total isolation, and early and rapid communication is learnt and used by the foal as a necessary means of integrating into the herd.

11.2   Good Husbandry of Domesticated Horses and Donkeys

In broad terms, good husbandry requires meeting the behavioural and physiological needs of animals. This section considers how to meet the needs of domesticated equidae: horses, donkeys and mules. Since most of our knowledge, at least in the developed world, relates to the horse, and many of the principles are common to all equidae, the word horse (rather than equid) will be used hereafter except in cases where the needs of donkeys or mules call for special attention. Horses owned and managed in captivity are completely dependent on humans for the delivery of their needs. This means that there is a requirement to balance the constraints imposed by particular types of animal use against the animals' welfare needs. The equine industries that we see today have grown out of humans identifying a purpose or use for horses (see Figure 11.1) as a result of their adaptability and versatility. This presents us with the challenge of examining their needs and determining whether, in the multitude of 'unnatural' situations in which horses find themselves, these needs are being met.

The first step is to use some form of structured approach to consider the general welfare needs of equids and then to extend this knowledge to consider welfare in the context of specific examples of equine use. A helpful general structure to use is the 'five freedoms' (Chapter 1). In the following sections welfare will be considered using this framework but with specific reference to particular types of equine use.

11.2.1 Nutrition and Digestion

Horses need to eat to provide themselves with nutrients to sustain maintenance, work, growth and reproduction, to maintain their overall health and that of their digestive tract; and to provide the behavioural satisfaction that the process of eating delivers. The essential constituents of any diet are water, energy (principally as carbohydrates and oils), proteins, minerals and vitamins. Horses evolved as herbivorous grazing animals but, unlike most other domestic grazing species that obtain much of their energy from the fermentation of plant fibre, they are not ruminants. Their digestive system is described as monogastric. Fermentation of fibre (principally cellulose) takes place in the large hindgut (caecum and colon).

The stomach is surprisingly small considering the large volumes of forage that these animals consume each day. Only a minimal amount of nutrient absorption occurs while food is in the stomach; its main role is to mix the food, begin the process of enzymatic digestion, then rapidly pass the food along to the small intestine. The horse is physiologically adapted to maintain a full (albeit small) stomach, which helps explain why in their wild state horses spend so much time consuming food. The small intestine is largely responsible for the enzymatic digestive process. This allows absorption of proteins and soluble carbohydrates (e.g. sugars and starch) which would destabilize the hindgut. The rate of food passage through the small intestine is rapid, moving the indigestible fibrous materials containing insoluble carbohydrates along to the hindgut. The large intestine, also known as the hindgut, makes up about 60% of the horse's digestive tract and comprises the caecum and the colon. It acts as a fermentation vat allowing microbial digestion of the fibrous plant material which leads to production of volatile fatty acids along with vitamins and microbial protein, some of which may be absorbed into the bloodstream as amino acids, although this is not proven. The hindgut also acts as a reservoir and the main absorption route for water and electrolytes which are needed for the maintenance of homeostasis. The water in the hindgut is also important in regulating the transit of solid materials.

Horses are well adapted to utilize forage-based diets and in a domestic situation these are usually presented in the form of grazing or conserved plants such as hay, silage or haylage which is a form of ensiled long-fibre grass. Horses and donkeys can survive very well on forage as a basic ration as long as they have access to water. Stabled horses that have limited access to fresh pasture may also require some form of mineral supplement. When grazing is not available or adverse weather conditions make it inaccessible, then conserved forages are offered in hay nets, mangers or, less commonly, on the ground. Supplying forages off the ground in hay nets and mangers is contrary to the normal grazing posture seen in horses and donkeys, and may have implications for both the behavioural satisfaction an animal derives from eating forage and the efficiency with which the digestive tract is able to receive and utilize the food. There is now a wider acceptance that whenever possible confined horses should be offered continuous access to forage. This is not always easy; in some cases either through tradition, received wisdom, or lack of resources animals still have limited or restricted access to forage during the course of a day. In other situations, owners of animals that are stabled or particularly prone to putting on weight find that they have to restrict access to forage to prevent their animals becoming obese.

Concentrate feeds are introduced into the diets primarily as a source of readily digestible, soluble carbohydrate, i.e. energy. This is sometimes done because the horses are being worked to such an extent that their energy requirements cannot be fully met by the provision of forage alone; in other circumstances limited supplies of forage may mean that it is more practical to feed concentrates. Most concentrates are based on cereals (maize, oats, barley or wheat) mixed with other ingredients such as soya bean meal to provide extra protein, beet pulp or dried grass to provided digestible fibre, vitamins and minerals. They may be sold as simple mixtures ('coarse mix') or in pelleted form. When offered concentrate feed most horses consume it rapidly and there is concern that they derive little behavioural satisfaction from eating concentrates and that such feeds deliver too much energy too quickly.

The most visible signs of inadequate nutrition are loss of weight and body condition. When this reaches extreme levels it is accompanied by deterioration in coat condition, a loss of skin elasticity, weakness, depression and compromised immune function. The term 'inadequate' may simply mean a shortage of feed or an imbalance between nutrient input (energy, protein, etc.) and requirements (maintenance, growth, work and reproduction). An entirely appropriate diet for a leisure horse living in a temperate climate doing a limited amount of work would be totally inadequate for a carriage or 'tonga' horse working for 12 hours a day in extremely hot conditions in Asia. Indeed, in some circumstances the level and duration of work performed by these animals so far outstrips their capacity to take in the nutrients they need that owners are advised to feed their animals supplements of oil, milk or cream as a source of energy-dense fats.

Problems can arise from inappropriate nutrition as well as from inadequate nutrition. In common with the modern disease of humans in the developed world, many horses and (especially) ponies can suffer from obesity resulting from a combination of lack of exercise and excessive nutrient intake. This may be coupled with the syndrome that afflicts many leisure horses, a perception by their owners that fat horses are happy, well-cared-for horses and a belief that treats such as polo mints, sugar cubes and carrots will make them happy. The consequences of obesity can be very serious and harmful. Overweight animals are prone to joint, heart and lung problems and it has been speculated that there may be a link between equine obesity and laminitis. Laminitis is an inflammation of the delicate structures that line the inside of the hooves suspending the internal apparatus of the hoof in its position. Laminitis it can cause extreme pain to the animal, may result in lifelong unsoundness and can often reoccur. Obesity in horses and particularly donkeys is also associated with an often-fatal condition called hyperlipemia, where the animal's fat reserves rapidly enter the bloodstream and overstress the liver.

The introduction of concentrate feeds into the diet poses some risk to digestive health. The nature of concentrate feeds means that they can be rapidly consumed rather than 'grazed' in the way that forages are eaten. Concentrate feeds increase the risk of creating an acidic environment in the stomach and have been linked to impaction colic. Colic is a generic term describing signs of abdominal pain, all too commonly associated with domesticated horses. The long and convoluted forms of the small and large intestines have been implicated as a risk in themselves for colic; in fact, at one point the large intestine folds right back on itself. Colic can take the form of mild through to severe bloating resulting from a build-up of gas (usually from microbial fermentation within the intestines) through to serious and life-threatening impactions (blockages) or twists in the intestine. Feeds containing large amounts of easily digestible soluble carbohydrates or which break down into very small particles which then have a tendency to clump together are often implicated in colic. Such characteristics can be easily attributed to concentrate feeds. Other well-recognized risks to digestive health include problems with teeth, most commonly overgrowth, as horses' teeth continue to grow throughout their life. The rate of wear of teeth is affected by the horse's diet and overgrown teeth can ultimately cause pain and difficulty in eating. Choke is not as commonly seen as colic but is extremely serious. Horses do not have the vomiting reflex that humans are familiar with; this means that they find it difficult to expel food which becomes lodged in their oesophagus. Insufficient chewing of feed, rapid eating and lack of water have all been suggested as causes of choke.

Welfare is as much about behavioural satisfaction as physical wellbeing. Behavioural satisfaction associated with eating and drinking is likely to have multiple components. As already discussed, the common practice of offering horses forage in hay nets or mangers asks the animal to 'graze' in a manner that does not mirror how it would be grazing in a free-ranging situation. Locomotion while eating and the process of selecting food are also both important components of the grazing process which are not available to the housed animal. It is difficult to gauge how significant these deviations from the natural grazing behaviours are to horses and donkeys but they may lead to frustration, anxiety or perhaps reduced satisfaction from eating. Observations of horses in the wild show that they expend considerable amounts of their daily time budget on grazing, including time spent grazing during the night. Restricted access to forage will reduce the amount of time the horse is able to devote to grazing each day, so feeding practices have been implicated both directly and indirectly in the development of behaviours that owners describe as undesirable. One example of an undesirable behaviour is the eating of bedding at night. Greet and Rossdale (1987) suggest that this behaviour may arise from restrictions in the availability of food and fibre, leading to horses consuming their straw bedding, which itself becomes a risk for colic. Owners often seek to ameliorate this problem by changing the type of bedding rather than addressing the underlying reason for the initiation of the behaviour. McDonnell (2002) suggests that the reduction in feeding duration imposed on many domesticated horses is a primary cause of behavioural problems, arising from inactivity or boredom. A final point to consider when looking at behavioural needs of equids, in particular horses, associated with feeding and drinking is the importance of having their herd around them. Many domesticated horses are stabled or tethered in isolation from other animals, and when they do live in groups these can be unstable and not constructed in the way that the bands of a herd would be, for example, mature females and castrated males housed collectively, or breeding-age females housed without a stallion. From the perspective of offering behavioural satisfaction associated with nutrition to horses, it is worth remembering that they are social eaters and drinkers; the presence of their group members offers them protection and security and may also offer cues, i.e. 'social facilitation' indicating when and where to begin eating.

Case Study: Elite Performance Horses: How Concentrate Feeds Affect Their Lives

Elite performance horse is the collective term describing top-level racehorses, show jumpers, event, endurance and dressage horses. They belong to an industry of the developed world and are often worth huge sums of money and represent enormous investments of time and skill on the part of their owners and trainers. The nutrient requirements of performance horses cannot be met from forage alone and so the normal practice is to feed high-quality, highly palatable concentrate diets in conjunction with limited but high-quality, low-fibre forages. There are a number of reported consequences associated with this particularly intensive form of dietary management (Henderson 2007). It is believed that high-concentrate, low-forage diets make horses vulnerable to gastric ulcers as a result of high gastric acidity. Stomach acid is buffered by saliva which is produced in response to eating forage and consistent gut fill. An endoscopic examination of US race horses in 1996 revealed that 93% had gastric ulcers (Murray et al. 1996). Gastric ulcers are probably painful; they are associated with weight loss, inappetance, reduced performance and colic. The speed with which concentrates are consumed can also present problems for the horse. Despite meeting the biological needs of the animal, the rapid completion of feeding will not address the horse's strong drive to forage over extended periods of time. Simply increasing the frequency of feeds rather than providing continuous foraging substrates does not appear to succeed in meeting horses' psychological needs. A further problem associated with such highly nutritious diets is that they provide horses with greater energy reserves, which often manifests in explosive and volatile behaviour. Not only can this be a problem for the handlers of these animals, but it leads to a reluctance to allow elite horses to mix with other horses because of the increased risk of injury. It is ironic that the management that helps these horses towards their 'elite' status in fact makes them less horse-like than their wild contemporaries.

11.2.2 Environment

Many horse management texts acknowledge that, from a behavioural perspective, horses and donkeys would be better off left outside all year round. This is obviously inconsistent with our aims for these domestic animals. In most practical circumstances it is also unlikely to be conducive to good welfare, since the quality and quantity of the pasture is likely to range from insufficient (leading to hunger and loss of condition) to dangerously rich (leading to obesity and laminitis). For practical reasons, enormous numbers of domesticated horses and other equine species are kept in stabling, or housing, or are restrained in some way as part of the management routine that surrounds them. This is an artificial environment which increases the animals' dependency on external provision of resources; food, water, bedding, light and companionship all have to be brought to them. When considering the welfare of horses kept in these artificial environments, it is useful, first, to consider why this management practice has gained such universal acceptance and then to look at how these environments perform in delivering needs such as comfort, protection and social contact.

In many urban areas of Asia owners can hire a space in a communal stable where the animals are tethered by the neck and/or forelimb and hindlimb in rows, rather like stalls without the divisions. All over the developing world the practice of tethering horses or donkeys, with or without shade, grazing or water, is extremely common. This is in part because many owners are very poor and have no land of their own. Traditional European and North American horse housing designs include single, high-walled loose-boxes with split doors that allow the horses to look out, or stalls in which they are tethered, usually by their halter. There are also more open designs emerging where a group of horses might be kept in a barn with divisions between animals created using bars or poles. The question to ask is: why are horses housed in this way? Eileen Gillen from World Horse Welfare (formerly ILPH) put it very well when she asked: 'Is it because they are in work and clipped out, so that they do not lose condition? Is it because they will poach the ground, causing more work and expense for the human to reclaim good grazing for the summer? Or is it because we feel sorry for them, as they cannot come into the house to sit by the fire so we stick them into a box to make us feel better?' To add to Eileen Gillen's list, other common reasons given for housing or tethering animals include:

- to make their capture easier or to stop them from wandering off (in Guatemala there are reported incidents of horses breaking free from their tethers and damaging neighbouring farmers' crops, resulting in these animals receiving slash wounds from machetes);
- to bring them closer to make inspection easier;
- to permit controlled feeding;
- to avoid having to carry resources (feed, water, saddles) out to their fields;
- to keep them clean, so they are not wet and muddy when they are wanted for work;
- to prevent conflicts between individuals and to reduce the risk of theft.

The important point to consider here is whether this list of reasons for stabling represents genuine benefit for the animals or greater expediency for the owners.

The comfort of the housed or tethered horse has multiple components. The most imme-diately obvious is to ensure an appropriate lying surface. A common and popular substrate is straw, but owners also use materials such as wood shavings, wood chips, peat, paper and mattresses. In dry areas, sand or dust is considered satisfactory. In some parts of the world very traditional stable practices are followed whereby horses are tethered by fore- and hindlimb on brick or paved floors during the day and only offered bedding at night. The selection criteria for bedding materials are influenced by their local availability and the ease with which the stable can be cleaned or mucked out. Horses seem to have a prefer-ence for straw and, as has already been discussed, they can also eat it. There is relatively little information available about the optimum depth of bedding but it has been observed that, when bedding material is sparse, horses will lie down as soon as new material is added (Houpt 2001). Comfort for the confined animal is also likely to be influenced by the space available and freedom of movement. Again, reflecting back to the evidence from wild and free-ranging herds of horses, much of their day is spent engaged in locomotor activity, in particular when they are eating. Both tethered and loose-housed horses have their capacity for movement severely restricted. A combination of space allowance and bedding substrate will also affect their capacity to roll. Both horses and donkeys are very strongly motivated to roll and they will try to establish a dusty area specifically to service this need. In stabled animals there is a risk of them becoming cast (stuck too close to a wall and unable to stand up) which can be associated with attempting to roll in a confined space. Further elements of comfort to be considered in a stable, stall or barn are the level of ventilation and lighting, both of which are likely to be altered in some way by the con-struction of a building.

The tethered horse is obliged to remain in the same space as its own faeces and urine. There are three potential issues arising from this: living among faeces and urine may be unpleasant and have health implications for the animal in terms of parasitic transmission, raised stable humidity and build-up of ammonia. Stallions in particular use faeces and urine as territorial markers and although it is not proven it must be considered that they may become confused or frustrated at being unable to position their markers and move away from them once placed, or alternatively may feel thwarted by having their carefully placed marks of territory regu-larly cleaned away. Finally, horses may perceive that strong concentrations of urine act as an olfactory indicator of their presence to potential predators.

From a human perspective we see stables as affording protection: from the weather, from theft, from agonistic interactions with unfamiliar conspecifics and from potentially injurious grazing environments. These are legitimate concerns when looked at from a purely human viewpoint. What we also need to do is look at them from the point of view of the horse. Horses appear to cope better with inclement weather than we think they do, they are unaware of the risk of theft, and when faced with any situation they perceive as threatening their instinctive response would be to initiate flight (run away) and seek the protection of other horses (if pos-sible). Horses frightened into bolting while out on a hack will attempt to return to their field mates (Summerhays 1975). What the stabled or tethered horse seems to experience is the opposite of what we think we are offering. The confined and isolated horse is unable to follow its natural instincts for self-protection. At best it may feel fearful when under immediate threat; at worst it may experience chronic frustration and anxiety at having its protective mechanisms compromised to such a degree.

A major welfare consideration for the housed and even paddock-grazed horse is social contact. It is very clear that horses and donkeys are social animals. Their social structures help keep them feeling secure and allow them to establish permanent societies, afford them companionship and facilitate relationships between individuals. Keeping a single horse isolated for long periods in a stable is a complete contradiction of its normal social situation. Mares held either in confinement with some social contact or in stalls allowing no social contact whatsoever demonstrated physiological changes indicative of stress (Mal et al. 1991). Many loose-box stables on yards are designed with split doors which allow horses to look out and may still affords horses some stress. This may be a consequence of knowing that others are close by but being thwarted from performing social activities such as mutual grooming and mutual, head to tail, fly swatting. Ironically, the converse may also be a source of stress to confined horses; they may find themselves housed next to animals with which they have no established social bonds or even have outright animosities towards. Many yards position horses in ways that offer greatest convenience and access for those looking after them, horses and ponies come and go regularly and are often popped into one another's stables when they are unoccupied. Similar problems may be experienced by horses during periods of turn-out to pasture; there may be a dynamic and changing group of animals and the balances of males, females and young may be inappropriate for forming social subgroups.

Stabling is recognized as one of the most commonly occurring risk factors for unwanted behaviours. Unwanted behaviours ranged from 'bad manners', pushing through doorways and fidgeting during mounting, through nipping and biting, to stereotypies. The problem with unwanted or undesirable behaviours is that because the human defines them as a problem they can elicit reprisals, attempts at discipline and even result in equids being frequently passed from owner to owner. These behaviours may or may not be of significance to the animal's welfare in their own right, but how they are perceived by owners can have a very great impact on their welfare.

11.2.3 Health

The physical condition of an animal is obviously an extremely important component of its welfare. It is the horse owner who has the greatest influence and responsibility in keeping their animal healthy because they spend the most time with it and make all the management decisions that affect its life. When considering animal health from a welfare perspective it is the management decisions that horse owner makes that are of particular interest, although of course, many other groups are involved in and advise on the health care of domesticated equidae including veterinary surgeons, farriers, alternative practitioners, feed suppliers, Ayurvedic compounders (traditional healers) and even welfare charities.

Case Study: Donkeys, horses and mules pulling carts around Delhi, India

There are an estimated 5000 horses, donkeys and mules working in and around Delhi in India. These animals pull either carriages used for carrying people or carts used for transporting commercial goods; these may be loads of scrap metal, bricks, hides, sanitary ware such as sinks and baths, fruit and vegetables, plastic chairs, filing cabinets or piles of refuse. They are also used to work in brick yards such as the one shown in Figure 11.3. It has been suggested that dense populations of working equidae provide a social environment that elevates their welfare above that of their European and North American counterparts. Many of these animals work up to 12 hours each day and, although there may be many periods during the day when they are waiting for loads, they are rarely released from the cart. In this type of environment the animals have many fleeting interactions with other horses, donkeys or mules each day and will regularly find themselves parked or pulled up beside an animal they have never met before. This constant interaction with strangers may well be stressful in itself. In such circumstances it would be normal for two animals to offer some behavioural signals to one another, take the opportunity to smell each other and generally size one another up. None of this is possible while restrained between the shafts of a cart. In this circumstance some animals may be experiencing regular bouts of fear and anxiety at being presented with strange and potentially threatening animals, many of which are stallions, while the more gregarious may be constantly frustrated at being unable to initiate communication with new animals, or even old acquaintances, that they meet. During the time the horse or donkey is held between the shafts of a cart, this defines its environment and largely reduces its capacity to make choices: to meet other animals, to stand in the shade, to scratch or swat flies, to eat or drink, or to lie down.

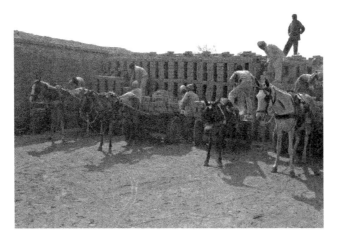

Figure 11.3   Loading carts at a brick works, Delhi, India.

In this section the issues that will be discussed are:

- preventive health care (stopping a problem before it starts);
- how modern management and animal use may lead to increased health risks.

To illustrate these points only four 'health themes' will be discussed here although in reality this topic is vast. The themes to be discussed are vaccination; parasite control; lameness; and skin lesions associated with work.

Vaccinations are used to protect individuals against specific infectious diseases, both viral and bacterial. When they are used widely within the population they can help prevent diseases spreading and in some cases have been used to eradicate diseases, such as human smallpox, from regions of the world. Vaccinations are particularly important for preventing infectious diseases for which treatment has poor success. They are conventionally made from a killed or weakened form of the bacterium or virus to be vaccinated against. When this is injected into a healthy horse, the horse's own immune system will learn to recognize the virus or bacteria and be able to mount a rapid and strong defence against it if the horse becomes infected at a future date. The most common diseases against which horses are vaccinated in the UK and Europe are tetanus, caused by the bacterium *Clostridium tetani* which lives in soil, and equine influenza, a contagious virus spread in an aerosol by coughing and sneezing animals. Worldwide, there are many other diseases for which vaccines are now available; e.g. equine encephalitis, herpes, strangles, botulism and Potomac horse fever. Clearly vaccination is a critical element of preventive health care. It is relatively easy to implement and does not require drastic changes in management routine. Some objections have been raised against the use of vaccinations on ethical and health grounds and there is a low risk of adverse reactions associated with vaccination, both at the injection site and systemically.

What cannot be in doubt, however, is the principle that preventing a disease or injury before it occurs is always preferable to presenting a suffering animal for treatment. However, it is also important to consider the reasons why a problem is sufficiently severe that preventive action, in this case vaccination, is required. Equine influenza is not a modern disease; reports of horses with flu-like signs have been traced back as far as 400 BC. However, as equine influenza is highly contagious and transmitted via aerosol it is worth considering whether management of the modern domestic equids facilitates transmission of the disease. In other words, is equine influenza a disease that has been allowed to flourish as a result of the way we use and keep domesticated horses? If this were the case then it would spark an ethical debate about the use of preventive steps, such as vaccination, to mitigate for poor animal management practices. In a wild or free-ranging situation, animals would be grouped in herds and would take steps to keep themselves segregated from other herds that would be considered a potential threat. Ever since horses have been domesticated it has been the practice to encourage mixing of animals, to move them from place to place, or even between countries, through competition, work or sale. The ways equidae are now used means that the giving of an equine influenza vaccine is a sensible measure to protect animal health because the way we choose to move and mix equids significantly increases the risk that a disease like equine influenza will flourish.

Horses are at risk from many parasites including flies and ticks; however, a particular problem are endoparasites that live in the large intestine, including large and small red worms, tapeworms, roundworms and pinworms (collectively classified as helminths). Roundworms are perhaps the most commonly experienced problem; once in the horse's gut they lay eggs that are flushed out in the faeces onto the grazing pasture where they can survive for a considerable time and infect or reinfect animals that graze the pasture. Roundworms can cause colic, loss of condition and in severe cases can be fatal. Older animals can develop a partial immunity to the worms but young foals are particularly susceptible.

The restrictions placed on domesticated equids increase the risk of picking up parasites (eating grass infected with worm eggs and larvae) because they are not continually moving onto new, fresh grazing land but are often kept on unchanging pasture which can become overburdened with parasites. For a considerable time now a cornerstone of worm management has been the use of anthelmintic drugs (de-wormers), the idea being that the drugs clear the animal of parasites and interrupt the cycle of shedding worm eggs into the environment via faeces. If deworming is accompanied by separation of the animal from likely areas of worm burden, for example the pasture they have just occupied, this should prevent reinfection and allow time for the pasture to become 'clean' of worm eggs. In many instances it appears that anthelmintic use has not been paired with careful pasture management, perhaps through lack of available land, and a heavy dependence on anthelmintics has developed. There is now evidence that this heavy, and somewhat irresponsible, use of de-wormers has led to parasites developing resistance to some classes of drugs. In a study of equines working in Moroccan souks (markets) it was found that there was no significant difference in faecal egg counts between animals that had been receiving routine anthelmintic treatment and control animals from a separate souk that were not part of the worm control programme. There was also no difference in the body condition score of the two groups, although the raw data showed a trend towards the untreated animals being in better condition (Wallace 2003). Evidence such as this that has led to the suggestion that in some situations animals are able to live in equilibrium with their gut parasites (a form of endemic stability); it is worth considering whether continuous attempts to scour away these parasites make animals more vulnerable to spikes in worm burden when they become reinfected.

Lameness seems to be a curse of domesticated horses. There is plenty of evidence that it is a painful condition, not least because it has been shown to improve following administration of analgesics or local anaesthetic. Lameness is the most commonly reported health problem in horses (Kaneene et al. 1997) and the risk increases with particular work types. Horse racing has long been recognized as being a high risk for limb injuries, a proportion of which are considered so severe, or untreatable, that the horse has to be killed. Among both horses and donkeys working in developing countries such as India and Pakistan, a lameness prevalence of 100% has been recorded, with most animals lame in all four of their limbs (Broster et al. 2009). Horses' feet and legs were well designed for their original purpose but the range of demands that have come with domestication have overwhelmed the initial design specifications of the limbs. Both carrying riders and pulling carts have changed the stresses and strains that act on the limbs. Activities of domesticated horses now include running and jumping to exhaustion when racing, using incredible agility and lift in show jumping, needing extremely controlled and fine movement in dressage, maintaining speed over very long distances in endurance riding, and pulling and turning during traction work. In addition, leisure horses are often worked infrequently and erratically so are unprepared for the sudden strain of enthusiastic exercise. In addition to the problems of pain and locomotor impairment associated with lameness, when treatment is offered the regimens often involve 'box rest', where the horse is kept shut in a loose-box for several weeks to restrict movement and exercise as much as possible. Rest is indeed extremely important for the healing of limbs but, as discussed previously, imposes the stress, frustration and anxiety of isolation on the patient and, ironically, some of the physiological responses associated with stress may in fact slow down healing.

The last health theme to be discussed in this section is skin lesions associated with work. Although not a very widely recognized problem in Europe and North America, it is very much a problem for equines working in developing countries in Central and South America, Asia and Africa. Historically, skin lesions were referred to as harness lesions, inferring that the cause was well understood and related to harnessing alone. This implies that the cause of these lesions is straightforward and consequently so too should be the solution. Although harness design and maintenance are very important, they are part of an interaction with the way in which the animal is driven, the weight of the load it is pulling, the standard to which the cart is maintained, the temperature, humidity and dustiness of the working environment and the general health and condition of the animal. In a recent communication with members of the Brazilian Mounted Police who use well-maintained, well-designed saddles and harnesses, they stated that they found it virtually impossible to prevent their horses developing skin lesions; such is the complexity of the problem. The results of recent work looking at risk factors for tail-base lesions in donkeys carrying tourists in Petra (Burn et al. 2008) indicated rather counter-intuitively that wide, well-padded rump straps posed the greatest risk for causing lesions. Skin lesions are likely to be painful for the animal, they seem to escalate over time if the animal continues to work and have the added annoyance of being very attractive to flies. Skin lesions are not only a function of poorly designed and maintained harnesses but a problem of animals being asked to work in difficult environments and beyond the point where they are able to maintain their own physical wellbeing. This clearly reflects the poverty and desperation of the owners who use these animals, but nonetheless represents an enormous preventive challenge to be resolved.

11.2.4 Emotion

It is safe to state, without recourse to anthropomorphism, that emotion – the internal experience of a sentient animal, how it 'feels' – has a significant *direct* influence on welfare. For example, a physical problem such as a fractured limb will be translated into an internal experience. The animal must experience the pain associated with the fracture, finds itself unable to move and then considers the implications of being unable to run if danger approaches. It is also important to bear in mind that in the context of welfare we are not only concerned

---

Case Study: Endurance and Performance Horses – a Problem Associated with Overexertion?

For a long time it has been recognized that, following bouts of strenuous exercise for training and competition, human athletes become more susceptible to common infectious diseases, particularly upper respiratory tract infections. This problem is attributed to the stress of strenuous exercise having a negative effect on immune function. The levels of exertion demanded of endurance and performance horses and working equidae are comparable to that of human athletes such as marathon runners and sprinters. Many researchers have reported an apparent link between strenuous exercise and the development of pleuropneumonia in horses and these findings have led to further studies of equine immune function following exercise. A study of the effect of exercise intensity using Standardbred horses found evidence of improved neutrophil function following moderate-intensity exercise but a reduction in neutrophil function following high-intensity exercise; a reduction which persisted across 17 weeks of training (Riadal et al. 2000). Neutrophils are phagocytic white blood cells which can consume harmful infectious cells which invade the body. They are part of the first line of immune defence and, although short lived, are very important in protecting against adventitious infections. The implication of this research is that horses' immune function may benefit from moderate-intensity exercise, but high-intensity exercise, which was described as a run to fatigue, exposes horses to an increased risk of infection. This knowledge can now be translated into examining the types of use to which horses and donkeys are put and asking ethical and welfare questions about the level of harm and risk animals should be exposed to, and how this risk can be controlled.

---

with negative emotions such as fear, distress, pain and anxiety but also with positive emotions such as happiness, anticipation and contentment. Three illustrations of components of domesticated equine lives that are to be considered here in the context of emotional welfare are the fulfilment of purpose (telos), isolation and human–animal interactions.

Telos is a term derived from the Greek word for purpose and refers to animals being allowed to live out the purpose for which they themselves evolved. The philosopher Bernie Rollin borrowed a line from a popular 1920s musical to explain telos as an animal welfare concept: 'Fish gotta swim, birds gotta fly'. The ethical principle of respect for autonomy (Chapter 1) requires us to allow a horse to be a horse and to 'do horsey things'. This raises some obvious conflicts between the concept of telos and domestication and animal use. Even a horse being galloped across the downs by its rider is being ridden by a human and therefore is less of a horse than a wild animal galloping with its herd. The ethical principle of justice requires us to seek a fair compromise between our needs and theirs. In relation to a horse's emotions it is worth looking at the myriad of constraints placed on their lives by humans and questioning how these constraints (stabling, environment, companionship and nutrition) might affect the animal's emotional state. David Fraser and co-workers (1997) have illustrated the problems faced by animals when they move from a wild state into a domesticated environment. They pointed out that there are some adaptations (physical or behavioural) which were useful in a wild environment but do not serve an important function in their new domesticated role; there are some adaptations that serve the animal equally well in both a wild and domesticated context; and there are demands of domestication for which the animal does not have adaptations. What this suggests is that animals, in this case horses, are likely to experience problems of unwanted adaptations and may well experience frustration and confusion at being unable to use these attributes. At the same time they may also be experiencing a lack of physical or behavioural skills needed to be able to cope in the domesticated environment and with the work given to them. This could not only lead to physical harms but emotional distress at not being able to understand, cope with or adapt to the demands being made.

Periods of isolation appear to be an integral part of the life of many domesticated horses and donkeys, whether this involves living alone in a stable or field, or being surrounded by other animals but isolated by the shafts of a cart or the walls of a stall. We know from their behaviour in the wild that horses are herd animals and would not normally spend prolonged periods in isolation. They also establish relatively stable social groupings so would not normally be subject to constantly changing or multiple transient interactions. Even short periods of isolation (6 hours) appear to evoke behavioural and physiological responses in mares separated from their established social groups. There is most evidence of the harm caused by isolation in young animals. Foals that are kept in isolation from conspecifics run the risk of failing to develop the social skills they will need throughout their lives, potentially leading to undesirable behaviours such as aggression, stereotypies or self-mutilation. In a study looking at the weaning of foals either as groups in paddocks or individually in solidly partitioned stalls, it was found that the weanlings kept in stalls spent more time engaged in aberrant behaviours such as licking or chewing the stall walls, kicking the walls, pawing, bucking and rearing, whereas the paddock-housed groups budgeted their time similarly to feral horses, including showing strong motivations to graze and spend time close to their colleagues (Heleski et al. 2002). A further risk of isolating young animals from their conspecifics is that they form strong attachments to their human owner. This can even reach the level of mal-imprinting where a foal may perceive a human to be its mate. This is potentially dangerous for the human but it also prevents the young foal from developing into a truly horsey horse. It is salutary to point out that the two domestic species most prone to behavioural disorders are the horse and the dog, the species that we have forced to become most emotionally dependent on ourselves.

The interaction between humans and their horses is a very important element of equine welfare. Many horses and donkeys are kept as pets and their human owners are looking for an emotional connection and a reciprocation of affection from their animal. This apparent return of affection from animals secures their status within a household and helps ensure their care and protection. Dogs have been particularly successful at learning to offer behaviours that humans interpret as emotions such as adoration, devotion and dependency. Horses and (particularly) donkeys are perhaps less adept than dogs with this skill but clearly form personal relationships with their owners. Humans, however, are inclined to anthropomorphism and attribute complex emotions and thought processes to their animals, who may view their owners simply as a resource and are trying to work out how best to extract offerings such as food, exercise and treats. An example of where this over-attribution of human characteristics can be problematic is in the training of horses and donkeys. Trainers will often make statements such as '*He did that wrong just to annoy me*' when an animal has simply misunderstood the question, or its consequences. Training succeeds when it is consistent, conducted in a minimally stressful environment and is based on an understanding of the way horses learn and communicate. Training exploits the animal's willingness to learn and adapt. It is a good survival strategy for a domestic animal to offer what is asked of it; however, the risk is that humans are inconsistent both in what they ask for and sometimes in what they give in return, both in terms of physical resources and behaviour. A human who demands an emotional relationship with their horse or donkey and then sells it on when it is outgrown, unable to perform at the level demanded or is chronically unwell betrays their side of the bargain.

Case Study: Riding School Horses and Ponies

Riding schools are establishments where a number of horses (and ponies) are kept and hired out to people who would like to ride a horse but may not have the money, resources, time or expertise to keep an animal of their own. Some people will hire an animal to ride out (hack) into the countryside and enjoy the experience of riding; others will have riding lessons where they learn the skills and signals needed to be a successful rider. Riding school horses often work long hours, working for a number of sessions each day. The horses will be ridden by a whole variety of people, with varying levels of competence. The variation in competence of riders means that on some occasions the horse will have a rider who gives very clear signals and directions, while at other times a less competent rider may give very unclear and contradictory signals to the horse. While at work the horse will find itself mixed with different groups of animals for each lesson or hack, and during rest it may not have one fixed stable which is its own domain. It is quite common for riding stables to have fewer saddles and harnesses than they have horses, so that animals will sometimes find themselves wearing a harness that smells of other, possibly unfamiliar, individuals. Clients of riding schools often feel a strong affection for a particular horse within the school and will either request a particular individual for their lessons or ensure that they visit their favourite horse to give it a treat before they leave. The objects of this favouritism are quite likely to find these gifts of affection unpredictable and confusing as they are not necessarily able to recognize the pattern which determines who will offer treats and attention and when this might occur, this can escalate into horses beginning to demand attention from everyone who visits the stable – these horses are then classified as badly behaved.

11.2.5 Behaviour

It is important to understand that animal behaviour results from an interaction between genotype and environment. Genotype may predispose towards certain behaviours but this will only be part of a complex which includes learning, environment and context. For example, a nervous and fearful horse may have had a genetic disposition towards fearfulness but this would not necessarily have resulted in a fearful animal had its training and life experiences acted to build up its confidence. Observation of behaviour is essential for gaining insight into an animal's experiences; it allows us to see what choices they make, what preferences they have, how they spend their time and with whom. However, interpreting behaviour is not always straightforward and sometimes humans can misunderstand animal behaviours. Male donkeys often display a reciprocal biting or nipping behaviour which can be accompanied by quite a lot of squealing and foot stamping. Humans often interpret this as aggression and rush to separate the protagonists. However, if left to themselves the donkeys will carry on with this behaviour for hours, either one reinitiating the activity when it has broken off. They do not cause injuries or retreat from each other and in fact the behaviour is much more akin to play than aggression. Humans often try to stop behaviours as a result of either not understanding their purpose or of classifying them as undesirable or inappropriate (from the human point of view); a playful young horse, excited about getting exercise, might be described as bad mannered as it fidgets and skips about in anticipation of going out. This chapter has used behavioural evidence in many of the welfare problems discussed, illustrating how important a knowledge of behaviour is when considering animal welfare. However, one huge topic of equine behaviour remains to be addressed: stereotypic behaviours.

Stereotypies are defined as repetitive behaviours that have no apparent purpose or function. However, in the context of the equidae, they have also been defined as 'variations on "normal" behaviour, developing as a result of a deficient environment, in which movement, diet, and social contact are restricted'. In this case they serve the very important function of signalling that something is wrong. The topic of stereotypic behaviour is extremely complex and this chapter can do no more than offer some uncertain generalizations taken from research into equine stereotypies, nearly all of which has involved the horse.

A substantial range of behaviours are classed as stereotypic (McGreevy 2004): these include:

- *oral and head-related behaviours* such as chewing, lip licking, licking the environment, wood-chewing, crib-biting, wind-sucking and head-nodding, shaking, tossing and circling.
- *locomotor behaviours* such as box (or stall)-walking, weaving, pawing, door-kicking with the front feet and box-kicking with the hind feet; and self-directed behaviours such as rubbing and self-biting.

The most commonly discussed and researched stereotypic behaviours are crib-biting, wind sucking, weaving and box-walking. Stereotypic behaviours are often colloquially termed 'stable vices' or 'abnormal behaviours' – terms that reflect how horse owners view them. Traditionally, owners report concern about horses with stereotypies because of reduced performance or work output, reduction in the financial value of the animal and possible associations with health problems including hoof damage, musculoskeletal problems and loss of condition. These repetitive behaviours can also be distressing to watch and can cause costly damage to stabling or fencing. However, the most important reason for concern should be that in some way, either directly or indirectly, these behaviours indicate that the horse is being subject to adverse management factors.

The reported prevalence of crib-biting, wind sucking, weaving and box-walking is between 0.4% and 5% among domesticated horses in developed countries. However, in Thoroughbred horses the prevalence of these stereotypies is as high as 11%. The majority of Thoroughbred horses are employed in the racing industry and are subject to intensive management practices specific to racing yards, so it has not yet been possible to determine whether this higher prevalence is a function of breed or management (or both). It has also been shown that the prevalence of stereotypic behaviours in horses increases with age, which suggests that stereotypies persist over long periods of time, and with time the behaviour may become detached from the original reason it first started. This has implications for curing stereotypic behaviours; despite changing a horse's environment or removing factors that are believed to contribute to the behaviours, the stereotypic activity may not stop because it is no longer linked to the original cause. This is borne out by the evidence that stereotypic behaviours are rarely cured.

Weaving and crib-biting/wind sucking are examples of stereotypies which demonstrate that the underlying causation is not straightforward or universal for all stereotypies. A weaving horse sways its head from side to side, often over the top of its stable door. In some cases the whole body can become involved with the swaying and it is not uncommon to see the horse stepping from one front foot to the other as it sways. This behaviour, along with other locomotor stereotypies, often coincides with feeding time or with a view of other horses being taken out for exercise. This suggests that, rather than a consequence of boredom, weaving is a consequence of frustration; as the horse anticipates walking forward and greeting a passing horse or moving towards a source of feed it is blocked by the stable door. This scenario associated with the onset of weaving is so common that it begs the question: 'Why don't all horses weave?' In a study of foals, Waters et al. (2002) found the median age at which weaving began was 60 weeks, long after the usual age for weaning foals. In fact 60 weeks coincides with the time when foals are sold from or moved away from the studs where they were born. This suggests that young horses are vulnerable to 'social disturbance', i.e. leaving behind familiar animals and being put into a new environment where they may feel vulnerable and need to rapidly form a new network of social support (make new friends). This then ties in with these young animals feeling a strong desire to greet other animals on their new yard but being thwarted from doing so by the constraints of being stabled or held in a distant paddock. The 'treatment' of stereotypies often centres on taking steps to physically prevent the activity. In the case of weaving, this involves restricting the space above the stable door to inhibit the side-to-side movement of the horse's head. In practice this is rarely successful as the horse simply withdraws inside the box to weave there instead. In fact, this idea of preventing the stereotypic behaviour as a form of treatment is a matter of considerable controversy. Put very simply, thwarting an 'unnatural' behaviour that arose as a consequence of thwarting a natural behaviour does not make much sense; two wrongs don't make a right.

It has been suggested that stereotypic behaviours are part of a coping strategy designed to reduce stress in circumstances where welfare may be compromised by environment or management. If so, then forcibly stopping an animal from using a strategy designed to cope with problems in the environment, rather than removing the cause of the behaviour, could be exceptionally cruel.

Crib-biting and wind sucking are believed to be closely related stereotypic behaviours. Crib-biting describes a horse which uses its front teeth to grab hold of a fixed object such as the top edge of a stable door, a manger or a fencing rail. The horse then leans backwards while holding on to the object and makes a grunting noise as air passes into the oesophagus. Wind sucking is thought to be an extension of crib-biting where the horse is able to take air into the oesophagus without having to hold onto any kind of fixed object. The environmental risk factors identified for crib-biting include feeding high concentrate diets with associated reductions in provision of forage, and housing horses in stables that do not allow communication with their neighbours. However, this may not be the entire story. Unlike weaving, which begins around about 60 weeks, crib-biting can begin as early as 20 weeks of age (Waters et al. 2002). This puts the timing of crib-biting development much closer to the time of weaning. Weaning, especially abrupt human-mediated weaning, is a stressful time for all young animals and foals are no exception. It is possible that crib-biting emerges as a redirected suckling behaviour, but it has also been linked to the feeding of concentrates at the time of weaning, a food source that would never be available to foals in wild herds. The role of concentrate feeds in the development of crib-biting may be through the increased risk of animals developing gastric ulcers. Over 50% of Thoroughbred foals aged three months or less have gastric lesions (Murray et al. 1998) and it is the feeding of concentrates with an associated reduction in forage provision or intake which has been identified as leading to increased gastric acidity and gastric ulceration. Saliva is used to buffer against gastric acidity and in horses this is produced by the process of chewing food. Horses and foals fed concentrates and offered only limited access to forage may not be able to produce sufficient saliva to adequately buffer against acidity in the stomach. So, one hypothesis for the initiation of crib-biting behaviour is that it acts to increase saliva flow, thus helping to counter gastric acidity. As with weaving, a physical means of preventing crib-biting is available. A tight metal collar can be fitted high up on the neck of the horse, which makes the act of crib-biting at best uncomfortable or at worst physically painful. This collar does often succeed in inhibiting the crib-biting behaviour, but as soon as it is removed horses will begin crib-biting again at a higher rate than before the collar was fitted (McGreevy and Nicol 1998). This suggests that the horse's motivation, or need, to crib-bite was increasing during the time that the behaviour was being thwarted by the collar. This strong motivation to crib-bite also explains the relative lack of success of other radical treatments such as electric shock collars and surgical removal of neck muscles and nerves.

There is also a widely held belief that horses learn to perform stereotypies through observation of each other, although the research evidence in this area is conflicting. The consequence of this belief is that horses with stereotypies may be isolated and kept out of visual contact with their conspecifics. This is a matter of considerable welfare concern, since isolation itself is a major source of distress.

It is clearly better to avoid stereotypic behaviour than to try to treat the problem once it has started. A greater understanding of the risk factors that predispose horses to develop stereotypies and knowledge of the high-risk periods in the horses' life will allow better targeted preventive activities. Once a horse has developed a stereotypy there are alternatives to imposing physical constrains on the animal to try to control the behaviour. Examples include managing the schedule of the stable so that weaving horses are fed first or taken out to exercise first in order to compensate for the factors that trigger a bout of weaving. Horses which crib-bite may be given diets and have forage delivered throughout the day to promote production of saliva. These are not cures, nor are they easy answers, but it is important to remember that wild horses do not have stereotypies. Whether they are indicators of coping or distress, they are unequivocal signs of human failure to match our husbandry to their physiological and behavioural needs.

Case Study: Stereotypic Behaviour in Working Equids

There is a general belief that horses and donkeys working as traction or pack animals in developing countries do not develop stereotypic behaviours. If this is true then investigating the reasons for this might shed further light on the causes of the problem in equines living in developed countries. It has been variously suggested that the reasons for this might be that they have considerable contact with other animals, they work long hours so are not subject to boredom or perhaps are simply too exhausted to go to the trouble of performing stereotypic behaviours.

During a research trip to Lahore, Pakistan, in September 2006 to study the behavioural repertoire of working donkeys, a young, 2-year-old, cart donkey was released into a 4 m by 4 m sand-filled pen enclosed with wooden post-and-rail fencing. From the moment the donkey was released into the pen it put its head between a set of horizontal railings and began to weave frantically. After waiting for a while to see whether the behaviour was transitory, it became clear that the weaving was not going to stop. It was not possible to keep the donkey on the study as the weaving masked all other behavioural activity. It was extremely distressing to see an already tired, thin donkey weaving with such vehemence. On talking to the owner of the donkey he confirmed that whenever it was released from the shafts of its cart it weaved continuously; unfortunately this meant it was rarely let out of the shafts. This was a one-off observation and one cannot construct a case around a single event; however it does illustrate two points: (1) that at least one working donkey shows signs of extreme stereotypic behaviour; (2) that researchers, veterinarians and welfare scientists working in developing countries should remain open to the possibility that working equids do show stereotypic behaviours and, if this is the case, we certainly need to know more about them and how equine owners are currently managing the problem.

11.3   Assessing Welfare in Practice

Welfare assessment is a tool used to capture data that can lead to judgements about the welfare of a single animal, a group of animals or even a population. Such judgements are made on the basis of both scientific knowledge and ethical reasoning. An animal's welfare is private and internal to itself. We as welfare assessors cannot know for certain how an animal feels and what it is experiencing so we use indicators of welfare, sometimes referred to as 'proxy indicators' because we are using them as a substitute for actually knowing what the animal is feeling. This section will look at the purpose of welfare assessment and how this can determine assessment structure. It will consider the components to be included in a welfare assessment and how these can be brought together to create a protocol for monitoring equine welfare in practical situations, whether for Thoroughbred racehorses or donkeys working in a brick factory. Finally, it will look at how welfare assessment can link with action for improvements in equine welfare.

The principles that underpin welfare assessment are described in Chapter 18. It is now widely believed that in order to know about an animal's welfare the assessment has to be carried out in the animal's own environment, and that all aspects of its life and welfare should be considered, not just single components. For example, to assess the welfare of a racehorse (or population of racehorses) we need measures to reflect the different elements of its life: yard or stable routine, training and exercise activities, travelling to and from racecourses, and time at the racecourse. We should also review the management decisions that surround the animal: who takes care of the animal and how, what veterinary services are provided and how, who decides what the horse eats, what social contact it is allowed, and on what basis are these decisions made. In addition we should look at the history of the animal: where it has been before, previous injuries, times when behavioural problems began to emerge. The assessment should also give some insight into future welfare and identify future risks. This is clearly a huge task; to make welfare assessment possible some rationalizing of objectives is needed.

If a protocol for assessing the welfare of a horse or population of horses is to succeed, it has to be feasible, practical and avoid infuriating owners and trainers. An essential first step is to ask the question: 'What is the purpose of this welfare assessment, what do we need the information for and how may it be put to use?' The aims may be general or specific. They include:

- Better understanding of the welfare needs of horses and how we can promote them in a domestic environment. Here the assessment would be directed towards consequences of domestication, looking at the lives of domesticated horses compared to their free-ranging counterparts.
- Provision of information for an equine industry, regulating body or policy-maker about specific problems associated with a specific type of use.
- Provision of information for owners about the welfare of their animals. This type of assessment would focus on individual horses or donkeys and the data collected would need to be useful and relevant to the owner, showing them opportunities for improving their animals' lives.
- Assessment of welfare in novel and little-known circumstances of domestication.

An example of this fourth case is provided by the industry to harvest pregnant mare urine, which has grown rapidly in the United States and Canada. The urine of pregnant female horses contains hormones that can be used in the production of hormone replacement therapies for menopausal women. Mares are kept in tie stalls in large barns and their movements are restricted in order to keep them attached to the urine collection apparatus. There has been huge debate about the ethics of this industry and the concerns about the welfare of these mares. In a case such as this, an initial welfare assessment is necessary in order to identify the main welfare issues and this might then become more focused and detailed once the main issues had been discovered.

Any welfare assessment on a specific establishment, be it a racing stable or a pregnant mare serum (PMS) 'ranch', needs to be built into a dynamic programme of welfare control that allows monitoring of a problem over time. The assessment should be sensitive enough to detect changes in welfare and broad enough to monitor whether improving one welfare parameter impacts positively or negatively on others.

Indicators of different types can be included within a welfare assessment. Measurements of the environment can be made; the dimensions of a stall, the thickness of the bedding, the visual range available to the horse, the levels of ventilation and airflow in a loose box, quantities and frequencies of feed given and so on. These are commonly referred to as measures of resource or provision and they help to build up a picture of the life the horse (or donkey) leads. From this the welfare assessor would have to infer how the animal feels about its situation. Further information could be added by interviewing the owner to bring in information about routines, how much exercise it receives, when it has access to companions, problems the owner might be concerned about and so on. Having obtained a record of husbandry (resources and management) it is then necessary to look at the animal itself, using direct or animal-based observations. This will involve measures of the animals' physical state including body condition scoring, counting the number of lesions on the body, examining the colour of the mucous membranes, checking for nasal discharge, looking for signs of limping, and so on. It might involve physiological measures such as measuring heart and respiratory rate, taking blood samples to test for cortisol and catecholamine concentrations, or collecting faecal samples to carry out faecal egg counts to check for endoparasites. The interpretation of these measures should be relatively straightforward. However, the measures that are likely to give the most direct insight into the horse or donkey's internal experiences are measures of behaviour since they are a result of the animal's own decision-making processes. Measures of behaviour might include observing the responsiveness of a horse or donkey to its environment, observing whether stereotypic behaviour is present, testing how a horse responds to a familiar and unfamiliar person, or observing how a donkey responds to being touched. Often a combination of approaches brings the most useful information.

Table 11.2 describes a set of welfare assessment measures made up entirely of animal-based observations. This welfare assessment was used among horses, donkeys and mules working in five developing countries: India, Pakistan, Egypt, Jordan and Afghanistan. The criteria which determined the design of this assessment were that:

- a large number of animals needed to be assessed (just under 5000) so time per assessment was limited;

Table 11.2 Examples of welfare parameters used to assess working horses, mules and donkeys.

Observations of behaviour	Observations of health
Alert/apathetic/severely depressed	Mucous membrane colour
Response to observer approach	Lesions at commissures of lips
Response to walk down side of animal	Molar hooks or sharp edges
Tail tuck (donkeys only)	Eyes
Accept/avoid chin contact	Coat staring/dry/matted/uneven
	Ectoparasites
General observation	Diarrhoea under tail
Body condition score (scale 1–5)	Heat stress
	Firing lesions or scars
Lesions of skin and deeper tissues	Tether/hobble lesions or scars
Head	Carpal lesions or scars
Ears	Hock lesions or scars
Neck	Swelling of tendons and joints
Breast and shoulders	Limb deformity
Withers	Cow-hocked conformation
Spine	Hoof walls length
Girth	Hoof horn quality
Belly	Sole surface
Ribs and flank	Gait
Hindquarters	
Tail and tail base	
Forelegs (except carpus)	
Hindlegs (except hock)	

Source: Pritchard et al. (2005).

- it was not culturally appropriate for observers to visit animals at home so observations of animals were made during work;
- stopping animals during their daily work would affect their owners' capacity to earn money so the assessment had to be for the minimum time possible;
- owner interviews were not possible because too many languages and dialects were involved to get reliable and consistent translation;
- the working animals led such complex lives that the assessment of their environment could not be comprehensive.

The animals in this study were involved in a number of different work types: pulling carts which carried goods or people, carrying packs or being ridden by tourists. From the data it was seen that in all three species 90% or more of the animals observed walked abnormally, between 18 and 28% had serious skin lesions in the region of the girth, up to 88% of donkeys had lesions associated with hobbling or tethering (79% in mules and 62% in horses) and the majority of animals were of low body condition score (either thin or very thin). Behavioural measures revealed that around 10% of all animals showed signs of apathy or severe depression, significantly more animals of all species showed aggressive or avoidance responses to the observers than friendly responses, and around 20% of all the animals avoided being touched on the chin.[2]

These data dramatically illustrate the many problems faced by horse, donkeys and mules working in developing countries. However, expensive horses in developed countries also have their problems, which include high prevalence of lameness and stereotypic behaviours. Many horses and donkeys live in social isolation, exercise is often limited or so excessive that immune function is compromised, and feeding regimes no longer reflect the patterns and time budgets of horses still living in the wild.

Addressing welfare problems of domesticated equidae is a considerable challenge. The result of domestication is that welfare problems, and remedies, are all mediated by humans. So resolving equine welfare problems is about changing human behaviour. The way that humans manage their animals, wherever they are in the world, is a synthesis of cultural norms, experience, learning, received wisdom and trial and error (and is, of course, dependent on income and access to resources). Many aspects of horse and donkey management are based around routines and these routines are often planned to deliver convenience for humans rather than to address the complex needs of the animals. Once routines are established they can be difficult to change, as the following, rather simplistic, example shows. The owner of a horse kept for recreational riding at weekends offers it food twice a day, morning and evening, because he or she has to work during the day to earn money to keep the horse. However, the horse is behaviourally driven to eat forage steadily for between 17 and 18 hours each day, and twice-a-day feeding does not allow this. To accommodate the horse's need the owner might have to travel home at lunchtime to provide more forage and go out late each night to give one last hay-net, hire pasture and spend extra time each day turning out, checking or grooming the horse, and extra time at weekends maintaining the pasture, or employ someone to offer additional forage to the horse during the day. Although all these options would improve the horse's welfare, none are as convenient for the owner as the current routine.

Owners should be aware of the inadequacies of such a routine and consider ways in which it might be improved. They must consider possible alternative strategies, perhaps talking to other owners to see how they have addressed the problem, and imagining how they might find the space in their daily schedule to introduce the new elements to the routine. This should be recognized as a fundamental responsibility of all owners to fulfil their duty of care. For people in developing countries, using horses and donkeys as a means to earn a meagre

---

2 This work was carried out on behalf of a working equine welfare charity, 'Brooke'; Brooke, 2nd Floor, The Hallmark Building, 52–56 Leadenhall Street, London.

living, making changes to improve the welfare of their animals may represent the difference between earning enough money to buy food or not.

Figures 11.4 and 11.5 illustrate a project to help working donkey owners in Lahore, Pakistan, make changes to their working practices and routines to improve the welfare of their donkeys.[3] The condition of many of these donkeys is very bad and donkey owners are extremely poor, marginalized and vulnerable. In order to promote improvements in the welfare of these working donkeys, meetings were held with a group of donkey owners who attended on behalf of the other donkey owners living in their communities. The owners identified a set of needs for their donkeys (Figure 11.4). These included provision of resources including food, water, veterinary treatment and opportunities to roll; animal care activities including grooming, washing and hoof picking; guidelines for the working day including maximum cart loads, driving adjustments for poor road surfaces and driving speeds; and guidance on owners' behaviours such as no beating, not putting donkeys in to work until four years of age, and resting female donkeys in late pregnancy. Although these needs failed to include such things as behavioural freedom, they became the priorities in order to give control of the project to the donkey owners themselves and allow them to take actions which they perceived as achievable within their own context.

The donkey owners in communities participating in the project were asked to assess how well each of the needs shown in Figure 11.4

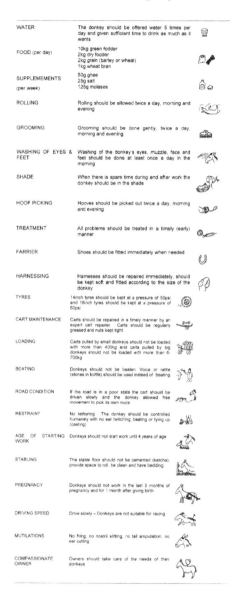

Figure 11.4 Welfare needs of donkeys working in Lahore, Pakistan; identified by owners' groups representing their communities.

---

3 This project was commissioned by The Brooke and carried out in conjunction with an Indian development organization called Praxis; Praxis Institute for Participatory Practices, 1st Floor, Maa Sharde Complex, East Boring Canal Road, Patna 800001, India.

	Jugnu			Rocket			Rani			Hira		
Food (fodder plus grain)	◆	☒	○	◆	○	○	○	○	○	☒	☒	◆
Water (5 times daily)	☒	☒	◆	☒	☒	☒	○	○	○	◆	☒	○
Washing (daily, AM)	○	○	○	☒	☒	◆	◆	○	○	◆	◆	◆
Hoof picking (twice daily)	◆	○	○	◆	◆	◆	○	○	○	◆	○	◆
Loading max 400 kg for small donkeys max 600–700 kg for large donkeys	☒	☒	☒	◆	☒	◆	◆	◆	○	☒	◆	○
Rolling (twice daily)	☒	◆	○	○	○	○	○	○	○	◆	◆	○
Tethering No tethering, twitching or casting	◆	◆	○	☒	○	○	☒	◆	○	☒	☒	☒

Key: Donkeys (Jugnu, Rocket, Rani and Hira) are monitored each month for welfare according to the needs described in Figure 11.4, and rated using a 'traffic light' system, where green is good, yellow is intermediate and red is bad. In this table red = ☒, yellow = ◆ and green = ○. Owners are given a clear explanation of the reasons for unsatisfactory ratings and advice as to appropriate action.

Figure 11.5 Example working donkey welfare monitoring chart for use on a monthly basis by owners of working donkeys in Lahore, Pakistan.

was being met for each donkey in their community. To do this a welfare monitoring chart (see Figure 11.5) was set up and the whole community was invited to join in the process of allocating red, yellow or green dots for each donkey in their community to indicate how well each need was being delivered. A red dot indicates that the need is not being met at all; a yellow dot indicates that the need is almost being met; and a green dot indicates that the need is being met completely. This process is repeated on a monthly basis so that all donkey owners can join in and owners who receive green dots can tell others how they have achieved this.

Processes such as the welfare intervention with the Lahore donkey owners are still experimental but they illustrate the effort and imagination needed to bring about welfare change. Although some of the changes identified by the donkey owners may seem modest, once the habit of making changes becomes familiar and the benefits to the donkeys can be seen, the owners will then be more likely to initiate further changes for themselves.

11.4 Final Notes

Today's domesticated equidae are important to humans for economic and commercial reasons as well as for providing pleasure to people who use them for leisure and view them as pets. The individual horse or donkey may find itself anywhere within a spectrum that ranges from that of loved companion to a mere commodity ('workhorse'). To the horse, donkey or mule, what is important is how our differing perceptions of their use and role are translated into actions that affect their welfare. Across the wide range of uses we find for our horses, ponies and donkeys, a common theme seems to be a continual demand for them to deliver and achieve more. They are expected to run faster, jump higher, live at greater convenience to their owners, pull heavier loads or work longer hours. Domestication is an ongoing process and there is a danger that it is being driven entirely by our needs, not theirs. People who care about horses and donkeys need to have both knowledge of the principles of animal welfare *and* a thorough understanding of how they live. Welfare themes that recur time and again include thwarting of normal behaviours, problems of isolation, risks of inappropriate feeding, unstable social groupings, and health problems associated with overwork. To make judgements about the welfare of horses or donkeys we must integrate information from all aspects of their lives. The huge diversity of roles and uses that they fulfil means that there is no simple single formula for assessing their welfare.

This chapter has considered equidae from all around the world, in acknowledgment of the fact that 85% of the world's horses, donkeys and mules can be found in developing countries. Each region and each task we set our equidae presents particular challenges. Nevertheless, the animals are equally important wherever they come from and all are vulnerable to compromises in their welfare. What domesticated horses, donkeys and mules give to humans through their versatility, adaptability and capacity to endure is truly amazing.

References and Further Reading

Anthony, D.W. and Brown, D.R. (1991). The origins of horseback riding. *Antiquity* 65: 22–38.

Broster, C.E., Burn, C.C., Barr, A.R.S., and Whay, H.R. (2009). The range and prevalence of pathological abnormalities associated with lameness in working horses from developing countries. *Equine Veterinary Journal* 41: 474–481.

Burn, C.C., Pritchard, J.C., Farajat, M., Twaissi, A.A.M., and Whay, H.R. (2008). Risk factors for strap-related lesions in working donkeys at the World Heritage Site of Petra and Jordan. *Veterinary Journal* 178: 261–269.

Fraser, D., Weary, D.M., Pajor, E.A., and Milligan, B.N. (1997). A scientific conception of animal welfare that reflects ethical concerns. *Animal Welfare* 6: 187–205.

Greet, T.C.R. and Rossdale, P.D. (1987). The digestive system. In: *Veterinary Notes for Horse Owners* (ed. M.H. Hayes and P.D. Rossdale), 5–24. London: Stanley Paul.

Heleski, C.R., Shelle, A.C., Nielsen, B.D., and Zanella, A.J. (2002). Influence of housing on weanling horse behaviour and subsequent welfare. *Applied Animal Behaviour Science* 78: 291–302.

Henderson, A.J.Z. (2007). Don't fence me in: managing psychological well being for elite performance horses. *Journal of Applied Animal Welfare Science* 10: 309–329.

Houpt, K.A. (2001). Equine welfare. In: *Recent Advances in Companion Animal Behaviour Problems*. Ithaca, NY: International Veterinary Information Services. http://www.ivis.org.

Kaneene, J.B., Whitney, R.A., and Miller, R.A. (1997). The Michigan equine monitoring system. II. Frequencies and impact of selected health problems. *Preventive Veterinary Medicine* 29: 277–292.

Mal, M.E., Friend, T.H., Lay, D.C., Vogelsang, S.G., and Jenkins, O.C. (1991). Physiological responses of mares to short term confinement and social isolation. *Journal of Equine Veterinary Science* 11: 96–102.

McDonnell, S.M. (2002). Behaviour of horses. In: *The Ethology of Domestic Animals: An Introductory Text* (ed. P. Jensen). Wallingford: CABI Publishing.

McGreevy, P. (2004). *Equine Behavior: A Guide for Veterinarians and Equine Scientists*. Philadelphia: W.B. Saunders.

McGreevy, P.D. and Nicol, C.J. (1998). The effect of short-term prevention on the subsequent rate of crib-biting in Thoroughbred horses. *Equine Veterinary Journal Supplement* 27: 30–34.

Murray, M.J., Schusser, G.F., Pipers, F.S., and Gross, S.F. (1996). Factors associated with gastric lesions in Thoroughbred racehorses. *Equine Veterinary Journal* 28: 368–374.

Pritchard, J.C., Lindberg, A.C., Main, D.C.J., and Whay, H.R. (2005). Assessment of the welfare of working horses, mules and donkeys using animal-based measures. *Preventive Veterinary Medicine* 69: 265–283.

Riadal, S.L., Love, D.N., Bailey, G.D., and Rose, R.J. (2000). Effects of single bouts of moderate and high intensity exercise and training on equine peripheral neutrophil function. *Research in Veterinary Science* 68: 141–146.

Rossel, S., Marshall, F., Peters, J., Pilgram, T., Adams, M.D., and O'Conner, D. (2008). Domestication of the donkey: timing, processes, and indicators. *Proceedings of the National Academy of Sciences* 105: 3715–3720.

Summerhays, R.S. (1975). *The Problem Horse*. London: Allen & Unwin.

van Dierendonck, M.C., Bandi, N., Batdorj, D., Dügerlham, S., and Munkhtsog, B. (1996). Behavioural observations of reintroduced Takhi or Przewalski horses (Equus ferus przewalskii) in Mongolia. *Applied Animal Behaviour Science* 50: 95–115.

Wallace, A.G. (2003). Assessing the efficacy of an anthelmintic programme on the health and welfare of working equines in Morocco. http:www.taws.org (accessed 28 October 2008).

Waters, A.W., Nicol, C.J., and French, N.P. (2002). Factors influencing the development of stereotypic and redirected behaviours in young horses: findings of a four-year prospective epidemiological study. *Equine Veterinary Journal* 34: 572–579.

12

Farmed Fish

Joy Becker

12.1   Introduction

Since the early 1980s, aquaculture is said to be the fastest growing food-producing sector and now accounts for about half of the world's food fish. Today, aquaculture is practiced in fresh, brackish and marine waters, in tropical through arctic conditions, in inland lakes and ponds

Management and Welfare of Farm Animals: The UFAW Farm Handbook, Sixth Edition.
Edited by John Webster and Jean Margerison.
© Universities Federation for Animal Welfare 2022. Published 2022 by John Wiley & Sons Ltd.

through to large offshore cage operations. In 2016, aquaculture production (including plants and animals) reached almost 110 million tonnes, valued at US$244 billion. The total production of farmed aquatic animals was 80 million tonnes (valued at US$232 billion), which consists of finfish, molluscs, crustaceans and other aquatic animals (e.g. turtles, sea cucumbers, sea urchins). Finfish make up half of global aquaculture production (by volume), with 70% of that consisting of freshwater species (such as grass carp, silver carp and common carp).

This chapter will introduce you to several animal management systems used in global aquaculture and will focus mainly on a wide variety of fish species used in aquaculture. Please see the previous edition of this book for a focused review on salmonids. The chapter will provide you with an overview of aquaculture and the importance of fish as a source of global protein. It is intended to help you assess the impact of aquaculture production systems on communities, the environment and the health and welfare of aquatic animals.

12.2 Defining Aquaculture

The Food and Agriculture Organization of the United Nations (FAO) defines aquaculture as the farming of aquatic organisms including fish, molluscs, crustaceans and aquatic plants with some sort of intervention in the rearing process to enhance production, such as regular stocking, feeding and protection from predators. Farming also implies individual or corporate ownership of the stock being cultivated. It is important to say that the FAO definition does not require absolute control over all aspects of the life cycle of cultivated organisms. In many aquaculture farming systems, there is often a need to harvest animals or plants from the wild for some aspect of the production cycle (e.g. wild collection of oysters spat or glass eels). When reading and considering the publications and statistics produced by the FAO and other global organizations, the term 'fish' refers to fish, crustaceans, molluscs and other aquatic animals and excludes aquatic plants, aquatic mammals and reptiles. Regardless of the definition, today's aquaculture practices include a wide variety of farming systems with little input from the wild (e.g. salmonid aquaculture) to wild input being central to the farming system (e.g. collection of juvenile tuna for fattening and future harvest).

12.3 Early History of Aquaculture

Aquaculture has been practiced for millennia. One of the earliest aquaculture sites from 30,000 years ago is found in Victoria, Australia, and is on the UNESCO World Heritage list. Known as The Budj Bim Cultural Landscape, the aboriginal people used and modified a series of channels and dams to keep and harvest eels. Similar examples of early aquaculture are found in other parts of Australia with large scale rock walls built by the indigenous people to trap fish (Figure 12.1). In other regions, aquaculture began in China as far back as 2000 BC, with the first known written account in about 475 BC. These early accounts began with the "intentional impoundment of aquatic species' also known as prototype aquaculture or proto aquaculture.

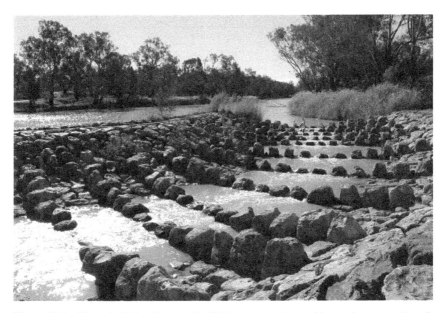

Figure 12.1 The refurbished Brewarrina fishing system, located in north-western New South Wales, Australia. The system is thought to be 30,000 years old and is an example of a large-scale fish trapping operation constructed by the indigenous Ngemba people. [Photo credit: Dr Greg Cronin].

Other early examples include:

- Pictographs from the tombs of Pharaohs of Egypt show people fishing for tilapia in apparent culture ponds (about 2500 BC)
- Japanese reportedly began farming oysters in the intertidal zones about 3000 years ago
- Romans cultured oysters 2000 years ago

In the USA during the late 1800s, some aquatic animal populations were already in decline, due in part to over-fishing. To maintain a supply of fish (mainly trout) for sport fishing activities, many fish culturists in the USA and Europe set out to develop the technology to mass produce, transport and stock various marine and freshwater fish. Initially, glass jars were used to incubate fish eggs and fry were being reared in raceways with devices to aerate the water. This allowed for a mass movement of fish eggs (mainly trout and salmon) to be moved around North America, Europe, Australia and New Zealand.

Commercial aquaculture was a cottage industry for the first half of the twentieth century with most fish being raised for the sport fishery. A defining moment in aquaculture, in 1934, was the demonstration that fish could be induced to spawn artificially. The development of methods for rearing larvae and controlling reproduction created huge diversity and an industry of significant economic value. The 1960s and 1970s brought entrepreneurs, industrialization of aquaculture industries, researchers and the public to the world of aquaculture.

12.4   Global View and Contributions to Food Security

Fish is a vital human food providing essential nutrients and is critical to global food security, with approx. 90% of the global aquaculture production is concentrated in the Asia-Pacific region, with the top producers being China, India and Indonesia. Fish farming in developing countries provides domestic food security and supports rural livelihoods with the production of high-value fish destined for export and according to the UN, more than 3 billion people depend on marine and coastal biodiversity for their livelihoods. In 2015 (FAO 2018) fish accounted for approx. 17% of animal protein consumed by the global population. This equates to one in six people gain all their animal protein from fish, while approx. 3.2 billion people gain almost 20% of their average per capita intake of animal protein from fish.

A key driver for the growth and expansion of the global aquaculture industry has been the increase in the annual per capita consumption of food fish, with the per capita consumption of food fish doubling over the last six decades to approx. 20.5 kg in 2017. This increase has been driven by increased production, technological advancements, better distribution channels and lower wastage due to growing demand. Overall, China by far is the world's largest consumer and producer of farmed fish.

12.5   The Aquatic Environment

Water is always a significant limiting factor in aquaculture production. Fish perform all their bodily functions in water, and they are totally dependent on water to breathe, feed, grow, excrete wastes, maintain a salt balance and reproduce. Water can hold large amounts of heat with a relatively small change in temperature, and this heat capacity has far-reaching implications. It permits a body of water to act as a buffer against wide fluctuations in temperature and the larger the body of water, the slower the rate of temperature change. Fish are ectothermic, meaning they take on the temperature of their environment. Aquaculture farming system can optimize production by changing thermal experiences to manipulate metabolic rates to increase appetite, growth and excretion rates as well as alter swimming activity and thus the demand for oxygen.

A key factor for all successful aquaculture farming systems is uninhibited access to a plentiful supply of suitable quality water for the species being farmed. The provision of water is a primary consideration in both the species and site selection and production schedule for a successful farm. Water can dissolve more substances than any other liquid. Over 50% of the known chemical elements have been found in natural waters and it is probable that traces of most others can be found in lakes, streams, estuaries or oceans. This feature can make the risk of chemical contamination high in aquaculture farms compared to terrestrial farms with equivalent land areas.

The main sources of water are surface, groundwater and occasionally municipal water sources. Surface water is used when the production system (e.g. net pen) is placed in the environment (e.g. oceans, lakes and rivers). Typically, surface water is inexpensive, but susceptible to interruptions of supply and a high risk of contamination, compared with groundwater or well water, which is often preferred source due to a lack of pathogen risk, contamination from urban or agriculture sources and usually at a constant temperature. The main disadvantages of ground water are the high cost of pumping it, the possibility of a well drying up and often the presence of strict regulations and licensing with daily maximum withdrawal volumes. A municipal water source is sometimes used in small recirculating systems (usually for research) but it tends to be relatively expensive to use and to remove the disinfectants it contains for human consumption.

12.5.1 Physical Factors and Ability to Support Fish Life

12.5.1.1 Temperature

After oxygen content, water temperature may be the single most important factor affecting the health and welfare of fish. The temperature of the water affects the animal's behaviour, feeding, growth and reproduction. Fish are generally separated into four loose non-discrete categories with respect to tolerable temperature regime including, cold water, warm water, cool water and tropical. As ectotherms, fish and other aquatic organisms used in farming (such as bivalves and crustaceans) typically cannot tolerate rapid temperature changes. Within the physiological range for each fish species, changes in water temperature should not exceed 1 to 2°C per day.

Water temperature should be measured continuously or at regular intervals at production and research facilities. Groundwater temperatures remain relatively constant year-round compared to surface water, where temperatures can rapidly fluctuate. Water temperature also determines the amount of dissolved gases, which include oxygen, carbon dioxide and nitrogen. The cooler the water, the more soluble the gas. Water temperature also plays a major role in the physical process called thermal stratification, whereby the mixing of warm and cool water is prevented by their different densities. This thermal stratification is an important consideration for pond culture as constant circulation of water may be necessary to avoid cold anoxic water moving through the stock that can result in events of high mortality.

12.5.1.2 Dissolved Gases

The most common gases are oxygen, carbon dioxide, nitrogen and ammonia, measured in parts per million or milligrams per litre. Dissolved oxygen (DO) is by far the most important chemical parameter in aquaculture and the amount of oxygen that can be dissolved in water decreases at higher water temperatures, greater altitudes and salinities. Water is 775 times denser than air and at saturation contains only 3% as much oxygen. As a result, fish must ventilate a volume of water, which is 10 to 30 times greater than the volume of air used by most terrestrial animals to obtain the same quantity of oxygen. The ventilation rate of fish is directly dependent on the amount of oxygen in that is available in the water.

Low dissolved oxygen levels are responsible for more fish kills, either directly or indirectly, than all other problems combined. The amount of oxygen required for respiration is dependent on the fish species, size, feeding rate, activity level and environmental temperature. Small fish consume more oxygen than an equal mass of larger fish because of their higher metabolic rate. As a rule, cold water fish require higher DO levels than warm water fish, e.g. salmonids require DO levels above 7–8 mg/litre compared to carps and tilapia which require levels above 4–6 mg/litre.

Oxygen dissolves in water through diffusion from the photosynthetic activity of land and aquatic plants. DO is under biological control in that daily fluctuations result from high levels during the day due to photosynthesis and lower levels at night due to respiration. Therefore, increases and decreases in DO over a 24-hour period are influenced by any activity which interferes with photosynthesis, respiration or mechanical mixing of the water (e.g. thermal stratification). Factors that can decrease DO are overstocking, increased activity, increased turbidity and increased temperature. Oxygen levels are depleted in several ways, but chiefly by respiration of fish and other organisms and by chemical reactions with organic waste composition (faeces build-up, excess feed, decayed plants and fish mortalities). Indications of dangerously low levels of DO include fish congregating at the intake or gasping behaviour at the surface of the water. Fish that die from oxygen deprivation often (not always!) have flared gills and open mouths. Oxygen levels can be increased by agitation of the surface water with paddlewheels, air compressors and blowers to produce small bubbles through diffusers, air stones and air lifts.

Fish release carbon dioxide (CO_2), which is also commonly detected in water sources originating from limestone bearing rock. Fish can tolerate concentrations of up to 10 ppm, provided DO concentrations are high. Water supporting good fish production has < 5 ppm of free CO_2. In recirculating aquaculture systems (RAS), CO_2 may regularly exceed 20 ppm, which may interfere with oxygen utilization by the fish. CO_2 is often removed by aeration or the use of degassing columns to blow off excess gas.

Gaseous nitrogen comes from the atmosphere and from the breakdown of nitrogenous compounds. Most of the nitrogen is converted to ammonia and ammonium, which exist in equilibrium. These are reduced to nitrites by the activity of nitrifying bacteria, *Nitrosomonas* sp. Nitrites are then oxidized to nitrates by the bacterium *Nitrobacter* sp. Nitrate acts as a fertilizer and is eventually recycled to gaseous nitrogen as organisms, which have used it die and decompose. Nitrogen and its intermediate forms have the potential to become toxic to aquatic organisms (especially in recirculating systems).

A critical constraint to RAS farming systems is that it requires three moles of oxygen to convert one mole of ammonia to nitrate. Furthermore, the nitrification process is acidifying, and pH must be constantly monitored and adjusted to meet the physiological requirements for the systems (e.g. the production species and the microbial community converting the nitrogen). Nitrite (NO_2^-) toxicity can be a common problem in RAS, where there is an imbalance in the bacterial flora in the biofilter prior to stocking fish or increasing organic loading caused by adding fish or feed). Nitrite competes with haemoglobin for oxygen to form methaemoglobin resulting in fish with chocolate-brown-coloured blood. When the oxygen carrying capacity declines below a critical level, fish die due to asphyxiation.

Fish excrete ionized ammonia mainly through the gill tissues and small amounts of urea into the water as waste. Increased ammonia interferes with respiration, disrupts osmoregulation and interferes with haemoglobin-mediated oxygen transfer. Lethal levels will destroy mucus membranes of the skin and intestine and cause external bleeding and haemorrhaging. Two forms of ammonia occur in aquaculture systems: ionized and un-ionized. The un-ionized form of ammonia (NH_3) is extremely toxic, while the ionized form (NH_4^+) is not. Both forms are grouped together as 'total ammonia' (TAN). The relative percentage of total ammonia that is in the toxic unionized form is controlled mainly by pH and, to a lesser extent, temperature. Through biological processes, toxic ammonia can be degraded to relatively harmless nitrates. The amount of un-ionized ammonia that is detrimental to fish varies with species, with the lethal limits for finfish between 0.2 and 0.5 mg/L of un-ionized ammonia in freshwater. Excess ammonia can be removed from the water using ion exchange columns, but denitrification is more commonly achieved simply through dilution. Biofilters should be big enough to cope with ammonia loads in recirculating systems.

12.5.1.3 pH

The optimal pH range for freshwater fish is between 6.5 and 7.5 and for marine culture fish; the optimum is 8.0 to 8.5. It is important to remain close to the optimum pH of the system since abrupt changes in pH are particularly detrimental to animals, plants and bacterial communities. Large pH changes can occur when there are changes in the buffering capacity of the water. Usually mineral carbonates (carbonate CO_3^- and bicarbonate HCO_3^-) buffer water and maintain constant pH. CO_2 from the atmosphere and from fish respiration will contribute to the acidity of water by dissociating to carbonic acid. Fish exposed to pH out of their normal range may spin near the surface of the water and an increase in jumping may also be observed. Problems with pH can be solved by management practices to stabilize the buffering capacity of the system. Avoiding organic loading and adding $CaCO_3$ are common practices.

12.5.1.4 Suspended Solids

Suspended fish wastes are a major concern for RAS. Large amounts of suspended and settleable solids are produced during fish production. Fish waste particles can be a major source of poor water quality since they may contain up to 70% of the nitrogen load in the system. These wastes not only irritate the gills of fish but also can cause several problems to the biological filter. The particulates can clog the biological filter, causing the nitrifying bacteria to die from lack of oxygen. Particulates can also promote the growth of bacteria that produce, rather than consume, ammonia.

12.5.2 Measuring and Recording

A single test at a given point in time is like taking a snapshot. The picture may capture the moment, but the stability of the moment is short-lived. Point sampling analysis of water, especially in heavily stocked systems, rarely provides a clear picture of the daily fluctuations in water quality and does little to predict impending or chronic stressors. Sampling at routine intervals throughout the day allows for the development of a fully integrated water quality profile and allows evaluation of the interaction between fish and the environment. For most systems best practice is multiple sampling and/or online continuous monitoring, which is more reflective of the entire management of the holding environment. However, when water testing is selective, test only where it is appropriate (e.g. not following feeding periods) and ensure that tests are performed regularly, if not continuously. It is important to remember that any sensor used to measure, and record water quality is only as accurate as the calibration!

12.6 Aquaculture Farming Systems

Every fish farm is different. Aquaculture systems are commonly described based on the species and life stage, the location, the type of infrastructure at the farm and the type of water exchange. There is close connection between the optimal choice for fish species and farm infrastructure based on the quality and volume of water available, and all of this is a balanced with the economics of a successful farming operation. Production stages are generally divided as:

1) Early life stage or hatchery phase consisting of rearing brood stock for egg production and hatching.
2) Nursery phase with the rearing of fry or juveniles.
3) Grow-out phase with on-growing of juveniles to harvest.

Fish species are often classified based on water temperature preference. Warmwater species (e.g. tilapia, carps, catfish) grow best at water temperatures above 25°C, cold water species (trout, salmon, cod) grow best below 18°C. Figures 12.2a and 12.2b illustrate two examples of aquaculture farming systems:Atlantic salmon (*Salmo salar*) intensively farmed in land-based tank systems for fingerling production and transferred to an open water system using sea cages for grow-out (Figure 12.2a): land-based nursery tanks intensively farming juvenile barramundi (*Lates calcarifer*) fingerlings using partial recirculation (Figure 12.2b).

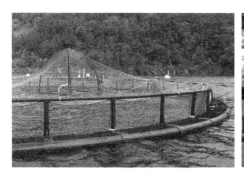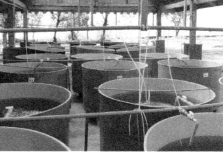

Figure 12.2 (a) Atlantic salmon at grow-out in sea cages, (b) juvenile barramundi in nursery tanks with partial recirculation of marine water. [Photo credit: Dr Joy Becker].

When deciding on an aquaculture species for farming, one must consider a range of biological and non-biological factors. The key biological factors for prioritizing species selection are often related to optimal thermal range, fecundity, ease of breeding in captivity, growth rates and feed choices, and ability to utilize non-animal protein sources. Other key factors for prioritizing species selection are consumer acceptance, market demand, availability of proven technologies (e.g. readily available 'off the shelf' systems) and regional or national priorities.

12.6.1 Ponds, Tanks and Net-pens

Common farming structures used for fish farms are ponds, tanks (and raceways) and net-pens (or sea cages). Ponds are the oldest form of aquaculture due to their relative simplicity and are usually constructed in close connection with the source of water (e.g. estuary or river). Ponds are earthen impoundments that are relatively inexpensive (compared to tanks and net-pens), commonly used for nursery and grow out production phases, and polyculture. Ponds are commonly constructed consecutively (especially if relying on tidal water exchange) so that water flows through each pond before leaving the site. This allows for easy movement of stock and maximal water usage. However, water quality level decreases with each passage and it is not possible to isolate individual ponds. This presents a major disadvantage with regard to disease prevention and control of spread. Small net-pens can also be placed within a pond to rear fish (Figure 12.3a).

Tanks and raceways are the second most common production structure in aquaculture (Figure 12.3b). Tanks are used in situations and locations when pond culture is not ideal, e.g. rearing early life stages and the grow-out stage for high-value fish species in RAS. Raceways are typically elongated tanks, whereby water enters at one end and leaves through the other. Raceways are narrow and shallow with a strong continuous water flow, perfect for swimming species, like trout and salmon. However, raceways require a large supply of water that is

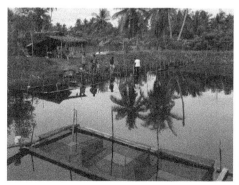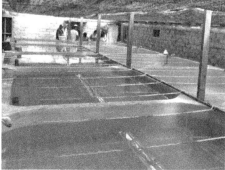

Figure 12.3 (a) net-pens placed inside a pond at a grouper (*Epinephelus* spp.) nursery, (b) larval rearing tanks containing barramundi (*Lates calcarifer*). [Photo credit: Dr Joy Becker].

usually pumped from a well or a river. Although tanks can be either flow through or recirculation, raceways are generally always flow through systems. Tanks and raceways are more expensive to construct (relative to ponds and net-pens), but they do offer increased stocking densities, stronger control on water quality (e.g. installation of UV or ozone systems) and biosecurity. Tanks and raceways are commonly made of concrete or fibreglass based on the required structure strength, cost, chemical residues, shape and risk of abrasion to the animals. The shape is very important and may dictate flow dynamics, solids removals and animal welfare.

Net-pens and sea cages are floating structures with a net suspended below and come in various shapes (round, rectangular or square) and are placed directly in the water body (also known as an open system). Typically, these structures are used for intensively farmed high-value fish species during the grow-out phase that can require months or years to reach market size. Net-pens are more expensive than ponds but cheaper than tanks and are relatively cheap to operate with no (or little) pumping costs. However, net-pen systems have no direct or immediate control over water quality other than through selecting optimal sites. Traditionally, net pens are located in protected inshore areas and they are subject to short-term and long-term changes in climate (e.g. algal blooms, fierce storms, jellyfish blooms). Net-pens consist of:

1) a float that keeps the cage at the surface and helps maintain shape
2) several nets to keep fish in and predators out
3) a mooring or anchor point.

Common production issues with net-pens include biofouling of the mesh nets with (e.g.) seaweeds, mussels and sponges that reduce water flow (and thus DO), escaped farmed fish if nets are damaged, predators, algal blooms, interaction between wild fish and farmed fish, potential exposure to pathogens or contamination from urban or agricultural runoff.

Net-pens are made up of (Figure 12.2a):

1) a float: keeps the cage at the surface of the water and helps to maintain shape
2) a collar: maintains the shape and assists in flotation
3) nets: multilayered with the main net to keep the fish in and a predator net

12.6.2 Recirculating Aquaculture Systems

Recirculating aquaculture systems (RAS) are a closed system and have minimal connection to the environment and their water source. Water is added to offset evaporation, incidental losses with cleaning and, most importantly, to maintain water quality. It is common to have up to 25% of the total volume of the water in the system exchanged each day to maintain water quality. The initial capital cost is quite high relative to other systems; however, the potential for high yield and year-round product is advantageous. Water quality is maintained in these systems by pumping the culture water through specialized filtration and aeration equipment. It is very important to build redundancy into the design of recirculating systems to allow for pumps and equipment to be cleaned and/or repaired. RAS design and technology is an advancing area and a review of current design practice can be reviewed in Malone (2013).

12.7 Fish Nutrition

Like other livestock animals, fish need the right diet in the correct quantities to maintain health. Adequate nutrition is required for body maintenance, optimal growth, energy expended in swimming and social interaction and, where applicable, reproduction. Additionally, the feed selected must be matched to the species, age and life stage for all aquatic organisms. Specific energy requirements and specific feed components vary across species. Fish are most commonly omnivores and carnivores, although some are detritivores and herbivores. Much of the fish nutrition research and subsequent diet formulations have been carried out on salmonids (carnivorous cold-water species) and then adjusted for other species.

12.7.1 Types of Feed

Small fish species and larval stages of larger fish (especially marine species) require several types of live feeds, including microalgae (phytoplankton), Artemia, rotifers (usually offered enriched with vitamins, and other commercial products) and copepods. Whenever possible, manufactured feeds are greatly preferred over live feeds because of increased control, they are less expensive and less intensive to produce. As for other animals, proteins, lipids and carbohydrates can all serve as energy sources. In the wild, most energy comes in the form of protein; however, in aquaculture, protein-rich feed components are expensive, require higher metabolic energy for oxidation and generate higher levels of nitrogenous metabolites. Protein concentrations in feed are levels are closely monitored and care is taken to ensure that the amino acid profile of the diet mimics the essential amino acid profile in fish muscle (which varies between species). Additional energy requirements are filled by carbohydrates and fat. Carbohydrates are not a good energy source in fish since they can utilize only 20% (cold water species) to 30% (warm water). Excessive amounts are harmful, producing high glycogen levels in the liver, slow growth and mortalities. Lipids can be used as an energy source, a carrier of fat-soluble vitamins and carotenoid pigments and supply essential fatty acids. Most freshwater fish require linoleic acid (18 : 2 n-6) and linolenic acid (18 : 3 n-3) in their diets and marine species require a supply of the longer highly unsaturated fatty acids (HUFA) like eicosapentaenoic acid (20 : 5 n-3) and/or docosahexanoic acid (22 : 6 n-3). Dietary phospholipids (e.g. lecithin) may be beneficial as well. Vitamins required are similar to those required in mammals. Minerals are largely taken up from the water via the gills and gastrointestinal tract. The use of low value ('trash fish') as a feed input for the production of marine fish occurs in some areas in the world where manufactured feed supply is of poor quality or if the supply of feed is variable (Figure 12.4).

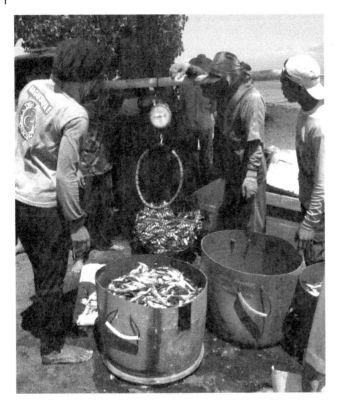

Figure 12.4 Low-value 'trash fish' being used as feed at a marine aquaculture grow out farm. [Photo credit: Dr Joy Becker].

12.7.2 Protein as an Energy Source

Dietary protein is the largest and most expensive component of aquaculture diets. The crude protein requirement can range from about 30% for some carps and cyprinids to about 50% for carnivorous species like yellowtail kingfish (*Seriola lalandi*) and red sea bream (*Pagrus major*). Fish meal has been the traditional protein source, but it is considered expensive, in demand from other animal production industries and has issues with regards to environmental sustainability. Therefore, researchers continue to explore alternative protein sources for aquaculture diets, such as soybean and cottonseed meal. Two of the biggest limitations to replacement protein sources are an imbalance of essential amino acid composition and the presence of anti-nutrient contents.

Nutritionists aim to formulate a least-cost diet so that as much of the energy required by the fish is provided by non-protein sources. This allows most of the protein to be directed towards protein synthesis and growth (which is commonly referred to as 'protein-sparing capability'). Fish species vary greatly in regard to the type and amount of protein sparing that is possible.

For example, it is necessary to provide lipids as a protein-sparing source for salmon whereas carbohydrates can be used for some eels. Optimal dietary protein-energy (P/E) ratios give an estimate of the optimal amount of energy required for efficient protein use for each species. For fish, the average is 22 mg/kJ protein but can range from as low as 17 mg/kJ protein for tilapia to almost 29 mg/kJ protein in channel catfish.

12.7.3 Feed Management

The number of feedings the fish will receive depends on the age and size of the fish, as well as water temperature. Most intensive production systems have mechanical equipment; however, it is important that at least one feeding per day is observed so that feeding behaviour can be monitored and recorded. Most problems in fish farming (e.g. poor water quality conditions, disease, stress) will initially manifest through reduction in appetite and changes in feeding behaviour. It is important to ensure the safe storage of feed so that it is kept cool, away from pests (such as mice, rats and insects) and used within the date stated by the manufacturer.

12.8 Biosecurity and Disease Management

It is often difficult to predict when a disease outbreak will occur at an aquaculture farming operation. The regular and consistent use of biosecurity measures can reduce the risk of pathogens entering a farm and causing high levels of fish mortality. Many biosecurity measures can be easily implemented at most aquaculture facilities, whereas other measures involve considerable planning and financial investment.

Many fish diseases are known to the aquaculture industry, and they continue to be one of the greatest causes of fish mortality, reduced production and economic loss. The total cost of fish diseases is the sum of direct costs due to fish mortalities as a result of a disease and indirect costs, such as reduced growth rates, feed efficiency, product quality, increased costs of labour and disease treatments. Biosecurity is the protection of living organisms from any type of infectious organism. Biosecurity in aquaculture is the protection of aquatic animals (fish or shellfish) from infectious pathogens, such as parasites, viruses, fungal agents or bacteria. One of the best ways to protect both the fish and the survival of the operation is by preventing disease with a good biosecurity program.

12.8.1 Developing a Biosecurity Program

Biosecurity involves a series of actions to stimulate and maintain fish health. A biosecurity program includes a variety of procedures and policies used on an aquaculture facility. The goal of a biosecurity program is to:

- reduce the risk that pathogens will enter an aquaculture facility
- reduce the risk that pathogens will spread through a facility if they are introduced

● reduce the conditions that are stressful to the fish which would make the fish more susceptible to disease if they meet a pathogen.

Every aquaculture farm is unique, and a biosecurity program needs to be created for each one. It must consider the entire aquaculture operation including the species of fish being produced, various fish life stages and the diseases that tend to occur in the geographical region. The biosecurity measures needed for each aquaculture facility are determined by identifying all the risks that would allow pathogens to enter the site. It is also important to consider which biosecurity measures are available to each facility and which measures would be the most cost effective.

12.8.2   Risk Factors for Pathogen Introduction and Spread in Aquaculture Facilities

There are five key risk factors for the introduction and spread of a pathogen in a fish farm. They are:

1) **Fish movements** – This represents the biggest risk for pathogen introduction and spread. It includes the movement of fish onto, within or off the farm. It also applies any fish that return to the farm, such as brood stock that are maintained at sea or a different location.
2) **The water source** – It is most desirable to use pathogen-free water sources, such as springs or wells. Surface water, such as rivers, lakes or oceans, has a high risk of carrying pathogens. Water used for aquaculture from this source should be disinfected.
3) **Fish health** – Optimum health is essential for disease prevention in fish. This is mainly done by minimizing stress with the use of appropriate stocking densities, maintaining a high level of water quality and proper nutrition. Dead and sick fish need to be removed on a regular basis (daily removal is ideal) as they are a high risk for containing pathogens.
4) **Equipment and vehicles** – Many aquatic pathogens can survive in the environment for long periods of time. It is important to clean and disinfect all equipment and vehicles that enter a farm or are used in more than one area. Examples of equipment that should be disinfected regularly include boots, nets, buckets, scales, fish tanks, pipes, pumps and harvesting equipment. Examples of vehicles include boats, barges, trucks for carrying live animals and passenger cars/trucks for transporting workers.
5) **Vectors** – Other animals may carry pathogens that will harm the stock, and it is important to reduce any contact with these animals. Vectors may include wild fish, domestic animals (dogs and cats), livestock (poultry) and other wildlife (seals, birds). People (including farm workers and visitors) can also be vectors for pathogens.

When designing a biosecurity program each of these risks should be evaluated for each aquaculture facility in consultation with a veterinarian or fish health scientist. After all the risks have been identified, biosecurity procedures and policies can be worked out and communicated to everyone at the farm. It is best for all workers at the farm to have regular 'hands-on' training in the biosecurity procedures used at the farm.

12.8.3   Components of a Biosecurity Program

A good biosecurity program (depending on the farm infrastructure and operations) should include procedures and policies related to:

1) **Disease Prevention** – to stop all potential pathogens from entering the farm. Some biosecurity measures include:
   - purchase stock from a producer that is certified as specific pathogen-free (if possible)
   - purchase stock from a known and trusted supplier
   - quarantine and isolate <u>all</u> new fish that enter the site for at least four weeks and monitor for clinical signs of disease
   - fish in quarantine should be maintained on a separate system and have dedicated equipment
   - completely depopulate a fish holding area before re-stocking ('all in – all out' policy)
   - vaccinate all fish (see section 12.9.4)
   - disinfect the water with UV and ozone to ensure it is pathogen-free
   - good husbandry practices (i.e. water quality, stocking rates, appropriate nutrition, reduce handling and fish movements) to reduce fish stress and ensure a strong immune system
   - secure fencing around the facility to keep unauthorized people out of the production area
   - use nets over outdoor tanks or cages to ensure that birds and other predators cannot access the fish
   - ensure that predators and birds cannot access dead fish carcasses
2) **Disease Monitoring** – to ensure a pathogen has not entered a facility. Some biosecurity measures include:
   - regularly scheduled health evaluation of all stock
   - health evaluation of all new stock entering a facility
   - health evaluation can include gill and skin sampling, blood sampling for immunological assays, bacterial cultures, virus isolation and histopathology
   - removal and inspection of sick fish
   - routine necropsy and health evaluation of sick fish
3) **Disease Treatment and Eradication** – a variety of chemicals are available to fish farmers once a veterinarian has diagnosed a disease caused by an invading pathogen. Biosecurity measures include:
   - alert the proper authorities (if required) of the disease outbreak
   - ensure all farm workers are aware of the disease outbreak and the procedures to be followed

- ensure the chemical is licensed for use in food fish (if applicable)
- complete all of the treatments set out by the veterinarian
- treat all the fish sharing 'common waters'
- depending on the pathogen, the system may need to be destocked for a thorough cleaning and disinfection and a fallowing period observed prior to re-stocking

4) **Cleaning and Disinfection** – to prevent the spread of a pathogen around a facility. Some commonly used biosecurity measures include:
- appropriate disinfectant for nets and other shared equipment (if separate equipment for each area is not possible)
- all disinfected equipment should be thoroughly dried, preferably in sunlight
- regularly maintain hand washes and foot baths
- area to clean and disinfect boats and trucks used to carry live fish that is away from the production area
- fish tanks and raceways should be disinfected between each stocking of fish
- avoid using wood in fish facilities as it is hard to disinfect and can harbour pathogens (e.g. viruses)
- minimize aerosols with the use of tanks lids or by placing barriers between the tanks
- accurate record keeping of all disinfection procedures
- ensure equipment is free of organic debris (such as fish mucous and faeces and algae) prior to disinfection as this will often inactivate the disinfectant.

5) **General Security Precautions** – applies to all facility operations. Biosecurity measures include:
- a manual of standard operating procedures
- on-site training to ensure everyone understands the biosecurity program
- clearly described procedures in case of a disease outbreak
- procedures to ensure up-to-date and accurate record keeping
- workers should wear clean clothes or coveralls and footwear
- perform tasks in areas from lowest risk (indoor tanks) to highest risk (outdoor tanks)
- perform tasks from the most susceptible life stages (fry or fingerlings) to the least (adults)
- access to brood stock, egg incubation and fry facilities should be highly restricted to a few well-trained people
- maintain a logbook for all visitors and deliveries to the facility
- visitors that have contact with other fish operations should change their clothes and boots and thoroughly disinfect hands prior to entering the site. It is best if they have no contact with fish.

Disease outbreaks can happen very quickly and usually result in high levels of mortalities. Preventing and controlling the spread of pathogens are significant economic and biological concerns for any aquaculture facility. It is extremely difficult and costly to completely eradicate a pathogen once it has become established in an aquaculture facility. When applying a biosecurity program, it is important to have both the formal description of the biosecurity procedures and the consistent application of the procedures by everyone involved.

12.9 Fish Health Management

One of the major problems encountered during the culture of aquatic organisms is the occurrence of disease. Outbreaks of disease may be related to adverse environmental conditions or occur where the cultured organism encounters a critical mass of a pathogen within the water column. Control of disease outbreaks in aquaculture, as in agriculture, demands a multidisciplinary approach. Thus, effective disease control programs should account for not only issues of quarantine, hygiene, treatment and vaccination, but also application of diagnostic methods to monitor health status of the farmed stock.

Numerous outbreaks of disease during intensive aquaculture are generally traceable back to inappropriate management practices. Since the treatment of disease is expensive, it remains obvious that prevention represents a major economic key in the profit-loss equation. Critical to all aquaculture operations is maintenance of good water quality, including oxygen levels, efficient feeding regimes and attention to sanitary procedures and biosecurity measures. One factor that is rarely considered during intensive aquaculture operations is that of facility architecture and design to minimize risks of contamination by control of personnel flow (including equipment, feed) to-and-from, and between production units. Appropriate use of disinfectants, for nets, feeding equipment, boots, machinery, throughout the facility, represents another measure that can reduce the risk of disease and disease transfers.

12.9.1 The Disease Triad

Before a disease outbreak occurs, there is usually a requirement for certain interactions to occur between the host, its environment and the pathogen. When these three separate components overlap, disease ensues. For example, a fish (host) may be stressed due to low water oxygen levels (environment) while in the presence of a high level of bacteria (pathogen). The stressor may lead to immunosuppression and decreased ability to combat invasive pathogens, giving rise to disease.

12.9.1.1 Factors Involving the Host

The gills consist of very delicate tissue often only one or two cell layers thick. The gill is the first line of defence against environmental effects like ammonia, pH changes or infectious agents (like ectoparasites). Bacterial, viral and fungal agents can also gain access and either colonize locally on the gill or cause systemic disease. The skin of fish varies much in thickness and mucous cell content both within different areas on the body and between different species. The mucous coating on the skin and gills is secreted by goblet cells in the epithelium and is continually produced. The mucous contains excretory antibodies and non-antibody humoral defence compounds. After irritation excess mucous production may occur.

As fish are ectothermic, the environmental temperature has significant effects on fish, both directly on the whole organism (tolerant vs. optimal range), but also on metabolic functions with the fish. Temperatures outside of tolerance levels may severely stress or kill fish, while less extreme values may still cause stress. Although some aspects of fish immunity are independent of temperature, the production and secretion of specific antibodies is significantly impaired at lower temperatures. Non-antibody humoral defences remain active at lower temperatures, although their production may be slower.

Stress has a profound effect on the fish's disease resistance. The stress response in fish follows the same general pattern of catecholamine and corticosteroid release in mammals under acute stress and may have positive effects on the immune response. Catecholamines cause an increase in heart rate and ventilation and the mobilization of glucose. Cortisol release stimulates the release of acute phase proteins (C-reactive), which may serve a protective function in the acute phase of stress. The long-term response to stress, however, is an immunosuppressive one with lymphopenia, reduced production of immunoglobulins and depressed synthesis of interferon.

12.9.1.2 Factors Involving the Environment

Environmental factors involve water quality parameters, mainly temperature and dissolved oxygen. Dissolved oxygen levels in water are negatively affected by increases in temperature, salinity and altitude. Aquatic plants and bacteria in the water will use oxygen, but plants will produce oxygen during the day. In RAS with active biofilters, the bacteria in the biofilter will use a significant amount of oxygen in their metabolism. Some chemicals by nature of being reducing agents have an oxygen demand as well (e.g. formalin). Fish vary in their requirements for oxygen, but lower than optimal DO levels lead to chronic stress, while very low levels cause death. Fish with unfavourable oxygen supply may exhibit the following signs: increase rate of ventilation or flared gills, loss of appetite, liver damage, failure to gain weight and reduced disease resistance. Acute and severe oxygen deprivation will cause agitation, swimming at the surface, gasping for air at the surface, followed by depression of the central nervous system and death.

12.9.1.3 Factors Involving the Pathogen

Biological agents are probably the most common cause of disease initiation and the primary focus of fish health professionals are infectious agents. Potential pathogens present in the environment include bacteria, viruses, fungi, protozoans, parasitic crustaceans, helminths and other worms. The virulence or pathogenicity of the agent is the relevant factor in the determination of health hazards. It depends upon the physical or biochemical attributes of the agent. For example, bacteria with flagella or with capsules are generally better equipped to invade the host and resist adverse conditions. Other bacteria are able to excrete toxins, which can cause haemorrhage or affect the nervous system. Penetration into the host is the first step for the pathogen to multiply and invade the target organs. This normally happens through digestion, rupture of the skin, transgression of the gill or penetration of the egg membrane.

12.9.2 Disease Treatment

The treatment of fish with chemotherapeutics is often necessary despite the most vigilant and strict hygiene protocols in aquatic animal rearing facilities. Treatment regimens must be adaptable to suit a specific production system to accommodate factors such as species, water temperature and quality, wastewater disposal and flow rates. Treatments should be prescribed by a veterinarian and part of health management plan following a complete diagnostic investigation. Depending on the type of disease, sick fish should be removed and treated in isolation or kept with the population and treated collectively. Entire populations are best treated for infectious diseases, but high-value fish (such as brood stock) may be treated individually.

Bath treatments of fish are very common. In general, it is the treatment approach of choice when fish are suffering from infections of the skin and gills. These types of infections are very common in both tropical fish and all species of farmed fish and if left untreated they are often fatal. Disadvantages include imprecise dosing and degradation of chemicals in water that may create an unwanted drug by-product.

Oral medications are often the best way to administer drugs to fish because they are the least stressful yet if consumed in the proper amounts and absorbed by the gastrointestinal tract, they are quite effective. Typically, fish are given a ratio of 1% of their biomass as medicated diet and the remainder of the daily ration (if accepted) of plain feed. In general, antibiotics are delivered via the feed, with the most common ones being oxytetracycline, amoxicillin, erythromycin and fumagillin. A few drugs can be commercially prepared at the feed mill, but most treatments are made at the farm by personnel (usually produced daily in smaller batches). However, there are some disadvantages: it can be cumbersome at commercial operations to produce medicated feeds, medicated feeds have short shelf life and may require special conditions (no light, refrigeration). Moreover, sick fish tend to stop eating.

Injection of drugs ensures a precise dose; however, it can be quite stressful to the animal and requires high levels of handling and anaesthesia. Fish should be fasted for 24 hrs prior to injection to reduce the risk of peritonitis by puncturing the stomach or bowel. Intra-peritoneal (IP) injections are given between pectoral and pelvic fins. This type of injection is often used for vaccinations and tagging (passive integrated transponder tags). Intra-muscular injections are best delivered to the dorsal musculature just lateral to the dorsal fin.

12.9.3 Use of Anaesthetics in Fish Production

Anaesthesia is generally used in aquaculture to provide immobilization of fish for tagging, weighing and measuring, during surgery, grading, collection of blood and transportation.

The choice of anaesthetic depends upon the nature of the procedure to be carried out, the species of fish and the duration of the process. Commonly used anaesthetics today are AQUI-S®, MS 222 (tricaine methanesulfonate), clove oil and 2-phenoxyethanol.

When choosing an anaesthetic, ensure compliance with the jurisdictional legislation for using veterinary medicines in food animals. The ideal anaesthetic for fish would include the following characteristics:

- fast acting: 1–15 minutes
- provides immobilization and muscle relaxation
- renders fish insensitive to pain
- easily administered with a wide range between safe and lethal dose
- quick recovery: ~ 5 minutes
- stable, biodegradable, non-toxic to humans
- cheap and long shelf-life

12.9.4 Vaccination

Vaccines provide the farmer with a means to combat disease and hence to become more profitable. A major factor governing the use of vaccines, especially for high numbers of animals (millions) of relatively low value, however, is cost. The antibody response of fish to an infection has been one of the most studied aspects of fish immunology. Teleost research indicated that similar mechanisms for antibody production to those observed in mammals. Most research efforts, however, have centred attention upon comparatively few species of teleosts (mainly cyprinids and salmonids). Nevertheless, the specific humoral defence mechanisms of fish appear to be broadly similar. After antigen stimulation, there is a large lag time before antibody appears in circulation (usually 10–15 days) and titres plateau around 20 to 30 days (dependent on temperature of course). Relative to mammals, the lag phase in fish is longer, but the antibody titres can be maintained for longer periods. Large-scale commercial production of fish vaccines is undertaken only for relatively few diseases and often those that occur in high-value species like salmonids.

12.10 Fish Welfare

Fish are sentient animals capable of experiencing pain (Braithwaite 2010). The sensory organs of fish are remarkably similar in structure and function to those of terrestrial vertebrates, as is the endocrine system, including the hormones involved in stress responses. Ray-finned, bony fish have a nociceptive system that is very similar to the nociceptive systems of mammals and birds Fish are similar to other vertebrates in terms of their general behavioural capacities: they show the same kinds of learning and navigate around their environment using similar cognitive processes. Fish can perceive their environment by vision, hearing, chemoreception and the mechanosensory lateral line. Like higher vertebrates, fish respond to environmental challenges with a series of adaptive neuroendocrine adjustments that are collectively termed 'the stress response'. Welfare indicators commonly used in fish farming include visible signs of injury or disease, changes in body colour, nutritional status such as anorexia, growth rate, reproductive capacity, changes in swimming pattern and frequency, and production of stress hormone (e.g. cortisol).

12.10.1 Physiological Stress Response

Fish have a hypothalamo-pituitary axis that mediates stress responses: following release of catecholamines (adrenaline and noradrenaline) from inter-renal tissue. Cortisol concentrations return to normal following brief exposure to stressors, but remain elevated if exposure is longer, and may take weeks to return to normal. Chronically elevated cortisol suppresses immunity and leads to increased infection and possibly death from fungal and bacterial infection. Cortisol can be measured in the blood but is affected by the stress of handling and taking blood; faecal cortisol provides a more stable measure and is useful for chronic stress measurement.

12.10.2 Behavioural Stress Response

Individual fish vary in both the cortisol response and behavioural responses. Changes in fish behaviour are often the first indicator of a problem. The behaviour of a fish represents its reaction to the environment around it. Common behaviours in response to stress include altered body colour (light or dark), shoaling to escape predators, hiding to escape predator or attack by conspecific, and altered speed and direction of swimming.

12.10.3 Transportation and Slaughter

Fish perceive both crowding and handling as a general stress. In 2009, the World Organization for Animal Health (OIE) first adopted recommendations to minimize the impact of transportation stress on the welfare of farmed fish. Since then, OIE has added further guidelines regarding the best practices for the killing of farmed fish during slaughter and emergency culling for disease control. It recognized that there is a critical relationship between fish health and welfare and improvements in farmed fish welfare can often improve productivity with economic benefits.

The killing of any fish should be carried out promptly and by humane means suitable for the species and numbers involved. The OIE guidelines do acknowledge that methods may vary between species and according to available technology and equipment. Currently, the recommended slaughter methods for best welfare outcome are electrical and mechanical stunning. Asphyxiation in air or ice or with carbon dioxide are associated with poor welfare outcomes and should not be used when stunning methods are feasible. Examples of common slaughter methods used are percussive stunning (e.g. a blow to the head) and electrical stunning in salmonid production and spiking of the brain in tuna and other marine species.

References and Further Reading

Braithwaite, V. (2010). *Do Fish Feel Pain?* Oxford, UK: Oxford University Press.

FAO. (2018). The State of World Fisheries and Aquaculture 2018 – meeting the sustainable development goals. Rome. www.fao.org/documents/card/en/c/I9540EN.

Huntingford, F., Jobling, M., and Kadri, S. (2012). *Aquaculture and Behaviour.* Oxford: Wiley-Blackwell Publishing Company.

Lucas, J.S. and Southgate, P.C. (eds.) (2019). *Aquaculture: Farming Aquatic Animals and Plants*, 3e. Oxford: Wiley-Blackwell Publishing Company.

Malone, R. (2013). Recirculating aquaculture tank production systems: a review of current design practice. In: Southern Regional Aquaculture Center (SRAC), Publication No. 453, Stoneville, Mississippi, USA.

Roberts, R. (ed.) (2012). *Fish Pathology*, 4e. Oxford: Wiley-Blackwell Publishing Company.

Wall, T. (2011). Farmed fish. In: *Management and Welfare of Farm Animals: The UFAW Farm Handbook*, 5e (ed. J. Webster), 452–476. Oxford: Wiley-Blackwell Publishing Company.

13

South American Camelids

Cristian Bonacic

KEY CONCEPTS

13.1 Introduction

The members of the camelid family are among the principal large herbivorous mammals of arid habitats; having evolved to cope with life in mountain areas, high plateaus, near-desert and desert conditions. They have made a crucial contribution to both human survival and development in these environments in Asia and South America. There are six types of camelid (Figure 13.1). The domesticated, one-humped dromedary of south-western Asia and north Africa, and the two-humped Bactrian camel, which is still found wild in the Mongolian steppes, are well known, but four more species in the New World are also classed as camelids: the llama (*Lama glama*), alpaca (*Lama pacos*), guanaco (*Lama guanicoe*) and vicuña (*Vicugna vicugna*). The vicuña is the smallest representative of the South American camelids and the llama the largest. The vicuña and guanaco are both wild species and live in South America (Table 13.1). Guanacos are by nature the most adaptable and thrive in a broad range of eco-systems from the Peruvian highlands to Chilean Patagonia. The range of the vicuña extends from a single site in Ecuador where it was reintroduced during the 1990s, through all the main Andean areas of Peru, extensive regions of the altiplano in Bolivia, the eastern side of

Management and Welfare of Farm Animals: The UFAW Farm Handbook, Sixth Edition.
Edited by John Webster and Jean Margerison.
© Universities Federation for Animal Welfare 2022. Published 2022 by John Wiley & Sons Ltd.

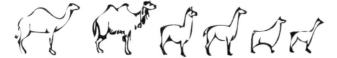

Figure 13.1 Camelid species, drawn to scale: from left, dromedary, Bactrian camel, llama, guanaco, alpaca, vicuna.

Table 13.1 Original distribution of South American camelids.

Name	Order	Family	Genus	Species	Habitat
Llama	Artiodactyla	Camelidae	Lama	*Lama glama* Linnaeus 1758	Central Andes Peru, W Bolivia, NE Chile, NW Argentina
Guanaco	Artiodactyla	Camelidae	Lama	*Lama guanicoe* Muller 1776	Andean foothills of Peru, Chile, Argentina and Patagonia
Alpaca	Artiodactyla	Camelidae	Vicuña	*Vicugna pacos* Linnaeus 1758	Central Andes Peru to W Bolivia
Vicuña[1]	Artiodactyla	Camelidae	Vicuña	*Vicugna vicugna* Molina 1758	High Andes Central Peru, W Bolivia, NE Chile, NW Argentina

[1]Also recently classified as *Paco vicugna*.

the North Andean region of Argentina and the western slopes and altiplano in the north of Chile, all areas above 3,500 m. The guanaco is found today from Peru (8°S) southward to the central east and western slopes of the Andes, and across Patagonia, including Tierra del Fuego and Navarino Island (55°S). This species inhabits arid, semi-arid, hilly, mountain, steppe and temperate forest environments. In this wide variety of open habitats, four subspecies of *Lama guanicoe* are recognized (*L. g. cacsilensis*, *L. g. huanacus*, *L. g. guanicoe* and *L. g. voglii*).

Llamas and alpacas have been successfully domesticated by Andean cultures around Lake Titicaca (the highest lake in the world, 4,000 m) and became abundant and a key livestock herd for the expansion of the Inca Empire 500 years ago. The alpaca population is estimated to be around 3–3.5 million animals and mostly concentrated in Peru, and 3.4 million llamas, with nearly 90% living in Bolivia. Wild South American Camelids are present in Argentina, Bolivia, Chile, Ecuador (where vicuñas were reintroduced) and Peru. The largest population of vicuñas lives in Peru (over 2000,0000 animals) and guanacos are concentrated in Argentina (1–1.5 million guanacos). A scattered population of guanacos still exists in the Paraguay and Bolivia Chaco region. Peru has a small and endangered guanaco population that has recovered from the brink of extinction during the last decade. Chile has the second largest population of guanacos scattered in the Andean region from the border with Peru and Bolivia and highly concentrated in Tierra del Fuego Island in Patagonia. The llama was among the world's earliest animals to be domesticated. While llamas are used mostly as a beast of burden in the Andes of Peru, Bolivia, Chile and Argentina, carrying things for the native herdsmen, they also provide local people with meat, wool, hides for shelter and manure pellets for fuel, and were used as sacrificial offerings to their gods.

Distinctive facial characteristics of the South American camelids (SACs) include prominent eyes and ears, and a lower lip with a central crevice. The feet are slender when compared to other members of the genus *Camelus* and present a soft pad instead of a hoof.

Wild animals within the genera *Lama* and *Vicugna* have persisted until the present, being represented by two species, the guanaco and vicuña, whereas llamas and alpacas originated from the domestication of their wild counterparts, a process which began approximately 7000 years ago. Because the process of domestication is closely related to the cultural actions of humans with their livestock, the distribution and radiation of llamas and alpacas occurred in the altiplano zones of the central Andes. Alpacas and llamas were domesticated several centuries before the beginning of the Inca Empire (fifteenth century) and played a major role in the success of the empire as pack and trade animals from the coast to the highlands. Under the Incas, the breeding of these animals was regulated as well as the use of their meat, hair and fur. In the sixteenth century, Europeans found millions of alpaca and a smaller number of llamas and other camelids in the Tahuantinsuyo (Titicaca Andean region). Beginning in 1539 these species were displaced towards marginal areas by sheep and cattle introduced by the Spanish conquerors. This process continued during colonial times and the republican era, so that the number of camelids was gradually reduced and remained mainly in the Peruvian and Bolivian highlands.

Llamas and alpacas currently reside in an area of 5 million hectares in the highest zones of Bolivia, Peru and border zones of the north of Chile and Argentina. These regions are mostly not suitable for intensive agriculture and traditional livestock production systems, but camelids are able to take advantage of the existing forages and survive in extremely dry and low productivity ecosystems. The rural population in the area under consideration is estimated at over 400,000 native Aymara and Quechua families, which depend mainly or entirely on raising alpacas or llamas and sheep for their subsistence because the climatic conditions allow no other alternative.

The origins of South America's domestic alpaca and llama remain controversial due to hybridization, near extirpation during the Spanish conquest and difficulties in archaeological interpretation. Traditionally, the ancestry of both forms is attributed to the guanaco, while the vicuña is assumed never to have been domesticated. Recent research has, however, linked the alpaca to the vicuña, dating domestication to 6,000 to 7,000 years ago in the Peruvian Andes.

South American camelids are considered an interesting new species for farming in the United Kingdom, Europe, North America, New Zealand and elsewhere. Worldwide the alpaca population is estimated to be 3 million, with the majority in the South American regions of Peru, Chile and Bolivia. North American farmers have an estimated of 73,000 llamas and close to 60,000, alpacas. Australia has an estimated population of more than 200,000 South American Camelids. In the UK, current estimates are around 10,000 domestic camelids. Camelids are attractive, small and appealing because of their fine fibre and in some cases recreational uses (backpacking, exotic pets). Domestic South American camelids were introduced into different ecosystems of Chile during the 1980s, from Mediterranean to temperate rainforest areas and Patagonian grassland. Nowadays, it is possible even to see small herds of llamas and alpacas side by side with wild guanacos in Southern Tierra del Fuego. South American camelids have been described as animals with the wool of a sheep, the strength of a horse and the brain of a dog. However, when contemplating South American camelids as potentially attractive species for hobby farming, we should not forget their origins and evolution. They all inhabit remotes areas of the Andes and Patagonia. Animal welfare recommendations should bear in mind the behaviour and natural adaptations of these four species that have developed in a region of the world where even the domesticated species are managed in an extensive way in open areas and have little contact with humans. South American camelids present a unique challenge for devising animal welfare criteria. These species have been historically interlinked with advanced ancient civilizations that developed sophisticated animal husbandry, practices domesticating the llama and alpaca and practising artificial selection before modern genetic knowledge. Alpaca mummies in archaeological sites show fine fibre and colour variations that are not present in current herds. Also, Andean cultures mastered sustainable ways of utilizing the vicuña, which was a sacred animal; every four years they were rounded up in a given region and brought into stone corrals for shearing and some for sacrifice. The finest wool in the world was considered a precious gift for the Inca and the four species of camelid played an important role in their traditions, trade and beliefs. Nowadays they still have an important place in their original distributional habitats, and also elsewhere. Different societies and individuals view South American camelids as pets, exotic animals, livestock animals, zoo animals and wild animals. Animal welfare recommendations need to recognize this variety of interactions between these species and humans and keep in mind that they can accomplish multiple roles rather than one single use by humans. Llamas and alpacas are now used for fibre or for meat, for showing, trekking or as companion animals (pets) in North America, Europe and Australasia. Often are kept in small herds of single species and Animal Welfare codes are produced locally in many countries.

13.1.1 Origin and Domestication

Camelids appeared in the late Eocene and were one of the first modern families of artiodactyls (even-toed ungulates), followed by pigs, peccaries and deer in the Oligocene, and giraffes, pronghorns and bovidae in the Miocene. The origin of camels, both those of South America and Asia/Africa, can be traced back to the ancestral camels of central North America. In fact, the camel family was entirely a North American group during most of the 40 to 45 million years of its evolution, with the critical dispersals to other continents occurring only 3 million years ago. The earliest camel (*Poebrotherium wilsoni*) stood only 30 cm at the shoulder and looked like a miniature, but slightly heavier-bodied, modern-day guanaco; this species of the upper Eocene period (40 million years before the present) had fours toes and a full set of 44 teeth with no gaps between them. From an ancestral Miocene form, evolutionary radiation in North America produced two important groups of advanced camelids. By the late Miocene

(5–10 million years ago) the genus *Pliauchenia* had evolved, exhibiting many llama-like characteristics.

During the late Pliocene (3 million years ago), camelids first emigrated to Asia via the Beringia land bridge. When camelines (probably in the large Paracamelus form) reached the Old World, they spread rapidly west along the dry belt of Eurasia, reaching into East Africa and eastward across the Gobi Desert and into China. These Old World camels (camelines) eventually differentiated into the two present-day species – the two-humped Bactrian camel (*Camelus bactrianus*) of the Mongolian steppes and mountains and the one-humped dromedary or Arabian camel (*Camelus dromedarius*) of the southwestern Asian and North African deserts.

Meanwhile, the long-limbed *Hemiauchenia* was diversifying in central and southern latitudes of North America. Then, about 3 million years before the present day, the Panamanian land bridge gradually formed, linking the North and South American continents. Subsequently, one of the most spectacular and best-documented faunal interchanges took place, including the invasion of the llama-like *Hemiauchenia* into the Andes and onto the pampas of South America by the beginning of the Pleistocene. The centre and evolutionary origin for *Paleoloma* and modern *Lama* appears to have been the rugged Andean mountains, where their shorter legs provided better jumping ability and manoeuvrability in the rough terrain. The *Hemiauchenia* was a grazer, whereas the Andean *Paleoloma* became both a grazer and browser. *Lama* rapidly dispersed from its Andean homeland and extended eastward and southward over most of southern South America, overlapping extensively with the already established distribution of *Hemiauchenia*. While *Lama* expanded its range east and south, *Paleoloma* ranged west and north from its Andean origin (spreading as far north as Central America and the gulf coast of present-day Texas and Florida).

Toward the end of the Pleistocene Ice Age, 10,000 to 12,000 years ago, both genera of large llamas (*Paleoloma* and *Hemiauchenia*) became extinct. All other North American camelids also became extinct at about this time. The cause of the sudden demise of camels and other members of the American megafauna are debated, but current theories include climatic change, habitat change as a result of human activity, and overkill by an efficient and newly arrived predator, the human. However, the origin of the domestic species has been a matter of debate. Recent studies of variations in chromosome G banding patterns and in two mitochondrial gene sequences have shown similar patterns in chromosome G band structure in all four lamini species, and these in turn are similar to the bands described for camels, *Camelus bactrianus*. The combined analysis of chromosomal and molecular variation showed close genetic similarity between alpacas and vicuñas, as well as between llamas and guanacos. Current molecular biology research suggests that the llama would have derived from *Lama guanicoe* and the alpaca from *Vicugna vicugna*, supporting reclassification as *Vicugna pacos*.

13.1.2 Camelid Species Description

Today there are approximately 21.5 million camelids in the world, with around 7.7 million in South America (Macdonald 2006). These comprise llamas (3.7 million), alpacas (3.3 million), guanacos (875,000) and vicuñas (250,000).

The llama is the largest of the South American camelids, has a slender shape, and may be found in up to 50 different colours. The llama has elongated legs, neck and face, and may reach as high as 1.5 to 2.0 metres from the ground to its head. Its long ears are erect and curve inward in a classic banana shape. Two breeds of llama are traditionally recognized – the woollier *Ch'aku* and those with less fibre on the neck and body, called *Q'ara*. Their fibre (technically it is 'fibre' and not 'wool') is less dense than that of alpacas, being an average of 26 microns on the undercoat and 70 microns on guard hair. Genetic selection produces distinctive fine fibre in llamas as it does in alpacas.

There are also two breeds of domestic alpaca distinguished by body size and wool characteristics. The more common *Huacaya* has shorter and more crimped and spongy fibre than the *Suri* with its long, straight or wavy wool fibres. The coat of Suri alpacas consists of long fibres with no crimp that hang down alongside the body in ringlets. Alpaca colouration varies from white to black with intermediate shades and combinations. The alpaca is the primary South American camelid fibre producer of the Andean highland. Alpaca wool (12–28 microns in diameter) is finer than that of the pack-carrying llama (20–80 microns) and body colour for both ranges from white to black, with some six intermediate shades of greys and browns. Dappled or spotty body colouration is more common in llamas than alpacas (Figure 13.2).

The vicuña is the smallest of the Andean camelids and has the finest fibre coat, the overall colour of the soft woolly coat is ochre, light cinnamon or reddish brown, with the under parts, insides of the legs, and underside of the head being dirty white. On the chest, at the base of the neck, is a peculiar, pompon-like 'mane' of silky white hairs which may be 20 to 30 cm (8 to 12 inches) in length. The vicuña is extremely slender, with long skinny limbs and neck. The head is small and wedge shaped, with small, triangular ears. Unique among living artiodactyls, the incisors of the vicuña are constantly growing, with enamel on only one side, to keep up with the wear caused by the tough grasses on which they feed. Vicuña fibre is the finest among all the animal fibres with an average diameter of 13–14 microns, but it is short, hardly reaching 3 cm. Its annual fleece can reach a maximum weight of 320 grams.

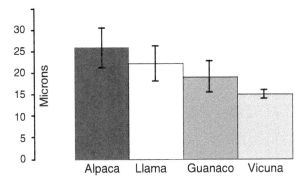

Figure 13.2 Comparison of fibre diameter (microns) between South American camelids. Error bars indicate standard deviation.

The guanaco has a similar silhouette to a llama, with a uniform colouration, with a dark brown upper body, neck and limbs; whitish fibre on the underside of the neck and belly; and greyish to black face. Guanaco fibre has a diameter of 18–24 microns.

13.2   Adaptation to the Environment

High altitudes, marked by intense solar radiation, extreme daily temperature variation, low oxygen concentrations and low quality of forages are the main environmental conditions to which South American camelids have adapted. The adaptive plasticity that camelids possess, due to their long evolution in arid climates, has made them very efficient in the use of vegetation present in marginal or low-productivity habitats (Box 13.1).

Box 13.1   Digestive Physiology: Main Adaptations of the South American Camelids

- Camelids are classified as functional ruminants. However, they have three compartments instead of four: C1 and C2 are equivalent to the rumen; the distal area of C3 contains secretory epithelium.
- The ability to select forage of high quality from natural pastures. This is based mainly on their feeding behaviour. Camelids have a highly diverse feeding niche from which they select on the basis of both availability and organoleptic forage quality.
- A high capacity to digest low-quality forage through prolonged particle retention time in the pseudo-rumen. The histological characteristics and motility of the digestive tract also differ from true ruminants.
- High efficiency in the use of water, especially when there is low consumption of feed.
- Longer foraging time than sheep and higher digestive efficiencies than goats in C4 when fed grass hay.
- Higher capacity to digest hemicellulose and more lignified grasses than other small ruminants.
- High nitrogen efficiency when recycling because of low renal excretion and high ruminal retention of the solid phase, allowing micro-organisms to process cell walls more efficiently.
- pH of the ruminal contents buffered by bicarbonate secretion from the first two compartments, closer to neutral, allowing more cellulotic digestion.
- Higher concentration of fatty acids in the first two compartments of the digestive system being available as energy source, compared to sheep and goat.
- Bloating is rare and all three ruminant compartments are glandular.
- Ulcers in the C3 are found in chronically stressed animals or after sudden stress episodes and in necropsies of stressed animals.

There are certain differences between South American camelids in terms of feeding behaviour. The guanaco and llama are considered to be grazers and browsers, while the vicuña and the alpaca are grazers only in their original habitats. This clarification is due to the fact that alpacas have developed browsing behaviour in more bushy environments, as has happened with individuals that have been transported from the altiplano to the Mediterranean zone in central Chile. The camelids' diet varies during the year, depending upon forage availability and quality. Llamas and alpacas vary their diet in the Puna, depending on the dry and rainy seasons (winter and summer, respectively), and have also developed the capacity to select forage in all sorts of ecosystems, choosing rough forages when they have options.

Low oxygen availability in their natural high-altitude habitats has been a major natural selection force, reflected by specialized adaptations within the respiratory and circulatory system of South American camelids. Lung morphology is similar to that of the horse, but there are no lobules except for an accessory lobule in the right lung. The mediastinum is complete. Tidal volume of llamas is 0.5 L and dead space is 0.33 L, compared with human (0.30 L) and camel (0.25 L). High-altitude adaptation comprises anatomical, physiological and behavioural traits making South American camelids the best adapted farm animals to highland. For example, the oxygen haemoglobin curve is more efficient and the oxygen-carrying capacity of the blood is greater in South American camelids compared to other small ruminants. Erythrocytes number over 13 million per mm^3 of blood, haemoglobin between 13 and 15 g/100 mL, and packed red cell volume between 35% and 40%. Erythrocytes are ellipsoid in shape and have small size in comparison with other mammals (28–28.8 μm) that results in a relatively lower packed cell volume (PCV) and resultant low viscosity. Low oxygen at high altitudes is thought to have brought about specialized adaptations within the circulatory system in alpacas. The heart and vascular system as well as the respiratory system present some differences compared to other ruminants and mammals. For example, llamas maintained at 4720 m above sea level did not show right ventricular hypertrophy, which indicates an adaptation to high altitude, suggesting that llamas and alpacas do not develop pulmonary hypertension.

The vicuña lives 3000 to 4600 metres above sea level and is well adapted to living in this harsh environment. It is clothed in a fleece of the finest known wool, one that has been valued and harvested since pre-Columbian times. This fleece protects the vicuña from the extreme cold and winds of the Puna and provides a cushion for its body when resting on the ground. In comparison to the Old-World camels, the vicuña has more deeply cloven feet, which allow it to walk and run more adeptly on the rocky slopes, cliffs and rockslides that are common on the Puna. Another important adaptation is the vicuña's open-rooted, continuously growing incisor teeth that allow the animal to graze upon small forbs and perennial grass close to the ground. The vicuña's dental formula is 1/3, C 1/1, PM 2–3/1–2 × 2 = 20–22 (deciduous teeth) and I 1/3, C1/1, PM 1–2/1–2, M 3/3 × 2 = 30–32 (permanent dentition). The vicuña shows interesting similarities to the pronghorn antelope (*Antilocapra americana*) of North America. Although unrelated, both of these inhabitants of windswept grasslands are of similar size and extremely swift of foot, running at incredible speeds to escape danger. Both are also strongly inquisitive, walking toward any moving object that is partly hidden, as if to identify it by closer inspection. Vicuñas and other South American camelids defecate and urinate on communal dung piles. All individuals of a band, whether it is a family group or a male troop, use the same dung piles.

Many native highland plants are generally poor in quality due to high lignin concentration and low energy content. Indigestible lignin is an important component of a plant's defence against harmful ultraviolet radiation at high elevations. Animals grazing Andean pastures must be capable of extracting sufficient nutrients from coarse, heavily lignified material. Due to the distinct Andean 'wet' and 'dry' seasons, alpacas and llamas must cope with dry mature forage for over six months of the year. Such evidence that is available suggests that alpacas and llamas are more efficient digesters of this type of vegetation than either sheep or cattle. This is probably due to slower passage of ingesta through the alimentary tract, thereby allowing more time for fermentation. In consequence, South American camelids tend to consume less forage per kg bodyweight than sheep or cattle. Contrary to these animals' natural adaptations to rough forage, farmers in Europe and North America tend to overfeed camelids with protein and energy-rich forages and feedstuffs that contribute to obesity and can be an animal welfare problem. Grain and other readily fermentable carbohydrates are not recommended and, if used to increase body weight in thin animals (body condition score below 2.5 or 3.0), should be added gradually over a week period. Pregnant females with a body condition over 4 may have birthing problems. Access to open areas is key for camelids welfare.

Alpacas on the Andean high plateau reach 50 to 60% of adult weight by six months of age. In the adult alpaca, mean weights differ between animals at pasture with extensive traditional management and those fed intensively in stables. Experimental studies have shown guanacos to be extremely resistant to water deprivation, and even able to drink seawater or capture most of the water from mist deposited on plant leaves. However, llamas and alpacas in hot, wet ecosystems experience welfare problems when they are unshorn, and heat stress, dehydration and death are likely to follow. Domestic South American camelids living in hot, wet regions of the world are particularly vulnerable to these conditions and those planning transport must take into consideration water, ventilation and resting time. Heat waves due to climate change have become more frequent worldwide and llamas and alpacas should have permanent open shaded areas and access to cold water day and night. All four species are not well adapted to heat and high humidity. Some areas of North America can be particularly unsuitable to maintain animals in open spaces without air conditioning during summer.

Even during the wet season in the Andean region, strong winds keep the ground arid and the vegetation sparse. Ponds and more humid terrains are the exception rather than the rule in the altiplano, and South American camelids are more adapted to intense solar radiation, cold weather at night and extremely dry air.

13.3 Reproduction and Social Organization

The South American camelids are social animals and in the wild form three basic social units during the breeding season: territorial family harems, non-reproductive male groups and solitary males. In captivity or on farms, juveniles and females are usually mixed together with crias (calves). Reproductive males are separated from herds and from each other to avoid fights and injuries. Guanacos and vicuñas are highly territorial but under extreme climatic conditions may displace to other areas.

South American camelids are naturally polygynous, meaning that an adult male defends a territory where females copulate with him. The guanaco or vicuña family group size in the wild ranges from 2 or 3 animals up to 13 (one leader male, five to seven females and yearlings). Males spend much time in active territorial defence against other males and drive their harem of females to more secure places and in the daily routine of grazing from resting places to grazing grounds. From the point of view of animal welfare, camelids are adapted to move in large open areas where visibility and group defence are closely interlinked.

In the wild, the reproductive cycle of birth, mating and early lactation coincides with the best environmental conditions during and after the rainy season. The timing of parturition varies with latitude. In the north of Peru, the offspring are born from April to June, while in Patagonia, births are delayed until between mid-November and the end of January. Guanacos in the Bolivian Chaco have their calving season earlier, between June and August, while on the arid coast of northern Chile it is possible to see neonates the whole year round, though births are more common between July and December. In the Andes of northern Chile, newborns begin to appear in August, but they are concentrated between November and February. In Torres del Paine National Park, female guanacos give birth between early December and January, with 49% of births occurring in early December. South of the park, guanacos in Tierra del Fuego give birth from mid-December to late February, with 85% of births occurring between mid-December and late January (Lichtenstein et al. 2008). Domestic camelids introduced in Patagonia closely resemble the natural annual cycle of the guanaco.

In South American camelids ovulation is induced by copulation. They deliver only one cria (calf) per year and females have no defined oestrous cycle but will ovulate 24–36 hours after copulation. Following copulation and subsequent ovulation, oestrus disappears within 8 days. If fertilization does not occur, follicles again become active and oestrus can be observed within 13 days. The absence of oestrus may be a diagnostic sign of ovulation or fertilization. Gestation period is approximately 11 months (340–350 days). This enables birth to occur when forage is green, nutritious and plentiful in early spring. Wild South American camelids shows a pregnancy rate between 50% and 60% and reabsortion and high juvenile mortality are the main constraints in the reproduction cycle. Llamas and alpacas in the altiplano also show a low fertility rate compared to other domestic species. Camelids tend to give birth during the day and guanacos show a synchrony with 78% of births being between 10.00 and 14.00 h. The concentration of births during the day, and in only a few weeks in the season, is an anti-predator strategy, producing an overabundance of prey during a very short period. Weight at birth is between 7 and 15 kg Low weight at birth is related to high rates of mortality. Neonates have follower behaviour, being able to stand up as early as 5 to 76 minutes postpartum and mothers exhibit aggressive behaviour towards predators.

The newborn llama and alpaca depend on milk during the first months of life. Alpaca milk is lower in lactose and higher in protein, fat and ash than llama milk. Forage intake begins as early as two to four weeks of age in the wild in the case of guanacos and vicuñas. The response is a high growth rate during the first month of life with weight gain decreasing over time up to the following spring. The young stay with mothers for one year, with the juvenile males being expelled aggressively from adult male territories before the females, despite their submissive behaviour. The forced dispersal of juvenile guanacos and vicuñas by territorial males is due to competition for food resources on territories, while sex and time of dispersion are related to future reproductive performance. Females reach maturity at two years old, and males at three years old. The males are able to defend a territory only when fully grown, at three to four years old, but many territorial males last only a few years defending a territory and the females in it.

In domestication, alpacas and llamas are not usually bred until they are two years old, although they are sexually receptive at one year. Breeding ratios are normally between 5 and 10 females per male. Reproductive parameters from other domestic species should not be considered a reference for South American camelids, given that they are considered closer to wild animals than to classic domestic and productive farm animals. Naturally, reproduction is limited by the extremely harsh conditions where they originally adapted.

Several factors contribute significantly to low fertility or birth rate under extensive conditions. These factors are associated with poor nutrition, harsh climatic conditions, rapid day/night changes in ambient temperatures, and possibly infectious and parasitic diseases. Inbreeding in small flocks may also contribute to the low reproductive rate. When South American camelids are kept outside their original distributional range and given excessive energy in the form of concentrate feeds, obesity may contribute to low reproductive success. In the wild, mortality during the first year may range from 50% to 90% in areas where harsh winter is combined with high predation rates by pumas and foxes. Under domestication, South American camelids are extremely sensitive to the presence of dogs, and even adult guanacos can be an easy prey for packs of feral dogs, and other carnivores. Any new farm that maintains llamas and alpacas in a new area should be extremely cautious about predation by dogs.

13.4 Attitudes Towards South American Camelids

People's attitude towards llamas and alpacas differ greatly between South America and Western countries, and this determines the kind of animal welfare problems that they may endure. Llamas comprise extensive herds grazing in open and poor grasslands with extreme temperature variation between day and night in the Andes. Poor indigenous farmers developed a traditional way of farming llamas even before the Inca Empire. Welfare problems such as cold stress after shearing, predation, abandonment of crias, and outbreaks of infectious diseases such us enterotoxaemia, mange and rotavirus in crias cause large mortalities and losses in Andean herds. Shearing also causes deep skin cuts and infections due to the use of broken glass or rusted pieces of metal cans in places where shearing equipment is not available. In conclusion, hunger and cold stress are the main animal welfare concerns in South American llamas. At the other extreme, llama farming in North American llama herds presents problems of overfeeding, heat stress in hot, humid summers and behavioural problems in bottle-fed animals in close contact with humans. Moreover, isolation when llamas are used as pets can cause stress and abnormal behaviours. Deaths and stress caused by dogs is a common agent of poor welfare in the Andes as well as in new farms in Western countries. Alpacas are particularly susceptible to predation and injuries by dogs and feral dogs.

Premature cria should be treated like sick babies. They are not mature internally or externally, so cannot be expected to run or digest milk as other cria do, nor will they grow quickly. Interventions should only attempt to sustain life until the cria starts acting as a normal and healthy young animal. If possible, *never separate* cria from the dam, even when you are responsible for feeding the cria. Cria should be encouraged to nurse from the dam and this can only be achieved by not overfeeding. Do not feed them during the night, 7 a.m. till 11 p.m. is sufficient, unless they need more intensive care. Bottle feeding will not, or seldom, affect the willingness of the cria to feed from the dam and, where possible, it is better to encourage cria to suck than to adopt tube feeding. Some cria that are born to term can still have problems (difficult or prolonged birth) or be dysmature. If this is the case they should be treated like premature cria (see appendix).

Breeding of camelids, even in the most progressive farms in Bolivia, Chile and Peru, is at a very low technical level, because of the lack of knowledge on the biology of these animals and consequently of the management they require. Many problems of economic importance remain unsolved. The problem of increased fertility and birth rate is of primary importance. On most of the alpaca and llama farms fertility or birth rate usually does not exceed 50%. This results in lower incomes and limits the selection possibilities. Most of the alpaca and llama farms are maintained without any definitive criteria of breed improvement. Neither qualitative nor quantitative selection for fibre, yield, animal weights and other economic features has been made. Little has been done in connection with nutrition; all food is derived from the natural high Andean pastures, most of which cannot be used for many other domesticated species. Pasture improvement and management are neglected practices and no systematic investigation has been achieved in this connection.

In the Andes, feeding practices are mainly extensive and involve low-contact management by farmers with no fenced areas and a daily routine of pastoralism and sometimes enclosure in stone corrals during the night. Aymara women and children drive animals from enclosures to wet and more productive patches of vegetation where animals roam freely during the day. The highland Aymara and Quechua human populations of South America are economically some of the poorest inhabitants of the continent, with a mean income of US$200 per family per year. Alpacas and llamas over much of their range suffer from disease, impaired hair production, low fertility and high mortality rates. These conditions are commonly attributed to poor nutrition due to overgrazing and improper herd management.

When domestic camelids are introduced into new ecosystems and are subjected to more close relationship with humans; rapid adaptation occurs involving significant physiological and behavioural adjustments. Captive-born animals reared under those conditions probably would not survive if returned to their original ecosystems. Therefore, animal welfare recommendations and husbandry procedures may differ dramatically for captive-born South American camelid in Europe or the USA compared to their original settlements in the high-altitude plains of South America. South American camelids are fast learners and adapt rapidly to human influences. However, some basic needs rooted in their genes should be kept in mind to avoid forcing animals into a complete deprivation of natural and social behaviours.

13.5 Handling and Management

Old World camels and New World llamas and alpacas are domestic animals that have been important contributors to the culture and economies of their native countries for thousands of years. When accustomed to being handled, they are tractable, but like any other domestic animal, they must be tamed and trained. Camelids are commonly kept in zoos, and if the zoo's policy is a no-hands-on relationship with the keeper, a different type of restraint may be necessary. Guanacos and vicuñas are wild animals and may be difficult to handle. However, guanacos may be tamed and handled similarly to llamas if procedures are carried out slowly and quietly. Camelids may kick in any direction. This includes kicking with a sweeping forward and outward motion, as a cow kicks. Llamas and alpacas may also kick with a quick jab back, or jump with forelegs semiflexed to hit an opponent or a human. Guanacos in farms or bottle-fed animals can be extremely dangerous and even fatal to humans by kicking and biting. The padded foot lessens the sharpness of a kick, but the potential for injury from a large llama should not be underestimated.

Llamas may swing the head and hit a person in the face when an attempt is made to halter them. Alpacas are more prone to kick than llamas but with less strength due to their smaller size. Wild vicuñas handled for shearing are less aggressive and responsive to human handling than guanacos and tend to adopt a submissive behaviour often misdiagnosed as lack of stress response. While handling wild vicuñas for shearing the lack of response is indeed a stressful response that relates closely to handling time, visual contact with humans and restraint (Bonacic et al. 2006).

Llama males have sharp canines, but they are rarely employed against humans, except by behaviourally maladjusted males (too much human attention during early development or imprinted animals). In contrast to the males of most ungulate species, mature llama males may be safely handled by adults or children. The best restraint from an animal welfare point of view is no restraint. Replacement of restraint by careful observation, collection of non-invasive samples and careful interview of the owner should be a priority. Diagnosis and veterinary procedures in trained animals are easier, safer and cause less stress in the animals. Sometimes, veterinary restraint is necessary for a given protocol. Sampling techniques, facilities, previous experiences and the experience of the owner should be considered before any attempt to restrain an animal is made. Males tend to be more responsive and aggressive than females in all four species. Moreover, males tend to be heavier, stronger and larger than females.

There are many ways to restrain a camelid depending on the farm and the way that farmers have trained or not trained their animals. If a camelid is being imported from South America to start a farm, veterinarians and farmers should be aware that restraint is not a regular activity for them, and more severe restraint should be used compared to an alpaca or llama born in captivity and reared in more direct contact with humans. Effective restraint requires understanding of camelid behaviour. All camelid species are social animals, which may be an advantage when driving the animal into a smaller enclosure for close observation or capture.

Alpacas are more flock oriented than llamas and llamas more than camels. Vicuñas and guanacos are less flock oriented and their territoriality and family group structure makes it more difficult to mix groups of animals.

Well-trained animals do not require some of the techniques that follow. Use the least amount of restraint necessary to perform a task. Llamas may be herded into a narrow alleyway, or chute. Llamas may also be herded into a corner with ropes, poles or humans with outstretched arms. The arms should not be waved exuberantly, for this may alarm the animals. Only one person should signal the team to move forward or retreat. Boma-like visual barriers and swinging gates also help to drive wild camelids into a corral.

Two people may hold a rope (minimum length of 6 m) between them and even 10 to 15 people can drive wild vicuñas into a capture facility with a rope with colourful bits of plastic mimicking a barrier 1 m above the ground. Most farmed llamas will not challenge the rope, but a guanaco or vicuña might, and may sometimes even challenge people facing them with a rope. Occasionally, an individual will run under the rope or try to charge through it or, in the case of guanacos and vicuñas, may try to escape through wires and posts into the wild, fracturing their necks or legs. Zoo animals unaccustomed to being handled can be extremely dangerous to themselves their and handlers, and sometimes certain individuals should be handled only after sedation by darting. A handler may not be able to enter an enclosure housing an aggressive imprinted male, either domestic or wild. A South American camelid responds to 'earing' (pulling an animal from the ears) as does a horse, but it is contrary to good welfare. Also, holding a vicuña or guanaco by the tail is extremely stressful and undesirable. Ears and the tail are important in communication between camelids, and earing can cause damage and extreme pain. Ask the owner how each individual has been handled, before deciding on the most appropriate means of restraint. Optimal veterinary care of camelids requires suitable restraint facilities. Chutes and/or stocks should be provided so that work on the animals may be done safely and efficiently. Blood collection, diagnostic examination and, particularly, reproductive tract examination necessitate a chute or some degree of sedation. Rectal palpation can be traumatic in alpacas and llamas and repeated manipulation should be avoided. Many homemade chutes function admirably, as do commercially available chutes designed for deer or larger animals.

One may assess the docility of individual llamas by observing the ear set and tail position plus the intensity and frequency of vocalizations. The aggressive or agitated animal pulls the ears rearward over the neck, similar to an agitated horse. Although the alpaca has shorter ears, their position is the same. The body language of camelids involves the ear position, tail position and head position. Their long neck and agility to move makes them clearly an animal closer to a horse in terms of agility and speed than a sheep.

Camelids may vocalize during restraint procedures. Llamas may scream during restraint even when no pain is involved. Alpacas tend to be quieter and more submissive than llamas. Vicuñas are more like alpacas in behaviour; however, guanacos are the least tame and most dangerous of the four species. Angry llamas and male guanacos can jump and oppose human handling with great intensity, and always scream as if they were fighting between males.

South American camelids are also known for their spitting behaviour. An anti-disturbance police vehicle in Chile that has a water cannon is known as the guanaco. The actual spit is a regurgitated stomach content with a strong liquor odour and chewed grass consistency. South American camelids usually regurgitate their food close to midday when they lie and rest but in stressful situations they spit with great energy not only at other animals that cross their safe space but also at humans trying to handle them. Sometimes the spit of camelids distressed during handling can contain traces of blood due to lips cut by contact with capture facilities or pens. Traces of blood or obviously bleeding lips should be considered a sign of poor welfare during management, and corrections should be made to handling protocols, stock density during handling, time of the day and staff training.

The optimal method for initial capture is to drive camelids into a small catch pen or enclosure where animals are usually fed, hence accustomed to entering. The availability of water and food also helps when driving South American camelids into a handling area. Patience, training and careful handling allow safe and fast handling where animals show little stress. Camelids are extremely intelligent and learn routines quite quickly. Guanacos are perhaps the most intelligent and least docile, followed by vicuñas, llamas and alpacas. But all of them can learn to be handled and driven safely with little restraint and effort to handlers. In the Andes of South America they usually forage and move quite a lot during the day, and restraint and handling are rarely needed other than for shearing.

Camelids may be restricted by running them through chutes and narrow corridors with at least 1.8 m height (Figure 13.3). The walls of the chute should be solid to prevent the animal from sticking a foot through a space and fracturing a leg, and free of any sharp elements. Also no space or window of light should be allowed at the bottom to avoid them poking their heads through.

Clinical examination is easily carried out. Blood samples may be collected from the jugular vein. Venous distention is accomplished by digital pressure over the vein; male guanacos and llamas may tighten the muscles of the neck, making it more difficult to bleed them than an alpaca or vicuña. The lateral processes of the cervical vertebrae of camelids have an inverted U shape. The vital structures of the neck (trachea, vessels and nerves) are encased within the

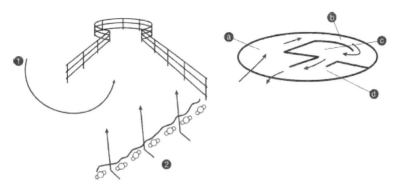

Figure 13.3 'The Chaku' handling facilities for camelids. 1 Funnel entrance. 2 People on foot driving vicunas into the corral; a, pre-handling corral; b, closed corridor and final enclosure; c, handling and shearing area; d, post handling corral.

inverted U, protected from bites during aggressive encounters between individuals. The jugular vein can be easily hidden by a stressed animal and even the most experienced veterinarians may fail to bleed an animal that is stressed or aggressive. A technique that has been used for centuries is to restrain camelids in the sternal recumbent position with a rope made from llama wool placed as a loop around the front limb and rear limb, with a knot on the animal's back. The skin of the legs is extremely thin and prone to bruises, so tightening of the ropes should be done with care to avoid erosions and pain. Ropes around their body are not appropriate for restraint during shearing. In this case, hobbles, in the form of ropes in the carpal and tarsal areas, may achieve effective restraint. In the case of wild camelids, restraint can also be accompanied with a blindfold.

13.6   Camelid Welfare

13.6.1   Camelid Community Standards of Care

A set of *Minimum Standards of Care for Llamas and Alpacas* has been developed (Box 13.2). These are the most basic requirements that all llamas and alpacas must have for physical welfare and, as such, define minimum requirements for animal control officers and government officials investigating questionable llama and alpaca care situations.

Box 13.2   Extract from Minimum Standards of Care for Llamas and Alpacas

1. *Water*: Animals should have continuous access to potable drinking water.
2. *Nutrition*: Animals should have nourishment adequate to sustain life and health.
3. *Shelter*: Animals should have natural or human-made shelter that enables them to find relief from extreme weather conditions. The sheltered area must allow the animals to stand, lie down, rest and reasonably move about.
4. *Mobility*: Animals should have a living area through which they can move freely and exercise independently.
5. *Neglect*: Animals should have a physical appearance free from signs of ambulation due to severely curled toenails, ingrown halters, or living conditions not meeting the minimums listed above.
6. *Safety*: Animals should be reasonably safeguarded from injury or death within their defined living environment and/or when travelling.
7. *Cruelty*: Animals should be reasonably safeguarded from cruel treatment and actions that endanger life or health or cause avoidable suffering.
8. *Socialization*: Llamas and alpacas are herd animals and should not live alone without a companion animal. A cria (a baby llama or alpaca under 6 months) should not be raised apart from other llamas or alpacas.

Source: Camelid Community Standards of Care Working Group © 2005.

Table 13.2 Reference values for South American camelids relevant to animal welfare assessment.

Parameter	Llama	Alpaca	Guanaco	Vicuña
Bodyweight (kg)	100–200	55–90	100–120	45–55
Body temperature (°C)	37.5–38.5	37.5–38.5	37.2–38.8	37–38.9
Respiratory frequency (/min)	10–30	15–40	20–50	20–50
Heart rate frequency (/min)	50–90	60–90	60–90	60.90
Blood glucose (mg/dL)	74–164	90–141	75–111	90–110
Leukocytes/μL	7,500–21,000	8,000–21,000	9,000–15,000	7,300–13,000
Neutrophil/lymphocyte ratio	1–2.5	1–2.5	1.9–3.5	1.1–2.8
Cortisol (nmol/L)	20–40	20–40	30–50	29
Packed cell volume (%)	29–39	27–45	33–37	39.5
AST (IU/L)	128–450	128–450	68–227	60–246
Creatine kinase (IU/L)	29–39	27–45	33–37	39.5

Source: Fowler (1998), Bonacic and Macdonald (2003), Hoffman (2006), Zapata et al. (2003).

Baseline values for a number of physiological parameters used to define welfare are given in Table 13.2.

13.6.2 Welfare of Vicuñas and Guanacos

Vicuñas and guanacos, which have no tradition of domestication, are managed now as zoo animals and as pets and are regularly captured and sheared in the wild in several South American countries. The so-called sustainable use programmes of capture for shearing wild camelids pay little attention to animal welfare standards, and a series of small enterprises are in place throughout the altiplano and Patagonia in Peru, Bolivia, Chile and Argentina for vicuñas and Argentina and Chile for guanaco. A special series of animal welfare considerations is necessary to ensure the welfare of these truly wild animals when brought into human contact. Both species offer challenges that are quite distinct compared to the domesticated cousins. Territoriality and group structure are both strong features in wild camelids. In order to handle them for shearing, large groups of vicuñas and guanacos are enclosed into corrals. This can cause social disruption, fights between males and crushing of crias while they wait to be handled. Accidents to humans are rare but can be fatal, particularly in the case of guanacos that can weight up to 120 kg.

Vicuña and guanacos have been captured, hunted, handled and shorn since the fifteenth century or before, when the Inca Empire conducted the 'chaku' throughout the Andes of South America for vicuñas, and South American tribes and hunters utilized the guanaco across many ecosystems where the species was abundant. The chaku consisted of herding thousands of vicuña into stone corrals for shearing. Local people surrounded vast areas and walked behind the animals, guiding them towards extensive corrals. Although large numbers of animals were shorn by this method, the associated morbidity and mortality probably had little effect on the population demographics because the process was conducted only once every four years in any given region. When Europeans arrived in South America, the traditional chaku was replaced by indiscriminate hunting. Current policies for vicuña and guanaco management include practices such as capture and shearing of wild animals, farming, ranching, and translocation and reintroduction. Little attention has been paid to the animal welfare implications of these interventions. It is reasonable to assume that both species become stressed by human contact in a similar way to other wild ungulates. The proposed sustainable use of vicuña and guanaco may result in an array of effects which could impact on their welfare: these include the introduction of new morbidity or mortality factors, increasing the risk of less efficient captures in the future, by affecting population dynamics, and the raising of concerns about the methods used to obtain the fleece, thus risking the economic viability of the programme. In the five South American countries there are estimated to be are more than 347,000 vicuñas, and more than 43 tonnes of fibre was sold at market in the last 10 years (McNeill et al. 2009). Guanacos are much more numerous and abundant in Patagonia, reaching more than 1 million (Argentina has the largest population of guanacos in the world). Many small enterprises are starting to capture animals for shearing and hunting quotas are allowed for guanacos in Tierra del Fuego (Chilean Patagonia).

The principles of the 'five freedoms' can be adapted to wild camelids as follows.

1) *Freedom from hunger and thirst*: Welfare could be compromised as a consequence of human action interfering with access to food, preventing access to watering points; or by limiting the access of the animals to those resources to which they are adapted.
2) *Freedom from discomfort and pain*: Discomfort and pain could be caused directly by humans due to the capture system, manipulation or captivity of a wild animal.
3) *Freedom from injury and disease*: Injury and disease could be directly attributable to humans as a consequence of hunting practices; due to an animal's exposure to an inadequate infrastructure, or an inappropriate management system; or by exposure, directly or indirectly, to contaminants or pathogens derived from domestic animals or humans. In addition, the close contact with conspecifics caused by confinement could also increase the risk of disease transmission and inter-animal aggression.
4) *Freedom to express their normal behaviour*: Animals should have adequate space and ecological niche resources that allow them to perform normal behaviours such as territorial defence, use of vantage points, sleeping and feeding sites, and so on.
5) *Freedom from fear and anxiety*: For a wild animal, this freedom implies that human contact must be kept to a minimum. There should be a protocol to assess any changes in the animal's behavioural and/or physiological expression as an indirect measure of potential suffering due to aversion, fear or anxiety during capture or captivity.

In general, capturing wild animals and placing them in captivity (either briefly in the case of wild harvesting or permanently when setting up a farm) exposes them to a variety of stressors grouped in three categories: physical, physiological and psychological. These stressors can result from the effects of capture, manipulation, restraint, drug immobilization, extreme temperatures, novel odours and noises, and so on. They might increase the risk of shock; capture myopathy and immunosuppression, among others. It is very important then to consider the current state of knowledge when a new species is going to be managed, for example: nutritional and habitat requirements, social organization, territorial behaviour, and so on. Neglecting these and failing to act upon them could cause high incidences of mortality during capture, disease post-capture and suffering during the entire process.

The impact of capture and restraint on animal welfare is influenced, to some extent, by the degree to which animals can adapt to human-designed environments, without experiencing any suffering. Since wild vicuña and guanaco are driven into human-made facilities, restrained, handled and shorn, it is reasonable to expect that animal welfare problems may occur. Vicuña management, both in the wild and in captivity, can produce immediate animal welfare problems including pain, injury, behavioural aversion, and other behavioural changes due to the effects of capture and manipulation. In captivity, there is the possibility of not having adequate access to food and water. There is also an increased risk of disease transmission from possible contact with domestic cattle and also through increased conspecific contact. Movement restrictions, limited ability to select habitat and changes in group composition due to human intervention also have the potential to impair welfare.

The stress of management, particularly shearing, has an exaggerated effect on the welfare and health of vicuñas by increasing the exposure to wind and low overnight temperatures in the extreme climate of the Puna ecosystem. The impact of capture and restraint on animal welfare is influenced, to some extent, by the degree of adaptation that animals can achieve in human-designed environments, without experiencing any suffering. Even when an animal has its basic needs fulfilled, such as food provision, and is physically healthy, the difficulty in adapting to captivity may be detrimental to its welfare and possibly affect aspects like reproduction that may indicate a long-term impairment. The opposite phenomenon also deserves attention: animals that adapt easily to the captive environment might not be able to cope in the wild again when released.

Whatever the chosen system of use for vicuñas and guanacos (shearing wild animals or farming them), the animals must be captured at some point. Studies with vicuña, conducted since 1995, have shown that five variables were affected by capture when compared with baseline values from captive animals. Rectal temperature, heart rate, respiratory rate, creatine kinase activity and plasma cortisol concentrations all increased as a result of capture, beyond the normal range described for vicuña and other South American camelids.

13.6.3 Animal Welfare Considerations and Future Challenges

The export of llamas and alpacas to various countries has only taken place to any extent since the early 1990s and is still in the order of only a few hundreds per year. This spread of herds around the world presents unique challenges to those concerned for their welfare, not least because of the wide range of human attitudes to camelids. They are variously considered as wild animals to be hunted for sport, domestic animals to be farmed for fibre or even 'man's best friend'. The rediscovery of South American camelids as multipurpose species and the fact that inter-species breeding is possible open the discussion for what are the limits of human management. 'Cama', an interbreed species between camel and llama by artificial insemination, is the single case of species manipulation that generates a new life form. Interbreeding alpacas and vicuñas for the paco-vicuña is also a matter for ethical discussion. The increased international expression of concern for animal welfare has extended to the South American camelids. It is clear, however, that much remains to be done to increase our understanding of their welfare and improve standards of husbandry for this group of species, unique in their physiology and behaviour and adapted to communal life in a unique habitat.

A new emerging problem in Latin America is the widespread population of domestic dogs that have become strays. Chile has a serious problem of protected populations of guanacos in the Atacama desert that are close to towns and small cities that have become a source of stray dogs that are hunting guanacos. Wild camelids are not well adapted to predators that act in packs like dogs. Puma as the main natural predator is a solitary and ambush style effective predator. Dogs tend to be very inefficient killers of camelids and domestic species and in many cases badly wounded guanacos are seen walking for hours before they die. Irresponsible ownership and poor legislation promoted by animal rights groups have led to outbreaks of stray dogs entering protected areas in Chile. Also in Argentinean Patagonia guanacos are illegally hunted using dogs and packs of stray dogs kills hundreds of guanacos without control.

13.6.4 South American Camelids, Bad Practices and Climate Change

Climate change consequences are affecting South American Camelids in their natural habitat as well as in the regions of the world where they thrive as pets, fine-fibre herds, burden animals for trekking and tourist attractions. Climate change is affecting the high Andes where the four species lives. During the recent decade mange has increased in domestic herds and is now widespread in wild vicuñas and guanacos in Argentina, Peru, Bolivia and Chile. The disease is caused by *Sarcoptes scabiei var. Aucheniae*. This disease affects vicuñas and guanacos in their white and less woolly areas of their body (ventral abdomen, lower chest, axillae and groin). The well-known Pampa Galeras Reserve where vicuña conservation began more than 50 years ago has a serious problem of mange as well as many other areas where local communities capture and shear vicuñas.

Chakus in different regions of Peru and Bolivia are reporting an increasing number of vicuñas affected by mange due to bad practices like: (i) mixing large numbers of vicuñas in a single capture, (ii) concentrating animals in small enclosures for several hours, (iii) utilizing the same shearing gear and shearing spots for sick and healthy animals and (iv) stressing the animals by not using a hood to cover their eyes. Lack of monitoring of groups re-union after release, unregistered mortality after capture and shearing, and the growing illegal poaching of semi-captive animals and wild populations should be a matter of animal welfare concern. Trans-border poaching occurs between Bolivia and Chile, as well as Bolivia and Argentina. The so called 'sustainable use of the vicuña' for fine fibre luxurious garments is not complying with animal welfare standards that are in place for domestic llamas and alpacas in Western societies. The end market of vicuña fibre production is Western fashion industry, where little care is taken about animal welfare standards as well as fair trade for local communities (rough fibre prices have not increased for over a decade in the Andean region).

Mange disrupts feeding behaviour by causing permanent pruritus. During reproduction males can transmit *Acari* to females and vice versa as they mount for several minutes with their medial thighs, prepuce, perineum and legs in close contact. Mange can also affect crias when feeding as their mouth rubs underneath their mothers (crias show face and pinnae skin lesions). Severe cases of mange in wild camelids cause skin erythema, skin bleeding and skin thickening. Sick animals tend to separate from their group and show walking difficulties when interdigital spaces are affected by mange (advanced stages of the disease). A pungent odour of decomposed powder milk can be detected when animals are handled. Severe skin damage also produces liquefaction of tissues under the skin and severe distress after animals suffer prolonged weight loss during winter time. Treatment is often not possible in wild camelids and some bad practices include the use of rubbing in burned diesel fuel after shearing vicuñas in Peru. Ivermectin treatment is regularly used in domestic llamas and alpacas. Treatment with two to four injections of Ivermectin at 0.2–0.4 mg/kg at intervals of 7–14 days has been reported to be effective, but a single dose in wild vicuñas is not effective.

Mixing groups during chaku and the spread of fenced areas to manage vicuñas in a semi-captive way have contributed to the spread of mange in wild animals in the altiplano of Peru. Unsafe and irresponsible captive management in an Italian zoo has created the first population of feral llamas in Europe. Rural emigration and poor husbandry have caused the interbreeding of llamas and guanacos in the Atacama desert of Chile and some areas of the Peruvian Andes. Rural to urban migration of local farmers is leaving domestic herds unattended outside their traditional extensive farming area. Where herds of llamas and alpacas are not rounded up at night or corrals are far from households, conflicts between natural predators and domestic camelids cause retaliatory killing of pumas and foxes. Recent advances using solar devices that emit random light flashes (fox lights) have proven effective to deter pumas in northern Chile, but failed to prevent foxes hunting alpaca or llama crias.

Climate change is affecting the altiplano of the Andean region as well as many ecosystems around the world. Severe long-term drought is affecting the altiplano and food shortages occur regularly. Dry and cold winters are also causing mortality between domestic and wild camelids. In Western countries heat stress and massive fires are more frequent and cause mortalities in domestic llamas and alpacas. Proper evacuation plans in case of fire should be implemented in the West coast of the US, Europe and Australia.

Llamas are often used as a tourist attraction in cities of Europe or parks in North America during summer. Animals are exposed to direct sunshine, high humidity and are not sheared. This condition may cause heat stress to those animals that are not able to cope with the weather combination of high temperature, low wind speed, high humidity and sun reflection in hard surfaces like walkways or paved roads.

It is good news that the international expression of concern for animal welfare has extended to the South American Camelids. Nevertheless, much remains to be done to increase our understanding of their welfare and improve standards of husbandry for this group of species, unique in their physiology and behaviour and adapted to communal life in a unique environment.

Appendix

Problems associated with premature births in camelid cria (calves).

Prematurity	Clinical signs	Complications	Actions
5–6 weeks	Weak, unable to stand, down on pastern, tremor in legs Sleepy, floppy ears, no teeth Sunken eyes, visually unaware Birth membrane attached to orifices (nose, mouth, anus) Raspy/wet/shallow breathing Body temp. < 37°C but *not* shivering, very short fleece	Systemic infection (mortality) risk Umbilical defect, herniation Respiratory infection No sucking reflex or unwilling to drink Retained meconium, constipation Overfeeding with bottle or tube No urine output	Keep cria on clean hay. Spray umbilical cord with iodine directly after birth. Wrap the cord in tissue and secure around belly with bandage until dry Monitor temp. daily: > 39°C can indicate infection Vitamin B complex injection. Hold cria upside down to drain lungs. Keep warm, rub body gently. Stomach tube feeding colostrum. Plasma infusion when unable to suck. Add liquid paraffin for constipation or give as enema. Substitute glucose and electrolytes. Monitor urine output (weigh dry and wet nappy).
3–4 weeks	As above but less extreme	Keep warm, monitor nursing. Good chance of survival after 2 weeks old, but still at high risk.	Expect slow weight gain only. Inject vitamin B complex.
>3 weeks	Floppy ears, can't straighten legs, shaky	Good chance of survival. Check for full, round soft belly. After 3 weeks cria is out of immediate danger.	Inject vitamin B complex.
Term			Cria that look premature should be treated as premature.

References and Further Reading

Alpaca World Magazine. http://www.alpacaworldmagazine.com.

Bonacic, C., Feber, R.E., and Macdonald, D.W. (2006). Capture of the vicuña (*Vicugna vicugna*) for sustainable use: Animal welfare implications. *Biological Conservation* 129: 543–550.

Bonacic, C. and Macdonald, D. (2003). The physiological impact of wool-harvesting procedures in vicuñas (*Vicugna vicugna*). *Animal Welfare* 12: 387–402.

Camelid Community Standards of Care Working Group. (2005). *Minimum Standards of Care for Llamas and Alpacas*. http://www.camelidcare.info/MinimumStandards.htm.

Camelids Quarterly. http://www.llamas-alpacas.com.

Fowler, M.E. (1998). *Medicine and Surgery of South American Camelids: Llama, Alpaca, Vicuña, Guanaco*. Oxford: Wiley-Blackwell.

Fowler, M.E. and Cubas, Z.S. (2001). *Biology, Medicine, and Surgery of South American Wild Animals*. Oxford: Wiley-Blackwell.

Hoffman, E. (2006). *The Complete Alpaca Book*, 2e. Santa Cruz, CA: Bonny Doon Press.

Lichtenstein, G., Baldi, R., Villaba, L., Hoces, D., Baiguin, R., and Laker, J. (2008). *Vicugna vicugna*. In *IUCN Red List of Theatened Species*. Version 2010.3. IUCN (2010). http://www.iucnredlist.org.

Macdonald, D. (ed.) (2006). *The Encyclopedia of Mammals*, 2e. Oxford: Oxford University Press.

McNeill, D., Lichtenstein, G., and Renaudeau d'Arc, N. (2009). International policies and national legislation concerning vicuña conservation and exploitation. In: *The Vicuña: The Theory and Practice of Community-based Wildlife Management* (ed. I. Gordon), 63–79. New York: Springer. *Manejo de Camelidos Silvestres* (MACS). http://www.macs.puc.cl.

Zapata, B., Fuentes, V., Bonacic, C., González, B., Villouta, G., and Bas, F. (2003). Haematological and clinical biochemistry findings in captive juvenile guanacos (*Lama guanicoe* Müller 1776) in central Chile. *Small Ruminant Research* 48: 15–21.

14

Turkeys

Stephen Lister

KEY CONCEPTS

14.1   Introduction

The current strains of turkey grown for meat production around the world are far removed from those which graced the table of the court of Emperor Montezuma. It was the Aztecs who first domesticated the turkey, prizing it for its decorative feathers as well as a source of meat. The turkey arrived in Europe in the sixteenth century, probably brought by merchants returning from the New World to Spain. From there, it found its way to the United Kingdom, into East Anglia, as the progenitors of the Norfolk Black, for many years remaining a specialty dish

Management and Welfare of Farm Animals: The UFAW Farm Handbook, Sixth Edition.
Edited by John Webster and Jean Margerison.
© Universities Federation for Animal Welfare 2022. Published 2022 by John Wiley & Sons Ltd.

for high society. As domestication continued, strains were reintroduced to the New World and were bred with existing wild turkey strains, giving rise to strains which survive today (e.g. the Narragansett from Rhode Island). A wide range of wild and 'domesticated' strains exist today, mainly for hobby breeders and showing. Some, such as the Norfolk Black and other heritage breeds, are bred commercially for niche sales in the commercial market, especially for seasonal whole bird production.

Globally, most of the turkey meat consumed today comes from commercial broad-breasted hybrids derived from various white breeds, offering markets a wide range of weight of finished birds as whole oven-ready carcasses or those for butchering and further processing. There is marked sexual dimorphism resulting in hens and stags (toms in the USA) being reared separately for specific weight band requirements.

Only a few primary breeding companies now supply most of the turkeys reared around the world, notably Aviagen Turkeys (incorporating British United Turkeys and Nicholas Turkeys) and Hybrid Turkeys (part of Hendrix Genetics). These companies maintain and develop genetic stock through pure line research and supply parent stock as poults or hatching eggs to breeder multipliers. These companies supply detailed management guides, which are a useful resource for practical information and guidance on management, nutrition and performance. Smaller breeders service the more specialist markets with strains used predominantly for free-range and seasonal production, e.g. KellyBronze, trademark name for Kelly Turkeys and Hockenhull Turkeys.

14.2   The UK Turkey Industry

There has been a considerable reduction in turkey meat production in the UK in recent years. Over the last 20 years production is estimated to have stabilized at around 155,000 tonnes carcass weight, through the slaughter of approximately 16 million turkeys in 2020. Reductions in UK production have been due to a combination of a lack of increase in domestic meat consumption and increased levels of imports. During the same period, the number of turkeys reared specifically for the Christmas market has remained buoyant at around 2 million per year. Therefore, although the traditional seasonal production is a significant market, the majority of sales are associated with year-round production with the sale of value-added products and portions greatly outstripping whole bird sales.

There are a few relatively large companies involved in all-year-round turkey production, accounting for approx. 90% of total output. They are vertically integrated, receiving day-old parent stock from the primary breeding companies for rearing and laying on company-controlled farms. Most operate their own hatcheries, hatching day-olds for growing on company or contract commercial farms to supply company slaughterhouses and processing facilities. Some independent breeders in the UK and mainland Europe supply day-old chicks as commercial stock, mostly as heritage breeds, to independent growing farms. These farms are contracted to supply processors or butchery outlets using on-farm slaughter, processing and marketing, to meet specific customer requirements, especially for seasonal consumption.

14.2.1   Farm Assurance and Animal Welfare Standards

Most production in the UK is now monitored under a number of farm assurance schemes, established by the industry, retailers or other bodies. The largest is the Red Tractor Farm Assurance Scheme for Turkeys, formed in 2017, while other standards exist, notably the RSPCA Welfare Standards for Turkeys. These schemes set specific standards for production methods, environmental control and stockpersonship, and all participating premises are subject to regular independent auditing for compliance with these standards. Retailers will often add further standards for compliance on management, welfare and include other aspects such as antimicrobial usage. This must be monitored and antibiotic usage reduction programmes are required, with emphasis on the application of management, biosecurity and vaccination to maintain good animal health and welfare. The government also sets welfare standards in general animal welfare legislation, which are specified in the DEFRA *Code of Recommendations for the Welfare of Livestock: Turkeys*. The last edition was published in 1987 and remains in need of updating to reflect current management practices and domestic and European recommendations (e.g. Council of Europe 2001).

14.3   Reproductive Physiology

Modern breeding turkeys (breeders) are brought into lay between 30 and 32 weeks of age, followed by a laying cycle of up to 25 weeks or longer. The onset of sexual maturity (semen production in stags and egg-laying in hens) is triggered by manipulation of daylength and, to a far lesser degree, point-of-lay body weight. Hens tend to be reared on 14 hours of light per day (minimum 60 lux) up until approx. 18 weeks of age. They are then conditioned using a shorter daylength of about 7 hours of light, again at 60 lux and where accommodation has effective light-proofing, hens can be held at this photoperiod until onset of lay is required.

The onset of lay is triggered by rapidly increasing the daylength to 14 hours at a minimum of 100 lux, which must be maintained throughout lay. Most accommodation for laying hens is in open, bird-proofed pole barns, but the maintenance of good egg production requires natural sunlight to be supplemented with uniform artificial light, which avoids the possibility of birds experiencing shortening daylength. Stags do not require the same initial conditioning, more simply commencing semen production at sexual maturity on a daylength of 14 hours of light at a minimum of 50 lux. Reproductive performance varies depending on the strain of bird, the body weight of the hen at point of lay and consistency of body weight through the laying period. Modern turkey strains aim to achieve fertility rates in excess of 90%, peak egg production above 80% and having produced up to 120 eggs per hen at 25 weeks of lay, which leads to around 95 poults per hen.

Due to significant sexual dimorphism in terms of body weight, breeding in commercial turkeys is achieved using artificial insemination. The stags are milked (stimulated to release semen) usually twice a week to maintain semen quality and quantity. The semen from several males is pooled and then extended by being added to specific volumes of diluent prior to insemination of the hens. The first insemination should usually be about 10 to 14 days after photo-stimulation, depending on the season, and should coincide with the first egg being laid. There should be three inseminations within the next 10 days, and then at least weekly throughout lay. This obviously requires regular handling of the hens and should be undertaken with care by fully trained stockpeople.

14.4 Nutrition

Turkeys are naturally omnivorous, feeding on plants, seeds, insects and worms. Commercially, nutrition is a major contributor to good health, performance and growth. The quality of the raw materials, consistency of supply, presentation and physical appearance of feed are all important factors that ensure the health and performance of the birds. The physical form of the feed can be as important as the nutrient content. Specialist nutritional advice should always be used and a planned feeding programme for breeders and commercial stock should be established. The expected targets for live-weight gain in breeder birds and 'commercials' (meat birds) are available from breeding company management guides.

14.4.1 Breeders

During rearing, feeding of breeders is aimed at increasing body weight in a controlled manner. This requires even, early growth to ensure the target growth curve is achieved but not exceeded, which is usually achieved by qualitative manipulation of energy and protein content of the ration rather than physical or quantitative restriction. Exceeding point-of-lay body weights and/or excessive amounts of body fat are likely to lead to poor laying performance by hens, as well as leading to potential health issues. This quantitative nutrient restriction tends to be far more problematic for laying turkeys than broiler breeders. Similarly, stags need to reach target body weight to stimulate good semen production and ensure good skeletal development. This is usually achieved by *ad libitum* feeding until about 16 weeks of age, along with regular checking of live weight against breed targets, which enables the expression of genetic potential and aids animal selection. Over 16 weeks of age, the live weight of stages needs to be controlled to avoid them becoming overweight, to avoid depressed semen output and poor health. This weight control can be achieved by qualitative and/or quantitative restriction, although the latter requires specialist feeding equipment and adequate feeding space to avoid competition. Stags and hens are reared separately to allow the control of photoperiod and feeding regimes to be tailored to suit their specific requirements.

14.4.2 Commercial Meat Birds

The market for turkeys requires the production of birds over a large weight range and this governs target growth curves. The larger stags are usually grown to allow butchery and further processing, while the hens and smaller stags are more often grown for oven ready whole bird production. Programmes for predicted growth rates must take account of these requirements in tandem with health and welfare requirements. Targets for metabolizable energy

(ME), protein and amino acid (quality and quantity) and vitamin/mineral specifications must be agreed, with well-organized input from a specialist nutritionist, taking account of the strain of turkey being grown to a specified slaughter weight at a specified age. The feed intake and performance will depend on animals having adequate feeder space, the feeder type, drinker availability and stocking density. In addition, placement dates for day-old poults for seasonal production can be adjusted to accommodate the predicted growth profiles for differing age of maturity at final expected slaughter age.

Most feeding programmes start with a crumbed feed or micro-pellets that are offered up to two to three weeks of age, moving gradually to an increase in pellet size for growing rations. Pellet quality (hardness and grist size) is very important, as are all aspects of feed presentation and feeder space allowance, with a minimum of 3 cm of feeding space per bird or one tube or pan feeder for approx. every 50 birds. Drinker availability is also significant in ensuring adequate feed intake along with a constant supply of fresh, clean water which is essential. Closed nipple watering systems have the advantage of offering cleaner water, however the water flow rate may be inadequate and result in insufficient water intake, especially in older birds, so open bell drinkers or reservoir cup systems are more commonly used.

14.5 Environment

14.5.1 Controlled-environment Housing

Conventional, enclosed, controlled-environment houses are usually windowless and power ventilated with control of heating, ventilation and lighting. Most have concrete floors for ease of cleansing and disinfection although some older units are based on compacted earth floors. Flock size can be up to 25,000 birds per house but is usually much smaller. No cages are currently used in the UK for turkey production. Birds are reared on litter, the substrate usually being shavings or straw. Most houses operate on an all-in, all-out basis but this may be operated on a site that has multiple ages of animals in differing houses. Some companies use a brood-and-move system using specialist rearing houses up to 6 weeks of age and then move the birds to pole barns or controlled-environment houses on the same site or a separate growing site. Typically, males and females are grown separately. Stags are usually slaughtered between 21 and 24 weeks of age, mostly as cut-ups for portioning or further processing, while hens are slaughtered in relation to specific weight requirements and market demand, often being processed between 9 and 16 weeks of age. The larger specialty and seasonal whole birds may be over 20 weeks of age at slaughter and these are usually sold as oven ready whole birds or crowns (white breast meat on the bone, with the legs removed).

The stocking density is adjusted by placement stocking rates (i.e. the number of day-olds placed in a defined floor area per house) and subsequent moving of birds to fattening sheds, or later selections and thinning. The final stocking density for stags in controlled-environment housing may reach 60 kg/m^2, which for 21-week-old stags would equate to about three birds per square metre. Injurious pecking may be controlled by reduced light intensity (around 10 lux) or through beak treatment using infrared techniques at day-old in the hatchery (see section 14.7.2).

14.5.2 Pole Barns

Most parent stock and some fattening birds, especially for the Christmas trade, are reared in open sided barns, mostly netted to avoid contact with wild birds. These sheds are naturally ventilated (Figure 14.1) with environmental control against the elements using side panels or mechanically operated shutters, which may or may not be linked to an internal house thermostat. In smaller farms, a range of naturally ventilated farm buildings or polytunnels may be used. Such flocks may have access to free range paddocks at certain times of the year, even if not marketed as fully free range. These birds may have been brooded in controlled-environment houses. The labour input is higher in naturally ventilated housing with the requirement for more regular littering down, usually with straw. Birds kept in such accommodation are usually routinely beak-trimmed. The maximum stocking densities vary from 25 kg/m^2 up to 38 kg/m^2.

14.5.3 Free Range Flocks

Many flocks, especially for the seasonal market, are reared as free range where pole barns or enclosed housing are used for overnight roosting, while birds have access to range during daylight hours. The minimum requirements for stocking density, free range access and slaughter age are outlined in the Defra Poultrymeat Special Marketing Regulations. There are important considerations in encouraging good ranging behaviour which include pasture management, land type and drainage, along with the provision of shelter. Care must be taken

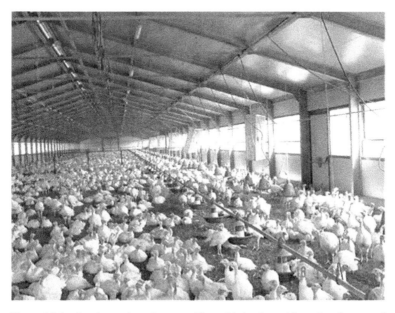

Figure 14.1 Rearing turkeys for meat. These birds, about 15 weeks of age, are housed on friable litter. The house is naturally ventilated and open sided with adjustable side curtains. Fans for circulation of air within the building hang from the roof.

to employ the highest biosecurity standard to protect flocks against diseases associated with contact with wild birds, vermin or other livestock. The most significant risks are from Avian influenza, Salmonella and Erysipelas infections.

14.6 Management

14.6.1 Young Stock

Day-old poults must be placed in clean, dry accommodation supplying a comfortable thermal environment and free access to feed and water. Heat is usually supplied by gas brooders suspended over the birds at a height designed to give a concentrated spot heat directly underneath with a thermal gradient from the centre to the edge of the brooder ring. This allows poults to seek their own comfort zone. Their behaviour and the distribution of birds within the ring should be assessed to determine their state of comfort. Birds are initially placed in circular or oval surrounds constructed of a solid board or wire netting fence, depending on house design and layout. Up to 500 poults may be placed under each brooder and the brooder surround may be enlarged as the birds grow, although there is some interest in whole house heating and brooding. Adequate bright lighting is essential for successful brooding. A light is often hung next to the brooder heater to attract birds and illuminate feed and water. Feed is usually initially presented as crumb or micro-pellets on shallow trays to allow easy access, which should be topped up regularly with small amounts of feed so that ample, fresh feed is always available. Small font drinkers or disposable apple trays may be used to supply additional cool, fresh drinking water in the first few days, in addition to the automatic nipple or reservoir cup systems set at a low height so that young poults can easily access them. The young turkeys are usually released from the ring surrounds at approx. six to seven days of age and are then given access to the whole house, or the area allocated in the surround may be more gradually increased over a three- to four-week period. Feed is supplied from a variety of feeder types, most usually suspended circular feed pans or hoppers that are filled by tube or auger. Fresh clean water is essential and is most often supplied by open bell-type or closed nipple and cup reservoir systems.

14.6.2 Breeding Stock

Breeders are mostly reared in light-proofed controlled environment housing to control photoperiod. Rearing is otherwise like that for commercial stock. Prior to point of lay, flocks are moved to specialist laying sites, usually of bird proofed pole barn design. During the laying period, hens and stags are housed or penned separately, both on floor systems, usually with straw as the litter substrate, although shavings may be preferred for stags. Hens are encouraged to lay in nest boxes placed around the pens. Trap nests are favoured which allow only one hen to enter a nest at any one time to allow privacy at egg-laying and reduce broodiness. The traps are usually hinged, such that the nest closes on entry, preventing a second bird entering, but then allows the bird in the nest to leave after egg-laying. Litter substrate for nests may be straw, sawdust or Astroturf. Automatic nest boxes are available which help to move birds off the nests at regular intervals, as a means of reducing the incidence of broodiness. In the case of manual nests, egg collectors will push hens off the nest at each egg collection, a minimum of six times per day. Any hens making repeated visits or spending long periods in nests can be identified as persistently broody, which occurs most frequently soon after peak production. These may be removed from the flock and are then placed in a sparsely littered, cool and brightly lit broody pen until regular nesting and laying behaviour has resumed. Stags are penned in separate accommodation and may be placed on a feed restriction programme to help control excessive weight gain throughout their breeding life.

14.6.3 Environmental Control

During the brooding period, heat is supplied to the day-old poults and after this period, the temperature of the house is gradually reduced and for older birds management is designed to remove metabolic heat produced by the turkeys themselves. This can be achieved by adequate, natural ventilation or forced (mechanical) fans. Adequate ventilation is also essential to maintain a constant supply of fresh air and oxygen while removing excessive carbon dioxide, ammonia, dust and moisture. The efficiency of the ventilation system in achieving these goals will limit the stocking density that can be successfully and comfortably used. Any mechanical ventilation system must have an effective back-up generator or high temperature alarm. In hot weather, additional recirculation fans may be needed in the house to assist evaporative cooling. Well-managed ventilation also contributes to good litter quality. As birds spend their lives in contact with litter, it is essential to maintain the substrate in a dry, friable state. This will help to avoid painful conditions such as pododermatitis and breast blisters as well as reducing the likelihood of respiratory problems. The management of stocking rates and effective drinker management are important factors in the management of animal health. There have been positive moves to closed, or semi-closed, nipple and nipple/cup drinker systems which help to improve water quality. Drinkers should be set at the right height for the age and size of birds. The depth of water in bell drinkers should be sufficient to allow drinking without restriction but not overfilled to avoid spillage when knocked. There should be at least two drinker points per 100 birds to avoid undue competition and, where possible, they should be movable to avoid litter under the drinkers becoming excessively wet or soiled. The quality of drinking water is as important as quantity, so the monitoring of water quality and the use of water sanitization are very important in the maintenance of bird health.

Lighting is important to turkeys in terms of its intensity, colour and quality as well as the photoperiod. Light intensity should be enough to allow birds to fully investigate their environment and undertake as many normal behaviours as possible. In brooder rings, a minimum of 25 lux is recommended. The Council of Europe (2001) [Standing Committee of the European Convention for the Protection of Animals kept for farming purposes – recommendations concerning turkeys (*Meleagris gallopavo* spp.)] recommended a minimum light intensity of 10 lux at bird eye level and, where possible, this should be supplied by natural light. With such light intensity, injurious pecking may be experienced and this may need to be controlled by reducing intensity to below 10 lux for short periods. The Red Tractor Farm Assurance standards require a minimum of 10 lux illuminating at least 80% of the useable bird area, while the RSPCA Farm Assurance standard requires a minimum of 20 lux across at least half of the available floor area. In some systems, beak trimming may be necessary to prevent injurious pecking if this level of light intensity is to be maintained, and informed decisions should be taken as to the necessity for trimming in specific circumstances. In breeder flocks, much higher light intensity (up to 100 lux) is required to maintain egg production, and in such situations beak trimming is regularly practiced to avoid injurious pecking, most usually as infrared beak treatment at day-old in the hatchery. A dark period in every 24 hours is considered advantageous for turkey health and welfare to allow birds to rest and sleep. The Council of Europe (2001) suggests that there is the need for an uninterrupted dark period of 8 hours as a guideline and recommends an absolute minimum of 4 hours.

Environmental enrichment is also important for floor-reared birds, allowing them to investigate and interact with their environment. The provision of low perches, platforms, straw bales and hanging toys or vegetation may be useful in promoting activity, which can avoid the likelihood of injurious pecking and improve leg strength and health.

14.6.4 Maintaining Health and Welfare

The importance of good stockpersonship cannot be over-emphasized. Effective staff training and empathy for livestock by all people involved with turkey breeding, rearing and slaughter are essential in ensuring the health and welfare of birds. All staff should be trained in all aspects of environmental control, management and husbandry. They should also be able to recognize the signs of good and ill health in the birds under their care. All stock should be inspected at least twice a day and preferably more often, taking time to walk within a metre of each bird in the house to assess general health of the flock as a whole, in addition to looking for any problems with individual birds. Any sick or injured birds should be removed promptly and either placed in a hospital pen for treatment or, if recovery is considered unlikely, they should be promptly and humanely culled. Smaller birds may be culled by neck dislocation; but for these and for heavier birds the use of concussive humane killers is recommended as neck dislocation may not cause instant loss of consciousness.

Detailed records should be kept for mortality, culling and for all treatments. Where practical, recording of feed and water intake should be made, as this can give the first indications to stockpersons of ill health in a flock. Where problems with the flock are identified, prompt veterinary advice should be sought. Where there is significant mortality or sickness, accurate diagnosis is essential to ensure that effective and appropriate treatment can be given. Health issues in commercial turkeys are predominantly associated with enteric disease, respiratory disease and skeletal health or lameness.

As with all intensive rearing systems, prevention strategies and the use of available vaccines are essential to avoid harmful disease challenges. This is especially important since there is a paucity of medicines specifically licensed for turkeys in the UK and many parts of Europe, where turkeys are classified as a 'minor' species. In addition, responsible use guidelines aimed at reducing the use of medicines is considered important in reducing contributions to antimicrobial resistance. Furthermore, some production assurance standards stipulate those specific antimicrobials which should not be used during the grow-out period. An effective written veterinary health and welfare plan and regular communication with a specialist veterinary surgeon is important in these processes. An important part of this plan must be to set up an effective and workable biosecurity plan to help prevent the introduction of disease to a flock or site, site set up and management, along with planned preventive programmes to reduce the impact of disease, and minimize antimicrobial use.

14.7   Welfare Issues

Commercial turkeys can grow to weights in excess of 20 kg and, as with all farmed animals, animal welfare considerations are important when such birds are used for meat production. Modern breeding programmes must take account of liveability, robustness and resistance to disease in developments for improved productivity. Programmes should be designed to avoid suffering or harm to parent stock and their progeny. At the farm level, the importance of effective stockpersonship cannot be over-emphasized. Historically, assessment of bird welfare has been based on welfare inputs (e.g. numbers of feeders/drinkers, stocking rates, and so on) whereas there is an increasing awareness that the best way to assess the suitability of any method of production for keeping of animals is better based on welfare outcomes. In turkeys, this may be assessed in terms of growth rates, feed efficiency, general health and mortality, although these may simply reflect how well a turkey is coping with its environment. There is a need to develop other factors on which to base this assessment. This may involve on-farm monitoring for pododermatitis, feather condition, injurious pecking or other signs and behaviours evident during rearing, factors identified at the processing plant such as the incidence of pododermatitis, injuries or other causes of condemnation or downgrading, which may enable an assessment of the quality of litter and environmental control as an indicator of general management and general stockpersonship on-farm. There is a need for further research in these areas to establish and monitor robust and meaningful assessments of welfare outcomes. Some specific welfare issues that merit more detailed consideration are discussed below.

14.7.1   Stocking Density

There is ample evidence in a variety of avian species of the importance of stocking rates and terminal stocking density in influencing bird welfare and expression of normal behaviour. The existing DEFRA Code of Recommendations for the Welfare of Livestock: Turkeys (1987) indicates a minimum floor area allowance of 260 cm^2/kg body weight. This equates to a stocking density maximum of 38 kg/m^2. The Council of Europe recommendations (2001) require enough space allowance to allow turkeys to exhibit as wide a range of normal social behaviours as possible, but do not state specific maximum stocking rates or density. Commercial experience over many years has demonstrated that modern controlled-environment housing utilizing efficient forced ventilation systems can allow turkeys to grow to breed targets and expectations at stocking densities significantly above 38 kg/m² for older birds, without compromising welfare. In such situations, it may be appropriate to recalculate a stocking density for turkeys to recognize the growth characteristics of larger birds on a three-dimensional basis rather than a simple weight per floor area assessment. The Farm Animal Welfare Council (FAWC 1995) concluded that when dealing with turkeys of different sizes, stocking densities should be scaled according to a two-thirds power of live weight. On this basis, they established that it was possible for terminal stocking densities as high as 59 kg/m² to be justified for 20-week-old commercial stags in appropriate accommodation, equating to about three stags per square metre close to slaughter. Despite this theoretical approach, it is still necessary for individual farms to demonstrate that environmental control under practical conditions can ensure turkeys are able to exhibit as wide a range of normal behaviours as possible and not to suffer unduly from excessive extremes of temperature or significant health issues. In naturally ventilated houses, stocking densities closer to 25 kg/m² are more suitable to prevent heat stress and maintain adequate litter quality. As indicated previously, welfare outcome assessments based on indices of performance: mortality rates, health and behaviour, and performed by a competent assessor, should reveal any harmful effects of overstocking in specific houses.

14.7.2 Beak Trimming

Beak trimming is used in virtually all turkey breeding stock and a proportion of commercial meat birds to control injurious pecking. In controlled-environment housing using artificial lighting, coupled with effective light-proofing, behaviour likely to lead to pecking injuries may be controlled by reducing light intensity at specific ages. Beak trimming is currently an allowable mutilation in the UK for turkeys. A mutilation is a procedure resulting in damage to, or loss of, a sensitive part of the body, in this case up to a third of the upper mandible. Such mutilations may cause pain and are considered by many to be an unnecessary welfare insult. Some production systems, e.g. free range at low stocking density and with certain breeds which appear to have a lower propensity to peck, eliminate the need for such a procedure.

Within the EU, beak trimming is permitted in situations where it is considered that a failure to do so would be likely to give rise to far more severe welfare issues, notably, injurious pecking. Currently it is legal to beak-trim up to 21 days of age, preferably using a cold-cutting technique for the upper mandible only. It is generally believed that the insult to the bird may be less if done at a younger age, i.e. less than 10 days of age, but there is then a greater risk of subsequent regrowth. As a result, the majority of poults will be individually treated at the hatchery at day-old. Infrared beak treatment (IRBT) requires that the bird's head is held gently on a carousel and the beak tip is exposed to an infra-red beam for about 5 seconds. The beam causes necrosis (death of cells) across the beak, the tip eventually falling off after 2 to 3 weeks, leaving a healed and altered (reduced) beak. This has the advantage of being performed in a controlled and consistent manner, no open wound should be created and regrowth is limited to a blunted beak which still allows the bird to effectively manipulate feed and other substrates in its environment

Beak trimming or treatment may be considered a justifiable trade-off if it enables birds to be reared under significantly higher light intensity sufficient to enable turkeys to exhibit a wide range of investigating behaviours with a greatly reduced likelihood of injurious pecking.

14.7.3   Catching and Transport

Turkeys should be caught and handled in a careful manner and only by trained, competent staff. Birds should be transported in containers appropriate for the size of bird, length of journey and expected weather conditions. Most transporters rely on natural ventilation to regulate the thermal environment for the birds. Problems may arise at high ambient temperatures, especially when vehicles are stationary. During inclement weather, side curtains can be used to prevent rain blowing in through the sides of perforated plastic crates.

Smaller turkeys should be picked up by placing a hand on either side of the body, holding the wings close to the bird's body. Turkeys should not be lifted by a single leg only. While larger turkeys may be carried by one leg and the diagonally opposite wing. In all cases, turkeys should be carried for the shortest period possible. They should then be transported without delay and be carried in crates at stocking densities appropriate to the size and age. The transport vehicles should be well ventilated and in any case journey times should be as short as is practical.

14.7.4   Slaughter

The processing of turkeys, especially large stags, requires careful handling of birds up to the point of slaughter. Transport to the processing plant and facilities at the lairage for birds awaiting slaughter should be designed and used to ensure the avoidance of injury or distress, and especially extremes of temperature. The lairage design and the use of trained personnel supervised by a dedicated poultry welfare officer throughout the time birds are present in the slaughterhouse are necessary to safeguard welfare. The live shackling of large stags as necessitated for electrical water bath stunning methods is likely to cause pain in the shackled legs and a degree of distress to inverted birds. In such systems, turkeys should be handled carefully by well-trained staff and should be inverted for the shortest time possible prior to death. As a result of these concerns, the vast majority of turkeys in UK are now slaughtered using controlled-atmosphere killing. This procedure allows birds to remain in their transport crates without inversion and to be culled by introduction into anoxic gas mixtures enough to kill the birds *in situ*. This equipment requires constant monitoring and maintenance to ensure effective killing of all birds in the system.

14.8   Conclusions

Turkey production within the UK, although showing a decline in recent years, remains a significant industry, presenting several welfare and management challenges. High standards of stockpersonship, with active veterinary input and the use of well-maintained and suitable accommodation can, with appropriate safeguards, ensure the welfare of birds reared in these systems. The challenge remains to establish meaningful welfare outcome assessments against which to monitor progress in all areas of the production process.

Further Reading

Council of Europe. (2001). Standing Committee of the European Convention for the Protection of Animals kept for farming purposes – recommendations concerning turkeys (*Meleagris gallopavo* spp).

DEFRA. (1987). *Code of Recommendations for the Welfare of Livestock: Turkeys*.

FAWC. (1995). *Farm Animal Welfare Council Report on the Welfare of Turkeys*.

Houghton Wallace, J. (2007). *Not Just for Christmas: A Complete Guide to Raising Turkeys*. Preston, UK: Farming Books and Videos Ltd.

Red Tractor Assurance for Farms Poultry Scheme: Turkey Standards. (2018).

RSPCA. (2017). *Welfare Standards for Turkeys*. Humane Slaughter Association (HSA). www.hsa.org.uk.

15

Ducks

Cormac O'Shea and Patrick Garland

KEY CONCEPTS

Management and Welfare of Farm Animals: The UFAW Farm Handbook, Sixth Edition.
Edited by John Webster and Jean Margerison.
© Universities Federation for Animal Welfare 2022. Published 2022 by John Wiley & Sons Ltd.

15.1 Introduction

The duck is a remarkably versatile and resilient animal and important source of meat, eggs and feathers. Contemporary duck production varies widely from backyard smallholdings to highly sophisticated, partially automated operations. Consumption of duck and eggs remains greatest in Asia but is a segment of the poultry which continues to grow steadily elsewhere. The more modern, genetically improved meat strains reach an impressive 3.5 kg in six weeks while egg-laying strains can produce in excess of 300 eggs per year. Regardless of the purpose or size of the operation, there are common approaches that should be considered to ensure optimal health and welfare of the animal, which will contribute to maximum productivity. A high welfare state in ducks kept for food production is a difficult concept to define and to assess at an operational level. An important foundation for achieving high welfare is ensuring ducks have the liberty of the five freedoms of welfare. Cherry and Morris (2008) remains an important source for more detailed account of domestic duck production.

15.2 Biology and Domestication

The common ancestors of the domestic duck are the Mallard (*Anas platyrhynchos*), which inhabit Europe, North Africa and North America and the Muscovy (*Cairina moschata*) that was found in South America. There is archaeological evidence that suggested domestication occurred independently in at least two regions, firstly in southern China and 1500 years later in Western Europe (Cherry and Morris 2008). The phylogenetic basis of duck domestication has recently been investigated with strong genetic evidence for a single domestication event approximately 2200 years ago followed by separate selection for eggs and meat production shortly thereafter. The discovery of duck bones from wild birds has been reported at various Roman sites in Britain where, it is assumed, they were important sources of meat, eggs and feathers. The wild mallard is a migratory water bird and therefore adapted to a range of environmental conditions and under wild conditions the mallard feeds on seeds, plants, insects and worms. They swim and walk efficiently. The Muscovy duck is a tropical bird, which in the wild lives in marshy forests; however, their robustness has allowed them to adapt to different climatic conditions and habitats. These ducks are sexually dimorphic with males being considerably larger and as with other food production species, genetic selection for economically important traits, such as egg production and meat yield gathered pace from the 1950s onwards. This has been enhanced by improvements in animal nutrition, husbandry and disease management. The breeds and strains of ducks that are popular for meat production are the Pekin, Muscovy and a crossbred between the two, which is a sterile mule that is fast growing. There are well-known egg-producing strains of ducks, which include the Khaki Campbell and the Indian Runner duck.

15.3   Market Outlook and Consumer Trends

Commercial duck production is an important source of meat, eggs and feathers. The demand for duck meat and eggs has grown substantially with duck production in 2010 being six times greater compared with production levels in 1961. In 2016 ducks were among the top five most numerous food animal species, having been estimated to consist of 1,241,388 thousand head of animals. The vast majority of the global duck population is based in China. It has been estimated that over 85% of the duck population are based in Asia, followed by Europe (6.8%), the Americas (2.5%; ~ 27 million slaughtered in the US in 2017), Africa (1.8%) and Oceania (0.1%) (FAOSTAT, 2018). Feathers are also an economically important output in various countries such as Taiwan, while duck production forms a relatively small portion of the poultry population in the United Kingdom, which has had a steady annual production rate of 30,000 tonnes of duck meat in recent years.

15.4   General Management Considerations

15.4.1   Meat Strains

The general management approach to ducks regardless of whether the focus is egg production or meat production will be similar, providing adequate housing, access to water and nutritious feed and optimal environmental control for temperature and air quality. The Pekin and Muscovy are the two most common strains used for meat production. Furthermore, a cross between the two strains, more commonly the offspring of a male Muscovy and a female Pekin called a mule, has become popular due to its rapid growth rate. These crossbreds are a sterile hybrid because of the difference in chromosome size and number between the two parents. Ducks, like other poultry, are amenable to the high stocking rates operated under intensive conditions due to the establishment of a relatively stable social hierarchy; a 'pecking order' that means they can live in large numbers. In Pekin ducks, genetic selection for traits such as growth rate has had a central role in leading to higher meat yield and lower rate of carcass fat deposition with animals reaching slaughter weight at around 6 weeks of age weighing around 3.5 kg In contrast, non-selected breeds may require 11 weeks of rearing to reach 1.7 kg Pekin ducks will grow between 60 and 80 g per day and are generally considered to be robust under intensive conditions. Mortality will be in the region of 5% which is comparable with broilers. A decline in physical scores such as gait and cleanliness are seen to a greater extent when life cycle is taken beyond 40 days of age.

15.4.2   Egg Strains

While the Pekin strain is a prolific egg producer, there are other strains that have been selected specifically for egg production, which include the Khaki Campbell and the Indian

Runner, both of which will have a small adult body size but still produce a good-sized egg and are therefore feed efficient. Khaki Campbells will lay approximately 300 eggs a year. As with meat, duck egg production and consumption are more concentrated in Asia. The critical considerations for ducks kept for eggs are the number, positioning and bedding of nest-boxes, appropriate nutrition with a focus on calcium and ensuring high levels of egg hygiene, whether they are destined for human consumption or incubation. In contrast with ducks reared for meat, egg strains will spend a great deal longer on the farm and so there is less opportunity periodically to depopulate and decontaminate the environment. This introduces an increased risk of disease associated with the persistent presence of ducks in the housing and any outdoor areas.

15.4.3 Environment

Housing of ducks may take different forms but generally must attempt to provide adequate temperature, ventilation and lighting to satisfy the environmental requirements for animal welfare, growth or egg production. Ducks are hardy in comparison with other domesticated poultry and capable of sustaining production under extreme environmental conditions due to a broad thermoneutral zone of approximately 7°C to 25°C. Regardless of this robustness, if the objective is to achieve a steady supply of eggs or meat production then optimizing temperature control must be achieved. Inadequate ventilation will contribute to an increase in temperature during warm weather and the accumulation of noxious gases which are a hazard for personnel and will negatively impact on the health and welfare of the animals. The source, intensity and duration of lighting are important considerations to simulate natural photoperiodism and the processes such as feeding behaviour and egg laying that are dependent on it.

15.4.4 Housing

Ducks kept for meat or egg production may be housed either wholly indoors or may have access to an outdoor range for part of the day. Indoor systems may be similar to broiler houses, incorporating litter, slats or cages. Research has shown that caged systems can produce heavier birds. This may be due to the lack of opportunities to exercise thus conserving energy. Caged ducks represent considerable welfare concerns and are increasingly rejected as a means of producing eggs by consumers; therefore, there is little merit to embarking on this type of housing system, particularly where future legislation is likely to prohibit it. Critical environmental variables in indoor operations are easier to monitor and control in comparison with accommodation with range access; however, there is a perception of improved welfare in the latter which may appeal to the consumer. Furthermore, the costs of housing may be reduced in outdoor systems as stocking rate can be alleviated by access to the range. Various housing systems will bring advantages and challenges which must be managed. There has been reported to be little difference in growth rate generally for various commonly used meat duck strains between non-caged housing systems with or without access to an outdoor range, but this may be subject to the range usage by the ducks and climatic conditions.

Stocking rate is an important consideration to ensure an adequate return on available housing space, but too high a stocking density will impact growth rate or egg production, welfare and the quality of the product (meat or eggs). Stocking rate guidelines will vary from region to region and be dependent on whether floors are solid or slatted and if there is access to an outdoor range. For example, in the UK, DEFRA guidelines permit a maximum of 50 ducklings up to 10 days old per m^2 on slatted floors and this decreases to 36 on solid floors. The maximum stocking rate for outdoor ducklings is 2500 per hectare, increasing to 5000 if grass can be maintained. These maximum stocking rates are not a target and a visual inspection of the feeding and other behaviours, plumage quality and general cleanliness of the ducks and the housing environment will provide important information on the suitability of the stocking rate.

15.4.5 Water

Water is an essential nutrition requirement provision for all animals. It is also needed to meet the special behavioural requirements of these waterfowl. Provision of a water source in the form of water lines can enable ducks access the water needed to meet their nutritional needs. Important considerations for the use of water lines are location and frequency on the site to ensure optimal consumption. Muscle and eggs are predominately composed of water and therefore bodyweight gain and egg number and size will suffer if water supply is inadequate. Furthermore, if water intake is insufficient, appetite for feed will also suffer as birds will eat and drink at similar times. A centralized water system is a useful vehicle for administering medicine to part or the whole flock if necessary. The intake of water will be impacted if the water temperature is too high or too low or has a detectable salinity to the birds. Providing water in a trough or similar open container can also meet their special behavioural needs such as bathing and preening behaviour. This is interpreted as a higher welfare state and some studies have reported improved bodyweight following provision of open water. However, access to water brings challenges including increased energy expenditure and the risk of contamination of water sources which can enhance the transfer of pathogens throughout the flock and increase mortality in younger ducks. In studies comparing water lines with troughs, it was found that ducks had higher (worse) scores for body cleanliness, increased contamination of water with potentially pathogenic bacteria and increased mortality. The wastage of water will also be far greater in line with provision of open troughs. Compromising solutions such as overhead showers to provide immersive opportunities might provide the best way to keep sanitation high and prevent contamination of water. In order to achieve satisfactory welfare it is necessary to strike a balance between productivity, health and welfare

15.4.6 Feeders

Feeders may be filled manually or automated for large operations. There are some important considerations for both. Feeders must be accessible to all birds, and this will be ensured through provision of enough feeders and ensuring enough feeder space per duck to accommodate the flock size, correct positioning and height. Ducks are communal feeders, eating small portions frequently and weaker animals will suffer if access is limited. Therefore, feed must be supplied continuously to match demand. Feed format, for example a mash or a pellet, has an impact on feed intake, feed hygiene and is discussed later in the nutrition section. Feed in pelleted form will flow better through an automated feeder system served by augers as there is less of a tendency for feed to 'bridge', resulting in periods where feed is not available to the flock. Trough space is an important consideration to ensure access to feed is comparable across the flock. The competition for trough space will lead to the stronger birds eating first and when feed is restricted, as may be the case with breeder ducks, there will be variability in feed intake leading to a lack of uniformity in body weight within the flock. There are guidelines for trough space for different countries, which in the UK, for example, recommends a feeding space of 0.5 m per 100 birds (DEFRA n.d.).

15.4.7 Bedding

There are various materials available that can be used for bedding and in nesting boxes. The selection of a suitable material will be dependent on availability, stage of production and local environmental conditions. In duck production systems, wet bedding is a significant problem due to usage of water and the production of liquid faeces. The excreta make the bedding degrade quickly, which results in the production of ammonia gas that contributes to poor air quality and facilitates the spread of disease. Poor bedding quality can contribute to the development of a group of foot lesions termed pododermatitis, also known as 'bumblefoot'. These vary in severity and constitute a health burden for ducks that compromises animal welfare and productivity. The occurrence of wet bedding litter is a complex problem, which is influenced by a variety of factors that includes building design, location of feeders and drinkers, along with the disease status and nutrition of the animals. The quality of the bed and ventilation is inextricably linked, with the provision of good ventilation improving bed quality by removing moisture and gases that build up as a result of respiration and the production of liquid faeces. Different bedding materials vary in their availability, price and ability to maintain the bed and environmental moisture content at appropriate levels. The bedding materials that are most commonly available include wood shavings, chopped straw and peat. Wood shavings have a greater capacity to absorb moisture compared with chopped straw. It is important to ensure that the wood shavings used create low amounts of dust, while it is important that straw is free from mould since both these are risk factors for respiratory diseases.

15.4.8 Nest Boxes

Provision and management of nest boxes are of critical importance, whether producing eggs for food or breeding. Some ducks may not habituate to laying in nest boxes for various reasons and such birds will lay on the floor, which produces lower quality eggs that may need cleaning, and can result in poorer outcomes from incubation. Laying outside the nest boxes is more common in younger flocks and tends to improve over time. The adaptation to nest boxes and their usage is a complex behaviour that is influenced by the availability and location of the nest boxes, social hierarchy and competition. Nest boxes should be introduced in advance of the onset of laying (24 to 28 weeks) a ratio of 4 to 5 birds per box and they should be bedded with a bedding material that readily absorbs moisture, such as wood shavings (Cherry and Morris 2008). The development of brooding behaviour will occur in some ducks, which have been given access to a nesting area and this leads to a pause in laying and egg production. The onset of brooding may be discouraged in some regions by restricting access to nest boxes after the peak lay period in the morning. This reduces the incidence of broodiness but may increase the prevalence of floor eggs.

15.4.9   Temperature

The body temperature of an adult duck is approximately 41°C and adult ducks exhibit various physiological and behavioural mechanisms that enable them to withstand a wide range of temperatures from as low as –8°C and as high as 40°C for sustained periods (Cherry and Morris 2008). The introduction of ducklings to a brooding area requires the temperature to be maintained at a constant 32°C, following which the temperature should be decreased progressively in small decrements of 0.5 to 1°C per day up until approx. 14 days of age. Once ducklings have developed their feathering, by approx. 20 days of age, the temperature should be maintained at approx. 15–17°C for optimal health and production. The behaviour of the birds should be monitored to assess suitability of temperature, especially during the brooding phase of ducklings. Ducklings that group together tightly and are noisy are clear indicators that they are too cold, whereas birds that lie far apart with legs extended, exhibit panting and/ or appear listless and sleepy are indicators that they are too hot. In either of these situations, this will lead to less productivity, greater rates of morbidity and mortality. Ducks that are feathered and well grown can withstand small fluctuations in environmental temperatures. However, ducks will need to expend energy to maintain homeostasis when they are maintained below their thermo-neutral range. Ducks maintained in excessively hot conditions exhibit panting known as gular fluttering and, in these situations such as during hot weather, the provision of access to open water sources that will enable them to dissipate heat. The lower limit of the thermoneutral range is influenced not only by air temperature but also the type of floor and the insulative properties of the bedding. The behaviour of ducks maintained below the thermoneutral zone is less apparent, but these animals use more energy to maintain homeothermy, which impacts negatively on productivity and/or feed conversion efficiency.

15.4.10   Ventilation

The purpose of ventilation is to assist with the regulation of temperature, introduce fresh air and remove water vapour, carbon dioxide (CO_2) and other gases that may impact negatively on the health and productivity of birds. The adequate removal of water vapour arising from respiration and liquid faeces from ducks is important in maintaining low relative humidity and litter quality. The production of noxious gas is generated from the excreta mingling with water and litter, which volatilizes over time. The rate of noxious gases release is much less pronounced at lower than higher environmental temperatures. Ventilation needs to be adequate to clear these noxious gasses, which include ammonia and hydrogen sulphide. There may be legal limits for ammonia and CO_2, and while these limits differ with region, the UK limit ammonia to 20 ppm and CO_2 to 3000 ppm (DEFRA n.d.). However, ammonia levels < 10 ppm should be applied as a target to avoid lower productivity and poor welfare and the occurrence of health issues such as poor gait, foot pad lesions, reduced growth rate and higher mortality rates that are associated with higher temperatures, greater relative humidity and higher ammonia concentrations. Therefore, the adequate removal of 'stale' air improves air quality, thus improving animal welfare and productivity and a ventilation rate of 1.2 m^3/s for each 1000 kg of body weight has been suggested. However, the actual ventilation rate required depends on various factors which include floor and bedding type, along with the ambient temperature. Ventilation may be provided naturally, through building siting and design and/or the addition of automated ventilation, each of which have their own merits and disadvantages (further details can be found in Cherry and Morris 2008).

15.4.11   Lighting

Ducks, like chickens, are photosensitive and have specific requirements for light intensity and duration to ensure normal development and reproduction. In the wild, ducks tend to exhibit greater feeding activity at twilight and their eyes are thus accustomed to feeding at low lux. A light intensity of 10 lux is sufficient to stimulate normal behaviour, but consideration must also be given for the ability of stockpersons to inspect animals and assess the environment. Greater activity is stimulated by greater light intensity, but this can lead to aggression and feather pulling. However, directly following hatching it may be advantageous to provide continuous light for the first 48 hours to facilitate orientation towards the feeders and drinkers, which encourages appetite and feed intake.

The regional guidance regarding lighting requirements should be consulted when designing lighting programs. In the UK for example, DEFRA guidelines state that ducklings should receive a period of reduced light intensity to allow them to become accustomed to the dark gradually and minimize panic if there is a power failure. A stepwise increase and decrease in lighting should be operated to avoid sudden changes in light intensity which might also create panic. At the onset of lay a stepwise increase in light duration to mimic increasing day length, as is used for chickens, will be suitable to prepare ducks for lay and maintain egg production. An example of a suggested lighting program can be viewed at the New South Wales Department of Primary Industries website (NSW). Research has shown that ducks exposed to seasonal light changes produce less eggs. Exposing them to a light duration and intensity typical to winter months (8 hours at 65 lux and 16 hours at 1 lux) compared with summer months (14.5 hours at 65 lux and 9.5 hours at 1 lux) can be avoided by increasing the duration and lux of lighting for ducks during the winter months.

15.5   Reproduction and Provision of Replacement Animals

The selection of breeding stock is based on whether ducks are being kept for egg or meat production. The specialist breeding companies are an important source of replacement livestock for commercial industry. These ducks have been selected to have maximum performance for a range of important traits and obtaining birds from this route provides the opportunity to take advantage of the latest genetic progress. These animal breeding companies provide guidance on the expected performance targets, best management practices and nutrition programme for the specific strains/lines of ducks. This prevents potential management issues, such as over-feeding of breeding birds from meat production lines, resulting in them becoming under or overweight for optimal laying performance and mating. Breeding replacement livestock from within the existing farm stock will lower the risk of introducing disease into the flock, but it will not allow the flock to benefit from the best contemporary genetics available. Furthermore, breeding companies tend to operate very high biosecurity standards, so the risk of introducing disease is relatively low.

15.5.1   Management of Breeding Ducks

Female ducks will commence laying eggs around 24 to 28 weeks of age. This can be controlled to some extent through the availability of feed and lighting (see previous section). Male birds should be placed with the female birds at a ratio of 1 male for every 5 females for meat line ducks and 1 male for every 7 to 8 females for egg-laying duck strains. Males should be reared separately from the females but in the early stages of rearing 1 female per 4.5/5 males should also be in the male pen from day old: these are known as imprinting females and this prevents homosexuality and a decline in fertile eggs. Unfortunately, ducks tend to bury their eggs in the litter and eggs that are visibly dirty should be decontaminated to lower the risk of the egg becoming infected by microbes. Younger laying flocks lay a greater proportion of eggs on the floor, rather in nest boxes, which results in a greater risk of microbial contamination and infection during incubation, leading to lower hatching performance. During incubation, the eggs should be inspected using a light (candling) at approximately the tenth day of incubation, so that infertile eggs and those that have been subject to early embryo mortality can be removed. In terms of hatching date, Mallard type duck eggs take approx. 28 days to hatch, while Muscovy eggs take between 32 and 35 days.

15.6   Livestock Monitoring

It is important to carry out livestock monitoring frequently to identify, intervene and thus prevent or mitigate problems that may occur. A knowledge and understanding of normal and abnormal behaviour in ducks is an important skill (see below). Livestock monitoring includes the assessment of the environment and the ducks to ensure conditions are optimal. The frequency of inspections should be greater for young ducklings, as suboptimal conditions can lead to morbidity and mortality more rapidly compared with older animals, which are more resilient. Technology in the form of temperature and humidity sensors and recording equipment such as cameras can be valuable tools for livestock monitoring. Such capabilities are improving and becoming cheaper, facilitating the collection of close to real-time data regarding the environment and animals. However, technology should be used as aid to, rather than a replacement for, direct inspections.

15.6.1 Normal and Abnormal Behaviour

The behaviour of ducks is strongly centred around their social nature, which is evident from the loud quacking of a single duck when it is separated from its pen-mates. The assessment of normal and abnormal behaviour focuses on the flock and how individual ducks behave in relation to each other. Ducks typically congregate together in large groups, except when engaging in feeding or reproductive behaviours. This contrasts with huddling and other behaviours seen in young ducklings and older ducks that are too cold. In duck production, abnormal behaviour may be observed as stereotypies (which describe repetitive, seemingly functionless behaviour) or in acts of aggression. Such aggression may influence the behaviour of other ducks, such as avoidance of areas within the enclosure such as nest boxes, or direct injury ranging from plumage damage to cannibalism. These behaviours are deviations from normal behaviour and therefore constitute indicators of poor welfare. It is important to modify the environment, management and nutrition to avoid abnormal behaviour. Feather pecking and cannibalism can be evident in flocks for no apparent reason and these behaviours are very difficult to resolve once learned. Such behaviours can be associated with specific strains or lines of ducks, and Muscovy ducks are particularly renowned for cannibalism. This cannibalism is a consequence of redirected foraging behaviour, which may not be fulfilled in intensive production and does not respond to provision of forage when introduced experimentally. Where permitted by local legislation the risk of aggression can be minimized or prevented through methods such as beak tipping and declawing to minimize the damage that birds can inflict. However, the beak is richly enervated and such procedures will be acutely painful around the time of the procedure and are likely to leave the animal with chronic pain. Toe clipping can affect birds to the extent of two days lost growth due to the discomfort and mobility reduction at time of insult.

15.7 Handling

There will frequently be a need to handle ducks, for example to conduct close examinations of health status and administer vaccinations or medicines. The approach adopted is dependent on the age of the animal and designed to protect the safety of the stockperson and animal. Ducks can initially be restrained briefly on the ground by placing a hand gently around the base of the neck, while taking great care not to put pressure on the trachea. Ducks should not be caught by the legs, which are prone to injuries such as hip dislocation. Once feathering has occurred, the wings must be restrained to avoid injury to the duck and the operator. Small to medium sized ducks can then be restrained by placing a thumb over each wing, while holding them in two hands by encircling the body. Larger ducks require picking up by putting one arm under the body while using your fingers to restrain the legs, by hooking your fingers around them. The head of the duck placed tucked under your arm and the other arm should be placed around the wings to provide support and avoid them flapping and causing injury. Muscovy ducks have claws, particularly the large males, which can cause injury if not handled carefully.

15.8   Euthanasia and Slaughter

At some point ducks will need to be euthanized, either on humane grounds for birds that are in poor health or for the purpose of consumption. In many countries slaughter is likely to take place in an abattoir. For these and birds euthanized outside of a licensed abattoir, the local legislation and guidelines must be followed in order to protect the welfare of the animal up until the point of loss of consciousness. Several online publications (United Nations (www.oie.int); European Member States (http://data.europa.eu/eli/reg/2009/1099/oj); United Kingdom (https://www.gov.uk/government/collections/welfare-of-animals-at-the-time-of-killing)) provide a good overview of the steps which should be taken to ensure animals are humanely dispatched with a minimum of stress, pain and discomfort. Slaughter methods are usually a two-step process involving (i) a loss of consciousness (stunning) and (ii) causing the death of the animal. For poultry including ducks, the main approaches to achieving loss of consciousness and death are (i) electrical stunning (followed by neck cutting and neck dislocation), (ii) concussion stunning, (iii) neck dislocation and (iv) gassing. In an emergency, cervical dislocation is performed by restraining the bird by the legs at chest height in one hand and, with the other hand placed behind the skull at the back of the neck, pressing rapidly downwards while tilting the bird's head back toward the tail, or by resting the bird's breast on the bent knee and then dislocating the head from the neck as above. It may be helpful to keep the arm straight and thrust down from the shoulder. Check that the operation has been successfully carried out by feeling for the gap in the vertebrae. Following successful dislocation, the duck may spasm and convulse for a short period. Death may be confirmed thereafter by lack of breathing and a heartbeat.

15.9   Nutrition

Ducks are omnivorous and in the wild they consume a range of plant and animal-based food sources, including seeds, plants and invertebrates. The duck, as with other poultry, has a simple digestive system that has implications for the range and digestibility of ingredients in order to support meat and egg production. The digestive system of the duck has some features that contrast with that of the chicken. Ducks do not possess a true crop: instead the oesophagus in the duck is modified to expand and facilitate the opportunistic consumption of substantial amounts of food. In intensive duck production the objective is to maximize the output of meat or eggs and nutrition focuses on providing enough carbohydrate, fat and protein to satisfy these requirements. These nutrients constitute the most expensive parts of the diet and may have the greatest impact on productivity. The feed conversion ratio (feed consumed/weight gained) of commercial strains of Pekin are approx. 1.8 to 2:1. Ducks that have access to pasture, consume grass enthusiastically. There is a lack of knowledge about the contribution this makes to the nutritional requirements of the animal, but excessive grass consumption may dilute the intake of a carefully formulated diet, while access to pasture may have beneficial effects on animal welfare by providing a source of enrichment.

Ducks require a species-specific balance of essential amino acids, vitamins and minerals that need to be supplied at the correct concentrations depending on the purpose (meat or eggs) and the physiological stage of production. There has been a tendency to rely on broiler chicken research to construct duck feed formulations, due to the lack of information about the nutrient requirements of ducks. In terms of limiting essential amino acids methionine is the first, followed by lysine, which is due to inadequate amounts found in the cereals that are used to formulate duck feeds. These limiting amino acids are added through inclusion of protein from feed resources such as soybean or rapeseed meal, or through addition of free amino acids. The dietary amino acid concentration lowers as ducks age, due to greater appetite and lower requirements, with the exception of the grower-finisher stage (~22 to 42 days of age) during which greater concentrations of methionine may be required to meet the demand for feather development. The main difference between laying and meat ducks is the much greater requirement for calcium by laying ducks, to support shell formation. In terms of the diet one of the important considerations is the format of the diet itself, which may be provided as a mash or in a pelleted form. Mash is usually less expensive but can cause caking around the beak and may deliver variable concentrations of nutrients due to settling of fine ingredients, while ducks may also be able to sort and select ingredients from feed provided. Pellets are usually more expensive than mash, but they are more likely to deliver a balanced nutrient supply and they tend not to bridge in silos or block augers compared to mash. Furthermore, the high temperatures which arise during the pelleting process will reduce the risk of microbial contamination of feedstuffs; an important consideration particularly for younger ducks.

15.10 Disease

Ducks are hardy relative to other poultry species. However, they can succumb to various diseases and much like other poultry, intensification may contribute to the incidence and spread of microbial infections (for a detailed discussion on diseases in ducks see Gooderham 1993). The main consideration and management factors critical to prevent outbreak and spread of disease include the selection and introduction of new stock into the flock, nutrition and welfare, hygiene and environmental control. Other important considerations are the prevention and control of disease transfer to humans. Waterfowl are an important reservoir for clinically relevant zoonoses for humans. Ducks may be contaminated with *Campylobacter*

Table 15.1 Suggested nutrient composition of diets for meat type (1 to 42 days of age) and egg-type ducks.

Nutrient	1 to 21 d	22 to 42 d	Laying period
Metabolizable energy MJ/kg	12.2	12.6	10.5
Met energy kcal/kg	2.9	3.0	2.5
Crude protein, g/kg	200	180	170
Methionine, g/kg	5	4.7–5	4
Lysine, g/kg	11	10	8
Threonine, g/kg	4.8 to 5	4.7 to 5	6
Tryptophan, g/kg	2.3	2.3	2.1
Calcium, g/kg	8.3	8.9	36
Non-phytate phosphorus, g/kg	4.6	3.8	3.5
Manganese, mg/kg	80 to 100	80 to 100	90
Zinc, mg/kg	60	60	90
Iron, mg/kg	60	60	50
Copper, mg/kg	10	10	10
Iodine, mg/kg	0.2	0.2	0.5
Selenium, mg/kg	0.3	0.3	0.4
Vitamin A, IU	10,000	8,000	12,000
Vitamin D3, IU	3,000	3,000	2,000
Vitamin E, IU	20	20	38
Vitamin K, IU	2	2	1
Thiamine, Vitamin B1, mg/kg	2	2	3
Riboflavin, Vitamin B2, mg/kg	10	8	9.6
Pyridoxine, Vitamin B6, mg/kg	4	4	6
Cyanocobalamin, Vitamin B12, mg/kg	0.02	0.02	0.03
Choline, mg/kg	1,000	750	500
Pantothenic acid, mg/kg	20	10	28.5
Folic acid, mg/kg	1	1	0.6
Biotin, mg/kg	0.2	0.2	0.15
Niacin, mg/kg	100	50	50

(Adapted from Whitehead 2001; Rodehutscord 2005; Fouad et al. 2018; Fan et al. 2019).

spp., *Salmonella* and *Listeria monocytogenes*, which display varying degrees of antibiotic resistance. While these microbes may not result in clinical symptoms of disease in ducks they can potentially cause serious illness in humans. A pathogen which causes serious disease for ducks is *Riemerella anatipesifer*. This is of primary concern in young ducks and may be precipitated by poor hygiene, which allows the pathogen to be inhaled or gain entry through foot lesions. In addition, stress has been implicated as a trigger to infection and *Riemeralla* infections can be accompanied by a secondary bacterial pathogen such as *Escherichia coli*. The preventative measures include good hygiene practices, which include disinfection between batches and operating all-in, all-out policies to lower bacterial load and in breeding farms, the washing of visibly contaminated eggs to prevent the risk of vertical infection.

Wet harvesting conditions can result in feed being contaminated with mycotoxins, which are fungal metabolites that develop in feed during crop growth, harvest and storage. Ducks and ducklings in particular, are more susceptible to mycotoxins than chickens and can develop mycotoxicosis. When sourcing and storing feeds the aim should be to maintain a low moisture content, which limits the development of fungus and greater concentrations of mycotoxins. Should feed be contaminated with mycotoxins there are various feed additives available that adsorb to the toxins and limit the toxicity post ingestion.

Ducks are vulnerable to several viral infections such as duck viral hepatitis-1, duck viral enteritis and bacterial infections such as *Streptococcal spp.*, *Pasteurella multocida* and *Erysipelothrix rhusiopathiae*. Good management of hygiene and prevention of stress should protect ducks from developing such infections, but veterinary consultation should be sought in the diagnosis and treatment of these. In addition to controlling the external environment, stimulating the natural microflora or microbiota of ducks is an important factor in limiting the subsequent onset of disease. The commensal and symbiotic members of the gut microbiota are valuable in combatting colonization and infection with potential pathogens. The process of microbiota development is stimulated by many differing factors, which include feed intake, antibiotics, supplements and other nutraceuticals, enzyme activities, age of the host, genetic modification and the whole environment. The gut microbial community is dynamic in the days immediately post hatching and is an opportune time to ensure ducklings don't become contaminated with pathogens by stimulating beneficial microbes, which can be achieved primarily through the dietary provision of pre- and probiotics.

15.11 Market Considerations

15.11.1 Duck Meat Production

Duck is a popular meat in many parts of the world, most notably Asia. While in parts of Europe, this sector is growing steadily, it remains a niche market relative to chicken meat consumption. Duck meat is a good source of protein, iron, selenium and niacin. Duck meat is lower in calories compared with many beef cuts and duck breast without skin is lower in calories (140 cal vs 165 cal), lower in fat (2.5 g vs. 4 g), and richer in iron (5 mg vs. 1 mg) compared to chicken breast without skin. Duck meat consumption in Europe and North America leads to a market in which in excess of 26 m ducks were slaughtered in 2017, of which Pekin type ducks weigh between 2.9 and 3.5 kg at six to seven weeks of age depending on various factors including genotype, housing system, nutrition and sex. Male ducks grow faster and have a greater final weight than females. The subsequent carcass components and some of the various organs are heavier from male compared with female ducks, including the gizzard, liver, breast and thighs. The major components of the saleable meats are, breast (~17%), back meat (~20%), thighs (~16%) and wings (8.5%) and the overall carcass yield is approx. 70 to 72%.

15.11.2 Duck Egg Production

Duck eggs are a good source of amino acids and various vitamins and minerals. Duck eggs are heavier than chicken eggs, weighing between 70 and 80 g, while a chicken egg will weigh between 60 and 65 g. As with chickens, the egg tends to increase in size as the duck ages, while the amount of eggshell and albumen decreases, and the yolk increases in size. Eggs have several mechanisms that repel microorganisms, of which the most important are the inner membranes that impede entry and the albumen which contains antimicrobial peptides retarding their growth. Duck eggs that have been contaminated with micro-organisms spoil faster than chicken eggs, although they have better storage ability, which is not worsened over time. Eggs remain an important source of human gastroenteritis and egg hygiene is an important consideration in their production.

15.12 Future Directions

The duck is a remarkably versatile food animal and the production sector is one that continues to expand. The genetic selection for growth and egg production has resulted in the production of high performing birds, with more specific management and nutrition requirements. Duck nutrition relies to a great extent on guidelines for broiler chicken and laying hens and would greatly benefit from more direct research on ducks. This should include a greater understanding of how to provide opportunities for ducks to exhibit more normal behaviour under intensive conditions to improve animal welfare and the perception of the industry.

References and Further Reading

Cherry, P. and Morris, T.R. (2008). *Domestic Duck Production: Science and Practice*. CABI.

DEFRA (Department for Environment, Food & Rural Affairs). (n.d.). https://www.gov.uk/government/publications/poultry-on-farm-welfare/ducks-mallard-and-pekin-welfare-recommendations.

Fan, L., He, Z.Z., Ao, X., Sun, W.L., Xiao, X., Zeng, F.K., Wang, Y.C., and He, J. (2019). Effects of residual superdoses of phytase on growth performance, tibia mineralization, and relative organ weight in ducks fed phosphorus-deficient diets. *Polutant Science* 98 (9): 3926–3936.

FAO. (2018). *World Food and Agriculture – Statistical Pocketbook*. Rome, 254 p.

Fouad, A.M., Ruan, D., Wang, S., Chen, W., Xia, W., and Zheng, C. (2018). Nutritional requirements of meat-type and egg-type ducks: what do we know? *Journal of Animal Science and Biotechnology* 9 (1): 1.

Gooderham, K.R. (1993). Disease prevention and control in ducks. In: *The Health of Poultry* (ed. M. Pattison). Harlow, UK: Longman.

Hrnčár, C., Weis, J., Petričová, L., and Bujko, J. (2014). Effect of housing system, slaughter age and sex on slaughter and carcass parameters of broiler ducks. *Scientific Papers: Animal Science and Biotechnologies* 47 (2): 254257.

Merck Veterinary Manual. (2016). 11e. Kenilworth, NJ: Merck & Co. INC.

NSW New South Wales Department of Primary Industries. https://www.dpi.nsw.gov.au/ animals-and-livestock/poultry-and-birds/species/duck-raising/egg-production.

Rodehutscord, M. (2005). Towards an optimal utilisation of phosphorus sources in growing meat ducks. 15th European Symposium on Poultry Nutrition, 86–96. Balatonfüred, Hungary.

Whitehead, C. (2001). Nicotinic acid in poultry nutrition. *Feed Mix* 9 (1): 32–34.

16

Game Birds

David Welchman

KEY CONCEPTS

16.1   Introduction

The term 'game birds' is broad and can be taken to include any bird shot for sport, whether wild or reared. This chapter will cover only those species that are bred and reared for shooting in the UK, namely pheasants and red-legged and grey partridges. It will not cover species such as red grouse (*Lagopus lagopus*) (which are managed and shot for sport in the UK but not reared artificially) and ducks (particularly mallard, *Anas platyrhynchos*) of which small numbers are bred and reared for game shooting but which are covered in Chapter 15. The approaches to game bird rearing and release vary in different countries and can differ from those used in the UK, for example, in the use of much shorter release periods in continental Europe and the US (Madden et al. 2018), but these other approaches are not covered in this chapter.

Management and Welfare of Farm Animals: The UFAW Farm Handbook, Sixth Edition.
Edited by John Webster and Jean Margerison.
© Universities Federation for Animal Welfare 2022. Published 2022 by John Wiley & Sons Ltd.

The principal game bird reared for shooting in Britain is the common or ring-necked pheasant (*Phasianus colchicus*) which was originally introduced in the eleventh century or possibly as far back as Roman times, has been reared artificially at least since Victorian times, and which is common in the wild or semi-wild state. Its preferred habitat is woodland and woodland edges with ample cover of long grass and other undergrowth. There are several different strains of the common pheasant, including more traditional strains such as the Chinese ringneck and recently introduced strains such as the Michigan Blue Back, and crosses between different strains. There are also heavier and lighter types of bird; although proponents of individual strains claim various advantages, particularly in flying ability compared with other strains, all are bred and reared in a similar way.

The second most common game bird is the red-legged or French partridge (*Alectoris rufa*). This species is also found in the wild and semi-wild state and was first introduced in the eighteenth century from southern Europe. In Britain its habitat in the wild is open fields and downland and birds gather together in small family groups called coveys. Accurate figures for the numbers of game birds reared in the UK are not available but one estimate is of 34.9 million birds (BASC 2015) of which 80% are pheasants and the remainder are partridges. The third species is the grey, English or common partridge (*Perdix perdix*) which is a native species of game bird whose numbers have been closely monitored in recent years as an example of a declining farmland species. Its natural habitat is fields and other open countryside with access to rough cover, and family parties stay together in coveys through the winter. Relatively small numbers of grey partridges, mainly of continental stock, are reared for shooting each year.

The purpose of game bird rearing in Britain is to produce a bird fit for release into the semiwild for shooting in the autumn and winter. For pheasants the shooting season in England, Wales and Scotland extends from 1 October to 1 February (31 January in Northern Ireland), and for partridges from 1 September to 1 February (31 January in Northern Ireland). The Game Act (1831) and other legislation enacted in the nineteenth century gives protection to birds during the closed season

The rearing of game birds is essentially a seasonal activity which is still based on the natural seasonal life cycle of the birds in the wild state. The seasonal cycle comprises the selection of adult breeding stock in the spring, egg production, incubation and hatching, the rearing of young birds and their eventual release into a semi-wild state in the autumn. The large numbers of birds that are now reared have necessitated the adoption of relatively intensive management and husbandry practices similar in principle to those used in commercial poultry, for example, for the incubation of eggs and the management of chicks during the critical first few days of life. The numbers of game birds bred and reared in this country are supplemented by imports, principally from France, and it is estimated that approximately half of the pheasants and 90% of the red-legged partridges reared are imported, mostly as eggs or day-old chicks, with a smaller number of poults at a few weeks of age.

Game birds are bred and reared in a wide variety of enterprises. These include game farms which have their own breeding stock and hatchery, and which may rear many tens of thousands of birds each year, and enterprises that buy in poults at a few weeks of age purely for release for shooting. Although the increase in the number of game birds reared has required greater intensification, nevertheless the important difference from commercial poultry keeping is that the end result is required to be a bird which is able to survive in a semi-wild or wild state. The seasonal nature of game bird rearing means that the capital and labour costs involved have to be met over a much shorter period than in the poultry industry, and the level of investment, for example, in hatcheries, is correspondingly lower except in the case of very large enterprises.

16.1.1 Welfare Legislation and Code of Practice

The Code of Practice for the welfare of game birds reared for sporting purposes was published by Defra in 2010, under the Animal Welfare Act 2006 and similar codes were also introduced in Scotland and Wales. The purpose of the Code is to provide practical guidance in relation to welfare legislation for birds bred and reared under controlled conditions for the purpose of shooting for sport, together with wild birds retained for breeding purposes. No specific legislation regulates the breeding and rearing of birds for sporting purposes but gamebird breeders and keepers must comply with the relevant legislation applying to their situation (Defra 2010). Game birds are covered up to their time of release into the wild by similar welfare legislation to poultry, including the Animal Welfare Act 2006, and the Welfare of Animals (Transport)(England) Order 2006 (and the equivalent legislation in Scotland, Wales and Northern Ireland). Game birds are also covered by notifiable disease legislation including the Avian Influenza (Preventative Measures) (England) Regulations 2006 (and equivalent legislation in Scotland, Wales and Northern Ireland) which includes the requirement that premises with over 50 game birds are registered in the same way as with all other types of poultry.

16.2 Pheasant Breeding and Rearing

16.2.1 Breeding and Egg Production

The pheasant season starts in January and February when adult birds are selected for breeding. These are usually birds hatched the previous year and are either kept in large covered pens over the winter or are sometimes 'caught up' from the wild (that is, they are adult birds that were released the previous autumn, and spent the intervening winter period in a semi-wild state, often relatively close to their point of release). Good-quality, healthy birds that are free from injuries or evidence of disease should be selected for breeding; however, the practice of catching up inevitably means that the disease status of such birds is unknown. By the end of February the birds are placed into breeding pens which are usually on grass and of two general types:

- large group (flock) pens with up to several hundred females (hens) and an approximately 1 : 8 ratio of males:females (cocks:hens);
- single harem pens containing seven to ten hens and one cock.

Flock pens on grass should have a space allowance of 4 to 5 m^2 per bird stocked although in practical terms this is more than is usually available (FAWC 2008). Egg production is generally better if flock size is less than 150 birds per pen. Flock pens should be arranged so that some cover is available to reduce aggression and fighting between the cocks and undue stress on the hens, poor egg production and infertility, and it is desirable that the pen should be subdivided into smaller areas to allow for the territorial nature of cocks. Perches should be provided for the birds, to allow for their natural roosting behaviour. Breeding pens are commonly enclosed with wire mesh sides up to approximately 1.5 m high. Single harem pens may be totally enclosed; if the breeding pens are open topped, the practice is to either clip the primary wing feathers of one wing or to fit an elastic 'braille' which prevents the bird stretching out one wing, in order to stop the birds flying out of the pen. Brailles should be removed when the birds leave the breeding pen. Adult breeding birds are sometimes fitted with 'spex' ('specs' or 'spectacles') which fit over the beak and are designed to obstruct forwards binocular vision to reduce aggression, cannibalism and egg pecking, but these can damage the nasal septum and should not be regarded as a substitute for good management. In some cases, larger anti-aggression masks or 'shrouds' are fitted over the head for the same purpose but the Code states that these should not generally be used as a form of bird management (Defra 2010). The space allowance required in single harem pens can be as low as 0.5 m^2 per bird. Single harem pens are more labour intensive and carry the obvious proviso that fertility should be monitored in the event of poor performance by the cock. During the breeding season the birds are fed a proprietary breeder ration with up to 20% protein content (Table 16.1).

The first eggs are normally produced in early April and the laying season extends until June, by which time a hen pheasant will have laid up to 50 to 55 eggs. The layout of the pen should allow hens to have undisturbed access to nesting areas or nest boxes with nesting material such as straw, and it is important that this should be kept as dry as possible to reduce

Table 16.1 Examples of descriptions, purpose and protein concentration (%) of commercial game bird feeds used at different production stages.

Feed type	Purpose	Protein concentration Pheasants Partridge
Pre-breeder pellets	From catching to 3 weeks pre-lay	13 13
Breeder pellets	From 3 weeks pre-lay and throughout lay	17.5–20 20
Chick starter crumbs	Chicks in first 2–3 weeks	28–30 28
Mini pellets	Chicks 2–6 weeks	25–28 25–28
Early grower pellets	Pheasants 4–12 W, Partridges 6–12 W	20–25 20–25
Poult release pellets	12 weeks onwards	16–18 16–18
Maintenance pellets	For use during the shooting season and over winter	14–15 16–18

fungal and bacterial contamination of the egg-shell. Eggs should be collected at least twice a day, in order to minimize the time the egg is left in the open. At least one collection should be made in the evening as the majority of eggs are laid in the afternoon and early evening. After collection, eggs should be sorted to remove any with cracked shells and other problems such as abnormal shell thickness and abnormally sized eggs; issues of this type may result in approximately 8% of eggs being rejected. The eggs should be washed (sanitized) promptly with a proprietary sanitizing agent following the manufacturer's instructions in order to prevent the entry into the egg of surface contaminants which may lead to death of the embryo. After sanitization and drying, the eggs are stored at 13 to 17°C before being set. However, there is a gradual loss of hatchability during storage, reaching approximately 10% by two weeks. Eggs are often set twice weekly to achieve a compromise between management requirements and viability of the embryo.

Game bird eggs are universally set in artificial incubators, which vary considerably in size and design, but are increasingly located in specialised hatcheries. The eggs are incubated at 37.6°C and at approximately 50% relative humidity, to achieve a target of 14% loss of weight over the incubation period which allows the airspace within the egg to develop. Large game farms and some smaller enterprises have access to their own incubators or hatcheries which enable them to maintain the traceability of the eggs. However sometimes eggs are sent away for incubation and an equivalent number of hatched chicks received back afterwards, which may not be from the same source, a practice known as 'custom hatching'. Custom hatching carries the risk of introducing disease from other sites. The principles of incubation and hatching, and the problems that can arise, are similar in game birds as in commercial poultry and outside the scope of this chapter, but further details can be found in references such as Game Conservancy Advisory Service (1993). It is essential to maintain high standards of hygiene within the hatchery, especially if eggs from multiple sources are being incubated. The incubation time for pheasant and grey partridge eggs is 21 days, and for red-legged partridges 20 days, after which eggs are transferred to the hatchery. Hatching should be complete within a further 3 days. Under optimal conditions a hatchability of at least 70% should be attained for the season as a whole, although the method of calculating the figure depends on the numbers of 'help outs' (chicks that require help breaking out of their shell during hatching) that are included, which may comprise 10% of the total (Wise 1993) but which may go on to rear as healthy chicks.

16.2.1.1 Alternative Breeding Systems

As an alternative to the grass-based system described above, some game breeding units house breeding pheasants in indoor flock or single harem pens, or accommodate the birds in cages in the form of raised laying units. In raised laying units only enriched cages should be used and not barren cages (Defra 2010). The birds in raised laying units can be stocked at higher densities than in conventional outdoor pens with examples quoted by FAWC allowing $0.33 \, \text{m}^2$ per bird (FAWC 2008). Such systems require a particularly high standard of management to control aggression between the birds but the claimed benefits include improved health of the birds, improved egg production and greater cleanliness of the eggs. Artificial lighting can be used to extend egg production earlier in the season. Whatever housing system is used, the

Code specifies that the accommodation should meet several criteria including being well constructed and managed and of sufficient size to ensure good health and welfare, capable of being maintained in a clean and hygienic condition to avoid the risk of disease transfer, be located so as to minimize disturbance to the birds and have sufficient shelter to provide protection for birds during periods of adverse weather (Defra 2010). Further comment is provided in section 16.10 at the end of this chapter.

16.2.2 Brooding and Rearing

After hatching, the chicks are placed in chick boxes for transfer to the brooding site. It is important that chicks get a good start, particularly if they have a long journey from the hatchery to their destination brooding site, which can result in chicks becoming dehydrated and heat stressed. Chicks are traditionally placed in brooders as 'day-olds', but delays in the taking off of chicks in the hatchery or a long journey to their destination can mean that chicks are up to three days old at the time of placement. Initially the chicks are usually confined to a brooder ring approximately 2 m in diameter, within a permanent or temporary building. The brooder ring should be circular in shape to avoid the chicks becoming trapped and smothered in corners and must be fully prepared in advance in terms of hygiene, bedding and ambient temperature. Scrupulous attention to hygiene is essential, particularly if the brooder accommodation is used for successive batches of chicks through the season, to minimize the transmission of disease such as rotavirus from one batch to the next or between different batches of chicks. Chicks are bedded at this stage on a variety of materials including wood shavings and shredded cardboard; sawdust should not be used because it creates dusty conditions and may be ingested by young chicks in mistake for feed. It is vital that the bedding materials are stored in a dry condition to prevent fungal growth which can result in outbreaks of aspergillosis in the birds. The background environmental temperature within the room must be carefully monitored and for the first six to seven days should be at least 20°C throughout the day and night, and artificial heat is provided by gas brooders or electrical heaters. More localized heat can be in the form of heated plates ('electric hens'; Figure 16.1) under which the chicks are brooded, and which need to be supplemented by a means of heating the entire air space such as infra-red heaters. The temperature underneath the heat source should not exceed 37°C, with a gentle gradient out to the background temperature. The room should be well ventilated but draught free. Lighting should be controlled so that sufficient light is available for the chicks to move about and find feed but, if the light is too bright, wing pecking may occur. A ready supply of palatable feed should be made available on open trays or chick paper on the floor, initially in the form of crumbs followed by a gradual transition to mini-pellets. Proprietary crumbs have a typical protein content of 28% (Table 16.1). In the initial period after hatching, chicks derive nourishment from their yolk sac but as this becomes utilized the chicks must start to find feed and water; failure to do so, or the ingestion of bedding material instead of feed, results in 'starve-out' and death in the first week of life. Water is supplied either from floor drinkers or from overhead nipple drinkers. There should be a minimum of one drinker per 100 chicks placed. The principles of managing young chicks in the first few days of life are the

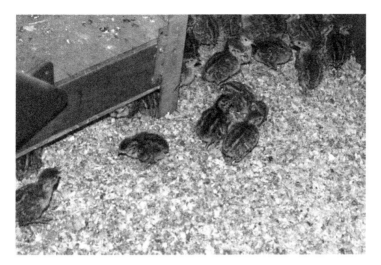

Figure 16.1 Young partridge chicks in a brooder ring. The chicks are bedded on wood shavings and can be seen emerging from beneath an 'electric hen' heater.

same as with commercial, artificially reared chicks of any domesticated species, and attention to detail is very important.

Over the next five to six days the brooder surround is removed to give the chicks more floor space, and in warm weather conditions they are gradually given access through a pop-hole to a covered ark which is partly exposed to the weather conditions outside. The growing chicks are still allowed access to the brooder area at night but, depending on the weather conditions, increasingly are allowed to spend more time in the covered ark or night shelter, and then in a grass run with wire-netted sides and roof which adjoins the ark. During this time, the availability of background heating in the brooder house is gradually reduced, in general by keeping the heaters on by night but off by day. However, poults should not be released until they have been without artificial heat for at least 10 days. Drinkers and feeders are positioned for the poults in the outside run (Figures 16.2, 16.3 and 16.4). This principle of brooder hut, night shelter and outside run

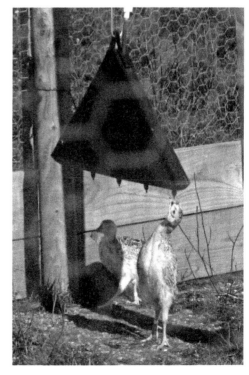

Figure 16.2 A pheasant poult drinking from a nipple drinker in an outside run. Note the correct height of the drinker above ground level.

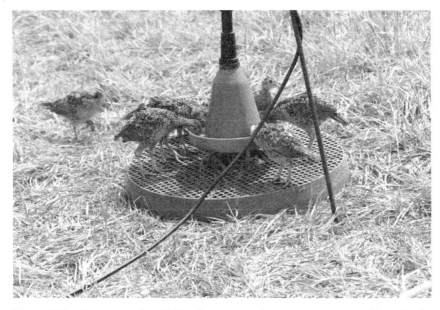

Figure 16.3 Pheasant poults drinking from a bell drinker in an outside run. Note the plastic mesh base which prevents the immediately surrounding area from getting muddy.

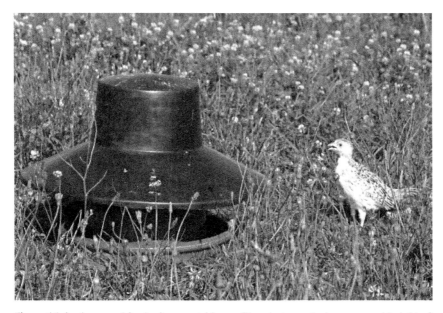

Figure 16.4 A covered feeder in an outside run. The photograph shows a good height of vegetation in the run which will help keep the birds occupied.

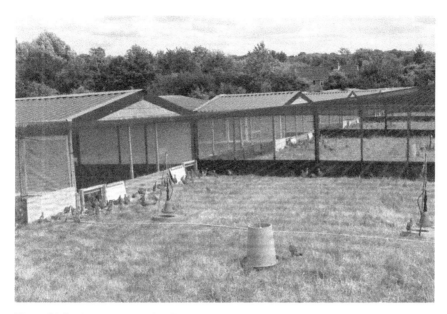

Figure 16.5 A pheasant rearing field showing the wire-netted runs and covered areas (night shelters), with pop-holes allowing the birds into and out of the covered and outside areas. The brooder huts are located behind the night shelters. A feeder is visible in the foreground with drinkers either side.

is very commonly used, but with variations in the layout on different units. Chicks in this system can be stocked at up to $70/m^2$ in the brooder hut and a minimum of $0.2\ m^2$ per bird should be allowed in the outside run. A recommended batch size is 250 birds, although up to 1000 birds can sometimes be stocked; further details of the measurements and stocking density of birds are available (Game Conservancy Advisory Services 2006). This type of accommodation is relatively easy to construct, can be used in both small and large enterprises and should ideally be moved to different positions or sites each year, which is important from a disease control point of view. Several brooder huts, night shelters and runs are often arranged side by side on the rearing field (Figure 16.5). There are also various alternatives to this system including totally enclosed housing, systems using a permanent brooder house with access to an outdoor run and systems where chicks are reared on wire mesh. Wire mesh rearing systems have benefits in terms of disease control and in some cases are designed to minimize the handling of the birds. In all types of rearing accommodation, strict attention to hygiene is of critical importance, as without it infectious agents such as rotavirus can build up in the environment, leading to disease outbreaks in successive batches of birds passing through the accommodation.

While on the rearing field, the young pheasants ('poults') must become adapted to outdoor life in preparation for entering release pens at six to eight weeks of age. This process of adaptation is referred to as 'hardening off', and for successful release the poult must have a good covering of feathers. Feather growth appears to be stimulated particularly by wetting, either from natural rainfall or by artificial means, and from the resulting preening activity of the birds. However, the emerging feathers can easily become a target for feather pecking by other birds, leaving areas of bare skin over the back of the bird, resulting in poor protection and insulation in the event of adverse weather conditions in subsequent weeks. Such birds will often fare badly if released before the feathers have re-grown. Feather pecking can be reduced by good management, for example, in the provision of stimulating surroundings with reasonably long (10 to 15 cm) vegetation and perches, to alleviate boredom. Perches also have the advantage of helping poults become accustomed to roosting above ground level, which is an important aid to their survival in the semi-wild situation after they have been released (Madden and others 2018). It has been shown that increasing the stocking density in the first six weeks of life from 0.7 to 4.0 birds per m^2 in an aviary environment is associated with a significant adverse effect on plumage quality and increased skin damage (Kjaer 2004). These are lower stocking densities than those used in commercial practice which may be up to 10 birds per m^2. It is also common for poults to be fitted with plastic 'bits' which clip into the nostrils and prevent feather pecking (Figure 16.6). The bits are fitted at approximately three weeks of age and initially can cause some difficulty in feeding, particularly if the pellet size is too large. It may therefore be preferable to keep the chicks on crumbs until two or three days after bitting before introducing mini-pellets unless the latter are of a very small size. Bits are usually removed when the poults are crated up, prior to being moved to the release pen. They should be removed with clippers,

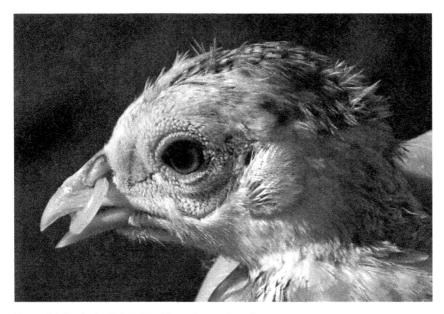

Figure 16.6   A plastic 'bit' fitted to a pheasant poult.

rather than pulled out, to reduce the risk of damage to the mucous membranes of the nasal cavity. Different sizes of bits are available which can be used for different sizes of birds. Some pheasant rearers are, however, able to manage their birds successfully without the use of bits. Bits are examples of management devices and their use should not be considered routine but should be justified on a flock by flock basis and regularly reviewed in a flock health plan (Defra 2010).

16.2.3 Pheasant Release

At approximately six to eight weeks of age the poults are caught and put into crates for transfer to the release pen. It is preferable to release birds as locally as possible to where they have been reared but in some cases poults reared by specialist game farmers have to be transported over long distances for release. They can become subject to heat stress and dehydration if attention is not given to their welfare and management during the journey and on arrival at their destination. Pheasant release pens are normally set in woodland and are surrounded by wire mesh fencing to a height of approximately 1.8 m, which must be secured to the ground and protected with an electric fence or other means around the perimeter in order to exclude predators, particularly foxes. A low stocking density within the pen of 10 m^2 per bird is recommended (see under sustainability below). The Game and Wildlife Conservation Trust (GWCT) recommends that the pen should have no square corners, to avoid birds becoming trapped, and it should comprise approximately one third each of open sunny ground, shrubby layer and trees for roosting (GWCT 2008). Feed and water are supplied to aid adaptation to this much more extensive existence. Proprietary feeds used in release pens have a protein content of 16 to 23.5% (Table 16.1) and are fed from hoppers, which should be covered to prevent the feed getting wet. It is preferable for the feeders and drinks in the release pen to be similar to those the poults have been accustomed to on the rearing field, to aid a smooth transition to the new environment. The poults are able to fly out of the pens and for the first few weeks can re-enter the pen for feeding through funnels in the fencing, designed in such a way as to exclude foxes. Growth of the birds is not complete until 18 to 20 weeks of age, by which time (October to November) they spend most or all of their life outside the release pen, although supplementary feed is still provided for them, either in the form of proprietary pellets or wheat, or a combination of the two. The pheasant shooting season starts in October.

16.3 Partridge Breeding and Rearing

The principles of red-legged and grey partridge management are similar to those for pheasants, and the aim is likewise to produce fit birds for release into the semi-wild for subsequent shooting, but there are some differences. The breeding season for partridges extends from April to July, and potentially for longer in the red-legged partridge. The two species are expected to produce 35 to 50 eggs through the season. Breeding adults are overwintered from

September in grass pens with the provision of additional cover for shelter and from January are paired off and remain in pair boxes for the remainder of the breeding season, after which they are either released or retained for a second breeding season. Pair boxes are used because of aggression between males and have been found to result in higher levels of egg production. The birds should preferably not be confined to the pair boxes for more than six months during a year, but in practice they are sometimes retained in pair boxes continually for up to three seasons. The pair boxes are raised above the ground and comprise an enclosed nest box and a small, covered exercise area with a floor of wire mesh and a feed area. The purpose of the wire mesh floor is to prevent the build-up of faecal material and enteric parasites, to which partridges are very susceptible. The box may typically measure approximately $1.4 \times 0.45 \times 0.3$ m overall (FAWC 2008) but smaller steel cages are also used. A larger floor area should be used if partridges are retained in the boxes for longer than six months in any year. The bedding for the nest box is in the form of fine grit, sand or 'Astroturf'. The incubation of the eggs and management of the young birds through the brooder and rearing phases are similar to pheasants, except that the birds are transferred at 12 to 14 weeks of age into moveable wire-mesh release pens within a cover crop and stocked at a typical density of 0.36 m^2 per bird. After 1 to 2 weeks (during August and September) the birds are then released into the cover crop, with feeders and drinkers placed in rides in the crop and in the release pens (Figure 16.7). Growth of the birds is complete at 14 weeks and the partridge shooting season starts in September.

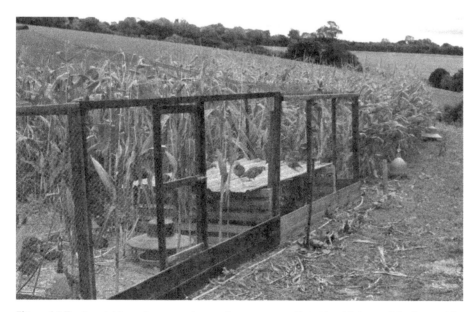

Figure 16.7 A partridge release pen in a maize cover crop. Note the drinker and feeder positioned in the ride nearby to the pen.

16.4   Sustainability of Game Bird Releasing

Releasing large numbers of game birds can adversely impact the environment in which they are released, through an adverse effect on wildlife biodiversity and damage to habitats. The GWCT has produced guidelines for sustainable releasing (GWCT 2007) which include advice on not positioning release pens within sensitive wildlife areas, limiting the numbers of pheasants within release pens to no more than 1,000/ha (700/ha in ancient woodland) and not moving release pens unless there are specific reasons for doing so. Pheasant release pens should not take up more than a third of woodland on an estate or shoot. Red-legged partridge release pens should be located on arable land rather than on natural grassland and should be located away from hedgerows of high wildlife value. However some game shooting estates take active measures to enhance wildlife diversity on their land, for example, through hedgerow management to encourage a greater variety of wild breeding birds, leaving uncultivated margins along field edges and leaving 'beetle banks' in fields which provide relatively undisturbed habitats for invertebrates and ground nesting birds such as the skylark (*Alauda arvensis*) and wild partridges.

Many gamebirds reared in the UK die for reasons other than being shot for sport. Most of the mortality occurs after release and is attributed to factors including predation (for example by foxes), disease, starvation and dispersal away from the release site. It is estimated that 60% of pheasants released do not end up being shot (Madden and others 2018). Actions that can mitigate against these losses include attention to management during the rearing period (for example by the provision of raised perches and a more varied diet, both of which may aid survival after release) and improved control of parasites, particularly nematodes. A more varied diet during the rearing period aids adaptation by reducing reliance on supplementary feeding and transition to a natural diet after release. Madden and others (2018) have suggested that undertaking actions such as these could benefit the survival rate of pheasants between two and five months of age, which could improve sustainability by reducing the numbers of birds needing to be reared, improving financial profitability and reducing the biomass of birds released into the wild.

16.5   Growth Rates of Game Birds

Table 16.2 (from Beer 1988) gives a guide to the weights of the three game bird species at different ages. Growth rates of young game birds are affected by various factors including management, diet and health, and the latter includes the effects of enteric disease and malabsorption, both of which are common. Therefore, the figures given should be taken only as approximate. There has been very little genetic selection of game birds, unlike in commercial chickens and turkeys, so the growth rates have changed little since the time they were originally published.

Table 16.2 Approximate weights (g) of game birds at different ages.

Age	Pheasant	Red-legged Partridge	Grey Partridge
Day-old	20	12	7
1 week	50	17	11
2 weeks	80	30	18
3 weeks	120	45	28
4 weeks	200	70	45
5 weeks	300	100	62
6 weeks	380	140	86
7 weeks	450	190	115
8 weeks	550	230	140
9 weeks	650	280	170
10 weeks	750	330	210
12 weeks	900	400	250
Adults: male	1400	540	390
Female	1100	480	330

Source: Beer (1988). Used with permission from the Game & Wildlife Conservation Trust (formerly The Game Conservancy Trust).

16.6 Water Intake by Game Birds

A supply of clean and palatable water must be available at all times to game birds. Figures for water intake at different ages of pheasant have been published (Beer 1988) and are reproduced in Table 16.3. Figures such as these are useful in calculating the amounts of medication that should be added to the water should this need arise, but the calculations need to take into account intake from other sources such as dew. These figures should be used only as a guide, as water intake varies with the method of feeding; intake rises in hand-fed birds after the feeding period but is more evenly spread through the day in birds fed *ad libitum* (Wise and Connan 1979). The physical consistency and water content of the feed may also affect water intake. There is little variation in water intake between ambient temperatures of 10 and 25°C. Water consumption follows a diurnal pattern with peak intake in the early hours of the morning. The water may be supplied in covered drinkers or via overhead nipple drinkers (Figures 16.2 and 16.3). When tray drinkers or bell drinkers are used it is essential that water spillage is minimized as this creates conditions suited to parasite and bacterial survival; e.g. the drinkers can be supported on raised mesh bases (Figure 16.3). The supply pipes and drinkers themselves must be kept clean by periodically flushing with a sanitising solution.

Table 16.3 Water intake (mL/day) of young pheasants.

Age	Water intake
A few days	10
3 weeks	28
4 weeks	41
5 weeks	57
6 weeks	62
7 weeks	67
8 weeks	72
9 weeks	74
12 weeks	77

Source: Beer (1988). Used with permission from the Game & Wildlife Conservation Trust (formerly The Game Conservancy Trust).

16.7 Nutrition

There has been little specific research into the nutrition of game birds but advances in the understanding of poultry nutrition have been applied to the formulation of commercial game bird diets. Several types of feed are used, varying in presentation and nutritional content appropriate to the age and perceived needs of the birds. Examples of commercially available feeds and their crude protein content are shown in Table 16.1. Feed is initially supplied on open trays or on chick papers to young chicks and then in covered feeders (Figure 16.4). Supplementary vitamins are commonly given via the water, particularly at times of potential stress such as transfer to release pens. Insoluble grit should be made available to birds that have access to grass and fibre, to reduce the risk of fibrous impaction of the gizzard. At all ages it is essential that the feed is stored and fed in a dry condition, as dampness can lead to fungal growth and outbreaks of aspergillosis in the birds.

16.8 Diseases of Game Birds

As with all livestock, good management and attention to detail are essential in minimizing the effects of disease in game birds and promoting good welfare. In situations where disease occurs it is important to achieve a veterinary diagnosis so that appropriate advice can be given to control the disease and minimize losses, which may require treatment to be administered. In addition, the biosecurity standards of game bird enterprises often fall short of those in the poultry industry and may adversely impact the success of disease control. Because of these and other factors the mortality rates between placing chicks as day-olds and transfer to release pens may reach 5% or more. Readers are referred for further information on game bird diseases to reviews such as those of Pennycott (2001) and Welchman (2008). Some important game bird diseases are summarized below.

The role of hygiene has already been mentioned and nowhere is this more important than in the control of enteric diseases, especially rotavirus and salmonellosis in young chicks, coccidiosis in rearing birds (particularly partridges) and spironucleosis (hexamitosis) in rearing and release pen birds. Rotavirus commonly causes enteritis (diarrhoea, dehydration and death) in chicks from 6 days to approximately 3 weeks of age and survives well in the environment, so strict attention to cleanliness between batches is essential if the same brooder accommodation is used repeatedly through the season. No specific treatment is available to control the disease. *Salmonella* infections occasionally lead to outbreaks of disease, sometimes accompanied by high mortality, most often in young chicks. *Spironucleus* (or *Hexamita*) is a motile protozoan parasite associated with watery diarrhoea, ill thrift and death in growing birds between approximately 3 and 12 weeks of age and is readily transmitted between birds in contaminated rearing accommodation. As with rotavirus, no specific treatment is available. Coccidia are also protozoan parasites which, unlike rotavirus and *Spironucleus*, are host specific and therefore cannot be transmitted between pheasants and partridges or vice-versa but can cause severe outbreaks of diarrhoea and mortality in partridges, in particular. The eggs (oocysts) produced by coccidia are particularly resistant in the environment. Some measure of control can be achieved by the use of in-feed coccidiostat drugs but it goes without saying that the efficacy of the product relies on the birds eating the medicated feed. Under current UK legislation, in-feed coccidiostats are supplied without veterinary prescription. Outbreaks of coccidiosis can also be treated by in-water medication with products licensed for use in poultry for this purpose. All three of these diseases are essentially associated with poor hygiene and can build up in areas of heavy contamination such as around feeders and drinkers, but this build-up can be reduced by the use of drinkers designed to reduce spillage.

A problem with using release pens, in particular, for birds in successive years can be a build-up of parasitic worms (nematodes), of which the best known is the gapeworm, *Syngamus trachea*, which is a parasite of the respiratory tract, particularly of pheasants. The eggs can survive for up to nine months in the soil and for longer periods in transport hosts, which include earthworms and other invertebrates. Other nematode parasites include *Heterakis* species (the caecal worm) and *Capillaria* and related species (hair worms), which parasitize the alimentary tract. Worm infections are routinely controlled by medication of the feed with anthelmintic products, and control programmes should include adult birds at the onset of the breeding season. *Heterakis* worms can carry the protozoan parasite *Histomonas* which is the cause of blackhead (histomonosis), a disease occasionally encountered, particularly in partridges. It has been recommended that release pens should be rested and/or rotated in successive years to control parasites such as *Syngamus*, which would also reduce the reliance on anthelmintic usage (Gethings and others 2014).

A commercially important disease of game birds is infectious sinusitis or mycoplasmosis, caused by *Mycoplasma gallisepticum* or mixed infections with this agent and other bacteria, or with viruses. Infection with this organism leads to a debilitating disease characterized by swelling of the sinuses of the head, giving a 'bulgy eye' appearance. *M. gallisepticum* can be transmitted from the breeding hen through the egg, so-called 'vertical transmission' and it is therefore particularly important that breeding birds should be as far as possible be free of the disease, and birds showing clinical signs of mycoplasmosis should not be used for breeding. *M. gallisepticum* can also be transmitted laterally (horizontally) between birds via the aerosol route and also indirectly, for example, via contaminated drinking water or clothing worn when handling birds. The hatching of eggs from infected parent birds in the same airspace as uninfected eggs also provides a ready means of transmission to previously disease-free chicks. Game birds are susceptible to the notifiable diseases, Newcastle disease and avian influenza. Outbreaks of both these diseases have been recorded in game birds in Britain, and outbreaks in captive game birds (i.e. prior to release into the wild) have been controlled under the statutory notifiable disease requirements in the same way as outbreaks in poultry, with the valuation and compulsory slaughter of birds on infected premises if disease is confirmed. Game birds are also subject to the rules covering protection and surveillance zones that surround infected premises where Newcastle disease or H5 or H7 strains of avian influenza have been confirmed, including movement restrictions, and in some situations this may include a ban on the release of gamebirds into the wild. A lack of adequate biosecurity may be a particular problem on game premises in the event of notifiable disease outbreaks.

16.9 Sustainable Disease Control in Game Birds

The control of disease in gamebirds primarily requires attention to good management of the birds, coupled with good standards of biosecurity and hygiene. Treatment may require the use of antibiotics, but only limited antibiotics are licensed for use in game birds and veterinarians may have to use products licensed for use in poultry for treating disease problems in pheasants and partridges. In the past much reliance was placed on the use of antibiotics to prevent and control disease. However, following the publication of the O'Neill report (O'Neill 2014), there has been a drive to reduce the use of antibiotics in all livestock, including game birds. A main purpose of this reduction was to reduce the development of antimicrobial resistance in bacteria, and the potential transfer of resistance to bacteria infecting humans. In the case of gamebirds, their proximity to the wild environment entails a particular risk of environmental contamination by antimicrobial resistant bacteria and transmission to wild birds and people (Díaz-Sánchez and others 2012). However there has been a considerable reduction in antibiotic use in game birds (Hammond and Tasker 2018) and it is essential that this is maintained, but it is also important that the opportunity to use antibiotics to treat disease outbreaks should continue to be available, under veterinary care, for the sake of bird welfare. It is considered good practice to produce a flock health and welfare plan with veterinary advice and to review this plan annually (Defra 2010).

16.10 Game Bird Welfare

With the considerable increase in the numbers of game birds reared since the mid-twentieth century, there has been a trend for increasing intensification particularly of the breeding, incubation, hatching, brooding and early rearing processes. This trend is largely driven by economic considerations and is likely to continue. It has raised concerns for the welfare of the birds which have been highlighted by the Farm Animal Welfare Council (FAWC 2008). The *raison d'être* of game bird breeding and rearing is the release of birds able to survive in a wild or semi-wild environment. The increased use in particular of raised laying units with wire mesh floors for breeding pheasants requires further research to assess their suitability for the welfare of the birds, for example, in allowing the expression of normal behaviour. Up to date recommendations are not readily available on the minimum requirements in terms of floor area and other measurements for these units, and the provision of perches sufficient for all the birds to roost comfortably at one time. Further research is needed on the provision of space and environmental enrichment to meet the physical and behavioural requirements of the birds in this system and is similarly needed to design improved accommodation for breeding partridges, bearing in mind that pair boxes have the benefit of reducing aggression and exposure to disease. In addition, many pheasants and the majority of partridges are derived from breeding units in continental Europe where intensive breeding systems have been more widely used than in Britain, and FAWC (2008) recommends that game owners should satisfy themselves that the health and welfare of the breeding stock meet the standards required in this country.

The use of particular types of management devices has also been highlighted by FAWC (2008), which has recommended that the use of bits (and other devices) should be assessed on an individual site basis as part of a farm health and welfare plan developed in consultation with the owner's veterinary surgeon. There appears to be little justification for the use of beak trimming which is occasionally carried out as an alternative to, or in addition to, the use of bits. The Code (Defra 2010) stipulates that 'bumpa-bits', which serve a similar purpose to 'specs' in breeding pens, should not be used except in response to a specific need in consultation with a veterinary surgeon. However, there appears to be some justification for the use of small conventional bits in controlling feather pecking in rearing birds.

Freedom from disease is an important component of animal welfare, and it is unfortunate that in the past relatively high mortality during the rearing and release periods were accepted almost as the norm. However, with increasing intensification has come a greater appreciation of the importance of biosecurity and hygiene in minimizing the exposure of the birds to disease agents, with consequential benefit to bird welfare, and mortality in the best-managed rearing systems has considerably improved.

References and Further Reading

BASC. (2015). https://basc.org.uk/blog/press-releases/latest-news/basc-statement-on-game-bird-release-numbers.

Beer, J.V. (1988). *Diseases of Gamebirds and Wildfowl*. Fordingbridge, UK: Game Conservancy Trust Ltd.

Defra. (2010). Codes of recommendations for the welfare of gamebirds reared for sporting purposes. http://www.defra.gov.uk/foodfarm/farmanimal/documents/copwelfaregamebirds100722.pdf.

Díaz-Sánchez, S., Sánchez, S., Ewers, C., and Höfle, U. (2012). Occurrence of avian pathogenic *Escherichia coli* and antimicrobial-resistant *E. coli* in red-legged partridges (*Alectoris rufa*): sanitary concerns of farming. *Avian Pathology* 41: 337–344.

Farm Animal Welfare Council. (2008). *Opinion on the Welfare of Farmed Gamebirds*. London: FAWC. http://www.fawc.org.uk.

Game and Wildlife Conservation Trust. (2007). Guidelines for sustainable gamebird releasing. www.gwct.org.uk.

Game and Wildlife Conservation Trust. (2008). Release pens. www.GWCT.org.uk.

Game Conservancy Advisory Service. (1993). *Egg Production and Incubation*. Fordingbridge, UK: The Game Conservancy Ltd.

Game Conservancy Advisory Service. (2006). *Gamebird Rearing*. Fordingbridge, UK: The Game Conservancy Ltd.

Gethings, O.J., Sage, R.B., and Leather, S.R. (2014). Spatio-temporal factors influencing the occurrence of Syngamus trachea within release pens in the South West of England. *Veterinary Parasitology* 207: 64–71.

Hammond, P. and Tasker, J. (2018). Gamebird antibiotic use reduction. *Veterinary Record* 183: 197. doi: 10.1136/vr.k2413

Kjaer, J.B. (2004). Effects of stocking density and group size on the condition of the skin and feathers of pheasant chicks. *Veterinary Record* 154: 556–558.

Madden, J.R., Hall, A., and Whiteside, M.A. (2018). Why do pheasants released in the UK die, and how can we best reduce their natural mortality? *European Journal of Wildlife Research* 64: 40.

O'Neill. (2014). Review on Antimicrobial Resistance – tackling drug-resistant infections globally. https://amr-review.org/sites/default/files/AMR%20Review%20Paper%20-%20Tackling%20a%20crisis%20for%20the%20health%20and%20wealth%20of%20nations_1.pdf

Pennycott, T.W. (2001). Disease control in adult pheasants. *In Practice* 23: 132–140.

Welchman, D. de B. (2008). Diseases in young pheasants. *In Practice* 30: 144–149.

Wise, D.R. (1993). *Pheasant Health and Welfare*. Published by the author.

Wise, D.R. and Connan, R.M. (1979). Water consumption in growing pheasants. *Veterinary Record* 104: 368–370.

17

Assessment, Implementation and Promotion of Farm Animal Welfare

John Webster

So far, this book has described, first in general terms and then on a species-by-species or group-by group basis, the principles and practice of good husbandry and its impact on the welfare of farm animals. In this final chapter we consider the broader picture: how to promote the cause of improved animal welfare through actions taken on the farm and within society at large. The steps in this process are:

1) Set high, but realistic, standards for husbandry and welfare on farms.
2) Establish robust protocols for monitoring husbandry and welfare on farms.
3) Implement and audit actions necessary to ensure overall welfare standards and address specific problems.
4) Provide incentives and rewards to farmers for complying with standards.
5) Promote public awareness and demand for food and other farm produce that demonstrably meets these standards.

Management and Welfare of Farm Animals: The UFAW Farm Handbook, Sixth Edition.
Edited by John Webster and Jean Margerison.
© Universities Federation for Animal Welfare 2022. Published 2022 by John Wiley & Sons Ltd.

17.1   Animal Welfare Standards

The aim of any set of standards for farm animal welfare is, of course, to ensure that the animals can sustain an acceptable quality of life, on-farm, in transit and at the point of slaughter, through the provision of adequate management and resources. Quality of life as perceived by the animals may be categorized and assessed in terms of paradigms such as the 'five freedoms' (Chapter 1). However, it is we humans who make the decisions as to the acceptability of specific practices (e.g. beak trimming of poultry, pregnancy stalls for sows) or the overall quality of life for the animals we use as sources of food and other utilities. Inevitably, therefore, it is our views of what constitutes good and bad welfare that determine how they live. Individuals from any background (farmers, veterinary surgeons, scientists, consumers and so on) would probably agree on broad descriptions of animals that were either clearly suffering or were obviously fit and well. However, the situation becomes less clear when describing the welfare implications of conventional husbandry systems or procedures. There is a clear diversity of views within public perceptions of animal welfare. Fraser (2008) has identified three 'world views'. Farmers and veterinarians may consider that health and productivity are most important (if not all-important). Ethologists may give highest priority to 'feelings', the emotional state of the animal. Those who consume meat, milk and eggs but have no direct contact with farm animals (i.e. the vast majority) may consider that good welfare can best be achieved by giving farm animals a 'natural' life. The increased demand for free-range eggs within affluent urban populations is a case in point. These three 'world views' are, of course, reflections of human feelings and attitudes and not necessarily consistent with the elements of welfare as perceived by the animals. However, the pressure of public opinion undoubtedly has a major influence on the laws and practices that affect farm animal welfare. The aim of those directly involved in the science and practice of animal husbandry must be to ensure that welfare needs as perceived by the public are as close as possible to of the animals. The simplest definition of animal wellbeing as 'fit and happy' (Chapter 1) embraces the first two world views but not the third. If the public is to buy into a high-welfare/high-price scheme for farm animals, then the scheme will almost certainly need to be seen to provide the animals with a reasonable approximation to the 'natural' life.

17.1.1   Farm Assurance Schemes

It has been said that when a man has plenty to eat, he has many problems, when he has nothing to eat, he has only one problem. Consumers who enjoy both spending power and the power of choice express a wide range of food concerns. These include provenance (country or even farm of origin), food safety, production methods (e.g. organic standards) and animal welfare. In response to these concerns producers, retailers and organizations such as the Royal Society for the Protection of Animals (RSPCA) have developed a series of farm assurance schemes that set, monitor and provide assurance with respect to standards in one or all of these areas of concern.

Farm assurance schemes have been developed for most livestock sectors in the UK and Europe. In UK these include 'Assured Food Standards' (the Red Tractor scheme), Organic Food Standards as set by the Soil Association, 'RSPCA Assured' (formerly Freedom Foods) and a number of schemes operated by individual supermarkets. Independent monitoring and surveillance of production units is a key requirement of all these schemes. This is to ensure that claims for quality assurance (QA) can be supported by evidence of independent quality control.

The central aim of all these schemes is to promote standards of good farming and consumer trust in these standards. They differ, inevitably, in emphasis and in requirements to meet their standards. The Assured Food Standards (Red Tractor), e.g. Assured Dairy Farms, are designed primarily by farmers for farmers (indeed, the red tractor logo has rather more appeal to working farmers than to green-minded consumers). RSPCA Assured (Freedom Foods) gives priority to animal welfare. The Organic Standards set by the Soil Association give priority (as the name implies) to protection and conservation of the environment but also set rigorous standards for animal welfare and food safety.

Compassion in Animal Welfare (CIWF 2012) compared these and other QA schemes. They rated the Soil Association standards first (and very good in absolute terms) on nearly all counts, RSPCA Assured standards were generally satisfactory to good, the Red Tractor scheme was good in parts but failed to meet several of the exacting criteria set by CIWF. This raises the question 'how good is good enough?'. The first requirement is, of course, to meet the requirements and standards set by legislation and Codes of Practice (e.g. DEFRA, http://www.defra.gov.uk, USDA, https://awic.usda.gov).

QA schemes such as those of the Soil Association and RSPCA standards are designed to encourage farmers to do better than simply comply with the law. The High Welfare schemes operated by the Soil Association, RSPCA and specific supermarkets are designed to give a financial reward to farmers who want to do better still. All these schemes are binary: i.e. a farm is in compliance with codes or it isn't. Other schemes, e.g. the pan-European Welfare Quality* scheme and the North American 'Global Animal Partnership' (GAP 2008) seek to rank farms from one to five stars or on a scale from unclassified, through basic, good to excellent. The attraction of this approach is that it seeks to encourage and reward continuous improvement. The problem arises when you attempt to arrive at an overall quality score based on performance according to different welfare criteria, assessed (e.g.) by the five freedoms. This will be discussed in in more detail in the next section.

17.2 On-Farm Assessment of Husbandry and Welfare

Standards in animal welfare may be assessed according to the following criteria (Figure 17.1):

- *Resources* – provision of the facilities necessary to ensure proper feeding, housing and handling of animals
- *Management* – provision of correct husbandry procedures and competent, sympathetic stewardship[1]

---

1 this is a sweeter-sounding gender-neutral alternative to 'stockmanship' than 'stockpersonship'

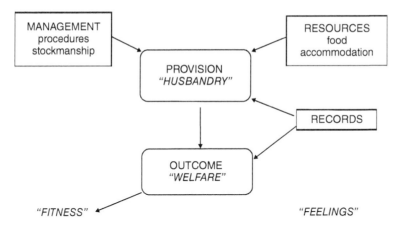

Figure 17.1 Elements necessary for assessment of the provision of good husbandry and welfare outcomes (from Webster 2005). Used with permission of UFAW.

- *Records* – written evidence of use of medicines, deaths and culls, incidence of disease and injury (etc.)
- *Welfare state* – evidence of physical fitness and mental wellbeing as perceived by the animals themselves

The following criteria are useful for assessing the effectiveness of the standards.

1) *Level of standards.* As a minimum, any QA scheme must include all legislation that is relevant to the stated objectives of the scheme. In the context of animal welfare and in the UK, these take as a baseline the DEFRA *Codes of Recommendation for the Welfare of Farm Animals.* However, the public appeal of a 'high-welfare' QA scheme, such as 'RSPCA Assured', will also depend on the extent to which it is perceived to improve upon minimal standards, especially in regard to issues such as barren environments for laying hens or confinement of sows in farrowing crates. A scheme whose standards are designed to allow any farmer entry is not likely to impress the discerning customer. The standards should, however, be achievable.

2) *Scope of the standards.* The standards should include all resources and husbandry practices on a farm that could affect the welfare of any individual of the species covered by the scheme. This should include all types of stock. For example, QA on a dairy unit should incorporate calf rearing and the management of cull animals.

3) *Formulation of the standards.* The standards should be clearly definable, understandable and unambiguous. They should be regularly and frequently updated. They should be auditable and enforceable since a standard that cannot be verified on-farm is unhelpful and could lead to false claims by the scheme. Most aspects of animal husbandry (*provisions*) can be assessed, provided the assessor has sufficient auditing and inspection skills. Assessment of Welfare state (*outcome*) is inherently more subjective so more difficult to assess in a way that can be incorporated into clearly defined standards. Past

protocols have placed most emphasis on measures of provision rather than measures of outcome. The current trend is to base most, or all reliance on animal-based measures of welfare outcomes (e.g. the Welfare Quality programme, www.welfarequality.net/ URI>). The emphasis on outcome measures is entirely laudable since outcomes are what matter. However, there are situations where a reliable measure of provision can be a better predictor of welfare than a subjective guess at an outcome measure such as emotional state.

Any farm assurance scheme can only deliver quality assurance to the consumer when there is a credible system for ensuring quality control. Typically, there are three key stages to this process.

1) Farmers are required to be fully aware of the detailed requirements of the standard. The farmer should receive updated copies of the standards. Some schemes use a self-assessment system partly to draw the attention of the farmer to the standard requirements and partly to provide evidence that the farmer is complying with the standards since an external auditor can verify the accuracy of the self-assessment.
2) Advisers can assist the producer to comply with the standard. The veterinary surgeon is well suited to perform this task, ideally in association with regular consultations on herd health and preventive medicine.
3) A representative of the scheme (assessor) will usually need to visit the farm to verify compliance with the standard. The assessor is looking to gather evidence (visual, verbal or written) that verifies compliance with the standard. The assessor gathers this evidence from observation of records, resources and management, structured dialogue with stockpersons and, of course, observation of the animals in their environment.

Key aspects of the assessment procedure include:

- *Robustness of the monitoring criteria*. The criteria used to assess husbandry and welfare need to be consistent, reproducible and not subject to observer bias. This is especially important in regard to animal-based measures of welfare outcomes, which are inevitably subjective. It is also important that observations made during visits by the assessor should, where possible, reflect long-term consequences of husbandry (e.g. body condition is a better measure of the adequacy of nutrition than presence of feed in the troughs at the time of the visit).
- *Competency of assessors*. This requires appropriate experience of the farming system under review and formal training in the conduct and report on the assessment.
- *Impartiality of the assessors*. This may be compromised if the assessor provides advice. It is necessary therefore to make a distinction between assessor and adviser.
- *Frequency and duration of visits*. Increasing the frequency and length of visits can increase the credibility of the assessment procedure. However, this obviously has a direct impact on the cost of the scheme and its nuisance value to the farmer. Assessors with suitable auditing and inspection skills (and suitable access to records) should be able to make some assessment of the management of the unit over a reasonable period such as one year prior

Table 17.1 The four principles and twelve criteria proposed by 'Welfare Quality' as elements of protocols for the direct, animal-based assessment of farm animal welfare (from Botreau et al. 2007).

Welfare principles	Welfare criteria
Good feeding	Absence of prolonged hunger
	Absence of prolonged thirst
Good housing	Comfort around resting
	Thermal comfort
	Ease of movement
Good health	Absence of injuries
	Absence of disease
	Absence of pain induced by management procedures
Appropriate behaviour	Expression of social behaviours
	Expression of other behaviours
	Good human–animal relationship
	Absence of general fear

to the visit. The assessments may need to be staggered to ensure that the farm is observed in different seasons.

The pan-European Welfare Quality Programme (www.welfarequality.com) has produced comprehensive protocols for assessment of welfare outcomes according to four principles of wellbeing: good feeding, good housing, good health and appropriate behaviour. These principles are, in essence, the same as those described by the 'five freedoms' (Table 17.1). The four principles are defined according to 12 more specific criteria, each amenable to direct monitoring under farm conditions. For example, 'good housing' is defined by the criteria of comfort around resting, thermal comfort and ease of movement.

Figure 17.2 illustrates how this information may be directed to the various interested parties: producers, legislators and retailers. Standards defined by the 12 welfare criteria are derived from a larger range of observations and measures appropriate to the species and farming system under review. These would include proven robust measures of physical and mental state (e.g. body condition, prevalence of lameness, incidence of mastitis, evidence of feather pecking). A report based on the evaluation according to these standards and the measures upon which they were based forms the basis of a general conclusion as to the acceptability and quality of the farm and more specific advice to the farmer and his adviser.

Welfare Quality has proposed that farms be given an overall ranking on a four-point scale: unclassified, basal, good and excellent. However, this is easier said than done. Even when reduced to four categories (Table 17.1) conclusions as to welfare standards are unlikely to be

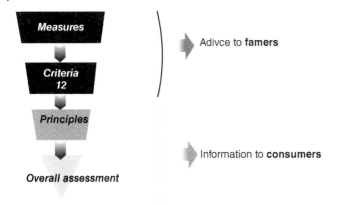

Figure 17.2 Characterization of measures and criteria used for the basis of on-farm monitoring of animal welfare and conveying information to farmers and consumers (adapted from Botreau et al. 2007).

clear-cut. Feeding may be good, health adequate but behaviour restricted (or any other combination of circumstances). Preliminary evidence would suggest that very few farms are likely to score 'excellent' according to all four principles. This poses several questions:

- How good is 'excellent'? Does it require evidence of positive welfare (e.g. happiness)?
- To what extent can excellence in one, two or three principles compensate for a score of basal or unclassified in another?
- Will retailers be prepared to accept a scheme whereby the majority of their produce is given a ranking lower than 'good'? It may be preferable to substitute a numerical ranking system (e.g. 0–3 stars).

The promotion of production and marketing systems that allow customers to express freedom of choice to decide what standard of welfare they wish to support is a matter for retailers and falls outside the scope of this chapter. Different retailers, especially the major supermarket chains, compete with one another to attract customers into their stores. Price is one element of competition but so too is quality, and increasingly supermarkets are promoting their concern for animal welfare as a mark of quality and demonstrating their commitment through their quality assurance schemes. Since consumers (and individual retailers) cannot possibly inspect every farm for themselves, they must take on trust both the standards and the audit of these QA schemes. Those of us who *care for*, rather than simply *care about* farm animals have a responsibility to develop the knowledge, skills and experience necessary to conduct a competent assessment of husbandry and welfare on farms and large production units, to make fair judgements as to standards, and (where appropriate) offer constructive advice as to actions necessary to promote and, where possible, improve welfare.

17.3   Welfare Monitoring Protocols

The exact details of an animal-based protocol for monitoring welfare will be governed by the species, the farming system, national legislation and the standards of value laid down by individual QA schemes. Approaches to monitoring welfare for the different species of farm animals have been described in previous chapters. Here I illustrate one approach to the direct, animal-based assessment of welfare based on protocols adopted by the Bristol Welfare Assurance Programme (www.vetschool.bris.ac.uk/animalwelfare). These protocols for monitoring welfare under farm conditions are based on the five freedoms. In each case we highlight one example of a welfare outcome measure within each of the five freedoms that can be assessed during a farm visit. The examples are taken from our dairy cattle welfare assessment protocol (Whay et al. 2003) and illustrate the information provided for each monitor. For each indicator of welfare within each welfare principle ('freedom'), we describe the criteria (what needs to be assessed) and the methodology (how the indicator should be assessed). This is followed by a brief explanation that can be used to explain the significance of each indicator to a farmer. Figures 17.3 to 17.6 present some of the illustrations that accompany these directions.

17.3.1   Freedom to Express Normal Behaviour

Example: rising restriction during housing

Observation

A cow will normally rock in a forward lunge of 60 cm, then raise the rear end first, moving a front foot forward, finally lifting the shoulders and head, all in a single fluid movement (Figure 17.3a). Record if cows show severe rising restriction, e.g. performing

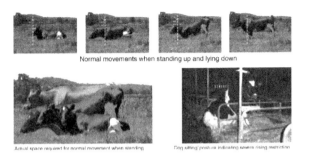

Normal movements when standing up and lying down

Actual space required for normal movement when standing

Dog sitting' posture indicating severe rising restriction

Figure 17.3   Freedom to express normal behaviour: example of assessment, standing up and lying down (source: www.vetschool.bris.ac.uk/animalwelfare).

behaviours such as rocking repeatedly, turning their heads sideways, dipping their heads as they stand, standing foot feet first, or hitting fittings during rising.

Methodology

If possible, observe 10 animals standing up. Try to observe cows that rise voluntarily; do not force the animals to stand. If more than one group is involved, take a representative sample of animals from each group.

Farmer significance

Are cows having difficulty when rising or lying down? Cows are more likely to sustain injuries in areas such as the hips and ribs when they are too large for the cubicles. Severe restriction in the lying area may discourage cows from lying down. Reduced lying time is known to be a high risk for lameness, especially in heifers. Space restriction may be caused by factors such as cubicle design, yard design or stocking density.

17.3.2   Freedom from Fear and Stress

Example: flight distance

Observation and methodology

Ensure the cow is standing still in an area where she has sufficient room to move away from you. Ideally this should be in the animal's habitual environment (cubicle house or barn). Walk quietly and steadily towards the cow at right angles to her shoulder. Do not look into her eyes. Estimate how close you can approach before the cow turns her head away or takes the first step away. Record the result in metres. Make observations on at least 10 animals.

Farmer significance

How far (in metres) is the flight distance? A short avoidance distance reflects reduced fearfulness, makes daily inspections and handling procedures less stressful and is a good indicator for 'positive health'. The test can be influenced by a variety of factors (lameness, social/environment for testing, previous experience, unfamiliar/familiar test person) but reflects in general the quality and quantity of handling and stockmanship.

17.3.3 Freedom from Hunger and Thirst

Example: body condition

Methodology

Stand behind and beside the cow and assess body condition by vision only. Look especially at the tailhead, spine and transverse processes. Refer to DEFRA publications on condition scoring (www.defra.gov.uk/animal welfare)

Recording thin cows
Record cows with body condition score (BCS) < 2.0. The tailhead area is a deep cavity with no fatty tissue under the skin (Figure 17.4). The spine is prominent and the horizontal spinous processes (transverse processes) sharp.

Recording – fat cows
Record cows with BCS 4–5. The tailhead is completely filled with fat and folds and patches of fat are evident. The vertebral processes are not visible and the animal appears completely rounded.

Farmer significance
Body condition scoring is a technique for assessing the condition of livestock at regular intervals. The purpose of condition scoring is to achieve a balance between economic feeding, good production and welfare.

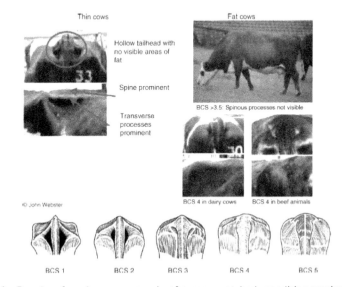

Figure 17.4 Freedom from hunger: example of assessment, body condition scoring (BCS) of cows.

Does the animal have a BCS of < 2? If it does then it is excessively thin. Dairy cows are under considerable nutritional stress, and adequate feeding is essential to avoid excessive weight loss. These animals can suffer discomfort (especially in cubicles). At service, cows should not be in energy deficit as this may result in low fertility.

Does the animal have a BCS > 3.5? If it does then it is overweight. Cows should not be excessively fat, especially before and at calving. Fat cows may develop fatty liver disease or ketosis and are more prone to milk fever, mastitis, lameness, infertility and calving difficulties. It is also not economical to feed excessively.

17.3.4   Freedom from Discomfort

Example: swollen hocks

Observation

Record if the cow has any obviously swollen hocks. This can be seen as an obvious increase in the hock diameter and may be caused by thickened skin, bursitis (hygromas) or increased fluid filling of the joints. The swelling can be seen on the lateral or medial side of the hindlimb (Figure 17.5).

Methodology

Assess both hindlimbs, standing behind and beside the animal, and include all swellings that are visible from a distance of 2 m. Compare to other animals in the herd and try to find a normal hock for comparison. In a normal hock all anatomical structures (bones, tendons) are visible.

Farmer significance

Does the animal have any swelling of the hock? This may indicate that the surface on which the cows are lying may not be comfortable. Swollen hocks are considered to be an indicator of discomfort in the lying area and are strongly associated with lameness.

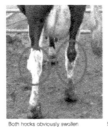
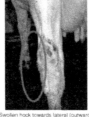
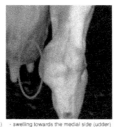

Both hocks obviously swollen   Swollen hock towards lateral (outwards)   swelling towards the medial side (udder)

Figure 17.5   Freedom from discomfort: example of assessment, swollen hocks.

17.3.5 Freedom from Pain, Injury and Disease

Example: lameness

Observation

Record number of cows seen lame (limping). Do not include those who appear only to have tender feet, or slight abnormalities of locomotion. Lame cows may display an arched spine when walking or standing (Figure 17.6), shortened stride and obvious head nods when moving. One or more limbs may be only partially weight-bearing or rested when standing. Lame cows may be reluctant to stand or move. Note, heifers that are lame do not usually arch their spines. All animals observed to be lame should be included in the count. This should include mild cases since these are the cows that would benefit from early treatment before lameness becomes severe and expensive through loss of milk, fertility and time.

Methodology

When walking through the cows make a preliminary note of any animals that are lame. If the number of lame cows is a cause for concern then the whole herd must be assessed for lameness. The most convenient way is to observe all cows walking as they leave the milking parlour. Alternatively ask the farmer to walk the whole herd past you, a few cows at a time.

Farmer significance

Are there any lame animals? Early recognition, investigation and treatment of lame animals are essential to reduce pain and provide effective control of the problem. Increased levels of lameness are also expensive to the farmer through loss of milk, fertility and time.

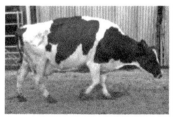 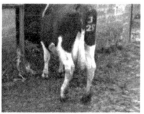

Lame cow: Walking with an uneven step rhythm, arched spine, nodding head and shortened stride length

Lame cow: reluctant to bear weight on left hind limb

Figure 17.6 Freedom from pain, injury and disease: example of assessment, lameness in dairy cows.

17.3.6 Interpretation of Observations

Figure 17.7 summarizes data from a survey of welfare on selected dairy farms in the UK (Whay et al. 2003) to illustrate the prevalence (%) of four of the conditions described by the above examples. The herd distribution for these observations is presented in quintiles (i.e. best 20% in black, worst 20% uncoloured, with patterns for the three middle quintiles). Figure 17.7 shows, for example, that for rising restriction, prevalence for the best quintile was below 10%; for the worst quintile it was 50–77% (i.e. the worst herd had a prevalence of 77%). For lameness, prevalence for the best quintile was below 14%; for the worst it was 30–50%. There were no fat cows in the best 60% of herds: the highest incidence of fat cows was 26%.

The information gathered from this set of animal-based indices of welfare in dairy cows was circulated to 50 experts who were asked to indicate the herd prevalence (in these examples) which would indicate a welfare problem sufficiently serious to justify intervention at herd level, both for the sake of the animals and to ensure compliance with welfare standards laid down by QA schemes. A herd problem was defined as one where the prevalence or incidence was such that 75% of experts recommended intervention. In the case of thin cows, 75% considered that intervention was necessary for farms in bands D and E (i.e. 40% of herds in which prevalence was > 21%). For lameness, intervention was recommended when prevalence was greater than 13% (bands B to E). Thus 75% of competent judges considered that lameness was a welfare problem that required attention in 80% of the recorded herds! Overall lameness prevalence in this study was similar to that in other contemporary reports from Europe and the USA. This puts the spotlight on two very important messages. Lameness is the major welfare problem for high-performance dairy cows in the developed world (Chapter 3). A quality assurance programme that simply records the prevalence of a welfare

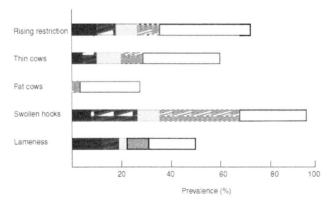

Figure 17.7 Prevalence of four indices of poor welfare in dairy cows (From Whay et al. 2003). Each index is divided into quintiles indicating the prevalence of these conditions from the best 20% (in black) to the worst 20% (unshaded).

problem such as lameness but does not lead to effective action is not providing the quality assurance it claims, either for the animals or for the public who are expected to put their trust in the system.

17.4   Simplified Monitoring Schemes: 'Iceberg' Indicators

Farm animal welfare monitoring and assurance protocols such as Welfare Quality and the Bristol Welfare Assurance Protocol can provide a fair and comprehensive indication of overall welfare standards on a farming unit *and* identify specific problems calling for specific remedies. However, these inspections must be carried out at some cost by a cadre of well-trained and experienced assessors and they are time-consuming. Farmers may reasonably conclude that their time and money will only be well spent if they can see a return in cash for their compliance with welfare standards higher than those defined by law, Codes of Practice and their own experience of the precepts of good husbandry. Moreover, for most of the people of the world there is little consumer demand for added welfare foods partly because they haven't given it much thought but mainly due to lack of money. In these circumstances, it is unrealistic to expect a widespread uptake of comprehensive, expensive welfare assurance protocols so there is a need to devise something cheaper and simpler for general application. One approach is to identify and implement a small number of 'iceberg' indicators: robust measures that can be carried out reasonably quickly by trained, but not expert, monitors. For example:

> Good feeding: body condition scores
> Good housing/environment: dirtiness, skin lesions
> Good health: lameness, diarrhoea, respiratory distress
> Appropriate behaviour: reaction to familiar handlers, approach, flight distance

Clearly, a brief inspection of this type cannot provide a complete picture of welfare state. However, the choice of a small number of robust, minimally subjective indicators means that there should be little variation between observers, and they should pick up, if not fully describe, any serious problems or concerns. If this preliminary inspection does raise one or more points of concern, then the managers of the surveillance scheme may recommend or insist upon a more comprehensive inspection, or a visit from a veterinary surgeon, or both.

17.5   Implementation and Promotion of Good Welfare

So far, this chapter has described the principles and practice that should govern the assessment of animal welfare under farm conditions. All the outlined protocols incorporate both measures of the elements of good husbandry (e.g. resources, records and stockmanship) and direct animal-based assessment of the physical ('fit') and emotional ('feeling good') elements of welfare, based on sound foundations of animal welfare science. This information can be used in several ways. It can be incorporated into a herd health and welfare plan tuned to the needs of the individual farmer. It can be used to set standards for QA schemes operated by producer groups, retailers or non-governmental organizations such as RSPCA. In extreme cases, it may be used to test compliance with minimal standards for legislative purposes.

A market-led scheme that seeks to add value on the basis of assured standards of animal welfare that surpass the statutory minimum will only succeed if this added value is recognized by both consumers and producers and receives due reward. If customers are to pay more, they need to be aware of, and trust, the assurances provided by the scheme. If retailers are to reward their suppliers for their compliance with superior standards, they need to promote the scheme, not least to achieve their own financial reward through increased market share. If farmers are to invest increased time and resources to animal welfare they need a financial incentive, since most of them are doing the best they can within the limits of what they can currently afford. The farm animals, the objects of these good intentions, will benefit only if all three responsible parties can be persuaded to act together. If it is to succeed, a welfare-based QA scheme (or the animal welfare element of a broader scheme incorporating health, welfare and provenance) needs to operate both on the farm and at the retail level; creating, in effect, two virtuous cycles of monitoring, action, review, reward and promotion, running together as elements of a single, continuous dynamic process. I have described this as a 'virtuous bicycle' (Webster 2009). The design and development of this whimsical, but conceptually sound, model are illustrated in Figure 17.8.

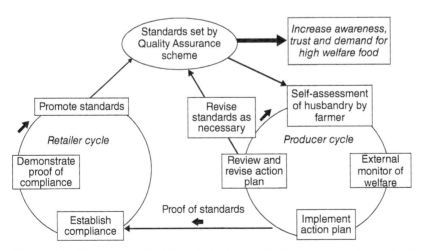

Figure 17.8 The 'virtuous bicycle': a vehicle designed to deliver improved animal welfare on-farm. The right wheel illustrates the process of self-assessment, external monitoring, action and review on-farm; the left wheel, the process of quality assurance and quality control at the retailer level (from Webster 2009).

17.5.1 Implementation of Good Welfare: The Producer Cycle

Guaranteed quality assurance requires a continuous process of welfare assessment, action to address specific problems, and review to address the effectiveness of the action. The right wheel, the 'producer cycle' in Figure 17.8, begins with a formal written self-assessment carried out by the farm owner with inputs from farm stewards and veterinarians as appropriate. The self-assessment should be based on the standards of husbandry and provision set by the QA scheme and will include: housing and hygiene; records of feed provision, health, use of medicines, etc.; stewardship and training; the existence and operation of a health and welfare plan. The farmer should be required to outline any specific welfare concerns and priorities for action to address these concerns. The second stage of the cycle is the visit by the independent monitor, trained for and operating to the standards of the assurance scheme. The visit will include an interview with the farmer, to discuss and review the self-assessment, and an inspection of the animals to assess welfare according to the animal-based criteria and principles described above. The report of the monitor will provide an assessment of compliance with the overall standards and the four principles (Table 17.1) or five freedoms. It should identify and rank areas where it is desirable or necessary to improve welfare. The next step is to identify critical control points and prioritize an action plan designed to address these welfare issues. The extent to which the assessor may or may not act as an adviser at this stage is a matter for the directors of the scheme to decide. As a general rule we would recommend that the farmer, having received the assessor's report, the farmer should consult an independent adviser such as a veterinary surgeon, then produce a written response to the report to include comments on any areas of disagreement and a prioritized plan of action. Copies of both assessment and response should be submitted to the supervisors of the QA scheme. After an appropriate interval (e.g. one year), there is a further review of welfare in general and the effectiveness of specific prioritized actions. This should, once again, be based first on self-assessment, then independent monitoring.

The aim of this approach – self-assessment, independent monitoring, action and review – is to create a dynamic cycle of continuous quality control. The first benefit of starting with self-assessment is that the farmer can address elements of husbandry, provision and records in his/her own time, thus reducing the amount of work that has to be done at the time of the visit from the external assessor. It also acknowledges that farmers also know most (if not necessarily best) the husbandry procedures that operate on their own farms and why they have evolved. The aim of the visit by the independent assessor is to mount a fair challenge to this self-assessment. While the first visit will have to be comprehensive, subsequent assessments can concentrate on the most important issues arising from previous assessments and the success or otherwise of the action plan. This may well take the form of a brief 'iceberg' inspection, restricted to a few robust markers of problems highlighted previously.

The practical merits of this approach are as follows:

- Elements of husbandry, including records of actions to ensure welfare, are included in the self-assessment. This recognizes that much of the information necessary to assure the quality of welfare on farm must be obtained from evidence relating to the provision of resources and management on-farm, records of these provisions and records of outcomes, e.g. relating to animal health and use of medicines.

- Compliance with the standards of the scheme would not normally be based on the results of a single monitoring exercise but on the effectiveness of actions to promote welfare and address specific problems.
- Once the cycle of self-assessment, monitoring, action and review has been established it should be possible for farmers and assessors to focus on the most important issues, thereby avoiding bureaucratic and time-wasting repetition of all elements of the assessment protocol at every visit.
- A scheme where compliance (and/or star rating) is based not on the assessment protocol but on evidence of the effectiveness of actions designed to promote welfare is sympathetic to the farmer, since it reduces the risk of subjective bias in the assessor's report (and variation in standards between assessors). It is also more challenging to the farmer since it does not allow him to file away the assessor's report and forget about it until next year. He must provide evidence of effective action.

17.5.2 Promotion of Good Welfare: Retailers and Consumers

The left wheel of the virtuous bicycle (Figure 17.8) is designed to improve the public awareness of, and demand for, food and other animal products from farms operating to proven high welfare standards. The aim is to create an improved, sustained, verifiable process of information transfer to the public and retailers relating to welfare standards and actions to ensure welfare standards on farms operating within the QA scheme. The welfare standards necessary for compliance within the scheme (or ranking within the scheme) are stated at the outset and freely available to all both in outline and in detail. Entry to the scheme occurs when the farmer can establish compliance based on evidence that he has established the action plan for welfare. Subsequent cycles require continuous proof of compliance based on evidence of attention to welfare standards. Proof of compliance, supported by evidence, can then be used by the retailer to promote the scheme. The aim of the scheme, the direction of the bicycle, is towards increased awareness, trust, demand and rewards for high welfare food.

17.5.3 Delivery of Good Welfare

Welfare-based quality schemes are now a fact of life, and they are likely to become even more prominent in the future. The tide of public opinion is in their favour. However, if these schemes fail to deliver on their assurances through piecemeal approaches that fail to complete the revolution of both cycles of challenge, action, promotion and reward, then consumers may lose trust, retailers and farmers lose faith. Farm animal welfare may go out of fashion, and the primary objective, quality of life for the farmed animals could be set back for years.

The approach illustrated by the 'virtuous bicycle' is more time-consuming and potentially costly to both producers and retailers than most conventional QA schemes that tend to operate on the basis of an annual inspection, involving one day or less and the probability that, unless the farm actually fails the assessment, no action will be required until next year. It is therefore unrealistic to expect it to succeed unless it brings real reward to all stakeholders, namely consumers, retailers, farmers and the animals themselves, through proper recognition of the added value accruing through better attention to animal welfare. Produce bearing the logo of a value-added scheme should retail at a price higher than that produced according to nationally approved (minimal) standards, and a fair proportion of this increased price should be passed to the producer. If it becomes pan-European policy to impose the monitoring standards and rating system proposed by Welfare Quality, then it would be logical to equate 'unclassified' (or zero star) with compliance with minimum legal standards assessed at annual inspection and not, in this case, impose an action plan to promote improved welfare. Awards of one to three stars (or rankings of basal to excellent) would reward increments of quality in terms of animal welfare, with commensurate increments in the cash value of the produce.

References and Further Reading

Assured Dairy Farms (UK). *Farm Assurance Protocol*. http://www.ndfas.org.uk.

Botreau, R., Veissier, I., Butterworth, A., Bracke, M.B.M., and Keeling, L. (2007). Definition of criteria for overall assessment of animal welfare. *Animal Welfare* 16: 225–228.

Bristol Welfare Assurance Programme. http://www.vetschool.bris.ac.uk/animalwelfare.

DEFRA. *Farm Assurance Schemes and Standards*. http://www.defra.gov.uk.

Fraser, D. (2008). *Understanding Animal Welfare: The Science in Its Cultural Context*. Oxford: Wiley-Blackwell.

Global Animal Partnership. https://globalanimalpartnership.org

RSPCA Assured (formerly Freedom Foods). http://www.rspca.org.uk.

Soil Association Standards (UK). *Animal Welfare*. http://www.soilassociation.org.

US Department of Agriculture. *Animal welfare audits and certification programmes*. https://awic.usda.gov.

Webster, A.J.F. (2009). The Virtuous Bicycle: A delivery vehicle for improved farm animal welfare. *Animal Welfare* 18: 141–147.

Webster, J. (2005). *Animal Welfare; Limping towards Eden*. Blackwell Publishing UK.

Whay, H.R., Main, D.C.J., Green, L.E., and Webster, A.J.F. (2003). Assessment of the welfare of dairy cattle using animal-based measurements: Direct observations and investigation of farm records. *Veterinary Record* 153: 197–202.

Index

Management and Welfare of Farm Animals: The UFAW Farm Handbook, Sixth Edition.
Edited by John Webster and Jean Margerison.
© Universities Federation for Animal Welfare 2022. Published 2022 by John Wiley & Sons Ltd.